Recent Advances in Quantitative Methods in Cancer and Human Health Risk Assessment

Recent Advances in Quantitative Methods in Cancer and Human Health Risk Assessment

Edited by

LUTZ EDLER

German Cancer Research Center, Germany

CHRISTOS P. KITSOS

Technological Educational Institute of Athens, Greece

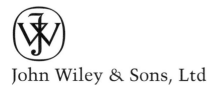

John Wiley & Sons, Ltd

Other Wiley Editorial Offices

John Wiley & Sons Inc., 111 River Street, Hoboken, NJ 07030, USA

Jossey-Bass, 989 Market Street, San Francisco, CA 94103-1741, USA

Wiley–VCH Verlag GmbH, Boschstr. 12, D-69469 Weinheim, Germany

John Wiley & Sons Australia Ltd, 33 Park Road, Milton, Queensland 4064, Australia

John Wiley & Sons (Asia) Pte Ltd, 2 Clementi Loop #02-01, Jin Xing Distripark, Singapore 129809

John Wiley & Sons Canada Ltd, 22 Worcester Road, Etobicoke, Ontario, Canada M9W 1L1

Library of Congress Cataloging-in-Publication Data

Quantitative methods for cancer and human health risk assessment/editors, Lutz Edler, Christos P. Kitsos.
    p. cm.
  ISBN-13 978-0-470-85756-4
  ISBN-10 0-470-85756-0
  1. Cancer–Risk factors–Mathematical models. I. Edler, Lutz, 1945- II. Kitsos, Christos Par., 1951-
  RC268.48.Q34   2004
  616.99'4071' 015118–dc22   2004028290

British Library Cataloguing in Publication Data

A catalogue record for this book is available from the British Library

  ISBN-13 978-0-470-85756-4 (HB)
  ISBN-10 0-470-85756-0 (HB)

To the memory all parents who leave before all thanks are given.

To my Father and Mother
who died from chronic disease.

To my Father and Mother
who both died from cancer.

L.E.

C.P.K

Contents

10. Modeling Lung Cancer Screening   161

Marek Kimmel, Olga Y. Gorlova and Claudia I. Henschke

18. Designs and Models for Mixtures: Assessing Cumulative Risk   299
James J. Chen, Ralph L. Kodell and Yi-Ju Chen

**19 Estimating the Natural History of Breast Cancer from Bivariate
Data on Age and Tumor Size at Diagnosis   317**
*Alexander V. Zorin, Lutz Edler, Leonid G. Hanin and
Andrej Y. Yakovlev*

VI CASE STUDIES

Introductory remarks

**20. Statistical Issues in the Search for Biomarkers of Colorectal Cancer
Using Microarray Experiments   333**
*Byung-Soo Kim, Sunho Lee, Inyoung Kim, Sangcheol Kim,
Sun Young Rha and Hyun Cheol Chung*

Contributors

Prof. Dr. Jose Jeronimo Amaral Mendes University of Évora, Dept. of Ecology, P-7000 Evora, Portugal, amaralm@netcabo.pt

Anastasia Apostolidou NCSR 'Demokritos', Institute of Biology, Lab. of Environmental Mutagenesis & Carcinogenesis, P.O. Box 60 228, GR-15310 Athens, Greece

Prof. Vilijandas B. Bagdonavičius Vilnius State University, Dept. of Statistics, Naugarduko 24, LT-2006 Vilnius, Lithuania, vilijandas.bagdonavicius@maf.vu.lt

Prof. Dr. Vladimír Bencko Charles University of Prague, Inst. of Hygiene & Epidemiology, First Faculty of Medicine, Studnickova 7, CZ-12800 Prague 2, Czech Republic, vladimir.bencko@lf1.cuni.cz

Dr. Milagros Bernal University of Zaragoza, C/Domingo Miral S/N, Medical School University Clinical Hospital, E-5009 Zaragoza, Spain, mibernal@posta.unizar.es

Dr. Frédéric Y. Bois INERIS, Delegue Scientifique des Risques Chroniques, Parc Alata, BP2, 5, Rue Taffanel, F-60550 Verneuil en Halatte, France, frederic.bois@ineris.fr

Dr. Iris Burkholder German Cancer Research Center, Biostatistics Unit C060, P.O. Box 101949, D-69009 Heidelberg, Germany, i.burkholder@dkfz.de

Dr. Chao W. Chen US Environmental Protection Agency, National Center of Environmental Assessment (Mail Drop 8623D), 1200 Pennsylvania Ave., NW, Washington, DC 20946, USA, chen.chao@epamail.epa.gov

Dr. James J. Chen US Food and Drug Administration, Div. of Biometry & Risk Assessment, National Center for Toxicological Research, 3900 NCTR Road, Jefferson, AR 72079, USA, jchen@nctr.fda.gov

Dr. Yi-Ju Chen US Food and Drug Administration, Div. of Biometry & Risk Assessment, National Center for Toxicological Research, 3900 NCTR Road, Jefferson, AR 72079, USA

Dr. Hyun Cheol Chung Yonsei University, Cancer Metastasis Research Center, College of Medicine, 134 Shinchon-Dong, Seodaemoon-Gu, KR-120-752 Seoul, S.Korea, unchung8@yumc.yonsei.ac.kr

Dr. Vincent James Cogliano IARC, Carcinogen Identification & Evaluation, 150 Cours Albert Thomas, F-69372 Lyon Cedex 08, France, cogliano@iarc.fr

Dr. Małgorzata Ćwiklińska-Jurkowska Nicolaus Copernicus University, Collegium Medicum, Dept. of Theoretical Basis of Biomedical Sciences & Medical Informatics, ul. Jagiellońska 13-15, PL-85-067 Bydgoszcz, Poland, mjurkowska@cm.umk.pl

Dr. Heike Dally German Cancer Research Center, Dept. of Toxicology C010, P.O. Box 101949, D-69009 Heidelberg, Germany, h.dally@dkfz.de

Dr. Cheikh Diack INERIS, Unité de Toxicologie Expérimentale, Parc Alata, BP2, 5, Rue Taffanel, F-60550 Verneuil en Halatte, France, cheikh.diack@ineris.fr

Dr. Lutz Edler German Cancer Research Center, Biostatistics Unit C060, P.O. Box 101949, D-69009 Heidelberg, Germany, edler@dkfz.de

Dr. Elenóra Fabiánová State Inst. of Public Health, Cesta k nemocnici 1, SK-97556 Banska Bystrica, Slovakia, fabianova@szubb.sk

Dr. Petr Franěk Charles University of Prague, Inst. of Hygiene & Epidemiology, First Faculty of Medicine, Studnickova 7, CZ-12800 Prague 2, Czech Republic, petr.franek@cnb.cz

Dr. Sandra Adelaida Garcet Rodriguez Universidad de Salamanca, Dept. Estadística, Facultad de Ciencias, Plaza de los Caidos s/n, E-37008 Salamanca, Spain, sandra_garcet@hotmail.com

Dr. Miloslav Götzl District Hospital of Bojnice, Dept. of Oncology, Komenskeho 10, SK-97201 Bojnice, Slovakia

Prof. Dr. Olga Y. Gorlova Anderson Cancer Center, Dept. of Epidemiology, 1155 Pressler Street Unit 1340, Houston, TX 77030-4089, USA, oygorlov@mdanderson.org

Dipl. Math. Jutta Groos German Cancer Research Center, Biostatistics Unit C060, P.O. Box 101949, D-69009 Heidelberg, Germany, j.groos@dkfz.de

Prof. Dr. Leonid Hanin Idaho State University, Dept. of Mathematics, Pocatello, ID 83209-8085, USA, hanin@isu.edu

Dr. Harald Heinzl Medical University of Vienna, Core Unit for Medical Statistics & Informatics, Spitalgasse 23, A-1090 Vienna, Austria, harald.heinzl@meduniwien.ac.at

Prof. Dr. Claudia I. Henschke Cornell University, Dept. of Radiology, Weill Medical College, 525 East 68th St., New York, NY 10021, USA, chensch@med.cornell.edu

Dr. hab. Piotr Jurkowski Nicolaus Copernicus University, Collegium Medicum, Dept. of Informatics & Research Methodology, ul. Technikow 3, PL-85-801, Bydgoszcz, Poland, jurkomal@mail.atr.bydgoszcz.pl

Prof. Dr. Byung-Soo Kim   Yonsei University, Dept. of Applied Statistics, 134 Shinchon-Dong, Seodaemoon-Gu, KR-120-749 Seoul, S.Korea, bskim@yonsei.ac.kr

Dr. Inyoung Kim   Yonsei University, Cancer Metastasis Research Center, College of Medicine, 134 Shinchon-Dong, Seodaemoon-Gu, KR-120-752 Seoul, S.Korea, kiy@yumc.yonsei.ac.kr

Dr. Sangchoel Kim   Yonsei University, Cancer Metastasis Research Center, College of Medicine, 134 Shinchon-Dong, Seodaemoon-Gu, KR-120-752 Seoul, S.Korea, kimsc77@yonsei.ac.kr

Prof. Dr. Marek Kimmel   Rice University, Dept. of Statistics MS138, 6100 Main Street, Houston, TX 77005, USA, kimmel@rice.edu

Prof. Dr. Christos P. Kitsos   Technological Educational Institute of Athens, Dept. of Mathematics, Ag Spyridonos and Palikaridi, GR-12210 Egaleo Athens, Greece, xkitsos@teiath.gr

Dr. Ralph L. Kodell   US Food and Drug Administration, Division of Biometry & Risk Assessment, National Center for Toxicological Research, 3900 NCTR Road, Jefferson, AR 72079, USA, rkodell@nctr.fda.gov

Dr. Andrzej Kołtan   Nicolaus Copernicus University, Collegium Medicum, Clinic of Pediatric Hematology and Oncology, ul. M. Sklodowskiej-Curie 9, PL-85-094 Bydgoszcz, Poland, akoltan@by.home.pl

PD Dr. Anette Kopp-Schneider   German Cancer Research Center, Biostatistics Unit C060, P.O. Box 101949, D-69009 Heidelberg, Germany, kopp@dkfz.de

Dr. Vassiliki Kotti   Demokritos University of Thrace, Dept. of Electrical & Computer Engineering, 12 Vas. Sofias Str, GR-67100 Xanthi, Greece, vkotti@ee.duth.gr

Dr. Sunho Lee   Sejong University, Dept. of Applied Statistics, 98 Gunjadong Kwangjinku, KR-143-747 Seoul, S.Korea, leesh@sejong.ac.kr

Prof. Dr. Jesus Fernando López Fidalgo   Universidad de Salamanca, Dept. Estadística, Facultad de Ciencias, Plaza de los Caidos s/n, E-37008 Salamanca, Spain, fidalgo@usal.es

Prof. Dr. E. Georg Luebeck   Fred Hutchinson Cancer Research Center, 1100 Fairview Avenue, MP-665, P.O. Box 19024, Seattle, WA 98109-1024, USA, gluebeck@fhcrc.org

Dr. Suresh H. Moolgavkar   Fred Hutchinson Cancer Research Center, 1100 Fairview Ave. North, MZ-B500, P.O. Box 19024, Seattle, WA 98109-1024, USA, smoolgav@fhcrc.org

Dr. Mikhail S. Nikouline   Universite Victor Segalen, UFR Sciences & Modelisation, 146 Rue Leo Saignat BP 26, F-33076 Bordeaux Cedex, France, nikou@sm.u-bordeaux2.fr

Dr. Fred Parham   National Institute of Environmental Health Sciences, MD A3-06, P.O.Box 12233, Research Triangle Park, NC 27709, USA, parham@niehs.nih.gov

Prof. Dr. Lyudmila V. Pavlova   St. Petersburg State Polytechnical University, Dept. of Applied Mathematics, ul. 29 Polytechnicheskaya, 195251 St. Petersburg, Russia, pavlova@stat.amd.stu.neva.ru

Dr. Eric Pluygers   Rue Jean Stobbaerts 81B, B-1030 Brussels, Belgium

Dr. Christopher J. Portier   National Institute of Environmental Health Sciences, Environmental Toxicology Program, MD A3-02, P.O. Box 12233, Research Triangle Park, NC 27709, USA, portier@niehs.nih.gov

Dr. Jiří Rameš   Charles University of Prague, First Faculty of Medicine, Inst. of Hygiene and Epidemiology, Studnickova 7, CZ-12800 Prague 2, Czech Republic, jrames@lf1.cuni.cz

Dr. Sun Young Rha   Yonsei University, Cancer Metastasis Research Center, College of Medicine, 134 Shinchon-Dong, Seodaemoon-Gu, KR-120-752 Seoul, S.Korea, rha7655@yumc.yonsei.ac.kr

Prof. Dr. Alexandros G. Rigas   Demokritos University of Thrace, School of Engineering, Dept. of Electrical & Computer Engineering, 12 Vas. Sofias Str, Building I, GR-67100 Xanthi, Greece, rigas@ee.duth.gr

Dr. Angela Risch   German Cancer Research Center, Dept. of Toxicology C010, P.O. Box 101949, D-69009 Heidelberg, Germany, a.risch@dkfz.de

Prof. Constantine E. Sekeris   National Hellenic Research Foundation (NHRF), Inst. of Biological Research, Vassileos Constantinou Ave. 48, GR-11635. Athens, Greece, sekeris@eie.gr

Dr. Sylvia Solakidi   National Hellenic Research Foundation, Inst. of Biological Research, Vassileos Constantinou Ave. 48, GR-11635 Athens, Greece, sylviamyrtia@yahoo.gr

Dr. Natalia Spyrou   NCSR 'Demokritos', Institute of Biology, P.O. Box 60 228, GR-15310 Athens, Greece

Prof. Dr. Gonzál Varela   University Hospital, School of Medicine, Thoracic Surgery Section, Avda. del Campo Charro s/n, E-37007 Salamanca, Spain, gvs@usal.es

Prof. Dr. Constantinos E. Vorgias   National & Kapodistrian University of Athens, Faculty of Biology, Department of Biochemistry-Molecular Biology, Panepistimiopolis-Zographou, GR-15784 Athens, Greece, cvorgias@biol.uoa.gr

Dr. Gerassimos Voutsinas   National Center for Scientific Research 'Demokritos', Institute of Biology, Lab. of Environmental Mutagenesis & Carcinogenesis, P.O. Box 60 228, GR-15310 Athens, Greece, mvoutsin@bio.demokritos.gr

Prof. Dr. Karen H. Watanabe   Oregon Health & Science University, OGI School of Science & Engineering, Department of Environmental and Biomolecular Systems, 20000 NW Walker Road, Beaverton, OR 97006-8921, USA watanabe@ebs.ogi.edu

Prof. Dr. Andrej Yakovlev   University of Rochester Medical Center, Dept. of Biostatistics & Computational Biology, 601 Elmwood Avenue, Box 630, Rochester, NY 14642, USA, yakovlev@bst.rochester.edu

Prof. Dr. Alexander Zorin   University of Rochester Medical Center, Dept. of Biostatistics & Computational Biology, 601 Elmwood Avenue, Box 630, Rochester, NY 14642, USA, alexander_zorin@urmc.rochester.edu

Preface

He who knows and knows he knows
He is wise – follow him.
He who knows not and knows he knows not
He is a child – teach him.
He who knows and knows not he knows
He is asleep – wake him.
He who knows not and knows not he knows not
He is fool – shun him.

Arabic proverb cited in Finkel (1990)

When we started planning the editing of the present text two streams flowed together which encouraged us forward. One was the scientific interest of both of us in risk assessment. One editor (L.E.) has been working in cancer research for most of his scientific career, with an engagement in the evaluation of *in vitro* and *in vivo* assay data and their use in risk assessment. Additionally, projects on the health effects of dioxins on workers in the German chemical industry, consultancy work for regulatory agencies on the assessment of chemical and environmental hazards, and a recent collaboration in an EU concerted action on food safety strengthened his interest in the methodology of risk assessment. The second editor (C.P.K.) has been working in the field of the design of experiments and its statistical theory for many years. This led him to the design and analysis of carcinogenicity bioassay data. His interest in risk assessment has been further strengthened since becoming an active member of a research project on biologically based cancer risk assessment, carried out as a pilot study within the CCMS NATO Program. Strongly engaged in teaching, he realized the necessity of making students familiar with real-life applications as early as possible.

A second stream was fed through our joint interest in statistical computing and our work in the International Association for Statistical Computing (IASC), a section of the International Statistical Institute (ISI). It was through the IASC that we first met, and we are indebted to the IASC for its support for meetings which allowed us to make our plans for this book. Without hiding our common origin in mathematical sciences, our approach to risk assessment has been undeniably influenced by the desire to quantify risks and thus to use mathematical and statistical methods. We strongly believe that risk assessment has to be quantitative and that it cannot develop properly without a correct appraisal of the stochastic nature of risk and its adequate mathematical treatment. Therefore probabilistic methods of modeling, methods of statistical inference, and mathematical thinking in general have to flow into a successful risk assessment. This credo on quantitative methods has been imprinted on this project from its very beginning.

As we proceeded, we realized that at least since the mid-1990s new ideas and new methods have been waiting to be incorporated into current risk assessment methodology. On the one hand, new biological data and new biological principles, for example genomic data, the notion of biomarkers and the idea of hormesis came up. On the other hand, new biostatistical methods became available which allowed further development and refinement of existing risk assessment methods. The availability of better statistical methods for model fit as well as the implementation of computational methods to perform model simulations should be mentioned. Finally, new data and analysis needs called for more appropriate quantitative approaches. We wanted to bring these new developments together in one volume in which researchers working in specialized risk assessment fields could find ideas and tools to improve their scientific contribution to cancer and human health risk assessment. Hence, the 25 chapters of this volume should not be considered as a closed compendium for risk assessment methods so much as a source of ideas and concepts for future studies and work.

The triggering event for our work on this book was the organization of the International Conference on Cancer Risk Assessment (ICCRA) – Mathematical, Statistical and Computational Methods held from August 23 to 25, 2003, in Athens, Greece, at the Department of Mathematics of the Technological Educational Institute. This meeting, planned during the ISI Session in Seoul (South Korea) in 2001 and supported by both IASC and ISI, was organized as a Satellite Conference to the 53rd Session of the ISI in Berlin (Germany) to provide a forum for the discussion and exchange of ideas on recent methods in cancer risk assessment. The stimulation of research at the interface between molecular biology and mathematical modeling of the carcinogenic process, and an improved transfer of risk assessment methodology to the risk management process, were further achievements of that meeting. During this conference many relevant topics were considered, such as biological carcinogenesis theories, stochastic carcinogenesis models, modeling for cancer survival and cancer screening studies, dose-response modeling, statistical evaluation methods, the Bayesian approach to uncertainty, design of experiments, the benchmark dose approach, biochemical and molecular biomarkers, genomic data, case studies for health risk assessment, regulatory affairs and quality standards. Related applied research on epidemiology, prognosis and prediction was also addressed. A large proportion of the authors and author teams invited to contribute to the volume attended the Athens conference where at last a time line for the production of the book was set up.

In parallel with the preparations for the ICCRA conference we found an encouraging interest of the part of John Wiley & Sons, Ltd in this book project. In particular, we wish to thank three persons from Wiley without whom this project would never been possible: first, Rob Calver with whom we discussed the scope of the volume and with whom we finally accomplished the project plan, its peer review and approval through Wiley authorities; secondly, we are as grateful to Kathryn Sharples who took over responsibility for this project in 2004 and who guided us through the production and printing with her expert knowledge in publishing; and finally, we have to thank Lucy Bryan for all the necessary technical advice for the production during the phase of the submission of the text and the final printing. We appreciate so much these persons' understanding of the two worlds of science and publishing business.

The present volume aims to present new concepts and methods for cancer and human health risk assessment which account for the wealth of new biological data and biological and medical concepts. This comprises mathematical, statistical and computational methods for exposure assessment, hazard identification, dose-response modeling and hazard characterization. We hope that the contributions brought together in this monograph will stimulate further research at the interface between molecular biology and mathematical modeling of diseases. We also hope to contribute to a better transfer of risk assessment methodology to the risk management process. Risk estimation is intimately connected to the availability of empirical data as well as the availability and use of quantitative methods which allow not only the estimation of risks but also the determination of the accuracy of those estimates.

It quickly became evident to us that this volume would naturally exhibit some heterogeneity not only because of the different scientific backgrounds of the various contributors but also because the complexity of the field itself. The more we worked on this project the more we came to understand why textbooks on risk assessment methods are rare and why others have restricted their work to specific aspects of risk assessment, such as specific mathematical models or specific applications.

We should mention that a number of valuable texts on risk assessment have appeared since the 1990s, for example, the volume on environmental risk assessment edited by Dennis Paustenbach (2002). Although not focused on mathematical and statistical methods, this multi-author monograph can be warmly recommended as secondary literature to our text, in particular for its large number of case studies on specific hazardous compounds. We should also mention that there are a number of other books on risk assessment available. These are cited below, mostly in the introductory remarks to each of the six parts of our book. We think that this volume is unique in that it covers a wide range of issues relevant at present and is directed explicitly to quantitative methods, thus having a genuinely statistical flavor. Therefore, we hope that this book offers the chance to see how 'statistics in action' behaves for the solution of a crucial problem of life sciences and that we have been able to bring important subjects close to a uniform comprehensive form. We would be pleased to see some of the topics in this book taken up in graduate courses such that this book may help to guide young researchers in this important field in public health.

In order to make the reader aware that there is a large amount of coherence between the topics and papers brought together in this book we decided to add a short introductory section to each of its six parts. As we see it, a comprehensive compendium on quantitative methods for risk assessment is neither possible nor actually needed. It is surely not easy to accomplish given the complexity of the subject, the vast amount of work done over the past 50 years, and the persisting basic scientific differences in meanings and understandings. Neither is it actually needed, because risk assessment is primarily a service task to support the risk manager and/or the risk regulator through the provision of best science. The methods presented below should enable the reader to extract the best possible information on risks from real-life examples. We should also remark that our introductory remarks are not intended to summarize or comment on the papers. We think that the collected papers speak eloquently enough for themselves. It would have been hard, anyway, to summarize the individual contributions without becoming repetitive. The remarks are simply intended to give some guidance on each topic and to give some additional information which we think might interest the reader and motivate future investigations.

All the papers in this volume were reviewed by both editors and by authors of other papers who are experts in the respective topic. We would like to thank all the reviewers, who worked hard to improve the submitted papers. We enjoyed further review support from Carina Ittrich (Heidelberg). Finally, we wish to thank all our staff members: in Heidelberg Renate Rausch, Regina Grunert, Daniel Czech and Kathrin Hilberath; and in Athens our students for their volunteer work, in particular, M. Paritsis, C. Fatseas, and A. Logothetis. Last but not least, we thank our wives for their understanding for the time we devoted to this work.

Introduction

This volume has been designed by Lutz Edler (Biostatistics Unit of the German Cancer Research Center in Heidelberg) and Christos P. Kitsos (Department of Mathematics of the Technical Educational Institute in Athens) to present concepts and methods for cancer and human health risk assessment. This comprehensive text accounts for the wealth of new biological data as well as new biological, toxicological and medical approaches to be used for risk assessment. Mathematical, statistical and computational methods are presented for exposure assessment, hazard identification, dose-response modelling and hazard characterization. This volume has been compiled with the intention of bridging different approaches to the risk assessment problem through 25 contributions written by a group of distinct expert authorities. The breadth of this approach is reflected in the number and the content of about 1000 references, a bibliographic source which may also bridge an existing gap in risk assessment literature.

Various topics such as *biological carcinogenesis theories, stochastic carcinogenesis models, modelling for cancer survival and cancer screening studies, dose-response modelling, statistical evaluation methods, the Bayesian approach to uncertainty, design of experiments, the benchmark dose approach, biochemical* and *molecular biomarkers, genomic data* and *case studies for health risk assessment* are addressed by well-known scientists who present recent work and points of view on the best risk assessment methodologies.

We believe that this book will contribute to a better transfer of risk assessment methodology to academic researchers as well as to risk assessors and regulators. This text should support all those interested in this challenging and exciting applied science: researchers in medical science, biology, toxicology, statistics or mathematics, risk assessors or stakeholders involved in the day-to-day process of risk assessment, and teachers of biomathematics and biostatistics planning a graduate–level course with real-life applications.

PART I

CANCER AND HUMAN HEALTH RISK ASSESSMENT

Introductory remarks

Lutz Edler and Christos P. Kitsos

In his comprehensive volume on environmental risk assessment, Paustenbach (2002) characterizes risk assessment as the description of the likelihood of adverse or unwanted responses to exposure and states as its goal the estimation of that likelihood after assembling and assessing all scientific information regarding toxicology, human experience, and environmental fate and exposure. It was not until the middle of the twentieth century that serious concern was expressed over the risks caused by synthetically manufactured chemicals and radiation, at least in industrialized countries (For a historical overview, from a US perspective, see the first chapter of Paustenbach's book.). Before that time infectious diseases had been the most feared threats to human health.

From the beginning of the risk assessment of chemicals in food and the environment, cancer risk assessment played the lead role in the development of quantitative methods. The very birth of cancer risk assessment was motivated and guided by the strong wish of most risk managers and regulators to determine threshold doses/ exposures. It was thought that a specific chemical should possess an absolute threshold value below which an exposure should not elicit an adverse health effect in humans. Setting a regulatory exposure limit at that threshold (or, when conservatively accounting for uncertainty, below it) would suffice to exclude any risk from humans. Consequently, research concentrated on the estimation of such a hypothesized threshold levels. The NOAEL (no observed adverse effect level) appeared as *the* natural estimate of that level. Therefore, experimental data were screened, either from human studies or from animal dose-response experiments, doses were

Recent Advances in Quantitative Methods in Cancer and Human Health Risk Assessment
Edited by L. Edler and C. Kitsos © 2005 John Wiley & Sons, Ltd

identified at which no differences compared to the unexposed control were observed, and the largest such dose was declared as the NOAEL value. For a thorough scientific discussion of the threshold concept and its consequences for risk assessment practice we refer to the work of Wout Slob (e.g. Slob, 2002). More formally, the NOAEL has been defined as the largest administered dose in a dose-response experiment which is not statistically significant at a predefined significance level of, say, 5 %. As such, it is a statistical estimate and is subject to the rules of statistical inference like any other parameter derived from dose-response data (see Part III below). However, insisting on the existence of an absolute threshold value or 'zero risk' as well as attempting to find 'no risk' levels of exposure would have led into a blind alley. Among the first quantitative methods for risk assessment which did not assume a threshold dose was the Mantel and Bryan (1961) procedure estimating the so-called virtually safe dose (VSD), an exposure or dose below which at maximum a very low incidence (above background), say, one in a million, would occur.

Fortunately, risk assessment has matured from a method deciding between the existence and non-existence of risk into a scientifically oriented methodology which comprises a number of life science disciplines, such as biology, toxicology, pharmacology, acute and chronic medicine, physiology, as well as chemistry, physical chemistry, mathematics and statistics. This maturation is by no means complete. Witness the barrage of new techniques, new data and new theories created in life sciences which call for recognition, as well as the further development of methodology for the analysis and interpretation of data. On the other hand, there is still a strong need to provide for the risk manager and the public adequate advice on the information content of risk measures such as the NOAEL, benchmark dose level, reference dose levels, etc. Statistics plays an important role in the transmission of correct information.

At the beginning of the twenty-first century, the discipline of risk assessment presents itself as scientific methodology which should guide and improve decision making in the sector of public health and environment, concerning pollution, contamination and accidental exposure to substances which may be hazardous for humans. The outcome of risk assessment is now increasingly becoming the basis of risk management decisions, and this fact is slowly being recognized by the public as well as by the media. Scientific risk assessment is the only rational approach to judging risks and developing measures to resolve their dangerous consequences to humans and their health.

The basics of current risk assessment were laid out in the USA by the National Research Council (1983). Since then, there has been overwhelming agreement that risk assessment consist of the four components

- *hazard identification*, involving all available valuable information to determine whether or not a substance is hazardous;

- *dose-response assessment*, replaced now by *hazard characterization*, using available quantitative information to estimate the response at exposure levels;

- *exposure assessment*, determining the sources, routes and amount of exposure;

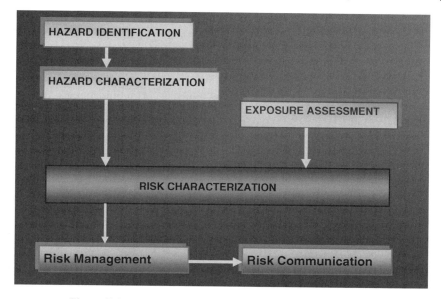

Figure I.1 Schematic view of the risk assessment paradigm.

- *risk characterization*, integrating the previous three components with a discussion of strengths and limitations; see Figure I.1 as well as Renwick *et al.* (2003).

The opening chapter of this volume, by V. J. Cogliano, provides a wealth of information and basic thoughts on the risk assessment paradigm and its present usage. That this risk assessment paradigm has not been adapted by different countries in the same way and that a large number of harmonization issues remain unresolved can be learned from an earlier article by the same author (Cogliano *et al.*, 2002).

There have been countless contributions on risk assessment in the scientific literature (in October 2004 PubMed returned more than 50 000 citations on 'risk assessment'). Less overwhelming is the flood of publications in the statistical literature (the CIS system of the American Statistical Association gave in its 2002 issue only about 300 citations on 'risk assessment'). The number of books on statistical and quantitative methods for risk assessment is not very large; see, for example, Travis (1989), Moolgavkar *et al.* (1999), Cox (2001), Chyczewski *et al.* (2002) and Cogliano *et al.* (1999b). For example, in the IARC monograph of Moolgavkar *et al.* (1999) 12 authors give a survey in nine chapters on the basic principles and the practice of quantitative estimation and prediction of cancer risks as used by the end of the 1990s at various regulatory agencies. This includes two chapters on epidemiological studies and two other chapters on mathematical modeling and statistics. In accordance with the editors primary scientific research interest, biological carcinogenesis theories and data available until the mid nineties are considered with strong a focus on the two-stage clonal expansion model also known as the Moolgavkar–Venzon–Knudson model. Some of chapters below will address more recent biological concepts and their respective sources of biological data as well as additional aspects relevant for risk assessment. Other monographs have focused on standard methods of animal bioassay for carcinogenicity, discussed the use of the maximum tolerated dose, and developed dose-response models on the basis of standard models of carcinogenesis. In contrast to this, our text will concentrate primarily on human data and their modeling.

A different view on risk assessment has been taken by Vose (2000), who uses the term 'risk analysis'. Actually, he applies methods of probability theory and statistics for the assessment of the variability and uncertainty of processes. A major focus is on Monte Carlo simulation and the Bayesian approach. This work is a valuable source of parametric statistical distributions. An even broader view on risk assessment has been taken by authors who also cover economic and societal risks, e.g. the water supply system. According to Hames (1998), risk analysis combines 'concepts, tools and technologies that have been developed and practiced in such areas as design, development, system integration, prototyping, and construction of physical infrastructure; in reliability, quality control, and maintenance; and in the estimation of cost and schedule and in project management'. These authors consider systems modeling and optimization, thereby emphasizing technical systems, extreme events, uncertainty and sensitivity. Their prominent risk analysis questions are: What can go wrong? What is the likelihood that it will go wrong? What are the consequences? When doing risk assessment in the life sciences, it may be prudent not to neglect those developments of risk analysis in the engineering and, in particular, in the economic sciences.

We hope that this short introduction to a very complex field has given a global point of view on the problems to be discussed in the following chapters. We are aware that the particular order of the chapters we have chosen is subjective, but we feel it is the most convenient. The experienced reader will doubtless choose his own way of working through the book.

CHAPTER 1

Principles of Cancer Risk Assessment: The Risk Assessment Paradigm

Vincent James Cogliano

International Agency for Research on Cancer[1]

1.1 THE RISK ASSESSMENT PARADIGM

The United States National Research Council has outlined a series of steps that many agencies follow in analysing risk (National Research Council, 1983, 1994). Although this chapter is focused on cancer risk assessment, the risk assessment paradigm can apply equally to other adverse effects.

- *Hazard identification* asks whether exposure to an agent can cause an increase in the incidence of an adverse effect. This involves consideration of the epidemiologic evidence in humans, the evidence in experimental animals, and other relevant data, including studies of toxicokinetics and mechanisms.

- *Dose-response assessment* characterises the relationship between the dose of an agent and the incidence of an adverse health effect. The fundamental activity of dose-response assessment is modelling, which can range from simple linear (proportionality) models to more complex toxicokinetic and mechanism-based models. The purpose of the modelling is to extrapolate from the conditions observed in the epidemiologic and experimental studies to the conditions that are of interest in a human exposure situation. It is common for risk assessments to extrapolate from high doses to lower doses, from experimental animals to humans, from one route of exposure to another, or

[1]The views expressed in this chapter are those of the author and do not necessarily reflect the views or policies of the International Agency for Research on Cancer.

Recent Advances in Quantitative Methods in Cancer and Human Health Risk Assessment
Edited by L. Edler and C. Kitsos © 2005 John Wiley & Sons, Ltd

from one pattern of exposure to another. There are also other extrapolations that have received less discussion.

- *Exposure assessment* determines the extent of human exposure to an agent. It identifies the *pathways* by which a population can be exposed, for example, through breathing contaminated air, eating contaminated fish, or swimming in a contaminated lake. For each pathway, an exposure assessment estimates how much of the agent the population is exposed to. This can depend on the magnitude, duration, and frequency of exposure.

- *Risk characterisation* describes the nature and magnitude of human risk, including attendant uncertainty. It integrates the hazard identification, dose-response assessment, and exposure assessment. It often emphasises a quantitative component that estimates risk by determining where an exposure estimate falls on the dose-response curve. The risk characterisation also includes a qualitative component that describes the assessment's strengths and limitations and identifies some key research needs.

The hazard identification and dose-response assessment steps are generally regarded as descriptive of the properties of a toxic agent. For example, health agencies may identify a hazard by describing a chemical agent as "carcinogenic to humans" or "possibly carcinogenic to humans". They may also estimate a dose-response curve for each agent (US Environmental Protection Agency (US EPA), 2003a). These steps are generally performed centrally, as toxic properties and dose-response curves are not thought of as varying from one location to another. In contrast to these centralised steps of a risk assessment, the exposure assessment and risk characterisation steps address a specific human population. These latter steps consider the various exposure pathways that may be involved, estimate the level of human exposure to the toxic agent, and then characterise the risk by determining where that level of exposure falls on the dose-response curve. Exposure assessment and risk characterisation often depend on specific knowledge of local populations and exposure conditions; accordingly, they are often performed at a more decentralised level.

In the future, this distinction between centralised hazard identification and dose-response assessment and decentralised exposure assessment and risk characterisation may break down as more is known about the distribution of genetic polymorphisms in different ethnic groups, and it becomes possible to estimate different dose-response curves for different segments of the population. Similarly, as more is known about the effects of one agent on the absorption, metabolism, and elimination of another agent, it may become possible to estimate different dose-response curves for different populations based on their level of exposure to other agents that modify the effects of the agent being assessed. At this time, however, because not enough is known about polymorphisms and the interactions of multiple agents to be able to estimate different dose-response curves for different populations and exposure conditions, dose-response assessment has generally estimated a single dose-response curve for each agent.

Because this chapter is focused on the assessment of potential carcinogens, the hazard identification and dose-response assessment steps are treated in greater detail.

1.2 HAZARD IDENTIFICATION

The data considered for hazard identification include human epidemiologic studies, long-term bioassays in experimental animals, and other relevant data on toxicokinetics and cancer mechanisms. Each source of data has a role in the hazard assessment. Epidemiologic studies can provide unequivocal evidence of carcinogenicity, but often are not sufficiently sensitive to identify a carcinogenic hazard except when the risk is high or involves an unusual form of cancer. For this reason, animal studies generally provide the best means of assessing potential risks to humans. To answer questions about the similarity of response between animals and humans, studies of toxicokinetics and mechanisms have been employed. Toxicokinetic studies investigate similarities and differences in absorption, distribution, metabolism, and elimination across species. Mechanistic studies can elucidate the chemical species and cellular processes involved in cancer initiation and development, including short-term tests to identify the potential for genetic toxicity.

The conclusion is often a judgement that weighs the evidence that an agent may or may not cause a specific adverse effect. For example, the International Agency for Research on Cancer uses the following terms to describe a cancer hazard:

- carcinogenic to humans (Group 1),

- probably carcinogenic to humans (Group 2A),

- possibly carcinogenic to humans (Group 2B),

- not classifiable as to its carcinogenicity to humans (Group 3),

- probably not carcinogenic to humans (Group 4).

Other agencies (for example, US EPA, 1986b, 2003a) have adopted similar descriptors for potential carcinogens.

A prominent trend in cancer hazard identification has been the greater availability and use of mechanistic information. Mechanistic studies attempt to identify the series of key precursor events that are involved in cancer development. This may permit a judgement about whether the mechanisms that cause cancer in experimental animals are likely to be operative in humans. Once the key precursor events involved in cancer development are identified, mechanistic studies also allow identification of sub-populations and life-stages that may be especially susceptible to cancer induced by the agent. In any use of mechanistic data, it is crucial to investigate whether more than one mechanism may be operating.

1.3 DOSE-RESPONSE ASSESSMENT

1.3.1 Different objectives, different data sets, different approaches

There have been two broad approaches to dose-response assessment. *Safety assessment* focuses on determining a safe dose for human exposure. This has generally involved identifying a dose that appears to be without adverse effects in the experimental studies and dividing that dose by several factors to arrive at a dose considered "safe" for human exposure. The other approach provides estimates of risk at low doses, by fitting dose-response models to data on the incidence of an adverse effect and using these models to estimate the incidence at lower levels of exposure. A large majority of cancer assessments have been of the latter variety, using models to estimate the cancer risk over a range of potential exposure levels.

The models used in dose-response assessment can be considered to belong to two broad classes. *Empirical models* are based on fitting a standard curve to data. (They are sometimes called *curve-fitting models*.) They are the least detailed models, describing the incidence of frankly observable adverse effects as a mathematical function of exposure to the agent. Such models are not based on specific knowledge about biological processes and mechanisms.

In contrast, *physiologically based toxicokinetic models* and *mechanism-based dose-response models* are based on specific knowledge about the biological processes and mechanisms leading from exposure to disease. (They are sometimes called *biologically based models*.) Toxicokinetic models simulate the relationship between external exposure and delivered dose at the target tissue. They can incorporate detailed information on an agent's absorption, distribution, metabolism, and elimination. Mechanism-based models simulate the relationship between cellular responses at the target tissue, precursor effects, and frankly observable adverse effects in the organism. These more detailed models require extensive knowledge of the disposition of a chemical in the body and the sequence of events leading to toxicity and disease.

Safety assessments, too, have begun to move toward increasing complexity. Formerly, dividing an apparently "safe" dose by a factor of 100 was believed to yield a dose fit for human exposure. This factor of 100 was later described as composed of a factor of 10 to account for differences between humans and experimental animals and another factor of 10 to account for differences between susceptible humans and the general population. More recently, these factors of 10 have in turn been described as being composed of a factor of 3 (being approximately the square root of 10) for toxicokinetic differences and another factor of 3 for toxicodynamic differences, or alternatively, a factor of 4 for toxicokinetic differences and a factor of 2.5 for toxicodynamic differences (assuming that these approximate factors can be refined to this level of precision). In addition, other factors have been used to account for differences between experimental conditions and human exposure conditions, for example, when a short-term animal study is used to infer a dose "safe" for lifetime human exposure, or when the experimental database lacks adequate studies of key adverse effects or studies that are pertinent to exposure during pre-natal and post-natal development. Another recent trend in safety assessment has been to replace the various factors of 10 by *data-derived factors* that attempt to reflect more precisely the degree of difference between humans and experimental animals.

Dose-response models can be developed for different objectives. For example, a dose-response model can serve as a framework for organising and synthesising the available data and identifying research needs. In this case, a rather detailed model might be appropriate, using default assumptions and parameter values as place-holders to indicate where further research is needed. A different objective of dose-response modelling would be to provide projections of the range of risks that populations can face under different actual or hypothetical exposure conditions. In this case, a model that is well supported by data and not overly detailed might be most useful when a government agency needs to reassure a community that they do not face an unsafe exposure condition. In this case, the more speculative compo-nents of a research-oriented model may not be useful in a governmental determina-tion of the risk that may be present.

1.3.2 Extrapolations in dose-response assessment

The fundamental objective of risk assessment, as with modelling generally, is extrapolation. Experimental data observed under specified conditions are extra-polated to human exposure conditions that may be similar in some respects and dissimilar in other respects from those in the experiments. Similarly, epidemiologic data observed in one human population exposed to certain conditions may be extrapolated to other human populations and other exposure conditions. The models developed as part of a dose-response assessment describe how these extrapolations are made and provide a basis for evaluating how well the extrapolations are supported by data. Several kinds of extrapolations are made in dose-response assessment.

- *Extrapolation from high doses to lower doses* is often a central objective of dose-response modelling. For example, studies in experimental animals generally use high doses to determine the effects that a specific agent can induce at some dose. This is often a practical necessity when fewer than, say, 100 animals are tested (and consequently a response rate of less than 1 percent cannot be observed), because government agencies are interested in ensuring that the risk to an exposed population is much less than 1 percent. This also happens when occupational studies are used to infer the potential for risk at environmental or occupational levels that are anticipated to be lower than those observed in prior occupational settings.

- *Extrapolation from experimental animals to humans* is also a common objective of dose-response modelling. Such extrapolation is often necessary just to compare modelling results from experiments involving different animal species. Although modelling can proceed using either animal dose metrics or human dose metrics, when the ultimate objective is a statement regarding risks to exposed humans, animal dose metrics must be converted into an *equivalent human dose.*

- *Route-to-route extrapolation* is the application of a dose-response relationship estimated from studies involving one exposure route (for example, ingestion, inhalation, or dermal exposure) to another exposure route. This form of extrapolation has both a qualitative and a quantitative component. Qualitatively, one must make a judgement about whether the effects observed following exposure by one route are pertinent to another exposure route. Such a judgement is generally warranted when effects are observed at a site distant from the site of entry and when absorption can occur by either exposure route to give an internal dose of the agent. Such a judgement is sometimes specified as a default option in the absence of adequate data to the contrary.

- *Extrapolation from one pattern of exposure to another* involves using information derived from occupational exposure patterns or experimental exposure protocols (for example, a single daily dose five days a week for 24 months) to make inferences about other human exposure patterns that are likely to be different. This common extrapolation, used in most dose-response assessments, has typically been handled by the use of default dose metrics such as average daily dose or cumulative dose.

- *Extrapolation from small samples to larger populations* generally has not been explicitly discussed in risk assessments. The experimental uncertainty inherent in using small experimental samples can be described by the confidence bounds associated with the estimates from the experimental studies. An important qualitative concern, however, with the use of small samples in experimental studies is the need to discuss the experiment's power to detect adverse effects. For example, a response that is not statistically significant does not indicate a threshold; rather, it can be consistent with a small risk that falls below the experiment's power of detection. A similar concern is that small samples generally do not include adequate numbers to make reliable inferences about safe doses for susceptible individuals.

- *Extrapolation from relatively homogeneous groups to more heterogeneous populations* also generally has not been explicitly discussed in risk assessments. It can, however, strongly influence the shape of a dose-response curve. This is particularly important in view of the fact that many experimental studies use relatively homogeneous, genetically similar animals. Similar animals may have a tendency to respond at similar dose levels, while a more heterogeneous population would not necessarily all respond at the same dose level. This may be true even when the mechanism of action suggests a threshold dose below which adverse effects would not occur, because the threshold could vary across a heterogeneous population and the population dose-response curve could become indistinguishable from those associated with non-threshold models. In the human population, genetic and lifestyle factors contribute to increased variation in susceptibility, which spreads the dose-response curve over a wider range of doses (Lutz, 1990).

- *Extrapolation to different life-stages* also generally has not been explicitly discussed in risk assessments. It is important to recognise, however, that many chronic experimental studies begin exposing the animals only after early-life developmental stages have passed, and that this can be a susceptible period of exposure for some diseases and agents. Similarly, many epidemiologic studies involve occupational exposure, which generally miss early-life and late-in-life stages. An analysis of the studies that investigated the effects of early-life exposure indicates that is a susceptible period of exposure that can lead to a higher incidence of cancer later in life (US EPA, 2003b). This suggests that the extrapolation to life-stages that are not covered by conventional experimental bioassays and epidemiologic studies deserves more explicit consideration.

- *Extrapolation from single-variable experiments to complex exposure situations* also generally has not been explicitly discussed in risk assessments. Conventional experimental study designs rightly try to minimise exposure to other toxic agents in order that the effects of the agent being studied can be unambiguously demonstrated. Human exposure circumstances, in contrast, involve a multitude of background and other exposures that can be toxicologically significant. Finding a safe dose in an otherwise unexposed population does not mean that that dose is safe when background and other common exposures are considered (US EPA, 2001b).

For those extrapolations that generally have not been addressed in past risk assessments, this implies that a particular source of human variation or uncertainty is not being considered. For example, the use of small samples to estimate rates of metabolism may mean that differences in metabolic polymorphisms are not being reflected in those estimates. Using the results of single-chemical experiments to estimate doses in more complex human exposure situations may mean that the effect of other exposures that can alter metabolic capacity (for example, consumption of alcoholic beverages or use of certain pharmaceuticals) is not being reflected in the dose estimates. Risk assessments could be improved by considering these factors when they may be important.

1.3.3 Safety assessment

Safety assessment is an approach to dose-response assessment that does not attempt to describe dose-response curves. Rather, its focus is to estimate an exposure level where there is little concern for adverse effects. Such a dose has been called, by various health agencies, an *acceptable daily intake* (ADI), a *tolerable daily intake* (TDI), a *minimal risk level* (MRL), or a *reference dose* (RfD). These approaches have generally not been used in cancer assessments, but EPA's recent draft final cancer guidelines (US EPA, 2003a) provide some discussion on subject.

Safety assessments generally are developed through a process that selects a critical precursor effect that occurs at the lowest doses, determines a dose where this precursor is either not observed or occurs at a specified incidence rate (for example, 5 % or 10 %), and reduces this dose by a factor that reflects the differences between study conditions and conditions of human exposure. The resulting dose is characterised as one where there is little concern for any adverse effects, but without an explicit characterisation of risk levels either above or below that dose.

1.3.3.1 Developing a safety assessment

A dose where the critical precursor effects are not observed is often called a *no observable adverse effect level* (NOAEL). Generally this is one of the doses in the experimental study. More recently, modelling has been used to derive a dose (sometimes called a *benchmark dose*) that would induce a specified observable level of adverse effects (for example, 5 % or 10 % incidence). Such a dose is generally not one of the doses used in the study, but is an interpolated dose that falls between study doses.

Because the study conditions associated with the NOAEL (or benchmark dose) can differ from conditions of human exposure, it would not be scientifically defensible to assume that exposure at the NOAEL would pose little concern for humans. The following are some of the ways in which study conditions can differ from the conditions of human exposure:

- *Uncertainty in extrapolating from animals to humans.* Although there are many physiological similarities that apply across mammalian species, there are also many quantitative differences to consider when using an animal NOAEL to make inferences about the safety of human doses. These differences can be toxicokinetic or toxicodynamic in nature. In the absence of specific data on the agent being assessed, a reduction factor of 10 is often used as a default to cover the differences between animals and humans.

- *Variation from average humans to susceptible humans.* Experimental or epidemiologic studies rarely target biologically susceptible individuals. Susceptible humans could be adversely affected at lower doses than a general study population (especially a healthy adult worker population); consequently, general-population NOAELs are reduced so that they would apply to more susceptible individuals. In the absence of specific data on the agent being assessed, a reduction factor of 10 is generally used as a default to cover the differences between average humans and susceptible humans.

- *Uncertainty in extrapolating from one exposure regimen to another.* Sometimes the experimental studies involve less-than-lifetime exposure. Lifetime exposure can have effects that do not appear after shorter exposure durations; consequently, a safe dose for lifetime exposure may be lower than the safe dose for less-than-lifetime exposure observed in the experimental studies. Similarly, sometimes the experimental studies use intermittent dosing, and a safe dose for continuous exposure may be lower than a safe dose for intermittent exposure observed in the experimental studies. An adjustment to the NOAEL may be appropriate when human exposure conditions are significantly different from the experimental exposure conditions. This may be complicated in the case of short-term intermittent human exposures to temporarily high levels. For example, one agent may act through a toxic metabolite that is preferentially formed at high doses, and another agent may act through toxic metabolites that are preferentially formed at lower doses. Depending on the toxicokinetics and the mechanisms of action, some short-term high-level exposures may pose significant risks, and others may pose much smaller risks.

Other factors are sometimes used to reflect a professional judgement about scientific uncertainties not explicitly treated above, including completeness of the overall database, minimal sample size, or poor exposure characterisation. An example would be an incomplete database that does not include adequate studies of some potential adverse effects. Another example would be a metal whose absorption or retention is reduced when ingested with food. If the animal study involved exposure in the feed while human exposure involves non-food pathways (for example, a child playing in contaminated dirt), then the animal NOAEL should be reduced to compensate for the higher absorption and retention expected in humans relative to the dietary exposure conditions in the animal study.

1.3.3.2 Characterising a safety assessment

The EPA's draft final cancer guidelines (US EPA, 2003a) note that a safety assessment is only a single point on the dose-response curve, and thus cannot by itself convey all the critical information present in the data from which it is derived. These guidelines list some points that should be discussed in safety assessments where cancer is an adverse effect being assessed:

- *Nature of the response.* Is the dose-response curve based on tumours or a precursor? Does it measure incidence or mortality? Is it a measure of lifetime risk, or was the study terminated earlier?

- *Level of the response.* What level of response was used to derive the safety assessment, for example, a 1 percent cancer risk, a 5 percent cancer risk, or a 10 percent change in a precursor measure? Obviously, different adjustment factors would apply depending on the level or nature of the response.

- *Nature of the study population.* Is the dose-response curve based on humans or animals? How large is the effective sample size? Is the study group representative of the general population, of healthy adult workers, or of a susceptible group? Are both sexes represented? Did exposure occur during a susceptible life-stage?

- *Slope of the observed dose-response curve.* At the low end of the dose-response curve, how rapidly does risk decrease as dose decreases?

- *Relationship of this assessment with those for other cancers.* For example, a safety assessment derived from data on male workers would not reflect the implications of mammary tumours in female rats or mice. It may be important to use both endpoints to provide a comprehensive picture of potential human risks.

- *Extent of the overall cancer database.* Is the database limited to particular cancers, population segments, or life-stages?

A safety assessment derived by calculating a NOAEL and dividing it by several factors is sometimes described as being based on the assumption that there exists a *threshold dose* below which an individual does not respond. This characterisation is not entirely appropriate, as experimental data are not able to estimate thresholds with much confidence. A response that is not statistically significant does not indicate a threshold; rather, it can be consistent with a small risk that falls below the experiment's power of detection. For example, if 50 animals are exposed and none develops an adverse effect, this result is completely consistent with a risk of, say, 1 in 100; consequently, a dose associated with zero incidence (in this case, 0/50) does not indicate a threshold. In addition, statistical significance is affected by study design and sample size; consequently, an NOAEL in one study may show a statistically significant adverse effect in a superior study with a different design or a larger sample size.

1.3.4 Modelling to estimate risk at low doses

The most common approach to dose-response assessment for potential carcinogens has been to fit models to the available data on a specific agent and to use those models to estimate the cancer risk in an exposed population.

The models discussed in this paper can be developed to varying levels of complexity as they consider the progression from:

(measures of dose)

1. exposure to an agent at some concentration in an external medium, to

2. internal dose, to

3. delivered dose at the target tissue or cell, to

(measures of response)

4. cellular response at the target, to

5. observable precursor effects, to

6. frankly observable adverse effects in the organism.

Models of the relationship between external exposure and either internal dose or delivered dose are discussed in Section 1.3.4.1. Models of the relationship between some measure of dose and some measure of response, at either the cellular, organ, or organism level are discussed in Section 1.3.4.2.

1.3.4.1 Dose modelling

Dose models consider the progression from exposure to an agent at some concentration in an external medium, through various intermediate measures of internal dose, to the delivered dose at the target tissue or cell.

Dose metrics

Dose-response assessment begins by determining an appropriate *dose metric* for each adverse effect that can be attributed to the agent. There are several components to a dose metric:

- *The agent.* Typically, this can be the administered agent, or it can be a metabolite or a reaction product that is produced internally.

- *The proximity to the target site.* Typically, this can be the administered dose, or it can be an internal dose such as the concentration of the agent in the blood or the concentration at some organ in the body.

- *A time component.* Typically can be the average dose, but it could also be the peak dose, the cumulative dose, or the average body burden.

The selection of an appropriate dose metric considers what is known about the agent and the mechanisms by which it produces each adverse effect.

The US EPA's Guidelines for Exposure Assessment contain useful definitions for different forms of dose (US EPA 1992a). *Exposure* is the contact of an agent with the outer boundary of an organism. *Exposure concentration* is the concentration of a chemical in its transport or carrier medium at the point of contact. *Dose* is the amount of a substance available for interaction with metabolic processes or biologically significant receptors after crossing the outer boundary of an organism. *Potential dose* is the amount ingested, inhaled, or applied to the skin. *Applied dose* is the amount of a substance presented to the absorption barrier and available for absorption (although not necessarily having yet crossed the outer boundary of the organism). *Absorbed dose* is the amount crossing a specific absorption barrier (for example, the exchange boundaries of skin, lung, and digestive tract) through uptake processes. *Internal dose* is a more general term without respect to specific absorption barriers or exchange boundaries. *Delivered dose* is the amount of the chemical available for interaction by any particular organ or cell.

The goal of dose modelling is to estimate, to the extent possible, the delivered dose of the *active agent* at the *target organ* or *target cell*. Having the knowledge about the active agent and the target site, plus the data to be able to estimate a dose metric at this level of detail, would allow one to estimate the level of exposure that is associated with the first organ or cellular response that can lead to an adverse effect. When the delivered dose cannot be determined with confidence, modelling often proceeds by using another less specific dose metric, for example, the average daily dose of the administered agent.

Standardising different exposure patterns

Complex exposure patterns are often present in the epidemiologic or experimental animal studies that are used for dose-response assessment. For example, workers can be exposed to intense but intermittent exposures during the workday. Experimental animals can receive a daily dose by gavage (that is, via a tube inserted through the mouth to the forestomach), or they can receive intermittent doses throughout the day via their food or drinking water. Doses also can vary from one time to another, or there can be brief or prolonged periods between times that exposure occurs. The resulting internal dose depends on many variables, including exposure concentration, duration of exposure, frequency of exposure, and duration of recovery periods between exposures. Dose-response models typically simplify these complex exposure patterns by estimating some *summary measure* of exposure, for example, an average daily dose.

When enough information is available, *toxicokinetic modelling* (discussed below) is the preferred approach for determining a summary measure for a complex exposure pattern. Toxicokinetic models are suited for this purpose because they generally consider an exposure profile over time and they can incorporate information about metabolism and target tissue. For example, if there is sufficient information to identify the active agent(s), a toxicokinetic model can be useful in modelling the internal concentrations of the active agent, whether it be the administered agent or a metabolite or a reaction product. When there is sufficient information to identify the target site(s) of biological interaction, a toxicokinetic model can be useful in modelling the concentration of the active agent at the target site, for example, the concentration in the blood or the liver or the brain. When there is sufficient information to identify which summary measure of dose is most relevant, for example, average concentration or peak concentration or cumulative dose, a toxicokinetic model can be useful for investigating the relationship between external exposure and the relevant internal measure of dose.

When there is not enough information to construct and fit a toxicokinetic model, or when the nature of the problem does not justify the time and effort to develop one, less detailed *default approaches* are used to estimate a summary measure of dose. These approaches generally involve computing a daily dose or concentration that is averaged over the duration of the study (US EPA, 2003a). In occupational studies, cumulative dose is often used. These practices make an implicit assumption that each unit of exposure carries an equal risk, so exposures can be averaged or summed across the duration of the study. Such approaches generally acknowledge that default approaches become less reliable as the duration of exposure becomes shorter or the intermittent doses become more intense.

Timing of exposure can also be important. When there is a susceptible life-stage, doses during the susceptible period are not equivalent to doses at other times, and they should be analysed separately (US EPA 2003a, 2003b).

Cross-species extrapolation

A milligram in a mouse is not the same as a milligram in a human. An appropriate measure of dose would consider the body size of the species, the size of the target organ, and the rates of pharmacokinetic processes. Large cross-species differences in dose can occur as a result of dissimilar rates of metabolism or elimination.

When enough information is available, toxicokinetic modelling is the preferred approach for extrapolating dose measures across species. This is because the models include many of the pertinent variables that differ across species, for example, organ sizes, blood volume, blood flow rates, intake rates, and metabolic rates. The values of many of these variables, with the exception of metabolic pathways and metabolic rates, are species-related (that is, independent of the agent being studied) and, hence, readily available to the model. Metabolic pathways and rates for humans, however, may not be available for toxic agents, due to ethical concerns about conducting experiments on humans to obtain such data.

When there is not enough information to construct and fit a toxicokinetic model, or when the nature of the problem doses not justify the time and effort to develop one, less detailed default approaches are used to extrapolate dose measures across species. One approach is to express experimental doses in terms of milligrams of the agent per kilogram of body weight per day (mg/kg-d) and to apply this metric directly to humans without further conversion; this makes an implicit assumption that mg/kg-d is the appropriate dose metric for cross-species extrapolation. Another approach in common use is to scale doses from animals to humans on the basis of equivalence of $mg/kg^{3/4}$ per day (US EPA, 1992b). This formula is supported by analyses of the allometric variation of key physiological parameters across mammalian species. Allometric scaling may be more appropriate for some toxic endpoints than for others. Other approaches that equate exposure concentrations in food or water are alternative versions of the same approach, because daily intakes of food or water are approximately proportional to the 3/4 power of body weight. Most cancer assessments use one of these default approaches for scaling dose across species.

Route extrapolation

Route-to-route extrapolation (that is, extrapolation between ingestion, inhalation, and dermal exposures) has both qualitative and quantitative components. The qualitative aspect involves a judgement that effects observed by one exposure route would be expected to occur if the agent were administered by another exposure route. This is likely to be the case if the agent (or the active metabolite or reaction product) can reach the systemic circulation and be transported to distal sites in the body. The goal of route extrapolation is to estimate the doses by each exposure route that result in equivalent delivered doses at the target site.

This can involve some rather complicated modelling. For example, ingested doses experience what is known as the *first-pass effect*, in which the agent is passed to the liver and is subject to metabolism before reaching the systemic circulation; this does not occur for the inhalation or dermal exposure routes. When enough information is available, toxicokinetic modelling is the preferred approach for determining equivalent doses across exposure routes. This is because the systemic circulation is at the core of a toxicokinetic model, so if the model includes components to simulate intake and differences in metabolism across exposure routes (including the first-pass effect), it can be used to estimate equivalent doses by different exposure routes.

When this is not the case, less detailed default approaches are sometimes used. Differences in intake rates (considering the fraction absorbed by each exposure route) can be used to estimate a rough equivalence across exposure routes. There are no generally applicable default methods for accounting for differences like the first-pass effect.

Toxicokinetic modelling

Toxicokinetic models simulate the relationship between applied dose and internal dose. They do this by tracing the flow of an administered chemical or its metabolites through the blood to different organs of the body (called *compartments*). Toxicokinetic models can range in level of detail from the simple to the complex. The least detailed *one-compartment model* is based on a simple relationship between intake, retention, and elimination from "the body" considered as a homogeneous whole. *Multi-compartment models* divide the body into several discrete components, for example, blood, liver, fatty tissue, and other tissue. More elaborate models simulate metabolism occurring in one or more compartments and trace the flow of both the administered chemical and its metabolites through the body.

Because toxicokinetic models are based on the flow of chemicals through the blood to different body compartments, they require information on the size of each compartment (known as the *volume of distribution*) and the rate of blood flow between compartments. These parameters, which generally do not depend on the chemicals being modelled, allow generic models to be developed for different animal strains or human populations. Chemical-specific rates of absorption and elimination are needed to adapt these generic models so that they can be used to describe the behaviour of a specific chemical in the body of a specific animal strain or human population. When metabolism occurs, chemical-specific descriptions of metabolism in different compartments are needed for an accurate model of the flow of the chemical and its metabolites through the body. The descriptions of metabolism are often complex; for example, there may be a maximal rate of metabolism that decreases as concentration increases.

Toxicokinetic models can improve dose-response assessment by revealing and describing complex relationships between applied and internal dose. Some dose-response relationships that are nonlinear at higher doses (for example, haemangiosarcomas induced in rats exposed to vinyl chloride) can be attributed to nonlinear toxicokinetics. These can involve, for example, saturation or induction of enzymatic processes at high doses.

Good modelling practice dictates that a discussion of confidence should accompany the presentation of modelling results. This would include consideration of model validation and sensitivity analysis, stressing the predictive performance of the model. Quantitative uncertainty analysis is important for evaluating the performance of a model. The uncertainty analysis covers questions of model uncertainty (is the model based on the appropriate dose metrics?) and parameter uncertainty (do the data support unbiased and stable estimates of the model parameters?); see Section 1.3.5.

When toxicokinetic modelling is used to make extrapolations across species (for example, from experimental animals to human populations), a key issue to consider is whether toxicity should be expected in the same tissues in different species. The objective of cross-species toxicokinetic modelling is to use differences in organ size and blood flow and metabolic rates between animals and humans to predict differences in tissue concentrations between animals and humans. This assumes that the same target sites are expected in animals and humans, an assumption that does not hold true in all cases.

1.3.4.2 Dose-response modelling

Empirical dose-response modelling

Empirical models generally have been used to fit tumour incidence data. These models express tumour incidence as an increasing function of dose. The functional form of the model can be a relatively simple mathematical expression, such as a polynomial model, or it can be based on a standard statistical distribution. These models are often sufficiently flexible to fit a wide variety of dose-response data sets and may be either linear or nonlinear at lower doses. When there is a choice between standard statistical models, there is often a preferred model (for example, the US EPA's linearised multistage model) to provide some consistency across analyses and because different empirical models can give different results at low doses with no scientific basis to choose among them (this is because empirical models are generally not grounded in the underlying biology leading to the disease). Goodness of fit to the experimental observations is not, by itself, an effective means of discriminating among models that adequately fit the data (US EPA, 1986b).

When the observed tumour incidences do not increase with dose, it is often because there is a competing mechanism of toxicity at the high doses. In this case, the high dose is dropped from the analysis and an attempt is made to fit the remaining data with the model. This approach is used because there is more value in a model that describes low-dose behaviour than that at high doses.

Sometimes the observed dose-response data are highly nonlinear, and it is difficult to fit them with any standard mathematical or statistical model. This can happen if the toxicokinetics of the agent are highly nonlinear. In this case, the analysis can be improved by using a toxicokinetic model to explain the nonlinearity that is attributable to dose. Similarly, when there are large survival differences across exposure groups and time-to-tumour data are available, the analysis can be improved by using an empirical time-to-tumour model.

Empirical dose-response models also can be fitted to data on a tumour precursor. Quantitative data on precursors can be used in conjunction with, or in lieu of, data on tumour incidence to extend the dose-response curve to lower doses. This generally implies that the relationship between tumours and key tumour precursors is known (see below).

Mechanism-based dose-response modelling

Mechanism-based toxicodynamic models simulate the relationship between responses at the target tissue or cell and frankly observable adverse effects in the organism. Toxicodynamic modelling is potentially the most comprehensive way to account for the biological processes involved in the development of adverse effects. These models reflect the sequence of key precursor events that lead to the adverse effect. Toxicodynamic modelling can be used when there are sufficient data to ascertain the agent's mechanism(s) of action and quantitatively estimate model parameters that represent rates and other quantities associated with the key precursor events of the mechanism.

As mechanisms of carcinogenesis are better understood, mechanism-based dose-response models can become more complex. For example, the Armitage–Doll multistage model (Armitage and Doll, 1954) can be considered to be a mechanism-based model: the hypothesis at the time was that cancer was the result of a sequence of finite number of mutations; the rate of each mutation could be parameterised as the sum of a fixed background rate plus a term that was proportional to the dose of the carcinogen; and the functional form of the model is a mathematical description of the probability of each mutation occurring in sequence. The Moolgavkar–Venzon–Knudson two-stage clonal-expansion model reflects a hypothesis that cancer is the result of two mutations, while cells altered by the first mutation can undergo clonal expansion to present a larger number of target cells that are susceptible to alteration by the second mutation (Moolgavkar and Knudson, 1981).

The events considered in these dose-response models are cellular events: for example, mutations, cell division, and cell death. The model, therefore, will include parameters that describe the rates of these events: rates of the first and second mutations, the rate of cell division for cells altered by the first mutation, and the rate of death of such cells. Numerous variations of the same basic model can be obtained by different choices of how to make these parameters depend on dose. For example, the mutation rates can be linear functions of dose, or the mutation rates can be constant independent of dose, and the cell division rate can be an increasing function of dose.

The extent to which the parameterisation is informed by laboratory data is a major factor in how well a model can be expected to perform below the high-dose range where there are data. It is possible for different models to provide equivalent fits to the observed data but to diverge substantially in their projections at lower doses. When model parameters are estimated from tumour incidence data, it is often the case that different combinations of parameter estimates can yield similar results in the observed range. For this reason, the critical parameters should ideally be estimated from laboratory studies and not by curve-fitting to tumour incidence data (Portier, 1987). This approach reduces model uncertainty (see Section 1.3.5) and ensures that the model does not give answers that are biologically unrealistic. This approach also provides a robustness of results, where the results are not likely to change substantially if fitted to slightly different data (US EPA, 2003a).

Mechanism-based modelling can provide insight into the relationship between tumours and key precursor events. To illustrate, a model that includes cell proliferation can be used to explore the relationship between changes in the rate of cell proliferation and the incidence of tumours – for example, what level of change in the cell proliferation rate is associated with a 10 percent increase in tumour incidence (Gaylor and Zheng, 1996). In this way, mechanism-based modelling can be used to select an appropriate precursor response level and characterise its relationship to tumour incidence.

1.3.4.3 Extrapolation below the range where data support dose-response modelling

Below the range of doses where data have been collected, alternative models that fit the data equally well in the observed range will begin to diverge. This form of *model uncertainty* (see Section 1.3.5) often applies at exposure levels that are of interest to decision-makers. In this case, health agencies often use a default procedure to provide an upper bound on the risk at lower doses where precise risk estimates may not be possible. One common approach is to use *linear extrapolation* to lower doses. Linear extrapolation has been justified in a variety of circumstances: as the most appropriate model when an agent is genotoxic; when human exposure or body burden is high and near the doses where key precursor events in the carcinogenic process can occur; or as a default approach that is not likely to underestimate risk at lower doses (US EPA, 2003a).

With linear extrapolation, a straight line is drawn from the modelled data to the origin (zero dose, zero risk, corrected for background). This implies a proportional (that is, linear) relationship between risk and dose at lower doses. (Note that this linear relationship is assumed only at lower doses; at higher doses, the dose-response curve generally does not have a linear shape.) The slope of the dose-response curve at lower doses (more commonly, an upper bound on this slope) is known as the *slope factor* and is used as an upper-bound estimate of risk per increment of dose at low doses. It is used to calculate an upper bound on risk over a range of exposure levels (US EPA, 2003a).

A different approach (one that provides less information) is not to estimate risk below the dose range supported by the available data. In this case, a *safety assessment* is often used to estimate a dose that might be safe for human exposure. This is the approach generally used for adverse effects other than cancer, but it is used in some cancer assessments. Although these safety assessments sometimes are described as being based on the assumption of biological thresholds, it is difficult to empirically distinguish a true threshold from a dose-response curve that is simply nonlinear at low doses (US EPA, 2003a).

1.3.5 Uncertainty and human variation

Model uncertainty refers to a lack of knowledge needed to determine whether the scientific theory on which the model is based is correct. There could be several alternative scientific theories, each giving rise to a different model, with no scientific basis for choosing among them. In risk assessment, model uncertainty is reflected in alternative choices for model structure, dose metrics, and extrapolation approaches. Other sources of model uncertainty concern whether surrogate data are appropriate, for example, using data on adults to make inferences about children. The full extent of model uncertainty cannot be quantified; a partial characterisation can be obtained by comparing the results of alternative models. Model uncertainty can be expressed through comparison of separate analyses from each model (US EPA, 2003a).

Some aspects of model uncertainty that should be addressed in an assessment include the use of animal models as a surrogate for humans, the consequences of using linear or nonlinear extrapolation to estimate risks at lower doses, and the use of a study sample to make inferences about the human population, including susceptible population segments and life-stages (US EPA, 2003a).

Toxicokinetic and toxicodynamic models are generally premised on *site concordance* across species, modelling, for example, the relationship between administered dose and liver tissue concentrations to predict increased incidences of liver cancer. Site concordance, however, does not hold true in general, as there are numerous examples of an agent causing different cancers in different species (US EPA, 2003a).

Parameter uncertainty refers to a lack of knowledge about the values of a model's parameters. This leads to a distribution of values for each parameter. Common sources of parameter uncertainty include random measurement errors, systematic measurement errors, use of surrogate data instead of direct measurements, misclassification of exposure status, random sampling errors, and use of an unrepresentative sample. Most types of parameter uncertainty can be quantified by statistical analysis (US EPA, 2003a).

Human variation refers to person-to-person differences in biological susceptibility or in exposure. Although both human variation and uncertainty can be characterised as ranges or distributions, they are fundamentally different concepts. Uncertainty can be reduced by further research that supports a model or improves a parameter estimate, but human variation is a reality that can be better characterised, but not reduced, by further research. Fields other than risk assessment use "variation" or "variability" to mean dispersion about a central value, including measurement errors and other random errors that risk assessors address as uncertainty (US EPA, 2003a).

Probabilistic risk assessment has been used in exposure assessment to estimate human variation and uncertainty in lifetime average daily dose. Probabilistic methods can be used in this exposure assessment context because the pertinent variables (for example, concentration, intake rate, exposure duration, and body weight) have been identified, their distributions can be observed, and the formula for combining the variables to estimate the lifetime average daily dose is well defined (US EPA, 1992a). Similarly, probabilistic methods can be applied in dose-response assessment when there is an understanding of the important parameters and their relationships, such as identification of the key determinants of human variation (for example, metabolic polymorphisms, hormone levels, and cell replication rates), observation of the distributions of these variables, and valid models for combining these variables. Specification of joint probability distributions is appropriate when the variables are not independent of each other. With appropriate data, formal approaches to probabilistic risk assessment can be applied to provide insight into the overall extent and dominant sources of human variation and uncertainty. On the other hand, there is little value in using probabilistic analyses to combine results of incompatible models or to bypass default options with alternatives that have no greater validity (National Research Council, 1994). It is important to note that analyses that omit or underestimate some principal sources of variation or uncertainty could provide a misleadingly narrow description of the true extent of variation and uncertainty and give decision-makers a false sense of confidence in estimates of risk (US EPA, 2003a).

PART II

BIOLOGICAL ASPECTS OF CARCINOGENESIS

Introductory remarks

Lutz Edler and Christos P. Kitsos

The biological basis of carcinogenesis has found increasing interest and attention in cancer risk assessment over the decades. The impact of biological carcinogenesis theories is obvious for the hazard identification step (see Figure I.1) when experimental *in vitro* and *in vivo* systems are used to detect effects and to find out about their mechanisms of action (see Eisenbrand *et al.*, 2002; Barlow *et al.*, 2002; Dybing *et al.*, 2002). During the 1960s and 1970s a large amount of biological information was collected such that more comprehensive theories on the origin of cancer could be developed. At that time the multistage theory of the origin of human cancer was shaped and the two-stage initiation–promotion or Moolgavkar–Venzon–Knudson model became popular (Moolgavkar and Knudson, 1981; Moolgavkar and Venzon, 1979); for a comprehensive presentation see Moolgavkar and Luebeck (1990). The transition from normal cells to malignant cells has been understood to take place as a biological multistage process, and the mathematics was developed to describe this process and to define characterizing functions to be fitted to epidemiological and experimental animal data. One should remark, however, that stochastic carcinogenesis modeling has roots going back to the late 1940s and the work of such famous statisticians as David Kendall (Kendall, 1948, 1960), Peter Armitage (Armitage and Doll, 1954, 1957) and Jerzy Neyman (Neyman and Scott, 1967). The toxicological classification of chemicals as genotoxic and non-genotoxic and, from a mechanistic point of view, as initiators and promoters clearly supported the line of thought leading to the concept of two-stage carcinogenesis, in particular for mouse skin. The implementation of two-stage clonal expansion (TSCE) as a biologically based model of carcinogenesis is described in detail in the monograph

Recent Advances in Quantitative Methods in Cancer and Human Health Risk Assessment
Edited by L. Edler and C. Kitsos   © 2005 John Wiley & Sons, Ltd

of Cogliano *et al.* (2002). Luebeck *et al.* (1999b) list five important points to be considered in carcinogenesis modelling:

1. Multistep process with clonal expansion of intermediate and malignant cell populations.

2. Biologically significant model parameters.

3. Unified modelling integrating both epidemiological and experimental data.

4. Account for all observed biological phenomena.

5. Incorporation of time and dose.

Beyond the special TSCE model, these steps may serve in general as a checklist for the use of biologically based modelling for risk assessment.

The contributions in Part II demonstrate convincingly how the biological basis of carcinogenesis has become more complicated during the past decade. It becomes obvious that the gap between biological theories and biological pathways on the one hand and mathematical modeling and statistical analysis on the other hand has widened. Bridging this gap requires new concepts which must simplify the biological theory in terms of its major constituents while being rich enough to be of value to biologists and medical researchers. Those theories must allow for the falsification of important biological hypotheses when checked with empirical data. The notion of biomarkers, illustrated in Figure II.1, can play an important role in future modeling approaches.

Recently biomedical researchers have explored the use of specific biological mechanisms for hazard identification as well as hazard characterization. This work can be seen as a reaction to the demand of the regulatory guidelines (US Environments Protection Agency, 1996) for a 'mode of action analysis based on physical, chemical, and biological information that helps to explain critical events in an agent's influence on development of tumors'. Two prominent biological modes of action were discussed more intensively during the last years: endocrine disrupture and hormesis. Endocrine disruptors and carcinogenic risk assessment were explicit topics of a conference at the Medical Academy in Bialystok (Poland) in 2000. The proceedings of this conference (Chyczewski *et al.*, 2002) are a valuable source for the study of endocrine-related effects on human health. They cover to a large extent the biological basis and medical consequences of endocrine disruptor mechanisms and provide basic information for these mechanisms at the general, cellular and molecular level. As far as we know, the present volume on risk assessment is the first to include the subject of hormesis, although it has been around as a biological concept for more than 100 years, since Hugo Schulz noticed in 1888 that many chemicals have the ability to stimulate growth at low doses (in yeast) and to inhibit growth at higher doses. This particular phenomenon was named hormesis by Southam and Ehrlich (1943). However, this idea had to wait another 50 years before becoming more seriously recognized by the risk assessment community; see Chapter 6 below.

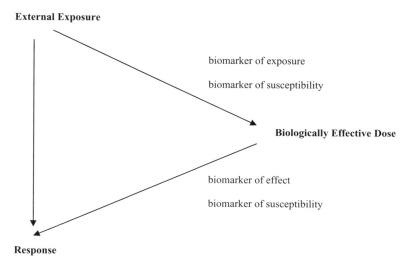

Figure II.1   The role of biomarkers in the hazard and risk characterization. *Biomarkers of exposure* are used as dose indicators, in contrast to *biomarkers of effect* which are used to predict response and which are useful as surrogate endpoints. The third class of *biomarkers of susceptibility* is useful to describe heterogeneity and effect modification, e.g. fast and slow metabolizers; see Amaral Mendes and Pluygers (1999).

Increased incorporation of biomarkers into risk assessment is expected to open another rich source of biological data, namely genomic and proteomic data available now through the high-throughput technology of microarrays and various gel-electrophoresis techniques which do a similar job at the protein level. It is interesting to look back in the history of science to when streams leading to this development started. When the Nobel prize in physics was shared in 1933 by the Briton M. Dirac and the Austrian E. Schrödinger, who laid the foundations for the nuclear age, the Nobel prize for medicine was awarded to T. Morgan who worked on chromosome genetics and after whom the unit of genomic distance was named. However, the advent of the genomic age had to await the discovery of the possibility of changing the genetic code by E. Tatum and J. Lederberg in 1946 (Nobel laureates in 1958 together with Beakle) and the discovery of the double helix in 1953 by F. Crick and J. D. Watson (Nobel Prize winners in 1962). Their four-letter alphabet, – A (for adenine), C (for cytosine), G (for guanine), T (for thymidine) – has become the dominant determinant of biomedical research. The impact of toxicogenomics on risk assessment is indicated by Kim *et al.* in Chapter 20 below; see also issue no. 4 of the journal *Environmental Health Perspectives* from 2004 where in a mini-monograph on genomics and risk assessment 13 papers report on various applications of genomic data for risk assessment. In order to make genomic and proteomic data as reliable as possible and fit for use in risk assessment, more development is needed not only on the biological side but also on the statistical and data analysis side. It is necessary that the many methods proposed today by various groups, in particular by data analysts from bioinformatics departments, be checked for their statistical properties (unbiasedness and efficiency), compared in order to find the best procedures, made transparent both to statisticians and to biologists.

CHAPTER 2

Molecular Epidemiology in Cancer Research

Gerassimos Voutsinas, Anastasia Apostolidou and Natalia Spyrou

Institute of Biology, NCSR 'Demokritos'

2.1 INTRODUCTION

Cancer is a genetic disease arising from an accumulation of mutations that promote clonal selection of cells with an increasingly malignant phenotype (Vogelstein and Kinzler, 1993). Exposure to natural or synthetic environmental agents may have a strong impact on biological systems. Depending on the biological system, therefore, on the genetic background considered, genotoxic or non-genotoxic environmental agents may elicit specific cellular responses (Furberg and Ambrosone, 2001; Pulford *et al.*, 1999). This may result in a variety of degenerative diseases, including cancer. Conventional epidemiology has provided a substantial amount of data that connect specific exposures to cancer manifestation. But the rather simplistic exposure–outcome concept cannot address questions regarding important inter-mediate steps in carcinogenesis. On the contrary, the development and use of molecular biomarkers in epidemiology has allowed a more precise unraveling of events occurring during cancer initiation and progression (Amaral Mendes and Pluygers, 1999).

Molecular epidemiology is a field where several disciplines meet: molecular genetics, cell biology, biochemistry, statistics, and bioethics were incorporated into traditional epidemiological research (Perera and Weinstein, 1982). Molecular dosimetry and cancer susceptibility are major issues in molecular epidemiology research, where biomarkers of exposure, susceptibility, and effect are being used for cancer risk estimation as well as for identification of sequential alterations in the carcinogenic process. For prediction of risk, the main parameters to be considered are: nature, dose, and duration of exposure; and genetic background variability,

Recent Advances in Quantitative Methods in Cancer and Human Health Risk Assessment
Edited by L. Edler and C. Kitsos   © 2005 John Wiley & Sons, Ltd

including the presence of gene variants for activation and detoxification of carcinogens, for efficient DNA repair, cell cycle control, and immune status (Furberg and Ambrosone, 2001).

Recently, the field of cancer genetics and epidemiology has been experiencing a revolutionary shift in approach. Researchers are looking at gene–environment relationships in cancer on a larger scale with new technologies and with more laboratories collaborating than ever before. New tools for high-throughput screening, such as cDNA or peptide microarray and proteome analysis, offer for the first time the possibility of closely studying changes in gene expression during all steps of the carcinogenic process to reveal the important alterations (Albertini, 2001).

2.2　FROM CARCINOGEN EXPOSURE TO CANCER

The effects of environmental agents on cell populations are dependent on the nature of the agent, the dose received, and the length of the exposure. After exposure, exogenous agents are usually metabolized for conjugation and excretion. Through oxidation, hydrolysis or reduction processes, phase I enzymes metabolize the agent to a reactive state. Then, detoxifying phase II enzymes catalyze conjugation of reactive intermediates, increase the water solubility of the product and enable excretion from the body. Excessive exposure or activation, or inefficient detoxification results in DNA or protein adduct formation.

At this stage, DNA repair enzymes (before or after temporary inhibition of the cell cycle) may successfully repair the damage. But if the damage is not repaired due to inefficiencies in DNA repair or cell cycle control or both, the cell enters the DNA replication process and the DNA damage becomes permanent. Genes important in growth control, apoptosis, as well as in immune recognition and function may additionally be involved in such mutational events, leading to unrestricted growth of cell clones with damaged DNA (Furberg and Ambrosone, 2001). Major steps in cancer development are depicted in Figure 2.1.

2.3　BIOMARKERS

After carcinogenic exposure, initiated cells acquiring some selective growth advantage undergo clonal expansion that may finally result in the formation of a malignant tumor. All stages from exposure to clinical disease may be assayed by a series of biological endpoints, each one corresponding to a specific step of the carcinogenic process. The biological endpoints used in molecular epidemiology studies have been termed biomarkers. The possibility of using biomarkers to substitute classical endpoints of traditional epidemiological investigations was a major advance that is highly likely to affect public health. Biomarkers of cancer risk may be subdivided in three categories: biomarkers of exposure, susceptibility, and effect.

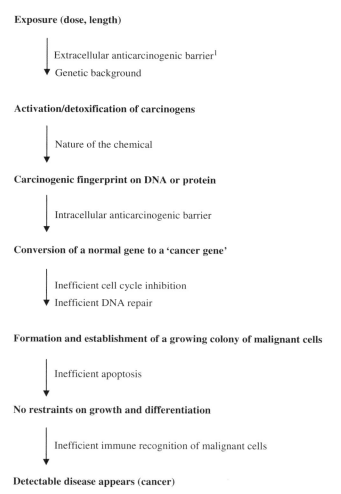

Exposure (dose, length)

      Extracellular anticarcinogenic barrier[1]
      Genetic background

Activation/detoxification of carcinogens

      Nature of the chemical

Carcinogenic fingerprint on DNA or protein

      Intracellular anticarcinogenic barrier

Conversion of a normal gene to a 'cancer gene'

      Inefficient cell cycle inhibition
      Inefficient DNA repair

Formation and establishment of a growing colony of malignant cells

      Inefficient apoptosis

No restraints on growth and differentiation

      Inefficient immune recognition of malignant cells

Detectable disease appears (cancer)

Figure 2.1 Steps in cancer development: from exposure to overt disease.

2.3.1 Biomarkers of exposure

Documentation of the exposure is an important piece of information that may arise from a molecular epidemiology study. Exposure information may be gathered using biomarkers of exposure, which are (a) exogenous substances or their metabolites or (b) the product of an interaction between a xenobiotic agent and some target molecule or cell that is measured in a compartment within an organism (National Academy of Sciences (NAS), 1989). Very important biomarkers of biologically

---

[1]Any mechanism resulting in the reduction of the carcinogenic effects of various intracellular or environmental factors is considered to be part of the anticarcinogenic barrier.

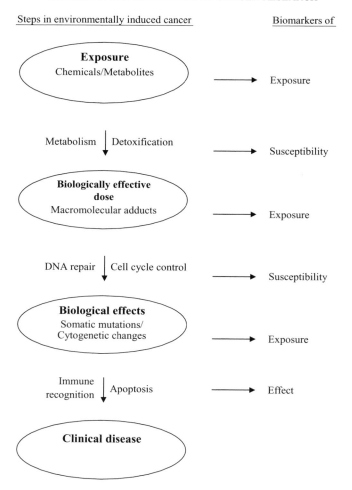

Figure 2.2 Biomarker responses during the sequential process of environmentally induced cancer.

effective dose are DNA adducts that are highly sensitive and specific to chemicals, while they can be related to specific DNA alterations that may drive carcinogenesis. Examples of other biomarkers in this category are DNA strand breaks and sister chromatid exchanges (Amaral Mendes and Pluygers, 1999); see Figure 2.2 for a schematic overview of biomarker responses.

2.3.2 Biomarkers of susceptibility

Genetic variations may modify associations between exposure and disease. Thus, the identification of allele variants has the potential to elucidate risk relationships more clearly and identify subsets of the population that are more vulnerable to specific exposures (Rothman *et al.*, 2001). A large number of high- or low-penetrance gene alleles have been proposed to play a role in cancer susceptibility and are being studied as potential indicators of individual susceptibility. Therefore, biomarkers of susceptibility are indicators of an inherent or acquired limitation of an organism's ability to respond to the challenge of exposure to a specific xenobiotic substance (NAS, 1989).

2.3.3 Biomarkers of effect

Exposure to mutagenic chemicals can cause damage to cellular macromolecules. A variety of responses can then be induced, including repair of the damage. Inefficient repair will certainly have health consequences. For this reason, several biomarkers of biological effects have been developed to document the damage or follow the consequences of the damage. Therefore, biomarkers of effect are measurable bio-chemical, physiological or other alterations within an organism that can be recognized as an established or potential health impairment or disease (NAS, 1989). Important biomarker assays in this category include the detection of chromosome aberrations, the formation of micronuclei, somatic cell mutation assays for *HPRT* or *glycophorin A* genes, as well as the detection of alterations in structure or function of important oncogenes or tumor suppressor genes (Hussain *et al.*, 2001; Bonassi and Au, 2002).

2.4 VALIDATION OF BIOMARKERS

A large number of biomarkers have been developed over the years. However, this does not mean that they will all be useful for human studies directed at public health issues. Before it can be used meaningfully, a biomarker must be validated. But although the characterization of valid biomarkers is a leading priority in environ-mental research, most biomarkers have still not been sufficiently validated, while the biological significance of some remains unclear (Albertini, 2001). Transitional epidemiology studies for biomarker validation bridging the gap between purely laboratory investigations and field studies are usually prospective cohort studies, where the external exposure and health outcome must be accurately determined. Prospective studies for validation of a biomarker of exposure are less complicated than similar studies for validation of a biomarker of effect. This is because in the latter the disease outcome is infrequent and often occurs long after the biomarker response. As for genetic susceptibility traits, validation studies must explore considerations of penetrance, heterozygous effects and the presence of compensa-tory genetic pathways (Schulte and Perera, 1997; Albertini, 2001). Finally, critical issues of strategy that need to be addressed when trying to identify the most effective epidemiological studies for evaluation of a cause–effect relationship in determining cancer risk in the general population are study design, genetic and statistical analysis, sample size requirements, and sources of potential bias

(Vineis *et al.*, 1999b; Rothman *et al.*, 2001). In most of these issues, requirements for obtaining valid data could be met by the establishment of population-based sample collections from different ethnicities for biomedical use, containing samples from large numbers of individuals, like the one funded by the Medical Research Council, the Wellcome Trust and the Department of Health in the United Kingdom. This collection will contain DNA samples from 500 000 individuals, the minimum duration for the collection will be 10–15 years and it is expected to cost more than £60 million (Wild *et al.*, 2002). Such collections would be ideal for use in large prospective studies.

2.4.1 Study design

Although high-penetrance mutations identified in family-based designs confer a high risk of tumors in cancer-prone families, they contribute to only a relatively small proportion of all cancers in the general population. On the other hand, polymorphisms with low penetrance and low relative risk, being common, may contribute a substantial fraction of attributable risk for cancer. Therefore, the primary approach to the study of common polymorphisms and their potential interactions with common environmental exposures should be through population-based epidemiological studies. There are two types of population-based epidemiological design: the case–control and the cohort study. The two approaches are complementary and both have relative strengths and weaknesses. For example, in case–control studies a large number of common or uncommon tumors can be enrolled in a relatively short period of time, a detailed assessment of specific exposures can be carried out, while it is possible to over sample population groups of special interest that are underrepresented in cohort studies. On the other hand, in prospective cohort studies both interview and exposure data are collected before cancer diagnosis, so they are considered to be unbiased, while in cohort studies there is no selection bias, unlike in case–control studies (Rothman *et al.*, 2001).

2.4.2 Genetic and statistical analysis

Critical issues in genetic analysis of samples include the large number of individual assays that must be performed, the amount of sample material required from an individual to conduct these assays, the need for a multiplicity of assays on large numbers of individuals, the cost per individual assay, and novel challenges in data management and analysis. Relatively recent advanced technological approaches, such as automated genetic analyzers, tissue arrays and microarray systems, which use only small amounts of sample material and promise to keep expenses per sample at a low level, are expected to address these points of consideration, but this remains to be proved.

The choice of the method used in statistical analysis depends on the study design. Such an analysis of environmental and genetic factors should begin with the assessment of their crude main effects and then proceed with the construction of a 2×2 interaction table. In this table the odds ratios are presented with individuals who lack both the exposure and the at-risk genotype as reference category. Specific questions that may be addressed from the table, as articulated by Rothman *et al.* (2001), are as follows:

> Is there an effect of the exposure, as measured by the odds ratio, in either of the genotype strata? Is the effect of exposure in one genetic stratum different from the effect of exposure in the other stratum? If an intervention successfully eliminated exposure in everyone, by what percentage would the cancer rate be reduced in each stratum? Is the potential reduction in cancer rate from an intervention that successfully eliminates exposure greater in one stratum than another?

An additional problem in statistical analysis, introduced by new high-throughput genetic studies, is multiple comparisons for the thousands of different genes included in these studies.

2.4.3   Sample size requirements

The estimation of the sample size needed to test for interactions is a complex process. Sample size estimates are highly dependent on assumptions that include the underlying interaction model (additive or multiplicative), the magnitude of the interaction, the effect of the genetic factor conditioned on the environmental factor and vice versa, etc. Just to give an idea, in an example from Rothman *et al.* (2001), the sample size needed to study an environmental exposure or a particular genotype with an odds ratio of 1.5 and prevalence 10 % in the general population, assuming 80 % power and performing a two-sided test at level 0.05, would be about 900 cases and 900 controls. And if one wished to evaluate and correct for 100 genotypes, then the sample size would need to be doubled.

2.4.4   Sources of potential bias

Some of the most important biases in molecular epidemiology study designs can be caused by incomplete ascertainment of cases, poor selection of controls, low response rates and any source of error in the collection and analysis of data causing different treatment of cases than controls. In addition, exposure and/or genotype misclassification will result in substantial increases in sample size requirements, while the use of unrelated controls may lead to confounding due to population stratification.

2.5   FACTORS INFLUENCING CANCER RISK

Prediction of cancer risk from environmental exposures is based on experimental and epidemiological studies addressing questions on the mode of action and tissue specificity of environmental agents, test system specificity, and dose range. In assessing risk a number of uncertainties arise. For example, mutational events cannot be attributed to single exposures but rather to complex mixtures, while there is differential susceptibility of individuals to additional stress. Other important issues include pathway-specific cancer development involving qualitative alterations that do not easily lend themselves to quantification, while in any tumor there are multiple expanding clones bearing different aberrations (Voutsinas, 2001).

2.5.1   Environmental factors

Carcinogenic substances have been documented since the middle of the eighteenth century. Mainly since World War II, epidemiology has successfully identified a number of major environmental risk factors for specific cancers, including a range of occupational hazards, tobacco smoke, high-levels of ionizing radiation, and a number of specific infections. Many of the high-risk exposures for cancer are already known. Nevertheless, together with studies aimed at identifying new agents that have unacceptable carcinogenic effects at levels of actual or anticipated human exposure, several types of low-risk exposure are currently being investigated, such as low levels of ionizing radiation, non-ionizing radiation, various aspects of dietary intake, endogenous and exogenous hormone exposures and a wide range of lifestyle factors. Additional issues of current interest in the field include chronic low-level exposures and threshold doses, interspecies extrapolations, mutation spectra for specific carcinogens, and exposures to complex mixtures (Holmquist, 1998; Hussain and Harris, 2000; Burkart and Jung, 1998).

2.5.2   Genetic factors

Genetic background is considered as a major contributor to cancer risk. Several genetic variants might modify the outcome of a specific exposure and contribute to disease appearance. Much attention has been given to the identification of alleles conferring susceptibility to specific types of cancer. Several genes, such as *APC, BRCA1,* and *BRCA2,* were identified as high-penetrance cancer susceptibility genes. However, predisposing mutations in these genes are rare and are likely to account for a small percentage of cancer cases. On the other hand, low-penetrance cancer susceptibility alleles with less direct impact on cancer risk may be of greater relevance to public health, since they may be present in significantly larger subgroups of the general population; therefore, their attributable risk may be higher, as they work in concert with related genes and environmental triggers. Such low-penetrance cancer susceptibility or modifier genes may be involved in carcinogen metabolism, DNA repair, cell cycle control and immune status (Furberg and Ambrosone, 2001).

2.5.3   Carcinogen metabolism

Several genes coding for phase I and phase II enzymes have been found to be polymorphic (Taningher *et al.*, 1999). A number of polymorphisms in genes of the cytochrome P450 family have been studied and some of them found to be associated with increased risk for a specific type of cancer (Thier *et al.*, 2002b). For example, a polymorphism in *CYP1A1* was associated with increased inducibility, producing a higher activation of carcinogens found in tobacco smoke, and thus lung cancer, while in some studies, the A2 polymorphic allele of the *CYP17* gene, which is associated with elevated levels of estrogens, was found to be associated with breast carcinogenesis in women with an earlier age at menarche (Kawajiri, 1999; Feigelson *et al.*, 1997). Phase II enzymes such as glutathione S-transferases (GSTs), N-acetyltransferases (NATs) and UDP-glucuronosyltransferases (UGTs) involved in the detoxification process were also found to be polymorphic. In some studies, the *GSTM1* null genotype was associated with increased risk for bladder, lung, and breast cancers (Dunning *et al.*, 1999), while the NAT2 slow-acetylation phenotype allele was found to be associated with bladder cancer. The UGT1A1 enzyme is involved in estradiol glucuronidation and anti-oxidant serum bilirubin conjugation. Therefore, low levels of the UGT enzyme might predict more oxidative damage and increased cancer risk. Regarding this latter hypothesis, opposite results were obtained in two different studies for breast cancer in African-American and Caucasian women (Guillemette *et al.*, 2000, 2001).

2.5.4 DNA repair

Base excision repair is particularly important in response to ionizing radiation exposure, which results in oxidation damage and strand breaks. Deficiencies in repair activities are suspected to increase susceptibility to cancer, while differential relative repair efficiencies might also play an additional role (Braithwaite *et al.*, 1999). *XRCC1* gene variant alleles have been found to show inferior base excision repair capacities and associated with increased risks of oral, pharyngeal, bladder, and breast cancers (Stern *et al.*, 2001).

2.5.5 Cell cycle control

Genes involved in cell cycle regulation, such as *H-ras1*, *p53*, *p21* and *p27*, are also candidates for cancer susceptibility. In two studies, two rare *H-ras1* alleles were found to be associated with increased risk for lung cancer, while *p53* gene polymorphisms were not consistently associated with cancer risk (Weston and Godbold, 1997; Pierce *et al.*, 2000). Regarding *p21* and *p27*, preliminary studies report an increased presence of *p21* variants in prostate cancer cells, squamous cell carcinoma of the head and neck and endometrial cancers (Hachiya *et al.*, 1999), whereas a codon 109 polymorphism in gene *p27* was associated with advanced prostate cancer in a European-American population (Kibel *et al.*, 2003).

2.5.6 Immune status

When immune response fails, a tumor may have more chance to develop. Based on this hypothesis, research was focused on polymorphic genes encoding HLA class I and II and tumor necrosis factor (TNF) alpha. It has been found that certain HLA alleles encoding HLA-DQB and HLA-DRB1, which have been associated with an increased immune response, are more common among controls than breast cancer cases, suggesting that these alleles have a protective role in breast carcinogenesis (Chaudhuri *et al.*, 2000). Regarding *TNF-alpha*, it is hypothesized that high levels of the protein result in greater inflammatory damage, which might have relevance to cancer risk. Thus, *TNF-alpha* variants were found to be associated with gastric, colorectal and breast cancers (Mestiri *et al.*, 2001).

2.6 NEW TOOLS IN MOLECULAR EPIDEMIOLOGY

Molecular techniques have revolutionized all fields of experimental biology. The first shift in traditional epidemiology was the substitution of classical endpoints by new markers of biological significance. Now, the oncoming completion of the human genome sequence, which will provide comprehensive information on the structure of human genes, has the potential to transform once more the methods of molecular epidemiology. The complete draft sequence of the 3.3 billion nucleotides comprising the human genome is now available on the Internet, including the location and nearly complete sequence of the 26 000 to 31 000 protein-encoding genes (International Human Genome Sequencing Consortium, 2001; Venter *et al.*, 2001). The wealth of human genome sequence information developed over the last few years is now being exploited to detect fundamental biological responses to toxic insults.

2.6.1 Microarrays and toxicogenomics

It has long been known that cells respond to noxious stimuli by altering gene expression. Alterations in gene expression have been studied at the mRNA or protein level for years using conventional molecular techniques. However, recent developments now allow extremely high-throughput analyses of RNA transcripts so that vast numbers of genes can be monitored for transcriptional activity in a relatively short period of time. Although several methods are becoming available for these analyses, the microarray approach is currently receiving most attention.

In a microarray setting, labeled cDNA or RNA probes obtained from test tissues are hybridized to the targets for the simultaneous expression monitoring of thousands of genes. The reverse technology is also in use, where synthetic oligonucleotides are hybridized to test RNA and allow determination of sequence as well as abundance changes in the affected tissues (Macgregor, 2003). Currently, custom microarray slides are being developed to monitor specific sets of genes involved in cell cycle control, DNA replication and repair, apoptosis, oxidative stress, dioxin/polycyclic hydrocarbon or estrogen responses, etc. Differential tissue-specific expression of genes makes it necessary to analyze a large number of tissues for candidate gene expression, so a new methodology termed tissue microarray was has recently been developed. In this method, hundreds of minute tissue samples

(0.6 mm diameter) can be placed on one microscope glass slide. This approach allows simultaneous analysis of all tissues with *in situ* methods (immunohisto-chemistry, fluorescence *in situ* hybridization, RNA *in situ* hybridization) of all tumors in one experiment under highly standardized conditions. In addition, tissue microarrays are not restricted to solid tumors but can be prepared from a variety of other sources, including cell lines, xenografts, and hematologic tissues. Thus, tissue microarray technology allows miniaturized high-throughput molecular epidemiology studies, and, it is thought that it will markedly accelerate the transition from basic research to clinical applications (Simon and Sauter, 2002).

2.6.2 Proteomics

Although the sequence of the human genome is of unquestioned scientific importance, the true value in the sequence information lies in the proteins. Proteomics is the study of proteins in a cell. Each cell type of an organism may present a different proteome, depending on the function and state of the cell. If changes in mRNA expression are to have functional significance they must be followed by alterations in protein expression. On the other hand, protein function and activity in cells are often regulated, modulated, or restricted by covalent modification of protein structure, by differential sequestration or localization of proteins, protein–protein interactions, or protein–small molecule interactions. To understand the functioning of proteins in biological systems, it is essential to use proteomic tools in the study of protein modifications and activity, changes in protein abundance, and protein–protein interactions (Hanash, 2003; Wulfkuhle *et al.*, 2003). When parts of the proteome are perturbed, malfunction or misfunction arises that may contribute to or cause disease.

Technologies such as two-dimensional gel electrophoresis or high-pressure liquid chromatography followed by mass spectrometry, protein microarrays, high-throughput two-hybrid systems, etc. are already or are becoming available to quantify protein expression comparing normal and disease states, to elucidate protein–protein interactions which may underlie disease, to determine localization of proteins within the cell since abnormal trafficking of proteins could have an inherited basis, and to characterize modifications of proteins which is relevant to modifier gene candidates (Thomas *et al.*, 2003). Therefore, the use of proteomics in the field of molecular epidemiology is of great importance since toxicogenomics and proteomics are complementary methods for monitoring large numbers of genes for response to environmental insults (Albertini, 2001).

2.6.3 Promising directions for cancer diagnosis and cancer biomarker discovery

The cellular proteome exhibits a dynamic profile and is subject to changes in response to various stimuli and disease progression (Sellers and Yates, 2003). Serum proteomic profiling, by using surface enhanced laser desorption/ionization time-of-flight mass spectrometry (SELDI-TOF MS), is one of the most promising new approaches for cancer diagnostics and the discovery of new biomarkers for cancer initiation and progression (Issaq *et al.*, 2002). Exceptional sensitivities and specificities have been reported for some cancer types, such as prostate, ovarian, breast, and bladder cancers, with these sensitivities and specificities being far superior to those obtained by using classical cancer biomarkers (Diamandis, 2004).

As an example, ovarian cancer has the highest mortality rate among cancers specific to women, and this is because patients typically present with late-stage disease. Several risk factors have been established; however, in aggregate, they have proved to be insufficient in identifying women at elevated risk for ovarian cancer. To date, the only marker available for the disease is cancer antigen 125 (CA125), which is present in high levels in most patients with advanced-stage disease, but is elevated in only 50–60 % of patients with stage I disease. Since women with stage I ovarian cancer have greater than 90 % survival, there is a critical need for additional biomarkers to identify early-stage disease. In a recent work, 50 plasma samples from patients diagnosed with ovarian cancer of stages I to IV and fifty samples from normal controls were analyzed using SELDI-TOF mass spectrometry (Petricoin *et al.*, 2002). Then an algorithm was created that could differentiate the profiles from ovarian cancer patients and normal individuals. With the use of this algorithm, 117 masked patient samples were analyzed, including 67 normal individuals and 50 patients diagnosed with ovarian cancer in stages I to IV. From the SELDI-TOF MS profiles, 63 of 66 (95 %) of the control samples were classified as non-cancerous, including 17 benign disease controls, while all 50 samples from cancer patients were correctly classified, including all 18 stage I cancers (Petricoin *et al.*, 2002). The remarkable accuracy of the analysis is very promising and, if verified, SELDI-TOF MS may well constitute a very useful diagnostic tool. On the other hand, the identification of individual proteins, which are responsible for the differences in protein pattern between normal controls and patients, would permit a series of studies aiming at determining genetic alterations in the genes that code for these proteins. Identification of mutations or polymorphisms in the genes coding for such proteins may be of particular relevance to molecular epidemiology in order to establish new cancer biomarkers, while identification of partner proteins may the genes that code for these partner proteins may be of major interest in the study of cell signaling in carcinogenesis (Sellers and Yates, 2003).

2.7   CONCLUSIONS

Over the past decade, the field of molecular epidemiology has undergone extensive development. Chemicals and their metabolites are now routinely measured, while macromolecular adducts and irreversible genetic changes such as mutations and chromosome aberrations *in vivo* are detected with ease. Additionally, the information available from the human genome sequencing project and the resulting high-throughput technologies are already spreading to molecular epidemiology. Advances in bioinformatics are expected to help in the control and interpretation of the resulting flood of data. In addition, transitional epidemiology is evolving to achieve biomarker validation. For this reason, molecular epidemiology is an expanding discipline with clearly defined objectives. Such objectives are: to increase the accuracy of external exposure assessments, to make predictions regarding individual health outcomes, to identify susceptible individuals, and to provide basic information for understanding the pathogenesis of cancer. The data derived from studies using the new technological tools should help in making more meaningful human cancer risk assessments, which is expected to have a strong impact on cancer prevention. Data on the mechanisms of carcinogenesis should provide molecular targets, which may prove useful in diagnosis, prognosis, as well as in decision-making for an appropriate individual therapy.

CHAPTER 3

Genetic Polymorphisms in Metabolising Enzymes as Lung Cancer Risk Factors

Angela Risch, Heike Dally and Lutz Edler

German Cancer Research Center

3.1 INTRODUCTION

Interindividual differences as a result of genetic polymorphisms have been shown to modulate the cancer risk caused by tobacco smoke. Studies further investigating the genetic basis of cancer susceptibility are required for a better understanding of the aetiology of different cancers and to provide clues to the mechanisms of carcinogenesis in humans. The information obtained from such genetic polymorphism studies in humans has the potential to improve cancer risk assessment substantially.

Genetic variability in metabolic enzymes, such as those metabolising carcinogens from cigarette smoke, may increase susceptibility to a number of human environment-related cancers. Xenobiotic metabolism of environmental carcinogens and DNA repair processes are two important ways in which individual susceptibility to environmental carcinogenesis can be affected. Genetic polymorphisms in enzymes involved in detoxification of procarcinogens, such as cytochrome P450 monooxygenases CYP1A1, CYP2A6, CYP2E1 (Bartsch *et al.*, 2000), CYP3A4, CYP3A5, glutathione S-transferases GSTM1, GSTT1 and GSTP1, N-acetyltransferases NAT1 and NAT2, and myeloperoxidase (MPO), as well as in DNA repair enzymes, may affect cancer susceptibility (for further references see Vineis *et al.*, 1999a).

Studies investigating the formation of DNA adducts and the possible modification of adduct levels by allelic variants indicate that certain polymorphisms have functional significance for metabolism and DNA-binding of carcinogens such as those present in tobacco smoke. The combination of homozygous mutated CYP1A1 and the *GSTM1*0/*0* genotypes, for instance, has been shown to lead to a stronger increase of anti-benzo[*a*]pyrene diol epoxide DNA adduct levels than CYP1A1 and GSTM1 wild type, in individuals with similar exposure levels (Rojas *et al.*, 1998). Also, a significantly lower level of benzo[*a*]pyrene diol epoxide DNA adducts in human skin after coal tar treatment was measured for *MPO-463A* allele carriers than for the *MPO-463GG* genotype (Rojas *et al.*, 2001). At-risk genotypes can therefore be used as susceptibility markers, with the aim of identifying high-risk individuals.

There are indications that interindividual differences as a result of genetic polymorphisms may be of particular importance to cancer risk at low-dose exposures. Among a group of smokers with low cigarette consumption (low nicotine/cotinine levels in blood), those with the slow *NAT2* genotype had higher adduct levels than fast acetylators, while this difference was much less marked in heavier smokers (Vineis *et al.*, 1994).

Worldwide, lung cancer has a very high incidence for men, and its incidence is increasing among females. Lung cancer has a bad prognosis, as therapeutic measures have only limited success. While tobacco smoking is strongly associated with lung cancer risk, only 12–20 % of heavy smokers develop lung cancer. Many genetic and molecular biological studies point towards a polygenic heritable predisposition for lung tumours. The purpose of this chapter is to summarize studies on genetic polymorphisms in metabolic genes as potential risk factors for lung cancer and to discuss methodological issues associated with such studies. Four examples are discussed in detail.

3.1.1   Studies investigating genetic polymorphisms as lung cancer risk factors

Given the strong aetiological link between environmental (mostly tobacco) exposure to carcinogens and human lung cancer, the study of genetic polymorphisms as possible modifiers of lung cancer risk has focused on enzymes involved in phase I/II xenobiotic metabolism and lately DNA-repair-relevant enzymes. Only the former will be discussed in this summary (for further information and references see Travis *et al.*, 2004).

CYP1A1 is involved in the bioactivation of polycyclic aromatic hydrocarbons (PAH) including benzo[*a*]pyrene. Several variant alleles of the *CYP1A1* gene have been described (http://www.imm.ki.se/CYPalleles/cyp1a1.htm). Two closely linked polymorphisms, *MspI* at 6235 nt and I462V, have been extensively studied in relation to lung cancer susceptibility, yielding inconsistent results. In a pooled analysis an odds ratio (OR) of 2.36 (95 % confidence interval (CI) 1.16–4.81) was found for the *MspI* homozygous variant genotype in Caucasians (Vineis *et al.*, 2003). PAH-exposed individuals with variant *CYP1A1* alleles have been associated with higher levels of PAH-DNA adducts in white blood cells and lung tissue (Alexandrov *et al.*, 2002), particularly in conjunction with *GSTM1 null*.

CYP1B1 has an important role in oestrogen (17β-oestradiol) metabolism. It also bioactivates many exogenous procarcinogens including PAH as well as aromatic and heterocyclic amines: it showed polymorphic inducibility in human (Japanese) lymphocytes (Toide *et al.*, 2003). CYP1B1 is commonly present in the lung. Several single nucleotide polymorphisms (SNPs) have been described: five result in amino acid substitutions (R48G, A119S, V432L, A443G and A453S). Ser119 has been shown to be associated with squamous cell carcinoma (SCC) in a Japanese study, but further studies are needed (Watanabe *et al.*, 2000). Ethnic variation in allelic frequency has been demonstrated, although a consensus on the biological significance of the alleles has not yet been reached. V432L and A453S located in the haem binding domain of CYP1B1 appear as likely candidates to be linked with biological effects (Thier *et al.*, 2002a).

CYP2D6 is involved in the metabolism of clinically important drugs, including the antihypertensive drug debrisoquine and the antiarrhythmic drug sparteine. It also bioactivates 4-methylnitrosamino-1,3-pyridyl-1-butanone (NNK, a tobacco-specific nitrosamine); however, this is a poor substrate. The expression of CYP2D6 in human lung has been reported to be absent or very low. CYP2D6 expression has been shown to exhibit interethnic variation, and phenotypic variation has been shown to have a genetic basis. At least 40 SNPs and different allelic variants of CYP2D6 have been identified, many of which have been associated with altered CYP2D6 activity. However, the much-studied association between incidence of lung cancer and polymorphic expression of CYP2D6 has remained inconsistent. A meta-analysis has reported a decrease in lung cancer risk for poor metabolisers (PMs)(OR 0.69; CI 0.52–0.90), but genotype analysis did not indicate such an effect (Rostami-Hodjegan *et al.*, 1998).

CYP2A13, a highly polymorphic gene, is expressed in the human lung and efficiently bioactivates NNK. More than 20 polymorphisms in *CYP2A13* (http://www.imm.ki.se/CYPalleles/cyp2a13.htm) have been reported but only two of these (R257C; R101Stop) are known to have functional consequences. The 257C variant has been shown to retain half the activitiy of the wild-type 257R protein (Zhang *et al.*, 2002) and has been correlated with a reduced risk for lung adenocarcinoma (Wang *et al.*, 2003). The *CYP2A13*7* allele results in a premature stop codon and leads to a severely truncated protein lacking CYP2A13 enzyme activity. An increased risk for small cell lung cancer (SCLC) in subjects heterozygous for the *CYP2A13*7* allele has been described (Cauffiez *et al.*, 2004).

Glutathione S-transferases (GSTs) detoxify tobacco carcinogens such as PAH by conjugation. Individuals lacking GSTM1 (null polymorphism, e.g. in 50% of Caucasians) appear to have a slightly elevated risk of lung cancer. A meta-analysis including the results from 43 studies (over 18 000 individuals) found an OR of 1.17 (CI 1.07–1.27) for the *GSTM1 null* genotype. When the original data pooled from 21 of the case–control studies (9500 subjects) were analysed no evidence of increased lung cancer risk among *GSTM1 null* carriers nor an interaction between *GSTM1* genotype and smoking was found (Benhamou *et al.*, 2002). Results on *GSTT1*, *GSTP1* and *GSTM3* remain inconsistent. *GSTM1* or *GSTT1 null* polymorphisms could lead to reduced carcinogen detoxification, and evidence that the *GSTM1* genotype affects internal carcinogen dose levels comes from studies on DNA adducts. Higher adduct levels were seen in lung tissue and white blood cells in *GSTM1 null* individuals exposed to PAH (reviewed in Alexandrov *et al.*, 2002). At present, GST study results are not consistent, probably because individual adduct levels will be affected by a range of genetic polymorphisms (Godschalk *et al.*, 2003).

N-acetyltransferases NAT1 and NAT2 with distinct but overlapping substrate specificities activate and/or detoxify aromatic amines. From 11 studies on lung cancer, ORs for fast versus slow NAT2 acetylators ranged from 0.5 to 3.0; most studies found no significant association, but in some, fast NAT2 acetylators were at increased risk, in one study only among heavy smokers (Zhou *et al.*, 2002). The *NAT1*10* allele, a putative fast acetylation allele with unresolved phenotype–genotype correlation, has inconsistently been associated with an increased risk for lung cancer, or certain subtypes of lung cancer.

Myeloperoxidase (MPO) is released by polymorphonuclear neutrophils when they are recruited into the lung for a local inflammatory response, such as may be caused by smoking. MPO catalyzes the conversion of H_2O_2 into the bactericidal compound hypochlorous acid, and is also involved in the metabolic activation of tobacco carcinogens. Eleven lung cancer case–control studies have reported ORs of 0.54–1.39 for the *GA* genotype, 0.20–1.34 for the *AA* genotype and 0.58–1.27 for the *(GA + AA)* genotypes. A large study did not find the *A*-allele to be protective for lung cancer (Xu *et al.*, 2002), while a meta-analysis (excluding this study) showed marginally significant inverse correlations of the *AA* and/or *GA* genotype prevalence and lung cancer risk (Feyler *et al.*, 2002). Carriers of the *A*-allele had a significantly reduced capacity to bioactivate benzo[*a*]pyrene (also found in tobacco smoke) into its diol epoxide DNA adducts in skin of coal tar treated patients (Rojas *et al.*, 2001). More recently, a similar significant association of both MPO activity and DNA adduct levels measured in human brochio-alveolar lavage samples with MPO genotype has been found (van Schooten *et al.*, 2004).

3.2 METHODOLOGICAL ASPECTS

The study results on genetic polymorphisms presented above show both their potential in identifying new risk factors as well as the difficulties of substantiating their findings in human studies. A multitude of issues apply to the investigation of variation in the frequency of allelic variants and of assessment of the magnitude of the associated disease risk; for a checklist and further references, see Little *et al.* (2002a). This section will address major aspects which may influence the results of genetic polymorphism studies and may be causes of heterogeneity.

3.2.1 Planning of the study

Genetic polymorphism studies are more complicated than clinical studies in general because their primary aim is to identify differences of effects between subgroups in the human population. The search for such gene–environment interaction effects requires particularly careful planning of these human studies.

3.2.1.1 Candidate genes/SNPs

In order to identify gene–environment interactions it is crucial to define clearly the biological hypothesis underlying the investigation, including the possible biochemical pathways involved and the known functional relevance of the genetic polymorphism to be investigated. Gene deletions and splice defects, as well as SNPs that lead to amino acid changes, are likely to affect enzyme activity, but other SNPs may also have an impact on the enzymatic phenotype (see Table 3.1). Where available, *in vitro* studies investigating the phenotype–genotype correlation may provide useful information: in certain cases *in vivo* data are also available. In the case of newly identified alleles, where such studies are lacking, it will be necessary to work on the basis of the likely functional relevance as deduced, for instance, from amino acid changes in combination with enzymatic models or from SNPs in the 5′ untranslated region (5′ UTR) in combination with identification of promoter regions.

Table 3.1 Examples of molecular mechanisms for enzyme polymorphisms.

Site of polymorphism	Genetic changes	Effect on enzyme	Example
5′ Promoter region	SNPs or deletion/ insertion; poly nucleotide repeats	Altered transcription or induction, can lead to altered enzyme levels	MPO, CYP1A1, MMP-1, MMP-9
Coding region	SNPs	Amino acid changes can lead to altered enzyme activity	NAT2
Coding region	Deletions	Inactive enzyme or complete loss of protein	GSTM1, GSTT1
Introns/coding region	SNPs change the splice site	Splice variants can have altered or missing enzyme activity	CYP3A5
3′ region	Changes in poly-adenylation	Changes in the half-life of the transcript can lead to altered enzyme expression	NAT1
Whole gene	Amplification of entire gene locus	Increased levels of enzyme	CYP2D6
Genomewide	Complex interactions, e.g. GSTM1 deficiency leads to increased induction of CYP1A1 and 1A2		

3.2.1.2 Combinations of genes and functional pathways

The risk-modifying effect of any one SNP may be more pronounced when it occurs in combination with other 'at risk' genotypes of biotransformation and/or repair enzymes, especially if both candidate genes are implicated in the same pathway of relevance to a given carcinogen. For example, in several studies the combined genotypes *CYP1A1-Val/Val* and *GSTM1-null* have shown an enhanced effect on lung cancer SCC risk, and an impact on intermediate end-points, that is, the formation of DNA adducts and mutations (Bartsch *et al.*, 2000). For the analyses of such gene–gene interactions very large populations are required.

3.2.1.3 Ethical considerations regarding the study population

The type and detail of information gathered on the study subjects varies between studies. In general, permission to conduct studies involving the archiving of DNA will have to be obtained from the local ethical committee and will have to follow guidelines such as the Helsinki Declaration (World Medical Association, 2002; http://www.wma.net/e/policy/b3.htm).

3.2.1.4 Study design

While in theory cohort studies have the benefit that study subjects are initially free of diseases, and preclinical diseases as confounders can therefore be excluded, in practice the huge populations and the long follow-up period required make them too expensive to conduct investigations on genetic polymorphisms as modifiers of cancer risk for most organ sites. Case–control studies, on the other hand, are susceptible to recall bias, selection bias and disease bias, making careful study design a prerequisite (see van den Brandt *et al.*, 2002). The standard approach in the area of lung cancer nevertheless has been to use case–control populations, though Begg and Berwick (1997) have argued for case-only study designs.

When planning a molecular epidemiological study on polymorphisms using the case–control design one has to distinguish both in design and analysis between matched and unmatched case–control studies. In the standard (unmatched) case–control study the two samples of cases and controls are each recruited independently. Cases are most often recruited in one or more hospitals, because of ease of recruitment at the place where they receive treatment. Another potential source of data is a disease registry which has the advantage of completely covering a large region. Non-diseased controls should be recruited, in as comparable a manner as possible to the cases in all aspects (except, of course, knowledge of the polymorphism). In practice, this can be very difficult and it is not always possible to fulfil all desirable requirements for an optimum design. For reasons of practicability, cost and convenience the control population is often recruited in the vicinity of the case population. Therefore, hospital controls have become a convenient choice as control population.

The matched case–control study aims at a high degree of comparability between the cases and the controls. This is attempted by stratifying the study population into strata within which the cases and controls are as similar as possible, a process referred to as 'matching'. A set of case characteristics $x = (x_1, \ldots, x_p)$ is defined, and for each case exhibiting the feature $u = (u_1, \ldots, u_p)$ a control is selected with a feature $v = (v_1, \ldots, v_p)$ such that the difference between u and v is either zero (totally matching) or very small. For 1:1 matching one control is matched to one case, while for m:1 matching m controls are matched to one case. Since the increase of efficiency decreases with the number of matches rather rapidly, the number of matches m ranges usually between 1 and 5.

In practice, it becomes rather difficult to conduct a matched case–control study for a pharmacogenetic hypothesis since one has to find a control matching for basic demographic factors, who must agree to donate samples for genotyping, and the laboratory analysis has to give evaluable results. Both the increased burden of recruitment and additional costs of matching when discarding cases (or controls) may have prevented researchers from designing matched pharmacogenetic studies. Indeed, this was the case in our studies on lung cancer risk factors where we recruited cases and controls from a population visiting a specialized clinic for pulmonary diseases. We considered the population of all patients visiting that clinic as the sample space and distinguished the patients with diagnosed lung cancer (cases) from those who visited the clinic for other reasons (controls). Instead of pre-adjustment through matching, we chose to post-adjust the ORs for possible confounding factors.

3.2.1.5 Definition of disease to be studied

Another important consideration in the planning phase of a study concerns possible clinical diversity of the disease to be studied. While the risk for all histological types of lung cancer is associated with duration and intensity of tobacco consumption, the strength of the association varies with different histological types of this disease. A meta-analysis including 28 studies evaluating the association between smoking and major histological types of lung cancer revealed a highly significantly increased risk, with the highest OR (72.5; CI 13.8–379) for SCLC and current smokers. The lowest OR was not significant, with 2.55 (CI 0.82–7.89) for adenocarcinoma and ex-smokers (Khuder, 2001). More peripheral tumours, such as adenocarcinoma and large cell carcinoma, show weaker associations with tobacco consumption than more central tumours such as SCC and SCLC (C. Yang *et al.*, 1989). Due to differences in the aetiology, the impact of genetic polymorphisms should be analysed separately for each histological type of lung cancer.

3.2.1.6 Power calculation

Another crucial question for appropriate study design concerns the required size of the study. The most convenient effect measure for power or sample size calculation is the odds ratio, that is, the chance of contracting the disease in the population of individuals exposed to the risk factor divided by the same chance in the population of individuals not exposed to the risk factor. Programs to calculate sample size are available for matched and unmatched studies. For their application one has to specify the size of the OR to be detected, the probability P_0 of exposure and a correlation φ which describes the correlation of exposure between a case and its corresponding control. A value of $\varphi = 0$ indicates independence between exposure rates for case and controls. It is often unrealistic to assume complete independence, so if no other information is available, a value of $\varphi = 0.2$ has been suggested. P_0 can be estimated as the expected relative frequency of high-risk persons in the control population. Note that P_0 is a critical parameter determined by the prevalence of the high-risk group defined by the genetic polymorphism. P_0 depends on the genes considered and may vary between 1 % and 50 %. The odds ratio to be detected in the study has to be set in a range which realistically can be assumed for those genes. Values around OR = 2.0 are more realistic than values around 5.0. The required sample size for an OR of 2.0 is much larger than for one of 5.0. Finally, the statistical error probabilities have to be defined. Standard values are a significance level of 5 % ($\alpha = 0.05$) and a power of 80 % ($\beta = 0.20$). If more than one gene is to be tested one may adjust for multiple comparisons by dividing the level α by the number of genes, or by the number of tests for the primary hypotheses.

3.2.1.7   Example of a power calculation

Assume that for a given gene the homozygous *variant* genotype is associated with a higher cancer risk than the *wild-type* (*wt*) homozygote or the *wt/variant* heterozygote. Prevalence is estimated at $P_0 = 20$ % for the *variant* homozygotes. Let us assume further that the same number of cases and controls can be recruited. We aim to detect an increase in the risk of *variant* homozygotes compared to the complementary group of *wt* homozygotes and *wt/variant* heterozygotes. To detect an OR of 2 at the significance level $\alpha = 0.05$ with a power of 80 % a total of $n = 269$ evaluable patients are needed, that is, $n = 135$ cases and $n = 135$ controls. Relaxing to OR = 3 would require only $n = 50$ cases and $n = 50$ controls. If the prevalence is higher than 20 %, say $P_0 = 40$ %, the sample sizes of 269 and 100 fall to 208 and 84, respectively. These calculations were performed using the logistic regression sample size program of PASS 2002.

3.2.2   Laboratory analyses

Before beginning the study it is important to consider sample banking issues (for further information and references, see Holland *et al.*, 2003), and any study reports should include information on the exact genotyping method used, including primer sequences and positions, the accession number for the DNA sequence their design was based on, and the exact position of the polymorphism, in relation to the base A (+1) in the start codon ATG. Importantly, where there is more than one variant allele for a gene, those tested should be specified, and where available it is helpful to use published nomenclatures, such as that for the N-acetyltransferases (http://www.louisville.edu/medschool/pharmacology/NAT.html). Frequently there is a high degree of homology between enzymes of interest, requiring careful checking of primer design using DNA sequence databases and sequence alignments.

Traditionally, many genotyping methods are based on the polymerase chain reaction (PCR) followed by restriction fragment length polymorphism analysis (PCR-RFLP). The gene fragment of interest is amplified using specific primers, and then subjected to digestion by a restriction endonuclease which is followed by agarose gel electrophoresis. The restriction endonuclease is specific to the region containing an SNP, which allows determination of whether a given SNP is present

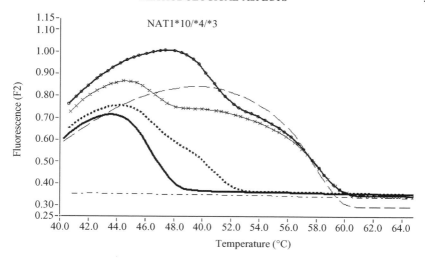

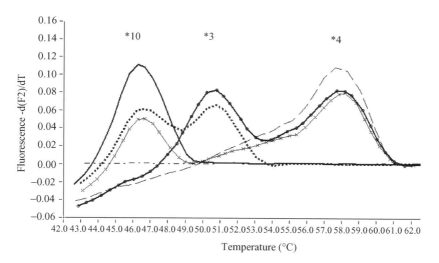

Figure 3.1 *NAT1*-melting curves and melting peaks obtained using *NAT1* specific primers in a capillary-based PCR followed by detection of the temperature at which allele-specific probes detach from the PCR amplicon – in combination with further melting curve analyses (not shown), this allows the unambiguous distinction of *NAT1* alleles.

from the pattern of fragments obtained. Given the ever larger sample numbers required to investigate gene–environment interactions, for example in histological subgroups or for more than one polymorphism, higher-throughput methods, such as those employing fluorescence-based probes, are becoming increasingly important (Figure 3.1).

Validation of genotyping results with a second method is the ideal. However, the validity of the results should at least be checked by independent retyping of a subset of samples, and the inclusion of positive control samples with known sequence in the analyses. This is especially important where newly described polymorphisms are being investigated, as other, not previously described polymorphisms in the vicinity could affect the results obtained with certain amplification methods or certain probes.

3.2.3   Statistical analyses

The statistical evaluation of pharmacogenetic (toxicogenetic, epigenetic, genetic epidemiology) studies is primarily determined by the design of the study and the data type observed in the subjects investigated. As explained above, most pharmacogenetic studies are non-matched case–control studies where a population of case patients of size n is compared with a control population of size m. Consequently, statistical methods of epidemiology for this study type should be applied. In this section we describe standard methods for the data analysis appropriate for this study type.

3.2.3.1   Odds ratio

Denote by AA the high-risk genotype and by non-AA the complementary group of low risk persons. Let the proportion of the controls showing AA be denoted by p_0 and that of the cases showing AA by p_1 (Table 3.2). The odds ratio OR is then formally defined as

$$\mathrm{OR} = \frac{p_1/(1 - p_1)}{p_0/(1 - p_0)} = \frac{p_1(1 - p_0)}{p_0(1 - p_1)}.$$

This odds ratio is also known as the crude odds ratio, indicating that it is obtained from the crude case/control and exposure/non-exposure data only.

Table 3.2   Scheme for the case–control study for the definition of the odds ratio.

Risk group	Case	Control
AA	p_1	p_0
non-AA	$1 - p_1$	$1 - p_0$

p_1 is the probability that a sample case patient is exposed to the risk factor, p_0 is the probability that a sample control patient is exposed to the risk factor.

A χ^2 test of the null hypothesis H_0: OR $= 1$ is identical to a test of equality of the two proportions $H_0 : p_0 = p_1$. The crude odds ratio can be biased due to population heterogeneity caused by (confounding) factors associated with the outcome. It is therefore a valid index of the association between the genetic polymorphism and the disease incidence only when constancy across all levels of the confounders (e.g. age, gender, smoking, occupational exposure) can be assumed.

Significance tests and confidence intervals for the crude OR were originally introduced by Mantel and Haenszel (1959); see Chapter 4 of Breslow and Day (1980). In the presence of confounding factors, one should stratify the population into subpopulations defined by individual levels of the confounder and calculate a stratified OR; see Section 4.6 of Breslow and Day (1980). In practice, this method can be applied only for one or two categorical confounders when each has only a few levels. Since our analyses have to account for several factors, including factors of continuous scale (e.g., age of the patients) we used the method of unconditional logistic regression to calculate ORs for the association between the genetic polymorphism and disease incidence. Confidence intervals (as standard at the level of 95 %) and statistical tests on the regression coefficients are calculated to explore which confounders have a significant (e.g., p-value less than 0.05) influence on the disease incidence, and to check for the presence of an interaction between the genetic polymorphism and specific demographic or environmental factors.

3.2.3.2 Unconditional logistic regression

To be more precise, the unconditional logistic model describes the disease probability as a function depending on the primary factor (the genetic polymorphism) and other factors which are considered as confounders. If x denotes the genetic polymorphism and $z = (z_1, \ldots, z_p)$ denote the confounders, the logistic model can be written as

$$P(\text{case}|x, z) = \frac{\exp\{a + bx + cz\}}{[1 + \exp\{a + bx + cz\}]}$$

or

$$\text{logit } P(\text{case}|x, z) = \ln \frac{P(\text{case}|x, z)}{1 - P(\text{case}|x, z)} = a + bx + cz.$$

If no confounders are considered and if the genetic polymorphism is dichotomously coded as $x = 1$ for the high-risk (AA) group and $x = 0$ for the low-risk (non-AA) group, in this notation the odds ratio is given by

$$\text{OR} = \exp(b).$$

Testing the hypothesis H_0: OR $= 1$ is equivalent to testing H_0: $b = 0$.

When examining the impact of a genetic polymorphism on cancer incidence one has to consider the possibility that the three genotypes AA, AB and BB each carry a different risk, and a combination of AB and BB into one class non-AA may a priori not be justified and could unduly average the different effects of AB and BB genotypes. Therefore, one should analyse the trichotomous factor AA versus AB versus BB by introducing two so-called dummy variables (x_1, x_2) into the logistic model defined as follows: $x_1 = 1$ if AA holds, and 0 otherwise; $x_2 = 1$ if AB holds, and 0 otherwise. *BB* is then the reference class of the genetic polymorphism and the logistic model equation is

$$\text{logit } P(\text{case}|x, z) = a + b_1 x_1 + b_2 x_2 + cz$$

and $OR_1 = \exp(b_1)$ provides the OR of *AA* versus *BB* and $OR_2 = \exp(b_2)$ the OR of *AB* versus *BB* (adjusted for the confounders z).

The applicability of the logistic model (originally developed for a prospective study design) to the retrospective case–control studies has been demonstrated in Section 6.3 of Breslow and Day (1980) using Bayes' theorem. This important theoretical result justifies the usage of the unconditional logistic regression model (e.g., implemented in SAS software packages as proc logistic) to analyse the association of the genetic polymorphism in the presence of confounders.

For the evaluation of genetic polymorphism studies it is important to note that the method of unconditional logistic regression allows testing for the presence of gene–environment interaction by including an interaction term in the model. In our analyses we routinely test for the presence of an interaction between genotype and smoking (z_1) and genotype and occupational exposure (z_2). Smoking is dichotomized as $z_1 = 1$ for more than 20 pack-years, otherwise $z_1 = 0$, and $z_2 = 1$ denotes possible occupational exposure to asbestos or strong carcinogenic chemicals such as benzene. This introduces additional model parameters γ_1, γ_2 into the logistic model:

$$\text{logit } P(\text{case}|x, z) = a + bx + c_1 z_1 + c_2 z_2 + \gamma_1 xz_1 + \gamma_2 xz_2.$$

Due to sample size restrictions in our studies, so far we have tested only for first-order interactions to avoid degenerate analyses and to preserve some power to detect at least those interactions. Interaction was considered worthwhile when the p-value of the γ-parameters was less than 0.1. When such interaction was present, we performed separate analyses for each stratum defined by the corresponding environmental factor and we compared the ORs of the different genotypes.

In order to investigate joint effects of two or more than two polymorphisms, for example joint effects of $X_1 = CYP3A4$ and $X_2 = CYP3A5$, we defined a combined factor CYP3A(4 + 5) either as product of the dichotomized single CYP factors X_1, X_2 or by explicit assignment of new categories

$$\text{CYP3A}(4 + 5) = \begin{cases} 0 & \text{if } X_1 \text{ and } X_2 \text{ at low risk,} \\ 1 & \text{if } X_1 \text{ at high and } X_2 \text{ at low risk,} \\ 2 & \text{if } X_1 \text{ at low and } X_2 \text{ at high risk,} \\ 3 & \text{if } X_1 \text{ and } X_2 \text{ at high risk risk.} \end{cases}$$

The evaluation using logistic regression then resulted in three ORs corresponding to '1 versus 0', '2 versus 0' and '3 versus 0'.

3.2.3.3 Polytomous logistic regression

The logistic regression technique described above was applied separately for NSCLC and controls and for SCLC and (the same) controls. Normally, we also pooled the samples of NSCLC and SCLC patients and investigated lung cancer as one disease. More appropriate would be a multivariate analysis where the response variable takes the three possible states (trichotomous response) NSCLC, SCLC and control. In the simplest case of a dichotomous risk factor $x = 1$ if AA and $x = 0$ if non-AA, one may consider the model given by the two equations

$$\ln \frac{P(\text{SCLC} \mid X)}{1 - P(\text{SCLC} \mid X)} = a_s + b_s x$$

$$\ln \frac{P(\text{NSCLC} \mid X)}{1 - P(\text{NSCLC} \mid X)} = a_n + b_n x$$

resulting in two ORs: $\text{OR}_s = \exp(b_s)$ and $\text{OR}_n = \exp(b_n)$, the subscripts s,n denoting SCLC and NSCLC. OR_s describes the relative odds of SCLC versus NSCLC combined with controls and OR_n that of NSCLC versus SCLC combined with controls. Notice that two equations suffice; a third model equation for controls would overparameterise the analysis.

More convenient is the application of a 'step down' modelling approach which first examines the combined effect of NSCLC and SCLC, and then the effect of NSCLC alone. This model is described by the two equations

$$\ln \frac{P(\text{NSCLC} + \text{SCLC} \mid x)}{1 - P(\text{NSCLC} + \text{SCLC} \mid x)} = a_{ns} + b_{ns} x,$$

$$\ln \frac{P(\text{NSCLC} \mid x)}{1 - P(\text{NSCLC} + \text{SCLC} \mid x)} = a_n + b_n x.$$

3.2.3.4 Hardy–Weinberg equilibrium

We finally remark that presentation of data on genotype distributions of biallelic polymorphisms of Mendelian inheritance should always include a test for the Hardy–Weinberg equilibrium (HWE); see Gyorffy et al. (2004). If the genotype distribution in the control population does not conform with the HWE, the results should be treated very cautiously. However, if HWE is not met in the diseased population, this may be an indication of a correlation between genotype and disease. The test for HWE is a simple χ^2 analysis comparing the expected genotype distribution based on the observed allele frequencies with the observed genotype distribution.

If an association between a certain allelic variant and cancer is identified, this may indicate functional relevance of the variant to carcinogenesis. However, due to linkage between different genetic polymorphisms within a certain gene, or even in different genes, it is also possible that the association is in fact not functional per se, but results from linkage with another (functional) locus (Smelt et al., 1998). Studies determining the degree of linkage between polymorphisms (Dally et al., 2004) are therefore required. If there is linkage between two sites, haplotype analyses may provide a more accurate picture of the disease association (Stephens et al., 2001).

3.3 EXAMPLES

3.3.1 N-acetyltransferases (NAT1 and NAT2) and lung cancer risk

The highly polymorphic N-acetyltransferases (NAT1 and NAT2) are involved in both activation and inactivation reactions of numerous carcinogens, such as tobacco-derived aromatic amines. The potential effect of the *NAT* genotypes in individual susceptibility to lung cancer was examined in a hospital-based case–control study consisting of 392 Caucasian lung cancer patients (152 adenocarcinomas, 173 SCCs, and 67 other primary lung tumours) and 351 controls (Wikman *et al.*, 2001). In addition to the wild-type allele *NAT1*4*, seven variant *NAT1* alleles (*NAT1*3, *10, *11, *14, *15, *17* and *22*) were analysed. A new method based on the LightCycler technology was applied to detect the polymorphic *NAT1* alleles at nt 1088 and nt 1095. The *NAT2* polymorphic sites at nt 481, 590, 803 and 857 were detected by PCR-RFLP or fluorescence-based melting-curve analysis using the LightCycler (Roche, Mannheim; Figure 3.1). Multivariate logistic regression analyses were performed taking into account levels of smoking, age, gender and occupational exposure. An increased risk for adenocarcinoma among the NAT1 putative fast acetylators (OR 1.92; CI 1.16–3.16) was found but could not be detected for SCC or the total case group (Figure 3.2). *NAT2* genotypes alone appeared not to modify individual lung cancer risk; however, individuals with combined *NAT1* fast and *NAT2* slow genotype had significantly elevated adenocarcinoma risk (OR 2.22; CI 1.03–4.81) compared to persons with other genotype combinations. These data clearly show the importance of separating different histological lung tumour subtypes in studies on genetic susceptibility factors and implicate the *NAT1*10* allele as a risk factor for adenocarcinoma (Wikman *et al.*, 2001).

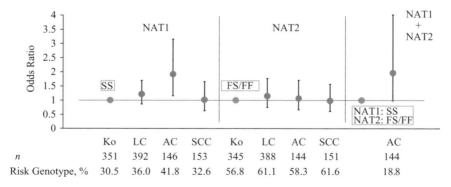

Figure 3.2 Odds ratios for NAT putative risk genotypes for lung cancer and different histological types of NSCLC; see also Wikman *et al.* (2001). Abbreviations: Ko: controls, LC: lung cancer, AC: adenocarcinoma, SCC: squamous cell carcinoma, SS: slow acetylator, FS: intermediate acetylator, FF: fast acetylator.

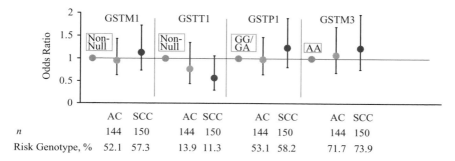

Figure 3.3 Odds ratios for carriers of different *GST* genotypes for adenocarcinoma and squamous cell carcinoma of the lung; see also Risch *et al.* (2001). Abbreviations: AC: adenocarcinoma, SCC: squamous cell carcinoma.

3.3.2 Glutathione-S-transferases and lung cancer risk

Polymorphism in glutathione-S-transferase genes which cause variations in enzyme activity may also influence individual susceptibility to lung cancer. In the case–control population described above, genotype frequencies for *GSTM1*, *GSTM3*, *GSTP1* and *GSTT1* were determined by PCR-RFLP-based methods (Risch *et al.*, 2001). While adjusted ORs indicated no significantly increased risk for lung cancer overall due to any single *GST* genotype, the risk alleles for *GSTM1*, *GSTM3* and *GSTP1*, conferring reduced enzyme activity, were present at higher frequency in SCC than among adenocarcinoma patients (Figure 3.3). This is consistent with a reduced detoxification of carcinogenic polycyclic aromatic hydrocarbons from cigarette smoke that are more important for the development of SCC than of adenocarcinoma. An explorative data analysis identified statistically significantly increased ORs for the combinations *GSTT1 non-null* and *GSTP1 GG* or *AG* for lung cancer overall (OR 2.23; CI 1.11–4.45), and for SCC (OR 2.69; CI 1.03–6.99). Additionally, in 28 patients with hamartomas (benign lung tumours) when compared to controls the *GSTT1 null* genotype was also protective ($p = 0.013$), while *GSTP1* variant allele carriers were overrepresented (OR 2.48; CI 1.06–6.51).

In conclusion, *GST* genotypes may act differently, by detoxifying harmful tobacco carcinogens and/or by eliminating lung cancer chemopreventive agents. The latter role for *GSTT1* would explain the observed lower risk of SCC and hamartoma associated with *GSTT1 null* (Risch *et al.*, 2001). Further confirmatory studies are required.

3.3.3 Myeloperoxidase and lung cancer risk

MPO participates in the metabolic activation of tobacco carcinogens such as PAHs. A frequent *MPO-463 G → A* polymorphism in the promotor region reduces MPO transcription and has been correlated with more than fourfold lower benzo[*a*]pyrene

DNA adduct levels in the skin of patients treated with coal tar. As described above, there was controversy about whether or not an association exists between lung cancer risk and the *MPO-463A* allele. Due to their different aetiology, we examined whether the *MPO* genotype affects histological lung cancer types differentially. A case–control study was conducted in 625 ever-smoking lung cancer patients that included 228 adenocarcinomas, 224 SCCs, 135 SCLCs, and 340 ever-smoking hospital controls (Dally *et al.*, 2002). *MPO* genotyping was performed with capillary PCR followed by fluorescence-based melting curve analysis. When combining the *MPO-463* (*G/A + A/A*) genotypes, a protective effect approaching significance (OR 0.75; CI 0.55–1.01) was observed on comparison of all lung cancer cases with controls. Among histological types of lung cancer, a weak protective effect was found for both adenocarcinoma (OR 0.81; CI 0.55–1.19) and SCC (OR 0.82; CI 0.56–1.21) which was stronger and significant for SCLC (OR 0.58; CI 0.36–0.95); see Figure 3.4. We also found evidence that the *MPO* genotype varies among inflammatory non-malignant lung diseases. In conclusion, our results emphasise the need for a separate analysis of lung cancer histological types and an adjustment for inflammatory non-malignant lung diseases in future MPO-related studies. We confirmed a previously observed (Cascorbi *et al.*, 2000) protective effect of the *MPO-463A* variant allele against lung cancer risk in smokers, which was strongest for SCLC patients (Dally *et al.*, 2002).

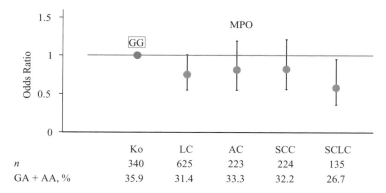

Figure 3.4 Odds ratios for carriers of the *MPO-463A* allele for different types of lung cancer among smokers; see also Dally *et al.* (2002). Abbreviations: Ko: controls, LC: lung cancer, AC: adenocarcinoma, SCC: squamous cell carcinoma, SCLC: small cell lung cancer.

3.3.4   CYP3A4 and CYP3A5 and lung cancer risk

CYP3A isozymes are involved in tobacco carcinogen and steroid metabolism, and are expressed in human lung tissue showing interindividual variation in expression and activity. The *CYP3A4*1B* allele has been associated with almost a doubling of

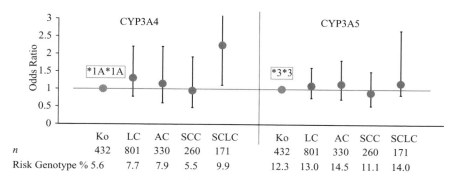

Figure 3.5 *CYP3A4* and *CYP3A5* genotype-dependent risk for lung cancer and different histological types; see also Dally *et al.* (2003). Abbreviations: Ko: controls, LC: lung cancer, AC: adenocarcinoma, SCC: squamous cell carcinoma, SCLC: small cell lung cancer.

luciferase expression in a reporter gene assay and with more advanced clinical stage and higher grade of prostate cancers. The very frequent intron 3 polymorphism in the *CYP3A5* gene (*CYP3A5*3*) results in decreased CYP3A5 protein levels. A case–control study was conducted in 801 Caucasian lung cancer patients that included 330 adenocarcinomas, 260 SCCs, 171 SCLCs, and 432 Caucasian hospital-based controls (Dally *et al.*, 2003). *CYP3A* genotyping was performed by capillary PCR followed by fluorescence-based melting curve analysis. A significantly increased SCLC risk for *CYP3A4*1B* allele carriers (OR 2.25; CI 1.11–4.55) was found (Figure 3.5). After dividing cases and controls by gender, an increased lung cancer risk for *CYP3A4*1B* carriers (OR 3.04; CI 0.94–9.90) for women but not for men (OR 1.00; CI 0.56–1.81) was revealed. Heavier-smoking men (at least 20 pack-years) with the *CYP3A4*1B* allele had a significant increased risk for lung cancer (OR 3.42; CI 1.65–7.14) compared to *1A/*1A* carriers with lower tobacco exposure (less than 20 pack-years). For women, the respective OR was 8.00 (CI 2.12–30.30). Genotype frequencies were generally in Hardy–Weinberg equilibrium, except for *CYP3A5* where a greater than expected number of *CYP3A5*1* homozygotes was observed among cases ($p = 0.006$). In addition, we observed linkage disequilibrium of *CYP3A4* and *CYP3A5* ($p < 10^{-5}$), but a non-significantly increased lung cancer risk was only found for homozygous *CYP3A5*1* allele carriers (OR 5.24; CI 0.85–102.28) but not for *CYP3A5*1/*3* heterozygotes (Dally *et al.*, 2003).

3.4 DISCUSSION

Our studies on GST genetic polymorphisms and lung cancer risk illustrate the importance of careful selection of the controls, and indicate that benign tumours must be excluded from the control group (Risch *et al.*, 2001). Population-based controls are seen by many as the gold standard in molecular epidemiology case–control studies today, but due to the difficulty and cost involved in their recruitment alternatives have to be considered, as described. For practical reasons sampling of cases and controls in our studies was confined to one hospital, which may restrict the generalisability of our results. Whether genetic risk factors identified for this subpopulation of individuals prone to some pulmonary problems hold for the general population remains to be explored. Genetic polymorphisms identified as relevant in the studies described above, however, should be first choice for further investigation.

Besides lung cancer, smoking is also related to the onset of non-malignant lung diseases and the individual risks of these diseases might also be influenced by the same genetic polymorphisms which are involved in lung cancer risk. Thus the use of hospital controls, as in our studies, may lead to an underestimation of lung cancer risk if the cause of hospitalization is also associated with smoking. Interestingly, a meta-analysis analysing the effect of smoking on the risk for SCC or adenocarcinoma could show differences in the relative risk when cases were either compared to hospital-based or population-based controls: among smokers and ex-smokers ORs were higher when cases were compared to hospital-based controls and lower when cases were compared to population-based controls. An inverse effect is observed for current smokers and SCLC risk: the OR was 37.9 (CI 18.5–77.9) with hospital-based controls, while with population-based controls the risk was increased by a factor of 72.5 (CI 13.8–379) (Khuder, 2001).

Among our hospital controls, an unequal *MPO (G/G)* genotype distribution was observed between different non-malignant lung diseases. Bronchitis and chronic obstructive pulmonary disease (COPD) seem to be associated with high *MPO (G/G)* genotype frequency, while alveolitis and pneumonia patients had a low proportion of *MPO (G/G)* genotype carriers. The development of some diseases, such as bronchitis, includes chronic or acute inflammatory processes in which *MPO* is highly active. The elevated level of the *(G/G)* genotype in some of the non-malignant lung diseases might indicate the involvement of the *MPO* genotype in their outcome. On the other hand, the onset of lung cancer has been associated with a history of certain lung diseases such as chronic bronchitis, emphysema, pneumonia and interstitial fibrosis (Pietra, 1990). The effect of the *MPO* genotype as a modifier of lung cancer risk may be strongest in individuals with chronic inflammatory processes. If this is the case, a disease-free control group may result in an incorrect estimate of the *MPO* genotype associated lung cancer risk because a direct impact of the *MPO* genotype on lung cancer risk cannot quite be separated from an indirect effect possibly caused by the *MPO* genotype affecting the onset of inflammatory diseases. In our study, data on concomitant lung diseases were available in tissue samples of 37 % ($n = 209$) of all lung cancer patients: most of them had bronchitis ($n = 40$) or bronchitis in combination with other non-malignant lung diseases ($n = 87$). Future studies on genotype-associated lung cancer risk should therefore recognise non-malignant lung diseases as potentially important confounders, especially in relation to inflammation-associated enzymes such as MPO. A recent study (Kantarci *et al.*, 2002) made a first step in this direction by adjusting for COPD in its statistical analyses.

In recent years industrialised countries have shown a rapid increase in lung cancer incidence and mortality amongst women at every level of smoking and for both high-tar and low-tar cigarettes, compared with decreases amongst men. In addition, the relative risk of specific types of lung cancer appears to differ for men and women. Women are less often diagnosed with those forms of lung cancer most closely associated with smoking. This may be due to socially constructed differences like smoking behaviour but also due to biologically determined factors (Payne, 2001). In comparison to male smokers, for female smokers, a significantly higher level of aromatic and hydrophobic DNA adducts per pack-year was found. This was significantly correlated to a higher expression level of lung CYP1A1 (Mollerup et al., 1999). Independent of smoking history, the combined variant CYP1A1 and GSTM1 genotypes conferred an approximately threefold increased lung cancer risk for women compared to men (Dresler et al., 2000). CYP3A isozymes are involved in oestrogen metabolism, thereby generating carcinogenic intermediates like 16α-hydroxyestrone. Metabolic studies showed a significantly higher CYP3A activity for certain clinical drugs in women than in men. We found an increased risk approaching significance for female CYP3A4*1B carriers, while male carriers were not affected (Dally et al., 2003).

In the past, genotyping of SNPs has been the most common tool for case–control studies investigating the impact of genetic variation on an individual's risk for certain diseases, including lung cancer. While some of the studies found significant associations with single SNPs, others could only be associated with a particular risk when several SNPs were combined. Recent studies could show that responses to certain drugs correlated with the patients' haplotype, rather than any individual SNP (Davidson, 2000). There are two main ways of identifying haplotypes. Molecular haplotyping, which involves the sequencing of the two homologous chromosomes independently to reveal which SNPs appear on the same DNA strand, is time-consuming and costly when it has to be performed on large populations. However, higher-throughput haplotyping methods have recently become available (Tost et al., 2002; Pettersson et al., 2003). The alternative is to use algorithms to infer haplotypes based on analysis of SNPs in patients and information on haplotype frequency in the population. This is cost-efficient but with the best available algorithms a success rate of only 80–90 % in correctly assigning haplotypes is achieved (Davidson, 2000). This implies that in the future molecular haplotyping will be necessary to check for previously unidentified disease-relevant haplotypes, requiring larger studies yet again.

In conclusion, studies investigating the genetic basis of cancer susceptibility should contribute to a better understanding of the aetiology of different cancers, and may provide clues to the mechanisms of activation of pro-carcinogens in humans. In order to tackle questions for which much larger subject numbers are required, anonymised genotype data will additionally have to be pooled for analysis in international collaborative studies (Benhamou et al., 2002). The better characterisation of the relevance of gene–environment interactions in the context of carcinogenesis is of great importance for preventive measures such as the setting of exposure threshold values and public health campaigns. Another medium-term aim is to evaluate their predictive value in connection with preventive measures such as chemoprevention and clinical applications such as chemotherapy, and, if applicable, to validate them for clinical use.

ACKNOWLEDGEMENTS

This chapter includes a summary of work carried out by the Division of Toxicology and Cancer Risk Factors at the German Cancer Research Centre and the Thoraxklinik Heidelberg. We are grateful to all patients and staff who helped to make these studies possible, and would particularly like to thank our collaborators P. Drings, H. Dienemann, K. Kayser, V. Schulz, P. Schmezer, B. Spiegelhalder and H. Bartsch. We thank C. Beynon, D. Bodemer, K. Gassner, M. Hoffmann, B. Jäger, N. Rajaee-Bebahani, C. Rohs, T. Ruf, U. von Seydlitz-Kurzbach, S. Stöckigt, S. Thiel and H. Wikman for their help with sample and/or data collection, archiving and genotyping, and R. Rausch for helping with the statistical analysis. We also thank O. Landt (TIB MOLBIOL, Berlin, Germany) for helping with the LightCycler probe design. This work was supported by Deutsche Krebshilfe (H.D.), and the Verein zur Förderung der Krebsforschung in Deutschland e.V.(A.R.).

CHAPTER 4

Biological Carcinogenesis: Theories and Models

Sylvia Solakidi

National Hellenic Research Foundation

Constantinos E. Vorgias

Faculty of Biology, University of Athens

Constantine E. Sekeris

National Hellenic Research Foundation

4.1 INTRODUCTION

All organisms are endowed with homeostatic mechanisms safeguarding the number of cells in a given tissue. Thus, cell replication and cell apoptosis are strongly regulated and coordinated, ensuring an equilibrium between these two processes. In cancer, the homeostatic mechanisms are deranged, cell replication is accelerated, apoptosis is decreased, and the cells acquire the capacity to infiltrate adjacent tissues and blood vessels and to metastasize (Hanahan and Weinberg, 2000; Vogelstein and Kinzler, 2004). These changes, characterizing the malignant phenotype, are due to defects in a variety of oncogenes and oncosuppressor genes involved in the many steps of the carcinogenic process – for example, replication, apoptosis, angiogenesis, cell–cell and cell–matrix interactions (Grana and Reddy, 1995; Weinberg, 1995; Hanahan and Folkman, 1996; Varner and Cherish, 1996; Christofori and Semb, 1999; Coussens and Werb, 1996). At least four or five gene mutations are required for the expression of the malignant phenotype. The gene defects encompass point mutations, deletions, insertions, amplifications and translocations, and result from the action of exogenous agents – physical, chemical and viral – and of endogenous metabolic products, such as reactive oxygen species. In addition, epigenetic events determine the transition from the normal to the malignant phenotype. The DNA repair machinery of the cell strives to repair the damage by means of stability (caretaker) genes, i.e. nucleotide mismatch repair genes, nucleotide-excision repair genes, base-excision repair genes and genes controlling processes involving large chromosomal segments, whose mutation leads to chromosomal instability and loss of heterozygosity. If the equilibrium between damage and repair shifts towards damage and enough deleterious mutations are accumulated, the cell takes the path of malignancy. The mutational concept of carcinogenesis predicts that tumors will have a monoclonal composition, which has been best demonstrated in colorectal tumors. Although the normal colon epithelium is polyclonal, arising from numerous stem cells, the tumors derived from these cells are monoclonal and are formed by clonal expansion of a cell provided with a growth advantage, due to a first somatic mutation of an oncogene or an oncosuppressor gene, over the other cells of the tissue. Subsequent somatic mutations will result in additional rounds of clonal expansion and thus in tumor progression.

To study the various steps of the carcinogenic process, experimental models are needed, in which the sequential events are amenable to detailed analysis. Information derived from the analysis of human tumors in various stages of carcinogenesis has also yielded important information but cannot cover all stages of this process. Both animal and cell models have been exploited to this end, each with its merits and its limitations (Balmain and Harris, 2000; Pories *et al.*, 1993; Herzig and Christofori, 2002; Bosland, 1992; Hann and Balmain, 2001; Mao and Balmain, 2003). The *in vivo* models are mostly cancers induced by carcinogens with or without parallel administration of promoter agents. Such models allow the reproducible isolation of all tumor stages (including normal tissue), which are then amenable to biochemical, genetic and pathological analysis and allow studies of the various steps of the carcinogenic process – initiation, promotion, progression and metastasis – in a defined time sequence.

Other models are based on the use of transgenic animals, in which defined genes can be either introduced in specific cells and tissues using cell specific promoters, or knocked out (Pories *et al.*, 1991; McDorman and Wolf, 2002). Cell-based models are principally of two types. In one, cells or tissue are exposed to chemical carcinogens or to one or more oncogenes usually using retroviral vectors to induce cell proliferation, and the sequence of events follows in cell culture or after grafting of the cells to animals. The other type of cell model is based on the isolation and stable culture of cells from tumors in the various stages of the carcinogenic process, which enables correlation of molecular changes with morphological and biochemical phenotypes. Combinations of animal- and cell-based models for various tumor types have appeared, rendering vital information on the sequence of events along the carcinogenic pathway.

4.2   MODELS OF HUMAN CARCINOGENESIS

The establishment of human genetic models of various cancers has permitted the correlation of genetic, molecular and biochemical defects with pathology.

Furthermore, the possibility of obtaining surgical specimens or needle biopsies of tumors in various stages of the carcinogenic process, in combination with the development of sensitive molecular techniques, has provided important additional information. Four models of carcinogenesis will be briefly reviewed: those of prostate, colorectal, endometrial and skin cancer.

4.2.1 Prostate cancer

The earliest precancerous lesion which can be detected in the prostate is intrae-pithelial neoplasia (PIN), which from its early (initiated) condition can proceed to its more advanced form, with characteristics of infiltrating cancers, known also as *in situ* carcinoma (Coffey, 1993; Bostwick *et al.*, 1995). During this transition from premalignant initiated to malignant localized (*in situ*) and then to infiltrating carcinoma, characteristic changes in many parameters – molecular, biochemical and morphological – are observed, which could be correlated etiologically to the carcino-genic process (Karp *et al.*, 1996). Although in half of the cases examined a genetic relationship between PIN lesions and cancer has been demonstrated, it seems that only a subset of PIN foci progresses to invasive prostate cancer. Furthermore, the analysis of PIN and contiguous foci of prostate cancer demonstrates the genetic and phenotypic heterogeneity among diverse PIN, cancer and metastatic lesions.

In apparently 'normal' cells, near the premalignant lesions, telomerase activity appears and glutathione thiotransferase activity is decreased, changes which are also observed in PIN lesions and carcinomas (Montironi *et al.*, 1999). As in other malignancies, prostate carcinogenesis represents a multistep process involving progression from small, low histologic grade tumors, to large, higher-grade metastasizing carcinomas. The introduction of rat and mouse models based on treatment of the animals with chemical carcinogens, sex hormones or a combination of both (Bosland, 1992) has yielded important information in this respect. Some of these induced animal tumors share a number of significant characteristics with human prostate cancer, with similar molecular and genetic alterations. Some of these models are low-incidence ones, adequate for study enhancement, whereas others are high-incidence models, better suited to the study of inhibition of carcinogenesis. Important information regarding molecular and biochemical changes during the carcinogenic process has also been gained from the study of clinical samples employing current microarray methodology, although no definitive proof has been provided to link specific genetic alterations with stages and grades of prostate cancer (Isaacs, 1995). The multicentric nature of the prostate carcinoma, its high variation in histological grade within the same prostate neoplasm and the possible association of different pathways with different etiologies necessitate the introduction of multiple model systems of prostate carcinogenesis.

The data stemming from clinical and animal model studies correlating molecular and genetic data with stages of carcinogenesis are summarized in Figure 4.1. The intraepithelial lesions consist of dysplastic, replicating cells, whereas the cells of the basal stroma lose the capacity to multiply. These changes have been correlated to increased expression of the oncogenes *c-erbB-2*, *c-erbB-3* and *c-met* and inactivation of the oncosuppressor gene *mn23H1*, which in normal epithelia are

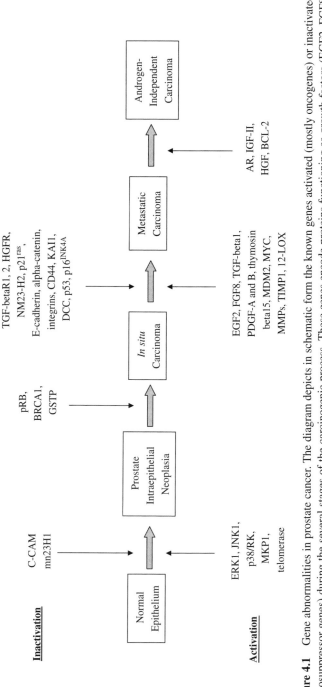

Figure 4.1 Gene abnormalities in prostate cancer. The diagram depicts in schematic form the known genes activated (mostly oncogenes) or inactivated (oncosuppressor genes) during the several stages of the carcinogenic process. These genes encode proteins functioning as growth factors (EGF2, FGF8, TGFβ1, PDGFA and B, IFGII, HGF) or growth factor receptors (TGFβR1 and 2, HGFR), metalloproteinases and their inhibitors (MMPs, TIMP1), cell adhesion (E-cadherin, alpha-catenin, integrins, KAI1) and signal transduction molecules (kinases and kinase inhibitors), cell-cycle regulators (pRB, p53, p16^{INK4A}), molecules involved in apoptosis (Bcl-2), telomerase, androgen receptor (AR) and enzymes involved in detoxification of carcinogens (GSTP).

expressed solely in the basal stroma cells. Furthermore, in 20 % of the lesions the expression of the *bcl-2* gene is deranged, leading to deregulation of apoptosis (Bonkhoff *et al.*, 1998). Chromosomal abnormalities are frequent in intraepithelial carcinoma (in 50 % of cases) and a similar percentage is observed also in infiltrating carcinoma (Emmert-Buck *et al.*, 1995). Ninety per cent of lesions show extensive methylation of deoxycytidine in the promoter region of the glutathione thiotransferase gene, leading to the lack of expression of the gene, apparently an early event in carcinogenesis (Lee *et al.*, 1994). In contrast to the total absence of telomerase in normal epithelium, 70 % of the precancerous lesions express the enzyme (Koeneman *et al.*, 1998).

In 70 % of prostate cancers, amplification of certain genes as well as loss of heterozygosity (LOH) is noted, correlated to the aggressive behavior of the tumor (Sandberg, 1992; Bova *et al.*, 1993) (Figure 4.1). Most defects are localized on chromosomes 7 and 8, but also on chromosomes 2q, 5q, 6q, 9p, 10p, 10q, 13q, 15q, 16q, 17p, 18q, 20q and Y. The chromosome regions lost could harbor oncosuppressor genes (Gao *et al.*, 1993, 1995, 1997; Dong *et al.*, 1995), whereas gene amplification probably involves oncogenes. Thus, the *hpc 1* gene is localized in the genetic locus 1q24-25, the oncosuppressor genes *Rb1*, *cdh1* and *DCC* in 13q, 16q, 17q and 18q, whereas gene *p53* and gene *hic-1* (hypermethylated in cancer) encoding a Zn-finger transcription factor are found in locus 17p13. An important role in prostate carcinogenesis is ascribed to the *Krev-1* oncosuppressor gene (Burney *et al.*, 1994), whereas *n33* and *mx11* seem to play a secondary role in this process. Gene amplification involves the oncogene *c-myc*, localized in locus 8q24. Microsatellite instability is observed in one-third of carcinomas, particularly in those with high Gleason scores and in advanced stages. It seems that the early stages of carcinogenesis are correlated with oncosuppressor gene inactivation, whereas later on activation of oncogenes is also observed, particularly of regions 8q, 7q, Xq and 18q. In one-third of hormone-resistant cancer cases, the androgen receptor gene is amplified.

Several proteins are increasingly expressed, correlated to carcinogenesis, acting through signal transduction mechanisms involving, among others, *src* and *ras*. These are EGF, TGF-α, c-erbB2, FGF7, FGF8, IGF-II, the IGF-1 receptor and TGF-β1, whereas TGF-β1 and TGF-β2 receptor expression is progressively decreased in aggressive carcinomas (Scher *et al.*, 1995; Kaltz-Wittmer *et al.*, 2000).

During the advanced, metastatic stage an increased mutation and amplification rate of the androgen receptor gene is observed, rendering the receptor sensitive to other steroid hormones and increasing its sensitivity to androgens, respectively. In advanced cases of prostate cancer low levels of expression of the NGF receptor are observed. Expression of IL-6 and IL-6R is also correlated to aggressive behavior of prostate cancer.

Loss of expression of the *E-cadherin* gene, located on chromosome 16q22, alpha-catenin and integrins, as well as of KAI1, encoding a transmembrane glycoprotein, is coupled with progressive disease (Morton *et al.*, 1993; Umbas *et al.*, 1994) and is linked to acquisition of a metastatic phenotype, as substantiated in a transgenic model of mouse carcinogenesis.

4.2.2   Colorectal cancer

One of the best-studied genetic models of human carcinogenesis is that of colorectal cancer. The 1990 model proposed by Fearon and Vogelstein has been the paradigm for the genetic alterations involved in the development of colorectal carcinoma (Fearon and Vogelstein, 1990). The change of the normal epithelium into malignant and metastatic proceeds, in the majority of cases, through intermediary adenoma stages. A series of genetic alterations involving oncogenes and oncosuppressor genes occur; some of the most significant are depicted in Figure 4.2 (Alitalo *et al.*, 1983, 1984; Ashton-Rickardt *et al.*, 1989; Baker *et al.*, 1989; Bos *et al.*, 1987; Calabretta *et al.*, 1985; D'Emilia *et al.*, 1989).

Although multiple stages of adenomas may exist in the process of adenoma progression to the malignant phenotype, three discrete stages of adenoma formation are shown in Figure 4.2. Colorectal cancer is thought to be initiated by the inactivation of the adenomatous polyposis coli (APC) gene. A further important somatic mutation in the appearance of colorectal carcinomas is the *K-ras* gene mutation found in 50 % of these tumors and in adenomas larger than 1 cm in size. Adenomas bearing *ras* gene mutations may be more likely to progress than adenomas without mutation. Hyperactive mutant *Ras* has been known to induce cellular proliferation. Recently, however, other effects of mutant *Ras* have been reported. Active *Ras* can phosphorylate pro-caspase-9, thereby inhibiting cytochrome-c-induced apoptosis (Cardone *et al.*, 1998). In mice, oncogenic *Ras* has been shown to cause cell-cycle arrest due to up-regulation of both tumor suppressors of the IKN4a-ARF locus, $p19^{ARF}$ and $p16^{INK4a}$, which in turn activate *p53* and *Rb*, respectively (Palmero *et al.*, 1998).

Allelic loss of chromosome 5p, harboring the APC locus has been observed in 20–25 % of colorectal carcinomas. APC has a role in the Wnt signalling pathway, acting as a partner molecule of beta-catenin, which is degraded and inactivated through binding to APC. The mutated and truncated APC product is unable to bind and titrate beta-catenin, so that Wnt signalling in an APC mutated cell becomes deranged (Ilyas and Tomlinson, 1997). Another molecular partner of beta-catenin is conductin, the mammalian homologue of axin, which seems to be involved in proper conduction of the complex formation of APC and beta-catenin (Behrens *et al.*, 1998). Furthermore, one of the genes inappropriately activated in a deranged Wnt signalling system turned out to be *c-myc* (He *et al.*, 1998).

Loss of specific chromosomal regions involving one of the two parental chromosomes (allele loss, LOH) occurs frequently in colorectal tumors and is interpreted as evidence that these regions contain tumor suppressor genes. In more than 75 % of these tumors, a large portion of chromosome 17p, which contains the *p53* gene, is lost. This event is rarely observed in adenomas. In addition, mutations resulting in amino acid substitutions in the *p53* gene product of the remaining *p53* allele are frequently found in colorectal carcinomas and render the p53 protein ineffective as tumor suppressor (Knudson, 1985).

The second most common region of allelic loss in colorectal tumors is chromosome 18q, lost in more than 70 % of the carcinomas and in 50 % of the late

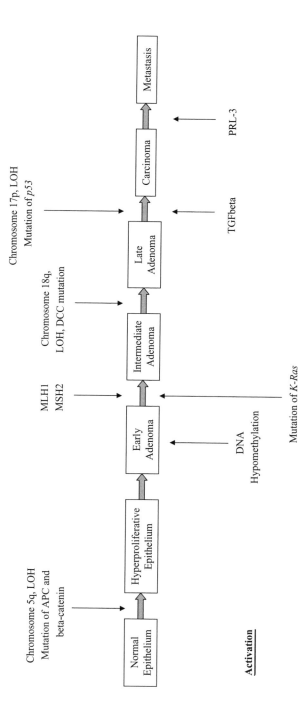

Figure 4.2 The Fearon–Vogelstein genetic model for colorectal carcinogenesis (38, modified). Colorectal cancer is thought to be initiated by inactivation of the *APC* tumor suppressor gene in a colon epithelial cell localized in crypts. In 85 % of cases the *APC* gene is mutated, while the beta-catenin gene is mutated in 50 % of cases. Cells become dysplastic and accumulate. Further mutations (*K-ras* and *DCC*) lead to formation of large polyps, whereas TGF-beta and *p53* gene mutations lead to the cancer phenotype. Chromosomal instability (CIN) seems to be an early event and accounts for LOH. Thirteen per cent of sporadic colon cancers show microsatellite instability (MIN), due to mutation in the mismatch repair enzymes MLH1 and MSH2. Mutations of the *PRL-3* (protein tyrosine phosphatase) gene are found in metastatic tumors.

adenomas, harboring the *DCC* (deleted in colorectal cancer) gene, encoding a transmembrane receptor for netrins, which shows strong homology to the family of adhesion molecules affecting cell–cell and cell–extracellular matrix interactions (Mehlen and Fearon, 2004). Although *DCC* was originally thought to be the oncosuppressor gene involved in 18q deletions, other tumor suppressors were found in this locus, including *SMAD-4*, one of the components involved in the TGFbeta signalling pathway. *SMAD-4* mutations have been observed in 6–30 % of colorectal carcinomas (Thiagalingam *et al.*, 1996). The *SMAD-2* gene, coding for another component of the TGFbeta signalling pathway, is positioned close to *SMAD-4* and can be induced by Ras (Eppert *et al.*, 1996). Since TGFbeta singalling normally results in cell-cycle inhibition and cellular differentiation, it appears that defects in this pathway may play an important role in tumorigenesis. Wnt and TGFbeta-signalling pathways converge on the p27^{Kip1} molecule, whose release from the cyclin E-cdk2 complex is induced by *c-myc* and inhibited by TGFbeta. It, therefore, appears that when the Wnt pathway is deranged resulting in upregulation of *c-myc* and the TGFbeta pathway is disrupted due to a *SMAD-4* mutation, a synergistic effect on the cell cycle ensues (Arends, 2000). This may be a crucial effect in colorectal tumorigenesis. Indeed, increased degradation of p27^{Kip1} has been reported in aggressive colorectal cancer (Loda *et al.*, 1997).

Many other chromosomal losses, in addition to those of chromosomes 5p, 17p and 18q, are detected in the colorectal carcinomas, involving chromosomes 1q, 4p, 6p, 6q, 8p, 9p and 22q. Such losses could either have no specific effect on the phenotype, arising coincidentally with the other genetic alterations, or could contain many suppressor genes present throughout the genome.

Another somatic alteration in colon carcinogenesis is the loss of DNA methyl groups. One-third of the DNA regions studied, even of small adenomas, have lost methyl groups present in normal DNA of colonic mucosa. This epigenetic change could contribute to the instability of the tumor cell genome and change the rate at which genetic alterations, such as allelic losses, occur. Some specific DNA regions, however, could be hypermethylated (Polyak and Higgins, 2001). Although the molecular and genetic defects usually occur at characteristic stages of tumor progression (as shown in Figure 4.2), the progressive accumulation of the defects is more important than the order of their occurrence.

Microsatellite instability is frequently seen in colon cancer tissue from patients with hereditary non-polyposis colorectal cancer (HNPCC), which is caused by a germline mutation of one of the mismatch repair genes. HNPCC-associated cancer exhibits microsatellite instability. Germline mutations of each of the six known mismatch repair genes have been identified in HNPCC kindreds. Mutations are most commonly seen in the *hMSH2* gene, found on chromosome 2p, or in the *hMLH1* gene, found on chromosome 3p. Mutations of *hPMS1*, *hPMS2*, *hMSH3* and *hMSH6* account for few reported cases (Calvert and Frucht, 2002). Individuals with germline mutations of a mismatch repair gene typically have high microsatellite instability, although the *hMSH6* mutation can be associated with low microsatellite instability (Parc *et al.*, 2000). Although 10–15 % of cases of sporadic colon cancer can exhibit microsatellite instability, it is usually of the low type (Boland *et al.*, 1998).

4.2.3 Endometrial cancer

The major known gene alterations during carcinogenesis of another well-studied cancer, endometrioid adenocarcinoma, are depicted in Figure 4.3 (Caduff *et al.*, 1997; Boyd and Risinger, 1991; Terakawa *et al.*, 1997).

Two different clinicopathological types of endometrial cancer can be distinguished: the estrogen-related or endometrioid type (type I) and the non-estrogen-related or non-endometrioid type (mainly papillary serous or clear cell carcinomas) (type II). Type I is a carcinoma of endometrioid type and low cellular grade, expressing estrogen and progesterone receptors, frequently preceded by endometrial hyperplasia and having a good prognosis. Type II endometrial cancers without associated hyperplasia are negative for estrogen and progesterone receptors and are characterized by high cellular grade and poor prognosis. Recent advances in the molecular genetics of endometrial cancer have shown that the molecular changes involved in its development differ in estrogen-dependent type I and non-estrogen-dependent type II. Type I carcinomas frequently show mutations of DNA mismatch repair genes (*MLH1*, *MSH2*, *MSH6*), *PTEN*, *k-ras* and beta-catenin genes, whereas type II malignancies are characterized by aneuploidy, *p53* mutations and her2/neu amplification. This dualistic model of type I and II endometrial cancers is not applicable in some cases, which show overlapping features. Mutations of the steroid receptor genes have not been linked with a distinct type of endometrial carcinoma (Oehler *et al.*, 2003).

Germline mutations in one of several identified DNA mismatch repair genes, most commonly in *MLH1*, *MSH2* or *MSH6*, are observed in approximately 60–80 % of patients with the HNPCC syndrome. Female carriers of such mutations have a 42 % risk of endometrial cancer by the age of 70 years (Dunlop *et al.*, 1997). Microsatellite instability, a characteristic of HNPCC, occurs also in 15–25 % of sporadic endometrial cancers, although it is very uncommon in uterine serous carcinomas (Tashiro *et al.*, 1997). MLH1 promoter hypermethylation has also been described in microsatellite instability-negative endometrial neoplasia coexisting with microsatellite instability-positive endometrioid endometrial cancers, suggesting that *MLH1* promoter hypermethylation occurs in the transition from hyperplasia to carcinoma. Furthermore, additional mismatch repair genes are secondary mutated, which accelerates genomic instability and the accumulation of additional genetic changes of oncogenes and tumor suppressor genes involved in early carcinogenesis (Inoue, 2001).

K-ras mutations have been identified in 11–31% of endometrial carcinomas. They are more frequent in endometrioid carcinomas and more common in mucinous subtypes, but almost absent in papillary serous and clear cell carcinomas (Lagarda *et al.*, 2001). *K-ras* mutations have also been demonstrated in about 15 % of endometrial hyperplasias, with a frequency similar to that seen in endometrial cancers. Thus a role of *K-ras* in the early steps of carcinogenesis seems very likely (Sasaki *et al.*, 1993).

Between 10 % and 30 % of all endometrial carcinomas and up to 80 % of uterine serous papillary malignancies show HER2/neu overexpression. As overexpression

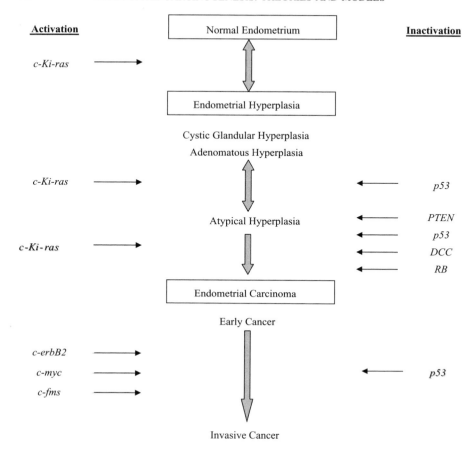

Figure 4.3 A genetic model for endometrial carcinogenesis. Type I carcinomas frequently show mutations of DNA mismatch repair genes (*MLH1*, *MSH2*, *MSH6*), PTEN, *K-ras* and beta-catenin genes, whereas type II malignancies are characterized by aneuploidy, *p53* mutations and *her2/neu* amplification.

of HER2/neu is also found in up to 15 % of normal and hyperplastic endometrial samples (Santin *et al.*, 2002), this may play a role in the early development of some endometrial cancers (Rasty *et al.*, 1998).

PTEN is a tumor suppressor gene encoding a phosphatase with homology to tensin. Loss of heterozygosity at the *PTEN* locus of 10q23.3 occurs in about 40 % of endometrial cancers (Matias-Guiu *et al.*, 2001). *PTEN* is also the most frequently mutated tumor suppressor gene in endometrial cancer (in 37–61% of these cancers), particularly in type I malignancies (Risinger *et al.*, 1997). *PTEN* mutations are found in up to 55 % of endometrial hyperplasias, but also in histologically normal-appearing endometrium exposed to estrogen (Mutter *et al.*, 1992). In addition, identical *PTEN* mutations occur in hyperplasias coexisting with microsatellite instability-positive endometrial cancers (Levine *et al.*, 1998). Inactivation of *PTEN* could therefore represent one of the earliest events in the multistep progression of endometrial carcinogenesis.

Mutations of the *p53* gene and accumulation of the p53 protein are detected in up to 90 % of serous papillary carcinomas, but only in about 20 % of endometrioid malignancies. Mutations are most common in high-grade tumors and are rarely found in endometrial hyperplasias. This finding suggests that *p53* mutations in endometrioid carcinomas are closely related to dedifferentiation and occur relatively late in tumor development. In contrast, the majority (78 %) of endometrial intraepithelial carcinomas, the putative precursor of serous carcinomas, have *p53* mutations, supporting a role of *p53* alterations in the early carcinogenesis of serous malignancies (Lax *et al.*, 2000).

The frequency of beta-catenin mutations in endometrial carcinomas ranges from 13 % to 50 %. However, stabilization of beta-catenin leading to accumulation in the cytoplasm and/or nucleus was also observed in endometrial carcinomas lacking mutations. This finding suggests that alterations in other genes of the beta-catenin/ Wnt pathway might be responsible for the stabilization of Wnt in these tumors (Fukuchi *et al.*, 1998).

As in the previously described cancer cases, the accumulation of the gene defects rather than the order of their appearance seems to be more important in carcinogenesis. Additional genetic changes, depicted in Figure 4.3, are correlated to the metastatic potential of the cancer cells.

4.3 THE MULTISTAGE MOUSE SKIN CARCINOGENESIS MODEL

Mouse skin has provided a paradigm for studies of multistage chemical carcinogenesis in epithelial cells. The chemical carcinogenesis regimen applied to mouse skin is the two-stage induction, which involves the administration of a single dose of the polycyclic aromatic hydrocarbon 7,12-dimethyl-benz[α]anthracene (DMBA), followed by weekly applications of the phorbol ester 12-*O*-tetradecanoylphorbol-13-acetate (TPA), which has the role of carcinogenesis promoter. This treatment results in the development of numerous benign papillomas, some of which progress to malignant squamous cell carcinomas 20–40 weeks after the first exposure to carcinogens. Because of the problems associated with studying biological mechanisms of carcinogenesis using *in vivo* tumour material, a series of cell lines has been developed in Allan Balmain's laboratory. They represent the development of the three distinct stages of mouse skin carcinogenesis – initiation, promotion and progression – thus covering the full spectrum of mouse skin carcinogenesis.

The mouse skin carcinogenesis model constitutes mainly of the following cell lines: the *C5N* immortalized, non-tumorigenic keratinocyte line derived form a Balb/c mouse (Kulesz-Martin *et al.*, 1983); the *P1* and *P6* benign papilloma cell lines, derived from a DMBA/TPA treated spretus X CBA F1 hybrid mouse (Haddow *et al.*, 1991); and the *B9* squamous cell line and the *A5* highly anaplastic, invasive spindle cell line, both isolated from the same primary tumour from a multiple DMBA/TPA treated spretus X CBA F1 hybrid mouse (Burns *et al.*, 1991). Furthermore, the *CarB* highly anaplastic, invasive spindle cell line, derived from a DMBA/TPA treated NIH mouse (Fusenig *et al.*, 1978), the *PDV* squamous cell line derived from a DMBA treated epidermal cell culture from a newborn mouse, and the *PDVC57* squamous cell line developed in one out of eight sites of injection of PDV cells in an adult syngeneic C57B1 mouse (Fusenig *et al.*, 1985). Although the *A5* spindle cell line was isolated from the same primary tumour as the *B9* cell line, it has different morphological and growth properties. The *C5N*, *P1*, *P6* and *B9* cells have a typical epithelial morphology, being cuboidal in shape, and are characterized by a cobblestone pattern of growth, while the *A5* and *CarB* cell lines show a fibroblastic morphology. The *C5N*, *P1*, *P6* and *B9* cell lines have a typical pattern of keratin and E-cadherin expression, whereas the *A5* cell line has an altered cytoskeleton and fails to express E-cadherin. The other spindle cell line, the CarB, does not express E-cadherin, but expresses vimentin. Compared with *PDV* cells, the *PDVC57* cell line has a more heterogeneous morphology, is characterized by an increased number of giant cells and is more tumorigenic when reinjected into adult syngeneic mice. *PDVC57* cells are eight times as invasive and secrete twice as much type IV collagenase compared to *PDV* cells, and are also more chemotactic.

The multistage mouse skin carcinogenesis model, although an artificial one, is an ideal system to study the timing of qualitative and quantitative alterations which take place during the different stages of chemical carcinogenesis, allowing analysis of the events that lead to the transition from the stage of initiation to the stage of promotion and finally to the progression of carcinogenesis. The following passage summarizes the main alterations observed in signal transduction molecules in the mouse carcinogenesis cell lines.

The *H-ras* mutations have a causal role in the initiation stage of carcinogenesis. Papillomas and carcinomas initiated with different carcinogens exhibit distinct spectra of point mutations in the *H-ras* gene (Quintanilla *et al.*, 1986). Furthermore, *H-ras* plays an important role in more advanced stages of carcinogenesis, in which the mutant allele is further duplicated and amplified. The squamous and spindle cell lines differ in the ratio of wild-type to mutant *H-ras* alleles: The *B9* cell line carries two wild-type and four mutant allels, the *A5* cells have 1 wild-type and 2 mutant alleles, the *CarB* cell line carries two mutant alleles and the ratio of wild-type to mutant *H-ras* alleles in *PDV* and *PDVC57* cell lines is 2:1 and 1:2, respectively.

Ras-mediated tumorigenesis depends on signalling pathways that act preferentially through cyclin D1, whose mRNA and protein levels are generally higher in mouse skin carcinomas than in papillomas. Cyclin D1 deficiency also results in up to an 80 % decrease in the development of squamous tumours generated through two-stage chemical carcinogenesis. Cyclin D1 participates, therefore, in the stage of promotion of carcinogenesis (Robles *et al.*, 1998).

Ras activates members of the JNK group of MAPKs, which are the major mediators of c-Jun and ATF-2 terminal phosphorylation, as well as the Raf/MEK/ERK branch of the MAPK pathway. The content of JNK1 and JNK2 isoforms, as well as JNK activity, is increased in the malignant mouse skin cell lines, with JNK2 elevated to a lesser extent than JNK1 in the spindle cell lines *A5* and *CarB*. The ERK1/2 isoforms are preferentially activated in advanced tumor stages, since phosphorylated ERK1 and ERK2 are elevated in the *A5* and *CarB* spindle cells, compared with the *P1* and *B9* epithelial cell lines. Studies in the *PDV:PDVC57* cell line pair revealed increased ERK1/2 phosphorylation in the *PDVC57* cells, which are more aggressive than the *PDV* cell line. This finding suggests that the biological characteristics of the squamous phenotype may depend on the activation of ERK1/2 (Katsanakis *et al.*, 2002).

The c-Jun and ATF-2 AP-1 transcription factor family members are likely to be involved in the progression of carcinogenesis in mouse epidermis. Increased levels of total and phosphorylated c-Jun are detected in the malignant cell lines, with maximum levels observed in the *A5* and *CarB* spindle cell lines. High levels of Fra-2, hyperphosphorylated Fra-1 and total and phosphorylated ATF-2 also characterize the malignant phenotypes. This increase probably takes place due to Ras protein overexpression, also observed in these cells. These changes in expression and post-translational modification of the AP-1 family members result in enhanced AP-1 DNA activity at the collagenase I TRE and Jun2 TRE in the metastatic cell lines *A5* and *CarB*. The major AP-1 components pariticipating in the AP-1/DNA binding complex are c-Jun and ATF-2 (Zoumpourlis *et al.*, 2000).

Increased serum response factor (SRF) protein levels and SRF DNA binding activity to the c-*fos* serum response element are observed in the mouse skin spindle cell lines. Furthermore, both total and active RhoA levels are significantly higher in *A5* than in *B9* cells. Transfection experiments with active and dominant negative forms of RhoA have shown that SRF overexpression has an important role in spindle phenotype formation and RhoA signalling regulates DNA binding activity of SRF (Psichari *et al.*, 2002).

A5 spindle cells, which are characterized by increased amounts of mutant H-ras protein, do not express any Tiam-1 (T lymphoma invasion and metastasis gene) protein, in contrast to *P1* cells, which express high levels of Tiam-1. Moreover, loss of Tiam-1 protein in *A5* cells is accompanied by a strong reduction in Rac basal activity. Tiam-1 function appears, therefore, to be essential for the initiation and promotion of Ras-induced skin tumours, but histological and biochemical data suggest that a subsequent loss of Tiam-1 increases the rate of malignant conversion of benign tumours (Malliri *et al.*, 2002).

High levels of the matrix metalloproteinase MMP-9 (which is regulated by the AP-1 and ets transcription factors) have been demonstrated in the invasive *A5* and *CarB* spindle cell lines, whereas MMP-2 levels are independent of tumorigenic and invasive cell properties (Papathoma *et al.*, 2001).

It has been suggested that *p53* alterations arise before the transition from squamous to spindle phenotype. In a study carried out on chemically induced mouse skin tumours, LOH at the *p53* locus is detected in approximately one-third of carcinomas, but not in papillomas. Furthermore, no loss of heterozygosity is detected in *PDV* and *PDVC57* cell lines. Moreover, the mutant p53 protein is present in the primary carcinoma which gives rise to *B9* and *A5* cell lines, but not in *CarB* cells (Burns *et al.*, 1991).

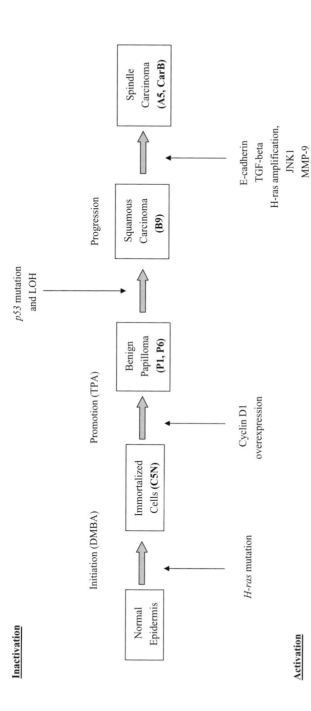

Figure 4.4 Gene abnormalities in the multistage mouse skin carcinogenesis model generated by application of a two-stage induction chemical carcinogenesis regimen, which involves the administration of a single dose of DMBA, followed by weekly applications of TPA, which has the role of carcinogenesis promoter. This treatment results in the development of numerous benign papillomas, some of which progress to malignant squamous cell carcinomas 20–40 weeks after the first exposure to carcinogens. *H-ras* is a critical target of chemical carcinogens and has a crucial role in initiation of carcinogenesis. Further mutations in *H-ras* target genes, as well as in oncosuppressor genes, guide the transition to advanced stages of carcinogenesis.

The immortalized, benign and malignant cell lines comprising the mouse skin carcinogenesis system have proved to be an ideal model for the study of multistage carcinogenesis, easy to manipulate and handle, and have been valuable tools in investigations that succeeded in correlating specific genetic alterations with specific stages of carcinogenesis (Figure 4.4). These observations were verified by *in vivo* experiments in knock-out and transgenic mice. These data could serve as a background for the identification of genes having a critical role in stage-to-stage transition in human multistage cancers.

4.4 EPILOGUE

Much of the data concerning the sequential genetic changes leading to the transformation of a normal cell into a cancer cell with metastasizing potential have been derived from the development of animal and animal cell models, although the analysis of surgically removed tumors or tissue biopsies has also contributed valuable information.

Objections have been raised concerning the value of animal models due to the discrepancies between human and rodent carcinogenesis (Balmain and Harris, 2000; Hann and Balmain, 2001). However, there is a high degree of genetic and biological similarity between development of cancer in human and rodent systems (Zoumpourlis *et al.*, 2003). Mice develop tumors in the same tissues as humans and with similar histopathological course, and the genetic events in humans are mostly also observed in rodents, with a similar stepwise progression from benign to malignant stages. Rodents have a short life span and develop tumors quite rapidly and rodent cells can be – in contrast to human cells – easily immortalized (Zoumpourlis *et al.*, 2003), which could be due to differences in telomerase activity and repair of chromosome ends (Rhyu, 1995). Independent of their possible shortcomings, the animal models serve the purpose of following the carcinogenic process from carcinogen exposure and genetic alterations afflicted, to the biological response and the malignant phenotype. The development of a series of animal and animal cell carcinogenesis models, taking into account the spectacular advances in molecular techniques – microarrays and proteomics – permitting the simultaneous analysis of thousands of genes and proteins, heralds important advances in our understanding of carcinogenesis, with significant impact on cancer risk assessment, tumor prevention, diagnosis, prognosis and therapy.

CHAPTER 5

Biological and Mathematical Aspects of Multistage Carcinogenesis

E. Georg Luebeck and Suresh H. Moolgavkar

Fred Hutchinson Cancer Research Center

5.1 INTRODUCTION

Mathematical models of multistage carcinogenesis have been in the making for half a century, starting with the early attempts by Nordling (1953) and by Armitage and Doll (1954) to provide biologically based descriptions of the cancer process. Even though progress in this area has been slow but steady, the efforts to quantify carcinogenesis and to model cancer risks in biological terms, rather than in pure statistical terms, have come a long way since. This evolution in our understanding of cancer is, at least in part, driven by the insights generated by modern molecular biology, which over the past two decades has dramatically increased our understanding of the genetic and epigenetic mechanisms involved in carcinogenesis (see Chapter 2 and 4, this volume).

In 1954 Armitage and Doll observed that the age-specific incidence of many solid tumors appeared to increase as a power of age, and that the power could be related mathematically (at some level of approximation of their model) to the number of rate-limiting steps required for the formation of a malignant tumor. However, they soon realized that this picture was too simplistic (Armitage and Doll, 1957) and that some adjustments had to be made for the possibility of clonal expansion of intermediate (say, dysplastic) cell populations which greatly amplifies the number of cells at risk for malignant transformation. Examples of such intermediate lesions are the dysplastic lesions found in the human lung (Park *et al.*, 1999; Wistuba *et al.*, 2000), adenomatous polyps in colon and rectum,

Recent Advances in Quantitative Methods in Cancer and Human Health Risk Assessment
Edited by L. Edler and C. Kitsos © 2005 John Wiley & Sons, Ltd

(pre)neoplastic lesions in Barrett's esophagus (Galipeau *et al.*, 1999; Prevo *et al.*, 1999; Wong *et al.*, 2001; Vaughan, 2002), and the enzyme-altered lesions in rodent hepatocarcinogenesis (see Lueback *et al.*, 1999b). Indeed, the action of most tumor promoters in chemical carcinogenesis can be attributed to an acceleration of growth of such intermediate lesions. Later models of carcinogenesis (Armitage and Doll, 1957; Kendall, 1960; Moolgavkar and Knudson, 1981) take explicit account of the clonal expansion of intermediate cells.

These considerations, combined with the idea of recessive oncogenesis formulated by Knudson (1971), led to the advent of the *two-stage clonal expansion* (TSCE) model which explicitly incorporates the role of clonal expansion (promotion) as a stochastic process during carcinogenesis (Moolgavkar and Venzon, 1979; Moolgavkar and Luebeck, 1990; Luebeck and Moolgavkar, 2002). Therefore, the TSCE model (and its multistage extensions) can be used to explicitly consider the action of agents that interact directly with DNA to produce mutations leading to *initiation*, that is, the formation of cells that have a propensity to proliferate, as well as the action of agents that modify the cell kinetics of such initiated cells. Examples of the latter are promoters that stimulate tumor growth, as well as growth inhibitors, such as non-steroidal anti-inflammatory drugs.

Although interesting hypotheses have been generated with the TSCE model concerning the interplay between *initiation* and *promotion*, and plausible explanations can be given for a number of specific exposure and age effects in occupational cohort studies (see Luebeck *et al.*, 1999a; Hazelton *et al.*, 2001), the TSCE model has also been criticized for being too simplistic, not accounting for the numerous mutations seen in many tumors and the causes and effects of genomic instability in the form of genome-wide allelic gains and losses (see Cahill *et al.*, 1999; Hanahan and Weinberg, 2000; Loeb and Loeb, 2000). Indeed, recent studies of the genetic profile of various cancers suggest the involvement of a number of genes in several signaling and regulatory pathways linked to tumorigenesis. While it is impossible in this space to review in detail the roles of various proto-oncogenes and tumor suppressor (TSP) genes in even the most common cancers (see Vogelstein and Kinzler, 2002), we will limit our discussion here to the salient features of colon cancer and esophageal cancer, and will make an attempt to sketch out some useful mathematical models that espouse the concept of multistage carcinogenesis.

5.2 FEATURES OF MULTISTAGE CARCINOGENESIS

5.2.1 Colorectal cancer

This cancer is perhaps the best-studied cancer in terms of the putative sequence of genetic events in its pathogenesis (Fearon and Vogelstein, 1990; Aaltonen *et al.*, 1993; Peltomäki *et al.*, 1993; Kinzler and Vogelstein, 1997; Hanahan and Weinberg, 2000). Over the last 15 years an impressive number of ground-breaking studies have been been carried out that identify a number of molecular pathways that are critically involved in the development of colorectal cancer. Among these pathways are the APC/β-catenin/T-cell (also known as the Wnt-signaling) pathway (Sparks *et al.*, 1998), the TGFβ (tumor growth factor β) signaling pathway and its intracellular SMAD components, and the G1/S checkpoint control system involving the *TP53* (tumor protein 53) gene and the *BAX* (*BCL-2*-associated X protein) gene products (Laurent-Puig *et al.*, 1999).

Disruption of the Wnt-signaling pathway, which may be caused by inactivation of APC (adenomatous polyposis coli) protein or direct mutation of CTNNB1 (β-catenin) at the glycogen synthase kinase (GSK)-3β phosphorylation site, appears to occur early in colorectal tumorigenesis. The net result of this disruption is the transcriptional activation of target genes involved in cell cycle progression (Fearnhead *et al.*, 2001) and the modification of cell adhesion properties via β-catenin binding to E-cadherin. The implication of the latter changes is less clear, but they are thought to result in abnormal cell migration and differentiation (van de Wetering *et al.*, 2002).

Abnormalities of the TGFβ receptors (type I and II) and associated SMAD components have been detected in various tumors, including colorectal cancers and pancreatic cancers. Inhibitory SMADs and transcriptional co-repressors, including c-Ski and SnoN, repress TGFβ/SMAD signaling. Defects in the TGFβ/SMAD signaling pathway may lead to tumor progression as tumorigenic cells become resistant to the growth inhibition induced by TGFβ cytokines. There is consensus that this pathway plays an important role in the adenoma–carcinoma transition in colon cancers (Grady *et al.*, 1998). Similarly, defects in the G1/S checkpoint control system appear late in the carcinogenic process, suggesting the sequential disruption of several critical signaling pathways in cancer development.

Colorectal cancers have been broadly categorized into two classes: so-called loss of heterozygosity (LOH) positive cancers (believed to comprise 70–80 % of all colorectal cancers), and so-called microsatellite instability (MIN) prone cancers (Ward *et al.*, 2001). These two categories appear to be mutually exclusive but are known to share common pathways, as discussed by Laurent-Puig *et al.* (1999). MIN positive cancers are usually associated with defects in the DNA mismatch repair system, involving mutations (or epigenetic silencing) in a number of genes, among them human homologues of the *MSH2, MLH1, MSH6* and *PMS2* genes. These defects are now known to give rise to a *mutator phenotype*, as postulated early on by Loeb (1998, 2001). The inheritance of a requisite step of this form of cancer (in colon) is referred to as heritable non-polyposis colon cancer (HNPCC). For a review, see Peltomaki and de la Chapelle (1997). In contrast, LOH positive cancers, which show abundant allelic losses and gains at numerous loci (Jen *et al.*, 1994; Boland *et al.*, 1995; Shih *et al.*, 2001), frequently present biallelic inactivation of the *APC* tumor suppressor gene, the gene that predisposes to *familial adenomatous polyposis* (FAP).

Although there are at least two distinct mechanisms by which colorectal cancers may arise – one of them involving a mutator phenotype leading to MIN, the other leading to chromosomal instability (CIN) – the same regulatory and signaling pathways appear to be affected for both types of colon cancer. To the extent that disruptions in these pathways are associated with early- or late-stage mutations, it is reasonable to model the pathogenesis of this cancer as a sequentially ordered multistage process involving a number of rate-limiting mutational events.

Among the earliest premalignant lesions observed in colorectal cancer are so-called aberrant crypt foci (ACF) of various histology. Dysplastic ACFs, also referred to as *adenomatous crypts* or *microadenomas*, appear to play an important role. These early lesions frequently show LOH on chromosome 5q, the locus of the *APC* gene (Takayama *et al.*, 1998; Otori *et al.*, 1998) and are believed to be precursors to the adenomatous polyps, the characteristic lesion in people afflicted with FAP. The transition from an adenoma to high-grade dysplasia (HGD) appears frequently accompanied by LOH events on 17p, implicating the *TP53* gene, generally considered a *guardian* of the genome. Once HGD is activated, 'genetic chaos' may ensue, setting the stage for malignant transformation (Boland *et al.*, 1995). In contrast, hyperplastic polyps in the colon have long been considered to have no or only low neoplastic potential. Recent studies, however, appear to contradict this view (Goldstein *et al.*, 2003; Jass, 2003).

Incidence rates of colorectal cancer are known to vary substantially worldwide (up to about 20-fold). Much of this variation is attributed to dietary and nutritional factors, in addition to lifestyle factors related to smoking and alcohol consumption. For a comprehensive review of these issues, especially in conjunction with genetic predispositions, see Potter (1999). Thus, in addition to the variability in the type of mutations involved and the components of pathways affected (as discussed above), there is considerable variability of factors that modulate the rate at which critical events occur and affect the clonal expansion rate of intermediate cell populations. Explicit mechanistic modeling of such effects is an outstanding challenge.

5.2.2   The role of genomic instability in colon cancer

As pointed out above, microsatellite instability has been linked to defects in the DNA mismatch repair system. However, the causes of CIN and of allelic imbalance (AI), representing losses or gains of particular chromosomal regions, are not well understood.

Shih *et al.* (2001) have undertaken a systematic study of AI in small adenomas in colon using single nucleotide polymorphisms (SNP) markers on chromosomes 5q (the APC locus), and also on chromosomes 1p, 8p, 15q, and 18q. They found that over 90 % of the tumors exhibited AI of at least one chromosome, and 67 % showed AI of a chromosome other than 5q. Therefore, AI appears to be a common phenomenon, even in lesions considered benign, suggesting that CIN occurs early in the development of a tumor.

An obvious question is whether loss of APC confers CIN to the cancer cell. A lead in this direction comes from the observation that the C-terminus of APC plays a crucial role in preserving chromosomal stability during mitosis in embryonal stem (ES) cells in mouse (Fodde *et al.*, 2001; Kaplan *et al.*, 2001). These studies showed that APC localizes at the kinetochore of metaphase chromosomes, involving an interaction between APC and EB1. Loss of APC is thought to lead to an abundance of spindle microtubules that fail to connect to kinetochores, resulting in chromosomal abnormalities such as (near)tetraploidy from non-disjunction, as well as structural rearrangements (e.g. chromosomal translocations) from chromosomal breakage and reunion after the formation of multipolar spindles (Fodde 2002).

However, the question has been raised whether the APC/EB1-related abnormalities observed in mouse ES cells really constitute CIN. It appears (see Nowak *et al.*, 2002) that the mutant ES cells actually undergo polyploidization in whole-genome increments rather than by elevated losses and gains of one or a few individual chromosomes (Fodde *et al.*, 2001) as would be typical for CIN-type cancers. It is therefore not clear whether loss of APC is the dominant force driving the cancer cells toward CIN. Moreover, as Nowak *et al.* point out, some well-characterized human colon cancer cell lines with APC mutations have chromosome complements that remain stable even after thousands of cell divisions *in vitro*, leading them to conclude that APC inactivation itself most likely does not trigger CIN in human colorectal cancers. Nowak *et al.* therefore propose a model that allows for the activation of CIN during initiation in parallel with the inactivation of a TSP gene such as the APC gene. According to this model, the activation of CIN may either occur in normal stem cells, or in mutated stem cells with an intact wild-type copy of the TSP, or in cells where the TSP is already fully mutated (i.e. with both copies inactivated). CIN-mediated losses are assumed to give rise to LOH at important TSP loci. However, cells are not likely to tolerate allelic losses involving both alleles of a TSP. A probable form of TSP mutation under CIN is therefore one that involves both LOH and a 'small' rare mutation at the TSP locus in question.

According to the calculations by Nowak *et al.* (2002), assuming that CIN cells are not selected for (over non-CIN cells), and assuming that there are about 10 stem cells per crypt in human colon, and that the rate of LOH in normal cells is about the same as the background mutation rate, five CIN conferring genes in the genome would be sufficient to make it more probable that the inactivation of APC in a dysplastic crypt is caused by CIN and not by sporadic background mutations. However, with the exception of the mitotic spindle checkpoint gene *hBUB1*, which appears to be mutated in a small fraction of colorectal cancers (Cahill *et al.*, 1998), few CIN gene candidates in human colorectal cancers have been identified so far. Whether or not CIN plays an important role in the early stages of colon cancer remains therefore an open question and further experimental studies are necessary to shed light on the mechanisms that facilitate CIN.

5.2.3 Barrett's esophagus

Esophageal cancer is another example for which the concept of multistage carcinogenesis is useful for understanding disease progression. The two common types of carcinoma in esophagus are squamous cell carcinoma and adenocarcinoma. Barrett's esophagus (BE), characterized by epithelial metaplasia in response to esophagitis, is a high-risk precursor lesion for adenocarcinoma of the esophagus. For a review see Levine (1994, 1995). *De novo* lesions within the BE segment can be detected by endoscopic biopsies taken throughout the BE segment (usually by quadrant, and every 1–2 cm along the segment). High-risk patients, that is, patients with HGD, may be examined endoscopically every 6 months. The accessibility of this organ to endoscopic surveillance is indeed a major advantage for studying the progression of this cancer, in addition to initiating treatment and/or surgery at the earliest point after a malignant cancer is detected. About 10 % of patients with BE develop esophageal adenocarcinoma.

There is some debate as to whether the metaplasia is clonal resulting from a critical mutation or whether it reflects a field effect as a reaction to acid and bile reflux from the stomach (Prevo *et al.*, 1999). Dysplastic lesions, which presumably arise clonally in BE, are considered the immediate precursors of adenocarcinomas (Galipeau *et al.*, 1999). The critical genetic changes preceding malignancy in patients with BE appear to be homozygous loss of *p16* INK4a, a cell cycle regulator (involving 9p LOH, p16 point mutations, or CpG hypermethylation of the p16 promoter) as well as loss of *p53* function (Barrett *et al.*, 1999; Prevo *et al.*, 1999). Figure 5.1 illustrates the sequence of histological and genetic abnormalities frequently observed in BE.

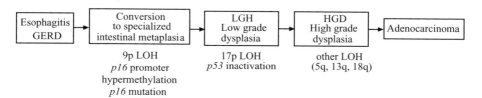

Figure 5.1   Sequence of histologic and genetic abnormalities in the development of esophageal adenocarcinoma (Vaughan, 2002).

Considering the prominent role of two TSP genes, *p16* and *p53*, in the pathogenesis of adenocarcinoma in BE, a minimum of three or four critical events may be required in esophageal cancer in patients with BE. There is some evidence that the same genetic changes are involved in adenocarcinomas without BE and in squamous cell carcinomas of the esophagus (Mandard *et al.*, 2000). However, it is believed that most esophageal adenocarcinomas arise in BE metaplasia. A comprehensive review and discussion of precursor lesions in esophagus can be found in Vaughan (2002).

5.2.4   Intermediate lesions

Models of multistage carcinogenesis provide a framework in which predictions with respect to the temporal development of premalignant lesions can be derived. Although these models describe the temporal growth of cell populations (lesions) on the pathway to cancer, they usually make no assumptions about the three-dimensional structure or shape of these lesions. However, for the quantitative analysis of real lesion data (say, the the number and sizes of adenomatous polyps in the colon, or the premalignant lesions in BE as identified by means of endoscopic screening biopsies, or the analysis of altered hepatic foci on histological liver sections, as discussed in the following chapter), spatial sampling occurs and statistical and stereological methods are needed to address it. For instance, in BE we may ask what is the probability of detecting one and the same clone in any two randomly placed biopsies. This sampling issue can be addressed using methods of spatial statistics.

5.3 GENERALIZED TSCE MODEL

The genetic and structural events associated with colorectal cancer are reflected by multistage models that describe cancer as the outcome of a series of rate-limiting events that change normal stem cells (and their progeny) via premalignant compartments into a state of malignancy. While premalignant cells sojourn in intermediate compartments, they may undergo clonal expansion and so may drastically amplify the carcinogenic risk.

5.3.1 Model building

The above considerations for colorectal cancer suggest the following extension of the two-stage clonal expansion model as a more general framework of multistage carcinogenesis: (colonic) stem cells may undergo a series of pre-initiation steps, accumulating allelic losses and/or mutations in genes participating in critical pathways. Although the cells do not proliferate *per se* until a later stage, they may gradually accumulate at various stages as the parental stem cells can be considered as quasi-immortal (as indicated in Figure 5.2). An important aspect of this model is that the rate-limiting events of the first step (considered to follow a Poisson process) are also 'Poisson' in space and occur independently (of location) in the organ, while subsequent events (e.g. aberrant stem cell divisions) occur in separate pre-initiated units of the organ (such as aberrant colonic crypts) tied to the immortal progenitors in which these events may occur.

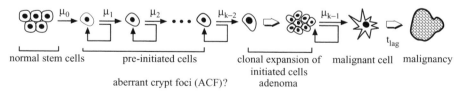

Figure 5.2 Extension of the two-stage clonal expansion (TSCE) model which describes the stepwise progression of a normal stem cell to an initiated cell via pre-initiation stages in which mutated stem cells may accumulate, but have not yet acquired the capacity to proliferate. Note that *pre-initiated* cells are considered immortal in this model. However, once initiated, stem cells may undergo clonal expansion which is modeled by a stochastic birth and death process. Initiated cells may also divide asymmetrically with rate μ_{k-1}, giving rise to a malignant cell. Cancer progression until detection may be modeled by a fixed or randomly distributed lag time t_{lag} (see Hazelton *et al.*, 2001).

In the case of colon, mutations that occur in normal transitional or terminally differentiated cells are most likely lost due to rapid crypt renewal. However, if a stem cell suffers a mutation, the mutation will propagate through the crypt in relatively short time (about one week). For the same reason, subsequent mutations, unless they also occur in a stem cell, or have led to the birth of an adenoma, will most likely also be lost. Thus, according to our model, all pre-initiation events occur exclusively in immortal stem cells.

Because the pool of normal susceptible stem cells in colon is large (in excess of 10^8 cells) usually one considers their number, say X, to be fixed and arrivals (of stem cell progeny) into the first intermediate compartment are modeled as simple Poisson arrivals with intensity $\mu_0 X$, where μ_0 is the rate of the first rate-limiting event in a cell.

After a cell is born into the penultimate stage it may undergo clonal expansion, increasing dramatically the risk of malignant transformation. Currently, this expansion process comprises the entire clonal evolution up to the point of malignant transformation of an initiated (premalignant) stem cell. More than a single distinct (clonally expanding) compartment can be considered in these models, naturally increasing both mathematical complexity and the number of free parameters. However, previous modeling work on colorectal cancer (Moolgavkar and Luebeck, 1992a; Herrero-Jimenez et al., 1998) suggests that a single proliferative compartment at the penultimate stage is sufficient to obtain fits that are consistent with the observed incidence of colorectal cancer.

With population data, where we want to model cancer incidence, we are naturally interested in the distribution of first arrival times of cells in a malignant compartment. This leads to the concept of the hazard function as an estimator of age-specific cancer incidence (see below). Obviously, modeling the subsequent process of malignant tumor development, up to clinical detection, adds another layer of complexity. We may incorporate a random lag time, accounting for the duration from the occurrence of the first malignant cell to detection of a malignant growth, in the following way: let f_{lag} be an appropriately chosen density function for the lag-time distribution, and let f_k represent the density function for the occurrence time of the first malignancy, using a k-stage model. Then the density function for the time of detection can be written as a convolution

$$f_{\text{detect}}(t) = \int_0^t du\, f_k(t - u) f_{\text{lag}}(u),$$

assuming that for $u > t, f_k \equiv 0$. The corresponding survival function for this model can be derived as

$$S(t) = 1 - \int_0^t du\, (1 - s_k(t - u)) f_{\text{lag}}(u),$$

where s_k represents the k-stage model survival function.

A particular advantage of the models formulated here (in contrast to purely statistical descriptions of carcinogenesis) is that one can compute the distribution of numbers and sizes of clones in intermediate compartments. This is of importance when data on premalignant lesions are also available and are to be analyzed quantitatively rather than descriptively. Examples are the adenomatous polyps in colon, the various histologic and genetic lesions observed in BE, and lesions in experimental models, such as the enzyme-altered liver foci in rodents (see Chapter 8, this volume).

5.3.2 Mathematical development and the hazard function

We briefly summarize the mathematical development for the multistage model represented in Figure 5.2. The hazard function is defined as the age-specific rate at which tumors occur in a previously tumor-free tissue. For simplicity, we identify the tumor with the first malignant cell in the tissue. However, a (random) lag time for the clinical detection of a tumor after the first malignant appears in the tissue can be incorporated as described in the previous section.

The hazard function for the class of models described here can be obtained by solving first the Kolmogorov–Chapman forward differential equation for the probability generating function, as shown in Luebeck and Moolgavkar (2002). For a model with $k \geq 3$ stages we can write the survival function (using the convolution theorem for a filtered Poisson process) as

$$S_k(t) = \exp\left\{\int_0^t ds_1 \mu_0 X \left[e^{\left\{\int_{s_1}^t ds_2 \mu_1 \left[\cdots \left[e^{\left\{\int_{s_{k-3}}^t ds_{k-2} \mu_{k-3}\left[y_{k-2}(s_{k-2},t)-1\right]\right\}} - 1\right]\cdots-1\right]\right\}} - 1\right]\right\},$$

where X is the (fixed) number of normal stem cells in the tissue, and where the function $y_{k-2}(s,t)$ is defined as

$$y_{k-2}(s,t) = \left[\frac{q-p}{f(s,t)}\right]^{\mu_{k-2}/\alpha},$$

with $f(s,t) = qe^{-p(t-s)} - pe^{-q(t-s)}$. The identifiable parameters p and q are related to the biological parameters α (the cell division rate), β (the cell death rate), and the malignant transformation rate μ_{k-1} via

$$p = \frac{1}{2}\left((-\alpha + \beta + \mu_{k-1}) - \sqrt{(\alpha + \beta + \mu_{k-1})^2 - 4\alpha\beta}\right),$$

$$q = \frac{1}{2}\left((-\alpha + \beta + \mu_{k-1}) + \sqrt{(\alpha + \beta + \mu_{k-1})^2 - 4\alpha\beta}\right).$$

For $k = 2$, the (TSCE) survival function can be identified with

$$S_2(t) = y_0(0,t) = \left[\frac{q-p}{f(0,t)}\right]^{\mu_0/\alpha}.$$

Note that $g \equiv -(p+q) = (\alpha - \beta - \mu_{k-1})$, which approximately is equal to the net cell proliferation rate in the penultimate stage (stage $k-1$) of the multistage process. The parameter q is approximately equal to $\mu_{k-1}/(1 - \beta/\alpha)$ which may be viewed as an upper bound for the malignant transformation rate. See Heidenreich *et al.* (1997) for more details.

Except for the two-stage model ($k = 2$), the survival function generally requires numerical evaluation of the nested integrals. The age-specific hazard function $h_k(t)$, which is required for the analysis of population data, can be derived from the survival function:

$$h_k(t) = -\frac{d}{dt} \ln S_k(t).$$

Explicit expressions for the hazard functions of the two-, three-, four- and five-stage models are derived in straightforward manner using the above expression for $S(t)$. For constant parameters we have the two-stage model

$$h_2(t) = \mu_0 X \left(\frac{d}{dt} \ln f(0, t) \right) / \alpha,$$

the three-stage model

$$h_3(t) = \mu_0 X \left(1 - \left[\frac{q-p}{f(0,t)} \right]^{\mu_1/\alpha} \right),$$

the four-stage model

$$h_4(t) = \mu_0 X \left(1 - \exp\left\{ \int_0^t du \, \mu_1 \left(\left[\frac{q-p}{f(u,t)} \right]^{\mu_2/\alpha} - 1 \right) \right\} \right),$$

and the five-stage model:

$$h_5(t) = \mu_0 X \left(1 - \exp\left\{ \int_0^t du \, \mu_1 \left[\exp\left\{ \int_0^{t-u} du' \, \mu_2 \left(\left[\frac{q-p}{f(u',t-u)} \right]^{\mu_3/\alpha} - 1 \right) \right\} - 1 \right] \right\} \right).$$

Note that X, the number of normal stem cells, appears always in a product with μ_0, and therefore cannot be estimated without further assumptions or constraints on other parameters.

It is easy to see that not all biological parameters of these models can be identified from incidence data alone (i.e. by using the hazard function or the survival function from which it can be derived). Only certain combinations of the biological parameters are identifiable (see Hanin and Yakovlev, 1996; Heidenreich *et al.*, 1997).

The hazard function for the two-stage model given here is equivalent to the one previously derived by Moolgavkar and Luebeck (1990). Our parameterization of the hazard function, which is a function of four biological parameters (μ_0, μ_1, α, and β), explicitly acknowledges the dependence of the hazard function on three identifiable parameters: say, $r = \mu_0/\alpha$, p and q. Obviously, other combinations can be chosen. For example, we may estimate the combination $-(p + q) = g$, which is approximately the net cell proliferation rate of initiated cells. Conversely, given identifiable parameters, certain sets of biological parameters can be computed by simple scaling. For example, we may assume that $\mu = \mu_0 = \mu_1$, and then use X, the number of normal stem cells, as a scaling factor to determine μ. All other biological parameters of the TSCE model can then be determined. Note, however, that certain constraints remain (such as $g \leq \alpha$) that limit the scaling freedom.

To summarize, for the type of models shown in Fig. 5.2, the following parameters can be estimated ($k = 2, 3, 4$ or 5): $\mu_0, \ldots, \mu_{k-3}$, the pre-initiation rates for models with three or more stages ($k \geq 3$); $r = \mu_{k-2}/\alpha$, the rate of initiation relative to the rate of cell division in adenoma (initiation index); $g \approx \alpha - \beta$, the net proliferation rate of initiated cells; and $q \approx \mu_{k-1}/(1 - \beta/\alpha)$, a parameter associated with malignant transformation.

To give an example, for the three-stage model, next to the parameters g and q, we may estimate $\mu_0 = \mu_1 = r \times \alpha$, assuming that the first two mutation rates are equal, either reflecting similar mutational targets or mutations that lead to the inactivation of both copies of a specific TSP gene. Therefore, to estimate μ_0 (or μ_1) in the three-stage model requires an estimate for α, the (symmetric) cell division rate in an initiated lesion (say an adenoma in the colon, or a dysplastic lesion in BE). A measurement of α in colonic adenomas is reported in Herrero-Jimenez *et al.* (1998), which is about 9 divisions per year. Although this value is likely to be associated with considerable uncertainty, our analysis of colorectal cancer data (see below) shows that the computed likelihoods are rather insensitive to a broad range of values for α. For colon cancer, this version of the three-stage model describes the recessive conversion of normal colonic stem cells into adenoma cells in two steps corresponding to biallelic inactivation of the APC gene. The third rate-limiting step then converts the adenoma into a malignant tumor.

It may appear plausible that the rate of the first locus-specific (recessive) event should be twice the rate of the second event (i.e. $\mu_0 = 2 \times \mu_1$), which acknowledges the fact that there are two target alleles for the first event. However, it is by no means clear whether the rate of the second event is actually not increased by mitotic recombinations that duplicate the defect caused by the first event. On the other hand, if the first event is a chromosomal deletion that brings about LOH, it is unlikely that the second hit is an allelic loss similar to the first (at the same locus) as this may render the cell inviable and cause apoptosis. In view of these uncertainties and the difficulties in measuring the rate of recessive mutations directly, we assume equality of the rates of the two events leading to biallelic inactivation of the locus, that is, we assume $\mu_0 = \mu_1$.

Two more interesting points are worth making here. First, all of the above hazard functions have finite asymptotes as age increases toward infinity. The two-stage model has an asymptote that is $\mu_0 X$ times the survival (non-extinction) probability of a clone of initiated cells, hence approaches a value below $\mu_0 X$, while all models of this type (shown in Fig. 5.2) with more than two stages approach the value $\mu_0 X$, because the stem cell from which initiated clones emerge are considered immortal for these cases. Empirical incidence rates may well reflect predicted asymptotic hazards generated from a two-stage model. However, this is unlikely to be the case with the other models. Assuming that μ_0 is of the order of 10^{-7} per year, and the number of stem cells larger than 10^7, the expected asymptotic incidence rate would be larger than 100 % per year, a value that is never attained, with the exception of rare familial cancers. The second point is that the models are not hierarchical (in the statistical sense), as they would be were the rate-limiting steps represented by simple transitions without stem cell replications. This issue is of importance in ranking and comparing models with different numbers of stages.

5.4 MODELING CANCER INCIDENCE

5.4.1 Age–cohort–period models

Important insights into age effects and temporal trends in cancer incidence and cancer mortality have been obtained from carefully collected data in high-quality population-based registries. The Surveillance, Epidemiology, and End Results (SEER) registry is but one excellent example. To isolate and identify temporal trends from such data has been difficult with traditional approaches such as the age-cohort-period models. It is well known that models of this type have a fundamental (and non-trivial) identifiability problem when age, cohort, and period are simultaneously included in analyses. Various approaches (Clayton and Schifflers, 1987; Holford, 1991, 1992) have been proposed to address the identifiability problem, none of them entirely satisfactory. In a couple papers in the early 1980s, Moolgavkar and Stevens (1981) and Stevens and Moolgavkar (1984) suggested that either cohort or period effects could be replaced in these models by specific information on important risk factors for the cancer under consideration. For example, cigarette smoking is known to have entered the population in a cohortwise fashion and, if good information is available on population smoking habits, this information could be used in lieu of non-specific cohort effects in a study of lung cancer.

5.4.2 Age-specific incidence

The inherent non-identifiability problem associated with the traditional age–cohort–period approach can be finessed in a way which recognizes age as the fundamental biological dimension that determines cancer incidence rates. In this case both cohort and period effects merely modulate the effects of age.

The basic idea is to replace the non-specific age effects in the traditional age–cohort–period models with the hazard functions generated by specific multistage models that reflect the salient features of carcinogenesis for the cancer under study. This approach allows flexible modeling of temporal trends. To be more precise, let $h(a)$ be the hazard function (as a function of age) associated with a specific multistage model. In analogy to age–cohort–period models, the non-specific temporal trends can then be isolated using a multiplicative (proportional) hazards model. That is, for a given age a, birth cohort b and period c, the hazard function can be written as $\theta_b \times \theta_c \times h(a)$, with coefficients $\theta_{b(c)}$ that adjust the incidence for non-specific birth cohort or period trends, respectively. Note, however, this approach also allows the incorporation of factors affecting temporal trends in a more biological way. If, for example, one is interested in investigating changes in smoking habits on lung cancer incidence, this can then be modeled directly by considering the impact of smoking on the biological parameters of the multistage model. This approach is tantamount to incorporating specific factors into the hazard function generated by the multistage model.

A requisite step in this new approach is the design of a biologically plausible baseline model for the cancer of interest, which is consistent with experimental evidence and reflects characteristic genetic events and cell proliferation processes involved in the neoplastic progression.

5.4.3 Colorectal cancer in the SEER registry

We describe a recent analysis of the incidence of colorectal cancer in the SEER database of the years 1973–1996 with the goal of identifying important temporal trends for this cancer (Luebeck and Moolgavkar, 2002). By using multistage models that reflect putative genetic events during colorectal carcinogenesis, we also hope to pinpoint models that make predictions that are consistent with the observed age-specific incidence in the SEER database (Ries *et al.*, 2001). From a comparison of the fits of these models, we gain insights into the nature of the underlying biological processes, the number and magnitude of the rate-limiting events involved, and the magnitude and stability of parameters describing the clonal expansion process as the number of stages is varied in these models.

In brief, for colorectal cancer the SEER data appear to be most consistent with a four-stage model that posits two rare events followed by a high-frequency event in the conversion of a normal stem cell into an initiated ($APC^{-/-}$) cell. An initiated cell is then free to expand clonally (via a stochastic birth–death process) to give rise to an adenomatous polyp. This model is shown schematically in Figure 5.2, assuming that $k = 4$, and the parameter estimates are given in Table 5.1.

Table 5.1 Maximum likelihood estimates (MLEs) of the four-stage model parameters from analyses of colorectal cancer incidence in SEER (1973–1996). With one exception (black females), the four-stage model gave the best fits. See Luebeck and Moolgavkar (2002) for details.

	APC mutation rate (per year)	Initiation index	Malignant transformation rate $\times \alpha$ (per year)^2	Adenoma growth rate (per year)
White males	1.4×10^{-6}	9.0	5.2×10^{-7}	0.15
Black males	1.2×10^{-6}	4.3	1.8×10^{-6}	0.15
White females	1.3×10^{-6}	0.7	1.2×10^{-5}	0.13
Black females	1.1×10^{-6}	2.9	5.2×10^{-6}	0.13

Several biological explanations can be given for the high-frequency event suggested by this model (referred to as the 'initiation index' in Table 5.1). One possible explanation relates to a positional process in the colon crypt. A colonic crypt is organized into a small stem cell compartment that may contain one or more stem cells (assumed in this model to be immortal), and a proliferative zone further up the crypt. The crucial idea here is that a stem cell that has suffered mutations on both copies of the APC gene remains a stem cell and serves as a progenitor (seed) for populating the proliferative zone, mainly through asymmetric divisions. Once an $APC^{-/-}$ cell arrives in the proliferative zone, it may undergo clonal expansion, dividing symmetrically (on occasion). Because of progenitor stem cell continues to be lodged in the stem cell compartment, the nascent clone (microadenoma) is protected from extinction and continues to be fed with mutant progeny at a high rate, possibly 50–100 times per year (Potten and Loeffler, 1990). However, other explanations may be possible. For instance, the high-frequency event may represent an epigenetic phenomenon involved in carcinogenesis.

The joint determination of age, cohort, and calendar-year effects under this model reveal that for colorectal cancers in the SEER database the calendar year effects were much stronger than the estimated cohort effects (Luebeck and

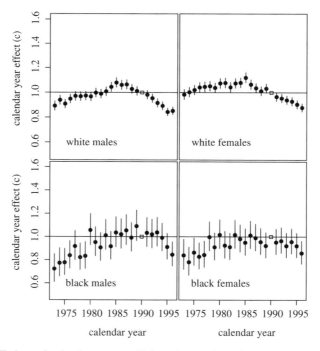

Figure 5.3   Estimated calendar-year coefficients by gender and race. Error bars reflect 95 % confidence intervals. Empty squares indicate normalization points where the coefficients were anchored to 1.

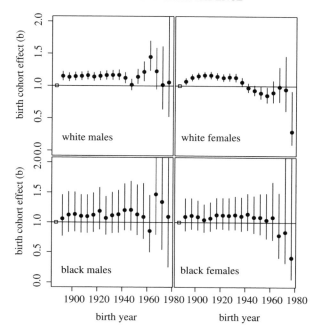

Figure 5.4 Estimated birth-cohort coefficients by gender and race using the four-stage model. Error bars reflect 95 % confidence intervals. Empty squares indicate normalization points where the coefficients were anchored to 1.

Moolgavkar, 2002). Indeed, inspection of the estimated birth cohort coefficients (the θ_bs) reveals no obvious temporal trend in this parameter. In contrast, for all population segments studied, we see the incidence of colorectal cancer rising significantly with calendar year until about 1985, and then decreasing modestly (see Figures 5.3 and 5.4). This increase in incidence by calendar year in the USA may possibly be related to improved population screening for colon cancer (related to fecal occult blood tests, and/or wider use of colonoscopies and sigmoidoscopies), while the drop seen after 1985 could be due to the gradual wearing off of a 'harvesting' effect (Mandel *et al.*, 2000), or alternatively to a reduction of cancers from increased opportunistic polypectomies following screening (A. Renehan, personal communication).

The model described here (Luebeck and Moolgavkar, 2002) is a refinement of earlier work and is broadly consistent with the findings by Moolgavkar and Luebeck (1992a), and with findings by Herrero-Jimenez *et al.* (1998) in their analyses of historical records of colon cancer mortality in the USA. It is worth pointing out that, when the clonal expansion in adenoma is modeled explicitly, all these analyses predict a small number of rate-limiting steps toward malignancy (or toward death from cancer).

5.4.4 Analysis of occupational cohort data

The TSCE model and its extensions also provide a framework in which occupational cohort study data can be analyzed for the purpose of quantitative cancer risk assessment, but with an added emphasis on gaining insights into the mechanisms of action of certain risk factors and occupational exposures. Prominant examples of such analyses (using the TSCE model) are the analyses of lung cancer mortality among underground miners exposed to radon in the USA (Colorado plateau) and in China (Yunnan province), including exposures to cigarette smoke and arsenic (see Luebeck *et al.*, 1999a; Hazelton *et al.*, 2001; Little *et al.*, 2002b; Heidenreich *et al.*, 2004), and the analysis of data on lung cancer mortality among coke oven workers exposed to coke oven emissions (Moolgavkar *et al.*, 1998).

The analysis of such data by means of traditional statistical methods frequently requires elaborate stratification to incorporate into the hazard function (or relative risk) age and exposure-pattern related covariates, such as age at first exposure, duration, time since last exposure, and exposure rate (as compared to cumulative exposure). For the TSCE model (and its extensions), however, many of these covariates are incorporated naturally into the model by assuming that the (biological) parameters of the model are certain functions of these covariates and follow the observed exposure pattern. For example, we may assume that the rate of net cell proliferation, g, is a function of exposure rate, or a function of cumulative exposure over time. The TSCE-based analysis of the Chinese tin miners cohort (Hazelton *et al.*, 2001) is a case in point: incorporation of the various patterns of exposure to radon, cigarette (pipe) smoke, and arsenic is easily achieved within the TSCE model and renders complicated stratification superfluous.

Furthermore, the models discussed here are 'predictive', in the sense that they allow for the prediction of individual risks under unique, but arbitrary, circumstances not necessarily typical of the studies used for risk estimation. For example, we may be interested in predicting the effect of dose protraction assuming that a given total dose is either fractionated or protracted over different time intervals and is starting (or ending) at different ages. In the case of radon, an important question concerns the quantitative estimation of lung cancer risks associated with residental radon at very low doses (and dose rates), but for durations that exceed the exposure duration of a typical underground mining experience.

5.5 SUMMARY

The extensions of the two-stage clonal expansion model described here are motivated by laboratory evidence implicating a number of rate-limiting genomic events in the carcinogenic process, in particular the realization that a least two rare events may be necessary to initiate a tumor, even in its benign state. Furthermore, as our results of analyses of colorectal cancer incidence with the multistage model suggest, positional and/or structural events in the organ of interest may also be of importance.

The ability to compute and predict the distribution of numbers and sizes of clones in intermediate compartments of the models described here is a major advantage over purely statistical descriptions of carcinogenesis which do not impose biological constraints on the predictions of one type of lesion given the observation of another type of lesion. To strengthen predictions and hypotheses that follow from the model, we hope to obtain data on intermediate lesions (say, their number and sizes) as well as data on malignant tumors (absence, presence, number, sizes, etc.) Therefore, multistage models that are consistent with both incidence and intermediate lesion data are also useful tools to predict risk (modification) in response to cancer screening (by conditioning on outcome), secondary preventions such as surgical removal of benign lesions, and chemopreventions using non-steroidal anti-inflammatory drugs, for example.

Here we take the view that the rate-limiting events occur in critical molecular pathways that can be isolated functionally, and that the different genotypic manifestations of a cancer (e.g. MIN versus CIN tumors in colon cancer) share defects in common pathways (see Laurent-Puig *et al.*, 1999). This view of multistage carcinogenesis offers the (perhaps best) opportunity to interface with new transcriptomic and proteomic data from a variety of cellular responses related to cancer for the purpose of modeling carcinogenesis and associated cancer risks. Our hope is that this approach will help fuse the genetic view of carcinogenesis with what is now referred to as systems biology.

CHAPTER 6

Risk Assessment and Chemical and Radiation Hormesis: A Short Commentary and Bibliographic Review

Jose J. Amaral Mendes

University of Évora

Eric Pluygers

Brussels

6.1   INTRODUCTION

The occurrence of hormetic effects has been known for more than a century. The concept of hormesis has long been marginalized in the belief that hormetic effects could be explained by a combination of poorly designed protocols and normal variability. Recent efforts have established that numerous reliable studies demonstrate that hormetic effects exist and that such observations appear to be generalized across biological models, endpoint measures and various classes of chemical agents and radiation. This chapter explores hormesis as a biological principle and its implementation in risk assessment as well as the relevance of hormesis for the assessment and understanding of low-dose behaviour. Hormesis may be defined as a dose-response relationship in which there is a stimulatory response at low doses but inhibitory response at high doses, resulting in a U-shaped or inverted ∩-shaped dose-response curve, depending on the endpoint measured.

Recent Advances in Quantitative Methods in Cancer and Human Health Risk Assessment
Edited by L. Edler and C. Kitsos   © 2005 John Wiley & Sons, Ltd

The hormesis hypothesis goes back to the nineteenth century, and is based on the factual observations of a phenomenon in every field of scientific research, both biomedical and non-biomedical. Yet it has been fiercely opposed by large sectors of the scientific community.

Edward J. Calabrese, from the University of Massachusetts, Amherst, USA, has produced a great deal of work on the hormesis hypothesis in papers, lectures and conferences. Since 1992 he has also edited the *BELLE Newsletter*. Calabrese has devoted his life to the hormesis hypothesis and has searched for hormetic evidence in thousands of scientific papers written since the end of the nineteenth century. He has analysed why chemical and radiation hormesis was marginalized by the scientific community, and pointed out the marked differences in the ways in which the hypotheses developed throughout the twentieth century, as well as the direction and accuracy of the research that supported them. According to Calabrese and Baldwin, hormesis is an adaptive response to low levels of stress or damage result-ing in improved fitness for some physiological systems for a limited period of time. In more specific terms, hormesis can been defined as a modest overcompensation to a disruption in homeostasis (Calabrese and Baldwin, 1999a, 1999c). In 1991, at the University of Massachusetts, Calabrese organized the first meeting on hormesis. The proceedings (Calabrese, 1992) constitute an excellent reference text.

Due to the scientific divulgation of hormesis, the *BELLE Newsletter* deserves special mention. Since July 1992 it has been published three times a year. The editorial of its first issue says:

> In May 1990 a group of scientists representing several federal agencies, the International Society of Regulatory Toxicology and Pharmacology, the private sector, and academia met to develop a strategy to encourage the study of the biological effects of low level exposures (BELLE) to chemical agents and radioactivity. The meeting was convened because of the recognition that most human exposures to chemical and physical agents are at relatively low levels, yet most toxicological studies assessing potential human health effects involve exposures to quite high levels, often orders of magnitude greater than actual human exposures.

The focus of *BELLE* thus encompasses dose-response relationships of toxic agents, pharmaceuticals and natural products over wide dosage ranges in *in vitro* systems and *in vivo* systems, including human populations. While a principal emphasis of *BELLE* is to promote the scientific understanding of low-level effects (especially seemingly paradoxical effects), the initial goal of *BELLE* is the scientific evaluation of the existing literature and of ways to improve research and assessment methods. It would be impossible to comment on the countless citations in the eleven *BELLE* volumes. Amongst the most paradigmatic issues containing thorough criticism, the following should, however, be mentioned: 'Alcohol and coronary heart disease' (Vol. **4**, No. 1); 'Cost of living with contaminants' **4**(3); 'The need for a new cancer risk assessment' **5**(2); 'Toxicological and societal implications' **7**(1); 'Implications for regulatory agencies' **8**(1); 'Hormesis and environmental regulation' **9**(2);

'Impacts on the ageing process' **9**(3); 'Ecological risk assessment' **10**(1); 'Hormesis and risk contamination' **11**(1); 'Recent developments in molecular radiobiology and in adaptive protection mechanisms' **11**(2); and 'Bystander Effects and the Dose Response' **11**(3).

This chapter is based on the vast bibliography on hormesis gathered by Calabrese over many years. It thus covers its historical inception at the end of the nineteenth century until the evolution of the concept in recent times, as well as the critical development of the dose-response relationship, characterized by the typical ∪-shaped or the inverted ∩-shaped dose-response curves.

6.2 THE CONCEPT OF HORMESIS

The concept of chemical hormesis goes back to the work of Hugo Schulz at the University of Greifswald, Germany, in the late 1880s. Schulz noted that many chemicals were able to stimulate growth and respiration of yeast at low doses, yet were inhibitory at higher doses (Schulz, 1888). Although establishing a scientific hypothesis, Schulz inadvertently created a major problem for the acceptance of his scientific theory by becoming associated with the homeopathic medical doctor Rudolph Arndt, in an attempt to provide an explanation for the homeopathic principle. This concept of a generalized low-dose stimulation/high-dose inhibition gradually gained supported from similar observations with other chemicals and eventually became known as the Arndt–Schulz law. Because of its association with homeopathy, the ∪-shaped dose-response theory became contested by medically oriented scientists (Clark, 1937). The phenomenon of low-dose stimulation observed by the early investigators was given the name *hormesis* by Southam and Ehrlich (1943). It is the name most widely used today.

The Arndt–Schulz law fell into disuse for several reasons. The most significant was the early association of hormesis with the practice of homeopathy (Southam and Erhlich, 1943). This negative association was a direct result of the hostility that existed between homeopaths and allopathic doctors. As a result, the concept of hormesis was virtually ignored by the scientific community. Another factor which contributed to the discarding of the Arndt–Schulz law was the emphasis on the toxicity of chemicals at high levels of exposure and the difficulty in determining the safe dose level.

Despite the widespread recognition of apparent hormetic effects into the early decades of the twentieth century, the Arndt–Schulz law gradually fell into disuse because it did not provide an adequately mechanism-based utility (Stebbing, 1981). Other relevant limitations were:

- lack of development of a coherent dose-response theory;

- difficulty in the reproduction of low-dose stimulatory responses without adequate bioassays;

- difficulty in distinguishing optimal experimental conditions from normal variations;

- lack of interest from practical technology and from commercial uses in the low-dose stimulation concepts.

Because of the close association of modern toxicology with traditional medicine and the age-old tension between traditional medicine and homeopathy, the Arndt–Schulz hormesis phenomenon did not achieve recognition as a legitimate scientific biological hypothesis, despite the support it has received from noteworthy investigators (for a review see Calabrese and Baldwin, 1999a).

6.3   CHEMICAL HORMESIS

Calabrese and Baldwin (1999a, 1999c), describe the principles of hormesis, its history, and how it became marginalized in society. In another paper they select published references from scientific material written over the past hundred years in order to promote public awareness of the hormesis phenomenon as a scientific hypothesis (Calabrese and Baldwin, 1997a). A comprehensive effort was undertaken to identify articles demonstrating chemical hormesis. A total of 350 studies were qualitatively judged to show high, moderate or low evidence of hormesis. A quantitative methodology was developed and criteria were established to classify the 350 studies (Calabrese and Baldwin, 1997b). These articles were gleaned from nearly 4000 potentially relevant articles retrieved from preliminary computer searches (Calabrese and Baldwin, 2001d). We do not intend to give a thorough review of the extensive bibliography, but want to mention only the most relevant references (see Calabrese, 2001a, 2001b; Calabrese and Baldwin, 1998c, 2001b, 2003a, 2003b).

In 1999 the Texas Institute for Advancement of Chemical Technology published a report that is an exhaustive account of chemical hormesis, and hormesis in plants, microbes and animals. It analyses the concept of hormesis and its generalization to carcinogenesis. It also questions why hormesis is not always observed and calls for the application of quantitative-based criteria for evidence of hormesis and its application (Charles, 1999). The same institution also published a booklet, *What are the Facts?* (Texas Institute for Advancement of Chemical Technology, 1999), on the public impact of hormesis.

On the subject of dose-response relationships in chemical carcinogenesis, six papers are worth mentioning:

- Lutz (1998) discusses the different mechanisms of action resulting in linear-sublinear curves, practical thresholds, J-shapes.

- Andersen *et al.* (2002) consider molecular circuits, biological switches and non-linear dose-response relationships.

- Conolly and Lutz, (2004) describe non-monotone increasing dose-response relationships and their mechanistic basis, kinetic modelling and risk assessment.

- Gaylor *et al.* (2004) analyse non-monotonic dose-response statistical relationships.

- Not directly releted to hormesis, Ashford and Miller (1996, 1998) discuss low-level chemical exposures as a challenge for science and policy.

6.3.1 The U-shaped and ∩-shaped dose-response curve

U-shaped curves are sometimes designated in the literature as J-shaped curves, while ∩-shaped curves are sometimes designated as β-shaped curves. In Figure 6.1 the U-shape is depicted showing response to a reference level (the control level) with a region of apparent improvement (reduction in dysfunction) as well as of toxic or adverse effects. The reciprocal of the same curve, the ∩-shaped curve, shows a region of apparent enhancement (increase above normal level of function) as well as region of toxic or adverse effects (Davis and Svendsgaard, 1992).

In Figure 6.2 a typical ∩-shaped dose-response curve depicts the characteristics of the chemical hormesis zone: Maximum Stimulation, no observable effect level (NOEL), zero equivalent point (ZEP) and lowest observed effect level (LOEL). The magnitude of stimulation is typically 30–60 % greater than the control value, while the zone of stimulation extends on average approximately over a 10-fold range (Calabrese and Baldwin, 1997b).

The definition of hormesis as derived from Stebbing (1981) refers to a low-dose stimulation followed by higher-dose inhibition. The most common form of hormesis follows the widely recognized ∩-curve (Figure 6.2). The use of the ∩-curve is mainly a consequence of the widespread use of growth as a principal endpoint in hormesis research. However, the term U-shaped as emphasized by Davis and Svendsgaard (1992) would most appropriately be applied when the endpoint relates to a traditional toxicologically based health endpoint such as cancer incidence.

Since hormesis is a scientific hypothesis, the question of whether hormesis is 'beneficial' or 'not beneficial' arises. In order to eliminate subjective decisions concerning 'beneficial' versus 'harmful' effects, the decision was made to evaluate model and endpoint responses with respect to 'stimulation' and 'inhibition' (Calabrese and Baldwin, 1997b, 1997c, 1998a, 1998d, 2000b, 2001c, 2001e). The criteria used to judge data for evidence of hormesis involved some of the following criteria and parameters:

- low-dose stimulation;

- consistency with ∩-curve;

- total number of doses;

- range of doses;

- number of doses in the hormetic zone;

- endpoint doses in the hormetic zone;

- statistical properties of effect estimates in the hormetic zone.

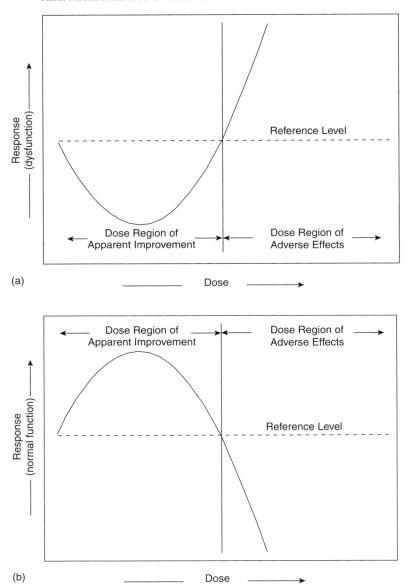

Figure 6.1 Shaped dose-response curves. (a) General form of a ∪-shaped dose-response curve showing response relative to a reference level (the control level) with a region of apparent improvement (reduction in dysfunction) as well as of toxic or adverse effects. (b) Reciprocal of the curve in (a) showing a region of apparent enhancement (increase above normal level of function) as well as region of toxic or adverse effects. From Calabrese and Baldwin (1997b, p. 547).

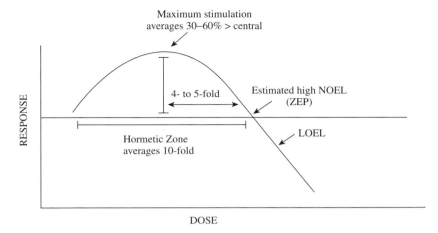

Figure 6.2 Dose-response curve depicting characteristics of the chemical hormesis zone: maximum stimulation, no observable effect level (NOEL), zero equivalent point (ZEP) and lowest observed effect level (LOEL). The magnitude of stimulation is typically 30–60 % greater than control values, while the zone of stimulation extends on average approximately over a 10-fold range. From Davis and Svendsgaard (1992).

Using these criteria, Calabrese and Baldwin (1997b) were able to determine whether the fundamental dose-response included a ∪-shaped response at the low end of the dose-response curve. They found according their criteria more than 130 articles displaying hormesis. They also found that the ∪-shaped response in toxicology and pharmacological experiments was highly generalized, regardless of chemical class and biological endpoint. Hormetic effects were seen in organisms from bacteria to humans and were caused by a variety of chemicals. These chemicals were classified into groups of low, low to moderate, and moderate to highly toxic substances, including heavy metals such as lead, cadmium and mercury and unintentional industrial by-products such as dioxin. The range of endpoints was extensive, included growth and a wide variety of behaviours, such as learning, eating and survival, as well as reproduction, incidence of birth defects, and diseases such as cancer.

The NOEL can be considered as the result of a biological/statistical artefact caused by the insensitivity of biological/statistical measurement, due to either insensitive biological experimental model or loss of statistical power. The dose-response curve parameters depicted in Figure 6.2 are relevant for the evaluation of chemical hormesis. Thus an experiment would be expected to have equal to or more than four doses distributed in a highly specific manner relative to the NOEL.

6.3.2 Critical issues in low-dose extrapolation

Although not objectively related to hormesis, the International Life Science Institute monograph, discussing the linearized multistage (LMS) model for use in regulatory applications of risk assessment and concerned with establishing safe exposure levels to various compounds and the improvement of public health, could be an important baseline contribution to the understanding of the hormetic phenomenon (International Life Science Institute, 1995). Thus, the reliability of LMS models, depending on whether low-dose linearity occurs in the true dose-response curve, is questionable in the absence of detailed chemical-specific data and other parameters. A number of regulatory agencies have accepted the assumption that low-dose linearity provides a plausible upper bound for estimating risk. Although the ILSI monograph's objective was to discuss the critical issues in cancer dose-response assessment, a number of conclusions allow an interpretation of low-dose effects in the light of hormesis (see also Chapters 13, 14, 15 this volume):

(a)   LMS models give similar low-dose results and yield linear and conservative upper-bound estimates of risk. In particular, for populations and for a wide range of chemicals they will overestimate risk with an unknown degree of conservatism more often than they will underestimate it. Because they overestimate with an unknown degree of conservatism, risks calculated from these models cannot be used in an actuarial sense to predict cancer. As a default procedure, however, the models have been a useful part of the process of setting regulatory standards. They identify exposure levels below which there is little basis for concern. The output of an LMS model that is generally used in the standard setting is the 95th percentile upper bound on the calculated risk for a given exposure. A more central estimate of the risk, the maximum likelihood estimate (MLE), would be more appropriate. The MLE of low-dose risks (10^{-3} to 10^{-6}) from the LMS model can in certain circumstances be highly sensitive to very small changes in the rodent bioassay data, and therefore, unstable. Thus the MLE, although the best estimate in a statistical sense, may not be useful as an upper-bound estimate in regulatory applications, owing to its potential instability. Estimates of central tendency can be quite informative when used in conjunctions with upper-bound estimates.

(b)   The most relevant question in risk assessment is related to the criteria of quality and reliability of data. It is known that in some instances, carcinogens may act indirectly, producing cancers only as secondary consequences by some kind of toxicity that has a threshold. From a hormetic point of view this concept is important because the existence of a threshold for the prior toxicity would imply that no cancer will develop unless that threshold is exceeded.

(c)   Another important conclusion in the regulatory application of dose-response models is the improvement by the use pharmacokinetic information.

(d)   More sophisticated mathematical representations that quantitatively relate the cancer risk to the underlying biological processes are necessary for advancing risk assessment methods.

(e) The use of biologically based models is limited by uncertainty regarding mechanisms of carcinogenesis and the inability to estimate important key parameters in the human population, or even in the experimental animals. Development of biological models is encouraged with the understanding that uncertainty will always remain in low-dose risk extrapolations. As the ability to characterize uncertainty improves, the present default methods in the risk assessment will be replaced and a better understanding of the biological and toxicological mechanisms will help to explain the phenomenon of hormesis.

6.3.3 The evaluation of dose-response relationships

For decades the shape of the dose-response curve for toxic substances has been the subject of fierce debate. The debate centred on whether there is a threshold below which no adverse effects would be expected, or whether the dose-response relationship is linear, with risk being proportional to dose. If a threshold response was assumed to exist, exposure below that level would have no effect, that is, it would be safe. However, if there was no threshold of response, then the potential for a risk could be expected regardless of how the doses were chosen.

Despite the apparent differences between the two concepts of dose-response relationships, both became accepted. The threshold concept has been principally applied to risk assessment from exposure to non-carcinogens. The non-threshold concept – in particular, the linear dose-response paradigm – has been used for carcinogens. The main public health implication with respect to carcinogens, the issue of what is an acceptable risk, arises because the linear concept assumes the potential for risk at all exposure levels, which implies that it is not possible to achieve zero risk (Calabrese *et al.*, 1999).

The risk estimation, especially for carcinogens, is typically based on the effects of exposing rodents to very high doses of compounds, often four to five orders of magnitude beyond normal human experience. A variety of biomathematical models extrapolate to low doses and estimates of risks of the order of one in a million (Calabrese, 1978, 1993; Calabrese and Baldwin 1998b).

However, it is necessary to understand how biological systems respond to low levels of a wide range of carcinogens and non-carcinogens. One unmistakable conclusion is that biological systems may have constitutive and inducible adaptive response mechanisms that help the organism to react to a wide range of stressor agents. These adaptive response mechanisms include stress protein responses, DNA repair mechanisms, and cell and tissue repair mechanisms (Hart and Frome, 1996). It is the interplay of these adaptive mechanisms with external stressor agents that determines the shape of the dose-response curves. Individuals or species with limited adaptive capacity are less fit to withstand lower doses of stressor agents than organisms or species with better adaptive mechanisms. These adaptive mechanisms help account for both interindividual and interspecies variation in responses to toxic compounds. It is important to recognize that adaptive responses may be affected by the dose of stressors. The key issue in hormesis is that there is significant biological activity below the traditional NOEL.

6.4   RADIATION HORMESIS

While chemical hormesis has been analysed over the past hundred years as a scientific hypothesis, radiation hormesis took longer to be defined, mainly due to the lack of interest on the part of radiation scientists in the concept of chemical hormesis.

The most critical factor affecting the 'demise' of radiation hormesis, according to Calabrese and Baldwin, was the lack of agreement over how to define the concept of hormesis and quantitatively describe its dose-response features (Calabrese and Baldwin, 1999b, 2000a, 2000c). If radiation hormesis had been defined as a modest overcompensation for a disruption in homeostasis, in accordance with the prevailing notion in the area of chemical hormesis, criticism of the hypothesis would have been avoided. A second critical factor undermining the radiation hormesis hypothesis was the lack of recognition by radiation scientists of the concept of chemical hormesis which was markedly more advanced. A third factor was that major scientific criticism of low-dose stimulatory response led the US National Research Council to exclude the hormetic hypothesis from its future plans for research.

Criticism of the leading scientists in the 1930s and 1940s was near-sighted and undermined the concept of radiation hormesis, by perpetuating early accepted reports throughout the decades. This atmosphere among the scientific community was linked to growing fear of the health effects produced by radiation from the atomic bomb. Supportive findings on hormetic effects in the 1940s by Soviet scientists were dismissed because of the atmosphere generated during the Cold War. Even a massive but poorly designed US Department of Agriculture experiment in the late 1940s on the capacity of low-dose plant stimulation by radionuclides failed to support the hormetic hypothesis. Thus the combination of a failed understanding of the hormetic hypothesis and its lack of linkage with chemical hormesis data, and reinforced by Cold War mentality, led to marginalization of a hypothesis that had substantial scientific foundations. Why did the radiation hormesis hypothesis become marginalized in the scientific community in the first half of the twentieth century? It appears that much of the blame can be placed on the lack of critical reviews by the scientific community of the available literature on low-dose stimulation by chemical agents and radiation. Apparently, there was also little communication among those researching the biological effects of chemicals and radiation at low levels. Also, underdeveloped biomathematical dose-response modelling supported the neglect of other than linear dose-response.

Calabrese and Baldwin (1999b) present a systematic effort to describe the historical foundations of radiation hormesis. The effort was designed not only to address the gap in current knowledge, but also to offer a toxicological basis for how the concept of hormetic dose-response relationship may affect the nature of the bioassay and its role in the risk assessment process. In this paper they opted for a broad search of the biological, radiobiological and toxicological literature, including responses to plants, bacteria, fungi, and other microorganisms, invertebrates and vertebrates, including epidemiological and clinical data. This broadly based, biologically oriented approach was designed to assess to what extent the concept of hormesis may be generalized. The approach sought mainly to provide an evaluation of radiation hormesis as a biological hypothesis rather than as an explanatory feature of medical practice. Later, Calabrese and Baldwin (2000a) examined underlying factors that contributed to the marginalization of radiation hormesis. There is little question that the radiation hormesis hypothesis had considerable support in the peer-reviewed, experimental and clinical literature during the first fifty years after the discovery of X-rays and radionuclides. This support was grounded in the quality of the findings and the remarkable similarities of the hormetic dose-response relationships in chemical and radiation effects.

Calabrese and Baldwin cite factors such as experimental design challenges that contributed to the 'demise' of radiation hormesis. They also refer to other factors such as lack of awareness of the research done on chemical hormesis, scientific criticism of radiation hormesis, the imprecise definition of the concept of hormesis, and the economic implications of hormesis. Most important, though, is the fact that radiation hormesis was rejected by science, medicine and society, and was therefore marginalized (Calabrese and Baldwin, 2000c).

A significant contribution to the hormesis hypothesis was provided by Myron Pollycove in a series of critical papers and lectures. One paper on 'Human epidemiology, biology and linear, no threshold, dose-response relationship (LNT)' was delivered at the Council of Scientific Society Presidents in Racine, Wisconsin, in 1997, and three lectures on epidemiology, radiation carcinogenesis, and human biology and non-linearity were delivered at the Annual Congress of the South African Radiation Protection Association, held in May 1998. At the same Congress, A.N. Tshaeche delivered a lecture analysing the extension of the linear hypothesis to low doses with the title 'Resolving the controversy over beneficial effect of ionizing radiation'. Jerry M. Cuttler presented a paper on the 'Effects of very low doses of ionizing radiation on health' at the WONUC Conference in Versailles, France, in 1999. Worth mentioning on radiation hormesis are the papers of S.M. Javad Mortazavi (2000), Shu-Zheng Liu (2003) and K.S. Parthasarathy (1998).

Important sources of radiation hormesis references can be found in the Proceedings of the 10th International Congress of the International Radiation Protection Association held in Hiroshima in 2000 on the theme of Harmonization of Radiation, Human Life and the Ecosystem. Radiation hormesis is cited in several communications presented at sessions this conference, in particular, in the sessions on Radiation Protection of Workers and the Public (Mitchel and Boreham, 2000; Kenigsberg, 2000); Radiation Adaptive Response (Mortazavi *et al.*, 2000; Mortazavi and Mozdarani, 2000; Zhu *et al.*, 2000); Evidence Supporting Non-Linear Effective Threshold Dose-Response Relationships for Radiation Carcinogenesis (Raabe, 2000; Persson, 2000); Tumour Suppressor p53 by Low-Dose-Rate Radiation (Ohnishi *et al.*, 2000; Yonezawa *et al.*, 2000); Harmonisation of Radiation for

Human Life (Hattori, 2000); also to mention the paper of Hornhardt *et al.* (2000) on the assessment of health risks at low levels from concomitant exposures to radiation and chemicals. We also want to mention several communications presented at the Non-linear Dose Response Relationships in Biology, Toxicology and Medicine conferences which were held on June 11–13, 2002 and May 28–30, 2003 at the University of Massachusetts, Amherst, USA.

6.5 CONCLUDING REMARKS

Hormesis has been a hotly contested concept and for some it still does not make sense. For years it has been a considered as a 'riddle' in toxicology. Despite having become more and more questionable, it was found that hormetic observations constitute a real physiological expression of living organisms against environmental stress. Homeostasis develops through molecular mechanisms, which are now being unravelled. No wonder that hormesis became a multidisciplinary field, recruiting not only toxicologists but also molecular biologists, epidemiologists, statisticians, radiobiologists, as well as medical doctors, not to speak of the recent emergence of risk assessment experts.

Perusing the huge amount of literature available from different sources, there seems to be scant discussion as to what hormesis actually is. This lack of information motivated the present summary review of a marginalized field of research that deserves more scientific insight. Our objective has been to uncover from the literature references where hormesis was identified.

A reflection on hormesis becomes appropriate, as endocrine disrupters become an important research field. Linking hormesis to endocrine disrupters is a logical step as endocrine molecular mechanisms depend on very low levels of exposure to environmental stressors (Amaral Mendes, 2002).

We would like to finish by citing eight scientists who have recently discussed the concept of hormesis in Calabrese (2001b). Chapman (2001) aims to 'provide encouragement and funding for biostatisticians to fully explore the concept of hormesis'. Harrison (2001) sets a path forward 'to observation and interpretation of gene expression, [which], coupled with cancer bioassay that included low-dose exposures, could provide a great deal of knowledge about hormesis'. Jonas (2001), on the other hand, questions the clinical relevance of hormesis and asks 'whether its future involves a new branch of pharmacology or simply an epiphenomenon of toxicology'. Olson *et al.* (2001) 'recognise hormesis and its implications to have potential to contribute to the improvement of the mechanistic understanding of drug action'. Rattan (2001), considering hormesis from the perspective of biogerontology, recognizes that 'hormesis appears to be the next step and represents a promising experimental approach in biogerontology'. Thomassen (2001) remarks that 'there is no question that BELLE's effort have made the scientific community more aware in acepting hormesis. However, the "literature-search" research strategy only will not help hormesis research become more acceptable'. Crump

(2001) evaluates the statistical perpsective, 'as there is ample evidence that hormesis occurs in many specific situations, the lack of a valid statistical test for hormesis being a major limitation when evaluating evidence for hormesis'. Finally, Upton (2001) acknowledges that 'the existence of stimulatory or "adaptive" responses [implies] that the dose-response relationships for genetic and carcinogenic effects of radiation may be similarly biphasic, or hormetic, in nature'.

We hope that this review on hormesis will become helpful to all those interested in familiarizing themselves with its nature, its pragmatic points of controversy, its acceptance by the scientific community and its perspectives to open future research areas.

PART III

MODELING FOR CANCER RISK ASSESSMENT

Introductory remarks

Lutz Edler and Christos P. Kitsos

According to the risk assessment paradigm (see Chapter 1, this volume), risk assessment has to address in the risk characterization step the determination of the dose-response relationship. At the beginning of a risk assessment, one usually has information on the existence of differences in responses between doses (e.g. due to an increase in exposure over a period of time), but one may not be at all certain about the size of the difference of the effects and whether critical response levels have been exceeded. A quantitative risk assessment, however, has to address 'how different' the effects are at different dose levels. More important from a regulatory point of view is, however, the inverse task, namely of inferring from a known difference in effects the respective difference in dose levels which may have caused this difference. Related to this task is the problem of low-dose extrapolation which has interested toxicologists and risk assessors for decades.

This part of the text presents basic modeling approaches. It covers an essential part of quantitative methodology in risk assessment where mathematical methods are linked with statistical procedures. Each chapter provides pointers to the literature to enable the reader to delve into the subject in greater depth. The five chapters address pharmacokinetic/toxicokinetic modeling for exposure assessment, two stochastic modeling approaches for carcinogenesis and two modeling approaches for the very relevant issue of cancer screening. Before the construction of a dose-response model, the notion of dose or exposure has to be clarified. A standard method of defining a dose metric for dose-response modeling has been the transformation of the administered amount of the toxic substance to a concentration, for example amount/body weight (in kilograms). The approach, however, almost completely ignores the toxicokinetics of the substance after intake, disregards the

Recent Advances in Quantitative Methods in Cancer and Human Health Risk Assessment
Edited by L. Edler and C. Kitsos © 2005 John Wiley & Sons, Ltd

physiology of the organism, and does not take into account any toxicodynamic or mechanistic information. Therefore it has been repeatedly criticized. An approach to filling this gap, at least partially, is achieved with the use of pharmacokinetic/ toxicokinetic models, as described in Chapter 7 by Karen Watanabe.

For some time researches have been developing stochastic mathematical models for cancer primarily for a better understanding of the process of carcinogenesis, but also for examining specific hypotheses on the origin of cancer and for obtaining models which could be fitted to experimental data; see Whittemore and Keller (1978). The first biologically based dose-response models were the multihit and multistage models. Hit models were originally derived from the quantum biological theory of interaction between particles and targets for the induction of a response influenced by radiation physics. In their *single-hit model*, Iverson and Arley (1950) used the biological idea that a single susceptible target has to be hit by a single biologically active unit of dose. This resulted in a dose-response model of the form $P(d) = p + (1 - p) \cdot (1 - \exp(-bd))$ which was used for a long time; were bd denotes the expected number of hits (in a fixed time interval) at the dose level d. Next, the *multi-hit model* was obtained by postulating that a single susceptible target has to be hit, say, m times by a single biologically active dose unit such that a response is elicited. The minimum number of hits required thus became a model parameter. The multi-hit dose-response model was characterized statistically by the tail of a Poisson distribution starting at the count number m with expectation bd. This model is equivalent to a tolerance distribution model where the cumulative distribution of the gamma distribution is used as model distribution. From the modeling point of view, the breakthrough came with the appearance of the *multistage models* based on multistage theory of carcinogenesis (see Whittemore and Keller, 1978). Occurrence of cellular events causing the stage transitions is assumed to be stochastically independently distributed according to an exponential distribution with constant rate, say $a_i + b_i d$, where d denotes the dose and a_i and b_i stage–specific model parameters. When time is constant, a risk function of the form $P(d) = 1 - \exp[-(q_0 + q_1 d + q_2 d^2 + \cdots + q_K d^K)]$ is obtained, which has served for low-dose extrapolation for regulatory agencies since the 1970s.

Later, when the multistage theory was developed further and when multistage models became used for low-dose extrapolation, the possible benefit of stochastic carcinogenesis models for risk assessment, in particular for dose-response modeling, became obvious. Several monographs, published since then, address stochastic carcinogenesis modeling and its applications. Tan (1991) discusses carcinogenesis modeling primarily from a mathematical point of view, with a strong affinity for the two-stage clonal expansion (TSCE) model. Focusing less on applications, this work is directed primarily at statisticians and mathematicians. In contrast, the multi-author monograph by Cogliano *et al.* (1999b) has risk assessment as its explicit goal. As a report on the outcome of a pilot study project of the NATO CCMS Science Program, started in the mid-1990s, various aspects relevant to risk assessment are covered, with the major focus again on the use of the TSCE model. The two papers by Kopp-Schneider and colleagues on stochastic carcinogenesis models and the state-space model approach presented by Chen demonstrate two modeling paradigms different from the TSCE approach and its extensions (see the contribution of Luebeck and Moolgavkar in Part II).

More specifically designed for the investigation of tumor growth and cancer screening is the book by Yakovlev and Tsodikov (1996) in which stochastic modeling and statistical and epidemiological methods are used. For readers interested in the basic theory of mathematical modeling of cancer screening, this work can be recommended as a further reference for the two chapters on current modeling practice by Marek Kimmel and colleagues (Chapter 10) and a the more theoretical paper by Leonid Hanin and Lyudmila Pavlova (Chapter 11).

Cancer screening aims at the early detection of a tumor, and it has been postulated that an earlier than standard detection would benefit the screened person in terms of an increased probability of cure, prolonged survival and improved quality of life after detection of the disease. From a disease management perspective, screening belongs to the diagnosis phase rather than the treatment phase. However, this distinction should not distract one from the critical point that any beneficial effect of screening depends on the availability of an effective treatment for the earlier detected disease. Both screening and standardized treatment have to be compared with detection during the natural history of the disease and subsequent treatment. One may expect that the benefits of screening will be large, when an efficient treatment is available and when the tumor is small, but no greater when the tumor is already large at the time of detection. In the absence of efficient treatment protocols, however, an improved diagnostic measure such as screening may be of minor or no benefit to the patient in terms of cure and prolonged survival. Prospective clinical intervention trials are required to resolve this question. At the end, only randomized trials may provide an unbiased evaluation of the efficacy of a screening measure in conjunction with a treatment strategy. Quality-of-life endpoint may then become another important endpoint in addition to the time intervals between first diagnosis and recurrence or death. The chapter by Kimmel *et al.* systematically discusses the most recent developments.

In order to demonstrate the beneficial effects of screening in a comparative clinical trial it will be necessary to design the screening optimally. Experimental design methods can be applied to find an optimal screening schedule defined by the number of screens and the interval between them. However, in order to find an optimal design one has to define an appropriate target function, named the efficiency functional by Hanin and Pavlova.

CHAPTER 7

Modeling Exposure and Target Organ Concentrations

K. H. Watanabe

Oregon Health & Science University

7.1 INTRODUCTION

The field of pharmacokinetics/toxicokinetics involves the study of how pharmaceuticals and toxicants are absorbed, distributed, metabolized, and eliminated from the body. In developing appropriate dosing regimens to achieve therapeutic effects, non-physiologically based compartmental pharmacokinetic models are used effectively to model the plasma concentration of a drug in the body. The needs in toxicology and risk assessment are slightly different, as data and results from animal studies must be extrapolated to humans. Physiologically based pharmacokinetic or toxicokinetic (PBPK) models have been developed for a large number of xenobiotics to predict target tissue concentrations from external exposure, to extrapolate from one set of conditions to another such as between species by modifying the anatomical and physiological parameters for the species of interest, from high to low exposure concentrations, and between routes of exposure.

7.1.1 Physiologically based pharmacokinetic models

Drawing upon chemical reactor theory and the concept of a continuously stirred tank reactor (Butt, 1980), PBPK models (Gibaldi and Perrier, 1982) attempt to simulate the processes governing xenobiotic disposition in the body including absorption, distribution, metabolism, and elimination (ADME) as shown in Figure 7.1. In the last two decades, PBPK models have been developed for medicinal compounds as reviewed by Nestorov (2003), individual xenobiotics as reviewed by Andersen (2003), and mixtures (Filser *et al.*, 1993; el-Masri *et al.*, 1995; Tardif *et al.*, 1995, 1997; Yang *et al.*, 1995; Leavens and Bond, 1996; Haddad *et al.*, 1999,

Recent Advances in Quantitative Methods in Cancer and Human Health Risk Assessment
Edited by L. Edler and C. Kitsos © 2005 John Wiley & Sons, Ltd

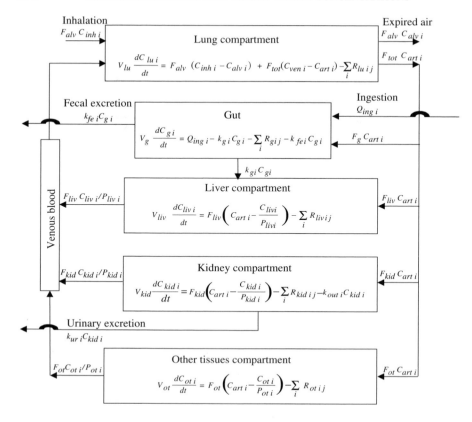

Figure 7.1 Structure and equations for a physiologically based toxicokinetic model that could be used to simulate concentrations of parent compound, i, and its reaction to metabolite, j. F_{alv} is alveolar ventilation rate (l/min). F_{tot} (l/min) is cardiac output. Concentrations (mg/l) are represented by C_x, with $x = inh$ for inhaled air, alv for alveolar air, lu for lung, g for gut, liv for liver, kid for kidney, ot for other tissues, b for the body. F_x denotes a blood flow rate (l/min) through the tissue compartments denoted previously. V_x represents compartment volumes (l). First-order elimination rate constants denoted by $k_{ur\ i}$, $k_{fe\ i}$, and $k_{g\ i}$ (min^{-1}). P_{xi} denotes a tissue–blood partition coefficient, and R_{xij} is the rate of formation of j from parent i in compartment x.

2000, 2001; Dobrev *et al.*, 2002; Klein *et al.*, 2002; Krishnan *et al.*, 2002; Liao *et al.*, 2002). The representation of organs and tissues in a compartmental sense is a highly idealized representation that can be modified to accommodate greater levels of detail as demonstrated in models for nasal passages (Frederick *et al.*, 2001) and liver (Andersen *et al.*, 1997b). Kohn (2000) summarizes physiologically based mathematical models that are formulated for different levels of biological realism. With respect to xenobiotic metabolism, some investigations modeled the formation of metabolites (Fisher *et al.*, 1989, 1991; Medinsky *et al.*, 1989; Watanabe *et al.*, 1994; Parham and Portier, 1998; Clewell *et al.*, 2000; Pastino *et al.*, 2000; Willems *et al.*, 2001) also in a relatively simplified framework. Yet with all the research devoted to such model development, no standardized, biologically based 'rules' exist for formulating PBPK models (i.e., determining the number and type of compartments) outside of individual expert opinion relying upon a known site of action, physicochemical dynamics, and curve fitting.

7.1.2   Model formulation

The PBPK model is formulated to represent the organs and tissues in the body that have an impact on toxicant disposition. It is a mathematical representation of the uptake, distribution, storage, and elimination of xenobiotics from the body. Simplifying assumptions are made about the physiological processes in the organs and tissues in order to create a tractable set of equations based on mass balance expressions for each organ or group of tissues represented in the model. Conceptually, the accumulation or time rate of change of the amount of toxicant equals the sum of all the flows into the tissue compartment minus the sum of all the flows out plus the sum of all production sources, minus the sum of all consumption processes:

$$\text{Accumulation} = \sum \text{Flow in} - \sum \text{Flow out} + \sum \text{Production} + \sum \text{Consumption.} \tag{7.1}$$

Determination of the tissue concentration from the blood concentration falls into two regimes (Lutz *et al.*, 1980; Gibaldi and Perrier, 1982; Medinsky and Klaassen, 1996; Nestorov, 2001): perfusion-limited or diffusion-limited. In the perfusion- or flow-limited case, the transport of chemical to the tissue in the bloodstream is the rate-limiting factor in how the chemical distributes. That is, the chemical-specific cell membrane permeability is much greater than the chemical perfusion rate by blood flow, and a simplifying assumption is made that the xenobiotic rapidly reaches equilibrium at the blood–tissue interface. Partition coefficients, measured ratios of the equilibrium concentrations of the xenobiotic in tissue and blood, are used in the mathematical formulation of the perfusion-limited model. In the diffusion-limited case, the cell membrane permeability is much lower than the flow of chemical to the tissue through the bloodstream, and transport of the xenobiotic across the cell membrane must be represented in the model. Willems *et al.* (2001) developed a diffusion-limited PBPK model for naphthalene that represented metabolism of naphthalene to naphthalene oxide in lung and liver. A flow-limited PBPK model for naphthalene oxide (Quick and Shuler, 1999) was linked with the naphthalene model to simulate its disposition.

Some tissues contain metabolizing enzymes that catalyze chemical reactions of the parent chemical at a rate, R_{xij}. This reaction term can be represented kinetically by a Michaelis–Menten type equation or any other appropriate chemical kinetic equation. Metabolizing enzymes are present in many constituents of the body; for example, the superfamily of enzymes collectively known as cytochrome P450 (CYP) can be found in virtually all tissues, although they are found at highest concentration in liver microsomes (Parkinson, 1996). Models that considered extra-hepatic metabolism include, for example, Kohn (1997) for 1,3-butadiene metabolism in lung, liver and kidney, and Willems *et al.* (2001) for naphthalene metabolism in lung. In many models, though, metabolism is represented in the liver alone, which does not reflect the true ability of the body to metabolize xenobiotics.

7.1.3   Data sources

A PBTK model requires anatomical, physiological, biochemical, and metabolic data in order to calculate the concentration of xenobiotic in each of the compartments over time. These input parameters include the alveolar ventilation rate, blood flow rates to each tissue compartment, organ and tissue volumes, blood to air and tissue to blood partition coefficients, and rate constants for metabolic reactions, absorption, and elimination. There are a number of sources compiling anatomical and physiological parameters measured in different species (Arms and Travis, 1988; Davies and Morris, 1993; Fiserova-Bergerova, 1995; Brown *et al.*, 1997) and authors often report the input parameter values used in their PBPK model. Since these parameters are dependent on the species and not the xenobiotic of interest, prior studies can be a good source of data. Interspecies extrapolation is a method of obtaining an unknown parameter value from measurements in other species (Davidson *et al.*, 1986; Mordenti, 1986; Ings, 1990; Chappell and Mordenti, 1991; Calabrese, 1993; Fiserova-Bergerova, 1995; Luebeck *et al.*, 1999b).

Partition coefficients between tissue and air (P_{xa}) or blood and air (P_{ba}) are chemical-specific. They can be determined experimentally *in vivo* and *in vitro* (Sato and Nakajima, 1979; Perbellini *et al.*, 1985; Fiserova-Bergerova and Diaz, 1986; Gargas *et al.*, 1989; Jepson *et al.*, 1994; Knaak *et al.*, 1995; Murphy *et al.*, 1995), or calculated from the octanol-water partition coefficient (Kamlet *et al.*, 1987; Connell *et al.*, 1993; Poulin and Krishnan, 1995). The tissue to blood partition coefficient (P_{xi}) is equal to P_{xa} divided by P_{ba}. The Hazardous Substances Data Bank (US National Library of Medicine), accessible through the United States National Library of Medicine website (http://www.nlm.nih.gov), provides peer-reviewed data and contains references for all data sources. Partition coefficients are generally constant across species, but some variation is observed in P_{ba} across species (Luebeck *et al.*, 1999b).

Diffusion coefficients or cell membrane permeability for diffusion-limited models need to be experimentally determined or approximated from values for similar compounds diffusing through the cell membrane. Andersen *et al.* (1993) developed a diffusion-limited PBTK model of dioxin in rats. Two mass balance equations, one for tissue blood and the other for tissue, represented each tissue compartment. The permeability–surface area product (liters per hour) used to represent transfer of dioxin from tissue blood into tissue was set as a fraction of the tissue compartment blood flow. Partition coefficients were used to determine the free (unbound) concentration of dioxin in tissues with initial values obtained from a prior study, and then adjusted to fit the data.

Uptake, elimination, and metabolic rate constants can be obtained from independent experimental studies. These rate constants are obtained by assuming a kinetic model (e.g., first-order or saturable, Michaelis–Menten kinetics) and estimating the rate constant from the data using regression analysis or a nonlinear estimation technique. Other methods of determining these rate constants from independent sources include interspecies extrapolation (Travis *et al.*, 1990) from animal data, extrapolation from *in vitro* studies which do not account for the feedback mechanisms controlling xenobiotic metabolism *in vivo* (Kedderis, 1997), and quantitative structure activity relationships (QSARs) which use physicochemical properties of chemicals to determine an activity or outcome, in this case rate constants. Related QSARs for chemical reductions of organic contaminants in the environment were reviewed by Tratnyek *et al.* (2003).

7.2 DATA FROM MOLECULAR BIOLOGY

Molecular biology through genomics, proteomics, and metabonomics has increased and will continue to increase our knowledge of the mechanisms controlling biological processes. Several biological databases, accessible through the internet (Baxevanis, 2003), connect genes, the macromolecules they encode, and the role of these macromolecules in cell function. This requires a tremendous effort, first in sequencing and gene identification, then associating the gene with its product and function in the body. In higher organisms, the activation of a gene is not indicative of a particular health effect due to the complex nature of both gene expression and regulatory control mechanisms in response to external stimuli. Since these data are discussed elsewhere in this volume, only examples relevant for physiological modeling are described here.

7.2.1 Metabonomics

Nicholson *et al.* (1999) defined metabonomics as 'the quantitative measurement of the dynamic multiparametric metabolic response of living systems to pathophysiological stimuli or genetic modification' and distinguished it from the 'metabolome' which refers to the small molecules within cells. They used nuclear magnetic resonance spectroscopy and pattern recognition techniques to analyze the metabonomic spectra observed in urine from rats following administration of individual toxicants. More recently, Nicholson and Wilson (2003) described the unique challenges that arise from a systems biology approach (i.e., integrating data from genomic, proteomic and metabolomic studies) in higher organisms due to cell differentiation and the spatial distribution of the different organs and tissues. They discuss the interrelationship of endogenous biological processes such as those necessary for life, and the reactions (i.e., phase I biotransformation and phase II conjugation) involved in xenobiotic metabolism. Highlighting the need for mathematical models that provide a comprehensive representation of the mammalian 'reactor', they propose a probabilistic model of metabolism (coined Pachinko[1] metabolism).

The Pachinko metabolism concept arises from Nicholson and Wilson's belief that the metabolic fate of a xenobiotic is not purely deterministic because the comprehensive underlying enzymatic state changes in time within an individual, and between individuals due to mutations and single nucleotide polymorphisms (SNPs). They explain that the pins represent key metabolizing enzymes or transporter molecules, and the location of the pins, whether one is missing, or a slightly different pin caused by genetic mutation or SNPs alters the path of the ball (i.e., the xenobiotic) to its ultimate fate. The fate of the ball is also affected by the presence of other balls (e.g., xenobiotics or metabolites originating from other endogenous biological processes) that compete for the pins and interact with the original ball. They conclude with the notion of 'global systems biology' to account for the interrelated and inseparable processes of 'normal' physiological function, xenobiotic metabolism and environmental factors that need to be measured and modeled to enhance our understanding of xenobiotics, their fate, efficacy or toxicity.

Nicholson and Wilson clearly describe the questions that a global systems biology framework should address and identify the challenges facing our understanding of higher organisms. In terms of the fate of xenobiotics in the body, the Pachinko metabolism concept accounts for an unknown initial metabonomic state, but fails to address the distribution of the xenobiotic or its metabolites within the body. Furthermore, urinary metabonomic analyses provide a picture of the hydrophilic chemicals eliminated from the body. Ideally, these same types of analyses of the major metabolizing tissues would provide a better picture of the state of the organism and its change over time. In lieu of these data, metabonomic analysis of samples from all routes of elimination (e.g., exhaled air, urine, feces) and blood could provide a reasonable picture of the state of the whole body. Metabonomic investigations provide an essential source of data for improving, calibrating and verifying physiological models that will require modification to accommodate data from molecular biology, but are needed to address the distribution of xenobiotics within higher organisms. This has tremendous potential for risk assessment since urine samples can be collected over an animal's lifetime with concurrent observation for the onset of disease. Comparative studies could be performed at high doses that may be necessary to observe disease effects and at low doses that are environmentally relevant.

With '-omics' data on molecular-level effects caused by xenobiotics, computational toxicology, a developing paradigm, will attempt to predict chemical toxicity using mathematical (e.g., numerical, *in silico*) models (Hogue, 2003). In order for this to succeed, a large database must be developed for existing chemicals containing observed molecular-level effects, perhaps at different exposure

[1]Pachinko a Japanese pinball game where a steel ball bounces off pins on a vertically oriented game board, eventually falling into a hole in the board.

concentrations, and chemical characteristics. However, in higher organisms, obtaining molecular-level data at the known site of action may be impeded by limitations in target tissue acquisition at the frequency needed to detect molecular-level changes, and the number of animals that can realistically be involved in the experiment due to cost and facility constraints. Furthermore, many of the questions regarding extrapolation between species, extrapolation from experiments conducted at high exposure concentrations to environmentally relevant concentration and routes of administration remain, and computational models will be needed to address these same questions. With these molecular-level capabilities and data in mind, this chapter outlines next how an old paradigm of physiologically based pharmacokinetic modeling can be modified to include new information that will allow it to better address the extrapolation questions above.

7.3   THE NEXT GENERATION OF PHYSIOLOGICAL MODELS

In the last 10 years, physiologically based pharmacokinetic models have been formulated with increasing levels of biological realism. In the study of 2,3,7,8-tetrachlorodibenzo-*p*-dioxin (TCDD), Kohn *et al.* (2001) developed a detailed PBPK model that extended past models (Kohn *et al.*, 1993, 1996) by including mathematical representations of: biliary secretion of TCDD due to liver cytotoxicity as a function of cumulative dose; first-order degradation (i.e., proteolysis) of the Ah receptor; a two-site model for transcriptional activation of *CYP1A1* and *CYP1B1* genes; mRNA stabilization by a nucleotide tail called poly(A) degraded according to first-order kinetics; and protein synthesis of CYP1A1, CYP1A2, and CYP1B1. They compare their predictions of the CYP1A2 ED_{01} (i.e., oral dose that produces in increase of 1% above the maximal response in the controls) with their earlier model (Kohn *et al.*, 1996) and the ED_{01} computed by the Andersen *et al.* (1997a, 1997b) model. Much lower levels were found by a factor of 3 and 10, respectively.

Andersen *et al.* (1997a, 1997b) developed a PBPK model with a multicompartment liver to simulate the induction of CYP. In their model, the total rate of production of CYP (dA_{CYPi}/dt) is equal to the basal production rate plus an increase in production proportional to the fractional occupancy, *FO*, of the DNA binding sites minus degradation of the CYP according to first-order kinetics:

$$\frac{dA_{CYPi}}{dt} = V_i \cdot \left\{ k_{0cyp} + \left(k_{mx} - k_{0cyp} \right) \cdot FO \right\} - k_{ee}A_{CYPi}, \qquad (7.2)$$

where A_{CYPi} (nmol) is the amount of CYP in compartment i, V_i is the volume of compartment i, k_{0cyp} (nmol/g/hr) is the basal rate of formation, k_{mx} (nmol/hr) is the maximum rate of induced transcription, k_{ee} (hr^{-1}) is the first-order elimination rate constant. The fractional occupancy of DNA binding sites is represented through a Hill-type equation (Segel, 1993) having the form

$$FO = \frac{v}{V_{max}} = \frac{[S]^n}{K_S^{*n} + [S]^n}. \qquad (7.3)$$

The substrate, S, in the Andersen *et al.* model is the ligand–receptor complex that is binding DNA, K_S^{*n} is equivalent to their dissociation constant, and n is the number of substrate binding sites per molecule of DNA. The Hill equation was used by Kohn *et al.* (1993) to represent CYP1A1 synthesis. They describe previous work by Leung *et al.* (1988, 1990) that first incorporated an inducible binding protein in the liver based on data (Abraham *et al.*, 1988) that showed high concentrations of TCDD in the liver relative to fat. Kohn *et al.* (1993) extended the PBPK model to allow for effects of TCDD on the aryl hydrocarbon, estrogen, and epidermal growth factor receptors.

The extension of the basic PBPK model to include receptor binding and CYP induction was driven by data (Abraham *et al.*, 1988) showing relatively high concentrations of TCDD in the liver compared to fat, and the diagnostic nature of PBPK model development in the context of risk assessment. Yet, a variety of enzymes involved in different biotransformation reactions can be induced and inhibited by xenobiotics (Park and Kitteringham, 1990; Ingelman-Sundberg *et al.*, 1994; Kedderis, 1997; Lin and Lu, 1998; Fuhr, 2000) complicating the pharmacokinetics where mixtures of drugs or environmental toxicants are concerned. As the mechanisms of xenobiotic metabolism are further elucidated through genomic, proteomic, and metabonomic studies where genes and receptors, such as pregnane X receptor (Zhang *et al.*, 1999), are identified that exert regulatory control over enzyme induction, PBPK model development can transition from a compound-by-compound, diagnostic method of development to a more biologically based model of the whole body that would be able to accommodate individual xenobiotic exposures and mixtures.

Induction of cytochrome P4502E1 (CYP2E1) by ethanol and other xenobiotics was described by Ingelman-Sundberg *et al.* (1994). Ethanol induction of CYP2E1 exhibits an interesting behavior called ligand stabilization, a phenomenon that occurs when the inducer retards the natural biphasic degradation of the enzyme to a single, slow degradation rate (Chien *et al.*, 1997). Chien *et al.* modeled the induction/inhibition of CYP2E1 by ligand stabilization using a compartmental approach. At high ethanol concentrations *in vivo*, CYP2E1 activity was found to decrease (Pantuck *et al.*, 1985). The assumption of two distinct pools of CYP2E1 was necessary to simulate the biphasic pattern of protein turnover observed *in vivo* in the absence of an inducer. Chien *et al.* modeled acetone and ethanol induction of CYP2E1 and assumed competitive inhibition of the inducer for the active binding site on the enzyme.

Kedderis (1997) extrapolated *in vitro* hepatocyte kinetic data to predict furan toxicokinetics *in vivo* and cited 11 other examples of *in vitro* to *in vivo* extrapolation for predicting metabolism kinetics. For rapidly metabolized xenobiotics he reported that blood flow to the liver actually limits metabolism of the compound, and thus CYP2E1 enzyme induction produces little or no effect in the metabolite tissue concentration; however, the time course of more slowly metabolized xenobiotics, such as therapeutic agents, may be affected by the enzyme induction. Kedderis' findings for rapidly metabolized compounds suggest that one could ignore enzyme induction in the formulation of the corresponding PBPK model.

However, while the extrapolated *in vitro* kinetic data predicted the *in vivo* furan pharmacokinetics, without measurements of CYP2E1 over the course of the experiment, a phenomenon like ligand stabilization may go unobserved and subsequent extrapolations of the model for risk assessment could yield erroneous predictions. Such examples underscore the need to move away from a Michaelis–Menten representation of xenobiotic metabolism reaction rates to a more generalized formulation where the concentration of enzymes involved in catalyzing biotransformation reactions are an integral part of the model.

A search of the recent literature reveals relatively little innovation in the development of physiological models to predict target tissue concentrations. For modeling chemical mixtures, Klein *et al.* (2002) describe BioMOL, a modeling software system under development based on reaction network modeling, as a means of handling all the biochemical reactions that occur in the body as a whole. Liao *et al.* (2002) describe how BioMOL would work for benzo[*a*]pyrene, although their example did not predict organ-specific concentrations. They propose to incorporate pharmacodynamics in 'critical compartments' of the PBPK model at the level of molecular mechanisms toward development of a 'second-generation PBPK/PD model'.

7.4 DISCUSSION AND CONCLUSIONS

As long as there is a need to predict target tissue concentrations, some type of physiological model will be necessary to account for ADME characteristics of xenobiotics in the body. In the last 25 years, PBPK models for different xenobiotics have been developed with varying numbers of compartments and levels of detail. To date, their development and formulation have been guided more by expert opinion and a need to fit measured data than by a formalized set of rules, a priori, that are biologically based.

There is a balance between keeping the model simple and imposing biological reality. Both paradigms can be informative; in fact, non-physiologically based compartmental modeling has been used for years in clinical pharmacokinetics. As molecular-level processes are elucidated through genomics, proteomics, and metabonomics, better representations of these processes (e.g., discovery of proteins and pathways that control the induction of enzymes) could be incorporated into the PBPK model. Additionally, current PBPK models establish their system boundaries around the processes of xenobiotic metabolism, and, as Nicholson and Wilson point out, in reality, xenobiotic metabolism is linked to normal metabolic functions in the body. Should this knowledge be incorporated into a PBPK model used in the context of risk assessment?

Certain levels of detail are required to meet the end-use of the model. Model extrapolations are somewhat less reliable than interpolations, and for the various types of extrapolations required by risk assessment, concurrent modeling of metabolic functions is probably not needed. However, receptor-mediated processes such as protein and DNA binding in the example of TCDD and enzyme induction are necessary details that could affect predictions from an extrapolated model. Thus, future advances in PBPK modeling may occur in the following ways: simulation of the enzymes that are involved in xenobiotic metabolism and incorporation of regulatory feedback mechanisms through the identification of regulatory control proteins; extension from pharmacokinetic aspects to include pharmacodynamics for multiple adverse effects in multiple target tissues; and modeling methods to address the mixtures question since an experimental approach is intractable.

In the long term, as biological mechanisms are better understood, a 'virtual' organism may eventually follow from the 'virtual' cell (University of Connecticut Health Center, 2004), which should accommodate both individual xenobiotics and mixtures. In the short term, -omics data will be crucial in elucidating biological mechanisms in cells, although where higher organisms are concerned, a physiologically based model will be needed to integrate the multitude of processes occurring within the body.

ACKNOWLEDGEMENTS

The author would like to acknowledge the NATO Committee on the Challenges of a Modern Society for providing fellowship support.

CHAPTER 8

Stochastic Carcinogenesis Models

Annette Kopp-Schneider, Iris Burkholder and Jutta Groos

German Cancer Research Center

8.1 INTRODUCTION

The quantitative description of the process of carcinogenesis is a rational basis for the assessment of cancer risk due to exogenous agents. Research in carcinogenesis is a field of interest not only for biological and medical scientists but also for mathematicians and statisticians who analyze data dealing with preneoplastic and neoplastic lesions. The focus of interest lies in the quantification of the time to tumor as it depends on environmental factors such as chemical substances or radiation. For 50 years, models have been used to describe the process of benign and malignant tumor formation. The process of carcinogenesis is inherently a stochastic process, at least as long as it is not known why certain individuals get cancer under conditions where others are unaffected. Therefore models of carcinogenesis are formulated in the framework of stochastic processes. There are two main reasons for formulating models of carcinogenesis. One is to elucidate the biological process of carcinogenesis, and the other is to provide a rational basis for risk assessment, to estimate risk due to environmental agents at the range of interest for regulating agencies.

In the course of development of cancer, preneoplastic lesions can be observed which represent precursors of the malignant tumor. This is a well-studied effect both in human carcinogenesis where precursor lesions have been identified amongst others for colon, prostate, endometrial, skin and liver cancer (Chapter 4, this volume) and in experimental carcinogenesis where the skin (Marks and Fürstenberger, 1987) and the liver (Bannasch, 1996) have been the preferred organs under study. The observation of precursor lesions of carcinomas has led to the development of biological hypotheses concerning the process of carcinogenesis which have been used to formulate stochastic carcinogenesis models.

Recent Advances in Quantitative Methods in Cancer and Human Health Risk Assessment
Edited by L. Edler and C. Kitsos   © 2005 John Wiley & Sons, Ltd

8.1.1 Classification of carcinogens

In experimental carcinogenesis, the process of carcinoma formation has been subdivided into at least three operationally defined stages: initiation, promotion and progression. In the special case of experimental skin carcinogenesis, these stages can be observed non-invasively. Initiation can be brought about by a single subcarcinogenic dose of a carcinogen. Repeated treatment with a promoting substance leads to the formation of benign tumors. Malignant progression of the benign lesions has been shown to occur at low frequency, independent of continuous promoter application.

Following these observations, carcinogenic compounds are in general classified as to their presumed predominant mode of action irrespective of the target organ (Thorslund *et al.*, 1986). A chemical which presumably increases the number of preneoplastic cells produced by normal cells is called an initiator. A chemical which increases the number of preneoplastic cells by stimulating clonal growth is called a promoter.

8.1.2 Foci of altered hepatocytes

Preneoplastic liver lesions have been identified as foci of altered hepatocytes characterized by specific morphological and biochemical changes. This is true both for humans and for animals, regardless of the way in which the liver carcinomas arise, be it by induction through chemical agents, viral infections, radiation or certain hormones (Bannasch, 1996). The occurrence of focal hepatic preneoplasia has proven to be a valuable indicator of the ability of a treatment to cause liver cancer. Although the number of liver cancers induced in rats by chemicals is orders of magnitude lower than that of liver foci, there is a clear correlation between the two endpoints. Focal hepatic preneoplasia, therefore, represents a sensitive marker of carcinogenic response and can be used to show the carcinogenic potential of a treatment.

The finding that a compound alters the number of foci or their size distribution may give indications about the mechanism of action of the compound. An initiating compound will increase the number of foci without changing their size distribution, whereas a promoting compound increases the size of existing foci without changing their number. Usually carcinogenic compounds will have a combination of initiating and promoting activities. One question of interest to toxicologists is whether the initiating or the promoting potential of a compound is the predominant mode of action. Another question discussed among pathologists concerns the mechanism of liver focal lesion formation and their growth.

8.1.3 Stereological aspects in the evaluation of liver focal lesions

The evaluation of a quantitative study on preneoplastic liver lesions induced by an oncogenic agent involves the morphometric analysis of stained liver sections. The result of this analysis is one data set per liver section which contains the total area of the liver section and each individual focal transection area. Depending on the stain used for detection of focal lesions, one or several phenotypes of foci can be distinguished. If more than one type of focus can be distinguished, a record is made of these types. As a rule, foci under a fixed minimum size are not recorded or discarded from the study.

From the raw data three variables are extracted for the statistical analysis. Adding all focal transection areas and dividing the result by the total liver section area yields the area fraction occupied by foci. According to the fundamental mean-value formula of stereology (cf. Stoyan et al., 1995), the area fraction is an unbiased estimate of the volume fraction whenever the foci are randomly distributed in the liver. The profile density is calculated by dividing the number of focal transections by the liver section area. The third variable for evaluation is the size of the transections which can be visualized by histograms or by empirical cumulative distribution functions.

The statistical evaluation of foci data can be used to investigate several questions. The question which is most directly answered is whether a treatment changes the volume fraction of foci because the area fraction can be calculated straightforwardly from the raw data and represents an unbiased estimate of the volume fraction. In addition, the evaluation of the area fraction is not affected by confluent foci, which may represent a serious problem at high doses of toxic chemicals. However, researchers are often interested in alterations in number of foci and their size induced by the treatment and in the mechanism of the treatment effect. Unfortunately, testing statistical hypotheses about the area fraction does not provide information about the number and sizes of foci because large area fractions may be due to small numbers of large foci, to large numbers of small foci or to large numbers of large foci (cf. Morris, 1989).

Measurements are made in two-dimensional liver sections and inference about reality in three-dimensional liver is limited by the stereological problem. This problem is described briefly by the fact that the probability of a focus being cut increases with its size. Therefore, large foci will be overrepresented in liver sections compared to small ones, and the number of transections observed in a liver section depends on both the number of foci in the liver and their size distribution. Observations on number and size distribution of focal transections therefore cannot be directly related to three-dimensional reality.

When cutting a sphere, the observed transection circle has a diameter depending on the distance of the section plane from the sphere center. The major assumption that has to be made for basic stereological considerations is that foci are randomly distributed in the liver and that they are spherical. However, preneoplastic liver foci are not always spherical and especially large foci have non-spherical shape (Imaida et al., 1989). The stereology of non-spherical foci will in any case involve the problems arising for spheres. Liver sections are about 2 μm thick. Compared to the diameter of single cells of about 24 μm, the thickness of the sections can be ignored and stereological methods for thin sections can be applied.

An example should illustrate the difficulty of drawing inference from two-dimensional data about three-dimensional reality. Consider the two populations of

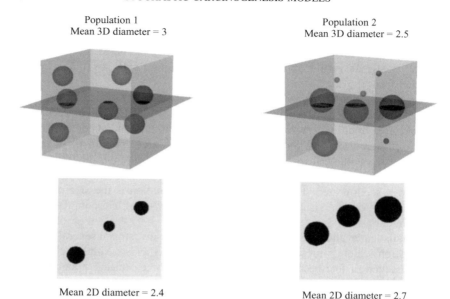

Figure 8.1   Two populations of spheres in three dimensions and their respective two-dimensional transections.

spheres displayed in Figure 8.1. The first population consists of spheres with diameter 3, whereas the second population consists of an equal mix of two subpopulations, small spheres with diameter 1 and large spheres with diameter 4. The mean diameter of the first population is 3, whereas the mean diameter of the second population is 2.5, the second population therefore being smaller in mean than the first. Considering the two-dimensional transections obtained from a section through the cube, their mean diameter is 2.4 for the first distribution, and 2.7 for the second distribution (Ohser and Lurz, 1994). Hence, an inversion in the order of the mean diameters is observed. It is also noticeable that in the second distribution, the mean diameter of the two-dimensional transections exceeds the mean diameter of the spheres. In addition, examples can be constructed to show that stochastically ordered transection size distributions do not in general originate from stochastically ordered distributions of foci (Kopp-Schneider, 2003).

Several methods have been proposed to reconstruct the three-dimensional size distribution of spherical objects from the observation of their transections (see Enzmann et al., 1987; Fullman, 1953; Ohser and Sandau, 2000; Pugh et al., 1983). All of these methods are based on Wicksell's (1925) formulas relating the distribution of the sphere diameters to the distribution of spherical transection diameters and vice versa. A number of methods concentrate on the estimation of the number of spheres in the volume – that is, the sphere density – from the observed number of transections and their diameters. Some approaches estimate a histogram for the sphere diameters from a histogram for the profiles using discretized versions of the

Wicksell formulas. Unfortunately, all approaches are unstable in the presence of a limited number of observed transections, which means that small changes in the data can result in large changes in the estimated sphere density and sphere size distribution. This is especially important when very small profiles are observed. Another unpleasant property of some of the estimates is their infinite variance. The number of focal transections observed in carcinogenicity studies, especially in short-term carcinogenicity studies, is often too low to use the reconstruction methods for reliable estimates of focal density and size distribution.

8.2 STOCHASTIC MODELS FOR HEPATOCARCINOGENESIS

Difficulties in the statistical analysis of hepatic preneoplasia can be eliminated by basing the analysis on a mechanistic model which describes the appearance and change in volume of foci. Several models have been developed to describe foci data. All of these models assume that foci appear randomly in space and time and use the concept of a Poisson process. The models are different as to how the change in volume and in phenotype of foci is described.

Two different hypotheses about the formation of preneoplastic lesions have been discussed in the scientific community. The first hypothesis assumes that single cells are transformed to the next phenotype by a mutational event. This hypothesis is depicted in the upper path of Figure 8.2 for the case of three different types of preneoplastic lesions. The lower path shows the alternative hypothesis, called the field effect hypothesis, that all cells in a preneoplastic lesion change their phenotype more or less simultaneously rather than by mutation of single cells.

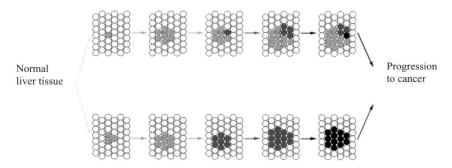

Figure 8.2 Two hypotheses about the formation and phenotypic changes of liver focal lesions. The upper path shows the mutation hypothesis and the lower path shows the field effect hypothesis.

8.2.1 The multistage model with clonal expansion

The most prominent biologically based models for carcinogenesis are the multistage models, which are formulated at the cellular level, describing the malignant transformation of normal cells as a process involving mutations, cell proliferation/ differentiation and occasionally repair. They commonly assume that a cell has to go through k (> 1) mutational changes and that intermediate cells are subject to a birth–death process. The basic assumption for this type of model is that cells act independently.

As an example of a multistage model we present here the four-stage model with clonal expansion. As depicted in Figure 8.3, a normal cell becomes malignant by sequentially passing through three intermediate (phenotypically different) cell types. Cells in the intermediate stages may proliferate according to a stochastic linear birth–death process with rate β_i, i denoting the intermediate cell type, they may die or differentiate with rate δ_i, or they may divide asymmetrically into one cell of the same type and one cell of the next type with rate $\mu\beta_i$. The birth rate of intermediate cells of type i, β_i, can be generalized to include recruitment of neighboring cells in addition to cell division. The cells in the normal stage are assumed to stay constant in number and are not subject to the stochastic birth–death process. As in all current multistage models, the malignant stage is assumed to be absorbing. However, this stage will not be considered in the current application because data about carcinomas were not evaluated.

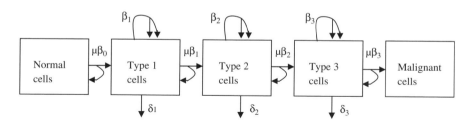

Figure 8.3   The four-stage model with clonal expansion.

Multistage models represent interconnected birth–death processes and as such are treated with Markov process methods. Unfortunately the model presented here cannot directly be used for application to data because the distribution of number and size of cell colonies of different phenotypes cannot be derived analytically. Therefore an approximation of the model was derived that describes the transition process between the different types of cells by a Poisson process with intensity depending upon the mean number of cells in the previous compartment. Details of the model and the approximation can be found in Geisler and Kopp-Schneider (2000).

The four-stage model describes the size of foci of altered hepatocytes in terms of number of cells. Under assumptions about the size of a cell and the packing of cells in a volume, the foci size distribution is translated into a distribution of foci radii in three-dimensional space.

8.2.2   The color-shift model

The field effect hypothesis is formalized in a model which describes the formation and fate of focal lesions in a three-dimensional situation and is shown in Figure 8.4. The centers of foci are generated according to a Poisson process. Foci start growing from the time point of formation onward according to a deterministic exponential law, initially starting from either a single cell or a whole cluster of cells. Growth occurs through clonal expansion of foci cells and/or recruitment of neighboring cells. It is assumed that the shape of every focus is spherical and therefore the size of a focus is given by its radius. When focal lesions are generated they all have the same phenotype. The phenotype changes sequentially over time, that is, each focal lesion may pass through a sequence of phenotypes. The changes in phenotype are irreversible. The phenotype will be called 'color' with reference to the method of detection of focal lesions by staining tissue. Details of the model can be found in Kopp-Schneider *et al.* (1998) and in Burkholder and Kopp-Schneider (2002).

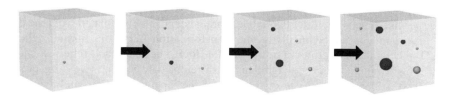

Figure 8.4   The color-shift model.

8.3   MODEL-BASED EVALUATION OF LIVER FOCAL LESION DATA

Both models presented in the previous section are applied to data by maximum likelihood methods. Corresponding to the experimental data, the log-likelihood for both models consists of a sum over all individual animal contributions where each contribution involves the number of foci of every phenotype, the area of the liver section and the size of all observed focal transections. The data obtained from experiments contain information from sections through a three-dimensional organ with three-dimensional preneoplastic lesions. For the application of both mechanistic models it is necessary to derive the two-dimensional size distribution of focal transections from the three-dimensional size distribution prediction for foci of the models. As proposed by Moolgavkar *et al.* (1990), the Wicksell transformation is used to translate the size distribution of foci into a size distribution of focal transections.

8.3.1   Model-based approach to study the mode of action of chemicals

As a first example we analyze liver focal lesion data to investigate whether the substance under study shows an effect on the size of the focal lesions. The data come from a study in which juvenile Wistar rats were given a single dose of N-nitrosodiethylamine (DEN) followed, after a two-week recovery period, by daily treatment with N-nitrosomorpholine (NNM) (8 animals) or vehicle (8 animals). Twelve weeks after the start of the study, liver sections were taken and stained for the placental form of glutathione S-transferase (GSTP). The data evaluated here represent a small subset of a large study involving 1600 rats and described in detail by Ittrich *et al.* (2003).

As a result of the staining procedure, focal liver lesions can be identified due to their increased expression of GSTP. The data set therefore contains information about focal lesions of only one type and the model-based description of the data requires a model allowing for one type of foci. Since the difference between the color-shift model and the multistage model lies mainly in the description of the process of phenotype change of foci, we evaluated the data with the two-stage model which allows for stochastic growth of foci of one type of intermediate cells.

The focus of the analysis presented here is to find out whether NNM has a promoting effect in the sense that foci sizes in DEN-initiated animals are increased by NNM compared to vehicle control. Due to the design of the study with only one sacrifice time point, only two model parameters can be estimated from the data by maximum likelihood methods: the transformation rate from normal cells to GSTP+ cells and the growth rate of GSTP+ foci. The likelihood ratio test shows that growth rates of foci are significantly different between the two dose groups ($p < 0.001$). The observed size distribution of the focal transections and the model fits for different growth rates are shown in Figure 8.5. Although the difference in size distribution is graphically obvious, we wish to stress here that application of a model describing the foci sizes is the only way for a rational test to answer the question whether NNM has promoting activity.

8.3.2 Model-based approach to study the process of formation and growth of liver foci

Both the four-stage model and the color-shift model were applied to another data set from a carcinogenicity study with NNM in which rats were continuously treated with NNM alone and liver sections were stained with hematoxylin and eosin (Weber and Bannasch, 1994). Several types of foci were identified and analyzed morphometrically. The analysis, however, was restricted to three types of foci. Application of the four-stage model to the data yielded maximum likelihood parameter estimates for the cell division rates which are biologically implausible (Geisler and Kopp-Schneider, 2000). In the following, the parameter range for the four-stage models was restricted to reflect biological reality. The four-stage model and the color-shift model are non-nested models and hence the comparison of fit cannot be tested by likelihood ratio methods. The size of the log-likelihood difference between the four-stage model with restricted parameters and the color-shift model, however, can be taken as an indication that the color-shift model may give a better explanation for the data than the four-stage model. Earlier simulation studies for the comparison of two non-nested carcinogenesis models have shown that

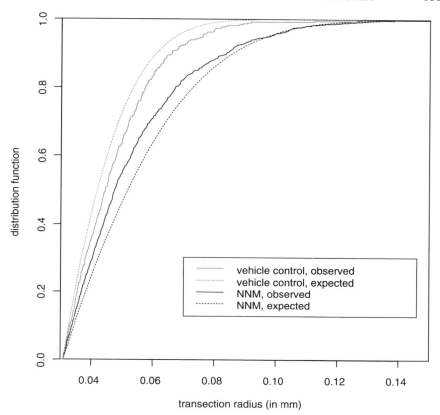

Figure 8.5 Observed vs. expected cumulative focal transection size distribution in a hepatocarcinogenicity study with DEN-initiated animals. Expected curves are derived from the two-stage model with maximum likelihood parameter estimates.

comparison of the maximal log-likelihood values may be taken as an indication for the appropriate model (Kopp-Schneider and Portier, 1991). Plots of experimental data and predictions of the two models can be compared graphically to give evidence as to which model is more appropriate in the present situation. Figure 8.6 shows the comparison of model fit for type 2 foci which indicates that the color-shift model explained the liver focal lesion data slightly better than the four-stage model. Drawing all the information together, the analysis suggests that for the type of preneoplastic foci observed in this study, the field effect hypothesis is a more likely explanation than the mutation hypothesis. This is intuitively appealing because the four-stage model predicts observation of many large early-stage foci and few small later-stage foci. Regarding the size distribution, the opposite is true for the color-shift model, which predicts many small early-stage foci and few large later-stage foci, this being the effect observed experimentally.

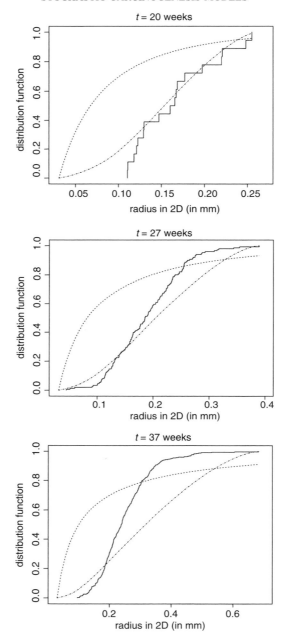

Figure 8.6 Observed vs. expected cumulative focal transection size distribution of type 2 foci in a hepatocarcinogenicity study with NNM 20, 27 and 37 weeks after start of treatment. Expected curves are derived from the four-stage model with maximum likelihood parameter estimates restricted to biologically realistic growth rates. The dot-dashed curves show the model fit of the color-shift model, while the dashed curves show the model fit of the four-stage model.

8.4 CONCLUSIONS

The example of the application of mechanistic models for hepatocarcinogenesis presented here shows their ability to contribute to cancer research. The models presented here can be treated with stochastic process theory and the quantities of interest for application to data can be derived analytically or calculated numerically. This allows formal maximum likelihood methods to be used for parameter estimation and for a comparison of model fit of nested models.

The models presented here are certainly oversimplifications of the biological process. It is obvious from Figures 8.5 and 8.6 that the fit of both models is only moderate. A number of future developments are necessary; this concerns multistage models as well as the color-shift model. The growth process in the color-shift model needs to be described in a more realistic fashion, and first investigations with altered growth processes of the lesions have been carried out.

CHAPTER 9

A Unified Modeling Approach: From Exposure to Disease Endpoints

Chao W. Chen

US Environmental Protection Agency[1]

9.1 BACKGROUND

One of the major objectives of incorporating available biological information into the quantitative risk assessment process is to reduce uncertainties in risk estimation. In assessing risk associated with exposure to a chemical, there are a number of uncertainties that lie along the continuum from source of exposure to adverse effects, including uptake, distribution, absorption, clearance, metabolism, receptor–ligand interaction, gene activation/protein production, signaling, cellular response, and systemic adverse effect, as articulated in a US Environmental Protection Agency computational toxicology conference report (US EPA, 2003d).

At present, only the first portion of this continuum is routinely considered in risk assessment. It is known as the physiologically based pharmacokinetic (PBPK) model, and it includes uptake, distribution, absorption, and metabolism. A PBPK model is usually represented by a set of deterministic differential equations. To a lesser extent, the last part of the continuum (cellular response and disease endpoint) has also been considered in some risk assessments – for example, trichloroethylene (Chen, 2000), inhaled particles (Chen and Oberdoster, 1996), radon-induced lung tumors (Luebeck *et al.*, 1996), and tumors in National Toxicology Program historical control animals (Portier and Bailer, 1989). These models are usually

[1]The views expressed in this article are those of the author and do not necessarily reflect the views of the US Environmental Protection Agency.

referred to as biologically based dose-response (BBDR) models, and they are constructed as stochastic processes. For BBDR models, although it is possible to construct a complicated model of a higher number of stages by numerical solution of partial differential equations (Little and Wright, 2003), most efforts have been limited to two-stage models of carcinogenesis, because it is difficult to obtain analytical solution beyond two stages. Furthermore, the modeling approach for BBDR models, as will be demonstrated, does not offer a conceptually unified procedure for risk assessment modeling. The main objective of this chapter is to present such a unified approach.

There is a large gap in the exposure-to-disease continuum that is not covered by either PBPK or BBDR models. Given the broad range of events involved in the continuum, it is desirable to have a unified modeling procedure that can incorporate information from the entire continuum. For example, 2,3,7,8-tetrachlorodibenzo-*p*-dioxin (TCDD) acts through Ah receptors, triggering a number of biological responses that can be divided into two broad categories: metabolic processes associated with uptake and subsequent binding with other proteins; and mitogenic processes associated with DNA replication, cell cycling, cell division, and differentiation. In this example, and in many others as well, more detailed modeling of the events occurring along the continuum of biological processes is necessary. Therefore, it is desirable to have a unified, flexible, and easy-to-use procedure. A natural way to model a biological process is to consider the process as a dynamic system in a state space model (to be defined) with input, output, and feedback, as is traditionally done in the engineering control system, that can be described by a system of deterministic differential equations. The challenge is how to extend this approach to include stochastic differential systems. The extension to stochastic processes is necessary because some events, such as cell dynamics, are stochastic in nature.

In this chapter a unified modeling approach is provided through state space modeling that takes advantage of recent advances in sampling techniques (e.g., rejection sampling and resampling, importance sampling, Markov chain iterations such as Gibbs sampling, and Metropolis–Hastings sampling) and increasing computing power. Application of these sampling techniques to state space modeling has been extensively investigated (e.g., Liu and Chen, 1998; Kitagawa, 1998). As will be demonstrated, many of the models used in risk assessment, including PBPK and BBDR models, can be described as state space models; some are obvious, and some require formidable mathematical manipulations. The advantage of state space modeling is that a great deal of research has been done over the last four decades in this field, and the technique has become more and more powerful because of improved statistical procedures and increasing computing power. These techniques have been developed out of practical needs in various scientific endeavors, such as creating navigational and guidance systems in the aerospace industry and target tracking and satellite orbit determination in civilian and military applications.

Modern state space modeling evolved from the concept of Kalman filtering, a mathematical tool for estimating and predicting state variables in a dynamic system on the basis of a noisy signal (data). An important feature of the Kalman filtering technique is that it not only allows for estimation (separation of noise and signal), as is the case for all the estimation methods (including least squares estimation) preceding the Kalman filter, but it also provides a solution for an 'inversion' problem, but predicting and updating from dependent (observation) to independent (state) variables and vice versa.

Historically, two papers by Kalman (1960, 1961) were the origin of the Kalman filtering (updating) techniques that helped man set foot on the moon in the late 1960s. Before that time, engineers were limping along with the Wiener filter, which was a method for obtaining best estimates by analyzing time series in the frequency domain. An interesting historical review of Kalman filtering can be found in Cipra (1993). For general state space modeling, the textbook by Grewal and Andrews (2001) is recommended. Recently, there has been a surge of interest in applying state space models to various problems, including DNA and protein sequence analysis (Liu *et al.*, 1997), some biomedical problems (Tan, 2002), and ecology (Wikle, 2003).

9.2   CONVENTIONAL APPROACH TO MODELING CARCINOGENESIS

To appreciate the difficulty of the conventional approach to carcinogenesis modeling, a brief derivation of the two-stage model is in order. It relies on the theory of Markov processes, first by using Kolmogorov forward equations to derive the probability generating function (PGF) of the number of cells in each stage and then deriving the hazard function from the PGF. Let us first consider a k-stage model of carcinogenesis. Let $N(t)$ be the number of normal stem cells at time t, $I_j(t)$ the number of the jth stage initiated cells at time t, $j = 1, 2, \ldots, k - 1$, $I_k(t)$: number of malignant cells at time t, and $T(t)$: number of malignant tumors at time t. We make the following assumptions:

1. $N(t)$ is assumed to be a deterministic function of t.

2. The first-stage initiation from normal (N) to initiation (I_1) is assumed to follow a Poisson distribution with intensity $\lambda_0(t) = N(t)\alpha_0(t)$, where $\alpha_0(t)$ is the rate of first initiation.

3. I_j cells follow a stochastic birth–death process, with birth rate $b_j(t)$ and death rate $d_j(t)$, and they can mutate to the next stage, I_{j+1}, with mutation rate $\alpha_j(t)$.

4. With probability 1, each I_k cell can instantaneously grow into a malignant tumor.

Denote the PGF of $\{I_j(t), j = 1, \ldots, k - 1, T(t)\}$ given $\{N(t_0) = N_0, I_j(t_0) = T(t_0) = 0, j = 1, \ldots, k - 1\}$ by

$$\psi(t_0, t) = \psi(y_j, j = 1, \ldots, k : t_0, t),$$

and the PGF of $\{I_j(t), j = i, \ldots, k - 1, T(t)\}$ given one I_i cell at time s by

$$\phi_i(y_j, j = 1, \ldots, k : s, t) = \phi_i(s, t).$$

By using Kolmogorov forward equations, $\psi(t_0, t)$, and $\phi_i(s, t)$ follow the partial differential equations

$$\frac{\partial}{\partial t} \psi(t_0, t) = \psi(t_0, t) N(t) \alpha_0(t) + \sum_{j=1}^{k-1} \{(y_j - 1)[y_j b_j(t) - d_j(t)]$$

$$+ y_j(y_{j+1} - 1)\alpha_j(t)\} \frac{\partial}{\partial y_j} \psi(t_0, t), \tag{9.1}$$

$$\frac{\partial}{\partial t} \phi_i(s, t) = \sum_{j=1}^{k-1} \{(y_j - 1)[y_j b_j(t) - d_j(t)] + y_j(y_{j+1} - 1)\alpha_j(t)\} \frac{\partial}{\partial t} \phi_i(s, t), \tag{9.2}$$

for $i = 1, \ldots, k - 1$, with $\phi_i(s, s) = y_i$, $\phi_k(s, t) = y_k$ and initial condition $\psi(t_0, t_0) = 1$. The hazard function for a malignant tumor at time t is given by

$$\lambda(t) = \frac{-\psi'(1, \ldots, 1, 0 : t_0, t)}{\psi(1, \ldots, 1, 0 : t_0, t)}, \tag{9.3}$$

where ψ' is the first derivative of ψ. If all the parameters are time homogeneous, then $\phi_i(s, t) = \phi_i(t - s)$, and the system of PGFs ϕ_i satisfies the Ricatti equations:

$$\frac{d}{dt} \phi_i(t) = b_i[\phi_i(t)]^2 + \{\alpha_i \phi_{i+1}(t) - [b_i + d_i + \alpha_i]\}\phi_i(t) + d_i, \tag{9.4}$$

with $\phi_i(0) = y_i$, for $i = 1, \ldots, k - 1$, and $\phi_k(t) = y_k$. For the case of $k = 2$, ψ has a solution

$$\psi(t_0, t) = \exp\left\{ \int_{t_0}^{t} N(x)\alpha_0(x)[\phi_1(x, t) - 1]dx \right\}. \tag{9.5}$$

Even in the time homogeneous case, when $k > 2$, an analytic solution for φ_i does not exist. For this reason, almost all models of carcinogenesis are limited to the two-stage model, which was made popular by Moolgavkar and colleagues (Moolgavkar and Venzon, 1979; Moolgavkar and Knudson, 1981), and subsequently investigated by many other authors (Chen and Farland, 1991; Yang and Chen, 1991; Tan, 1991; Yakolev and Tsodikov, 1996; Zheng, 1997; Kopp-Schneider *et al.*, 1998).

9.3   STATE SPACE MODELING USING SAMPLING TECHNIQUES

The general state space model consists of two equations: the system (state) equation of a Markov process,

$$X_t = f_t(X_{t-1}, \theta, \varepsilon_t), \tag{9.6}$$

and the observation equation,

$$Y_t = g_t(X_t, \theta, e_t), \tag{9.7}$$

where X_t is a vector of state variables at time t and Y_t is a vector of observed data, θ is a vector of parameters, ε_t and e_t are assumed to be independently distributed random errors, and f_t and g_t are known functions. It is interesting to note that ε_t (variability of the dynamic system) and e_t (measurement error) allow one to separately estimate system variability and measurement error, which are currently of great interest to risk assessors. Thus, the state space modeling provides, at least theoretically, a means to estimate these two quantities separately.

The state space model may also specify the two conditional densities, $P(X_i \mid X_{i-1})$ and $P(Y_i \mid X_i)$, which will play an essential role in estimating state variables and unknown parameters for a stochastic state space model. As will become clear, PBPK models represent a class of deterministic state space models, and BBDR and many other applications belong to the class of stochastic state space models. It should also be noted that a continuous time model can always be expressed in discrete time. For instance, a differential, dZ/dt, can always be expressed as a difference, $[Z(t + \Delta t) - Z(t)]/\Delta t$, with a small time interval $\Delta t > 0$.

Most problems in risk assessment can be represented by a state space model with state variables $X = (X_1, \ldots, X_m)$, where X_i is a vector of state variables at time i, noting that the time interval $(0, t_m)$ is divided into equal subintervals, with $t_m = m\Delta t$, and observations $Y = [Y_1, \ldots, Y_k]$, the collection of vectors of observations at fixed time points $0 \le t_1 \le \ldots \le t_k \le t_m$.

For example, in a PBPK model of five compartments, X may represent a vector of tissue concentrations in five organs over time t (or over discrete time, $t = 1, \ldots, t_m$), and Y may represent observed values of blood and urinary concentrations at times $0 \le t_1 \le \ldots \le t_k$. Y can also be observations on a state variable (i.e., organ tissue concentration) at some fixed time points.

In a state space problem, state variables, X, and parameters, θ, are unknown and need to be estimated. Given observations Y, a conventional statistical approach is to maximize the likelihood function using probability distribution $P[Y \mid \theta]$. However, as will become clear, maximum likelihood estimatioin method not only is impractical for estimating unknown parameters, but also fails to estimate unknown state variables because it only uses information $P[Y \mid \theta]$, the conditional probability of Y given θ. At an intuitive level, one can gain an insight into this problem by noting that in a state space model, Y is a function of the independent variables X that is random, and may not be measurable, unlike a general regression problem where the independent variable is known. Recent advances in sampling techniques have made solutions feasible using only a desktop computer. Because the focus of this chapter is not on sampling techniques for state space models, only a basic concept for a class of procedures that are most relevant to the problems in risk assessment modeling is considered here.

Generally speaking, all the sampling techniques available are applicable to most problems, but some may be more efficient than others for a particular application. For instance, Gibbs sampling (along with its extended sampling procedure) is a powerful tool for most biological applications, but it is not efficient when real-time prediction and updating for the dynamic system are required. For real-time prediction and updating of a dynamic system (e.g., navigation), the sequential importance sampling proposed by Liu and Chen (1998) would be more appropriate.

In most applications, there is a need to estimate state variables, X, and parameters, θ, for prediction, filtering, and smoothing, each of which is defined by a conditional density:

1. Predictive density: $P(X_t \mid \gamma_{t-1})$, the conditional probability of the state at time t, given observations up to time $t - 1$, where $\gamma_{t-1} = \{Y_1, \ldots, Y_{t-1}\}$, all observations up to time $t - 1$.

2. Filtering (updating) density: $P(X_t \mid \gamma_t)$, the conditional probability of the state at time t, given observations up to time t.

3. Smoothing density: $P(X_t \mid \gamma_T)$, $t < T$, the conditional probability of the state at time t, given observations over time $T > t$.

First let us consider the likelihood

$$L(\theta) = P(\theta \mid \gamma_N) = \prod_{i=1}^{N} P(Y_i \mid \gamma_{i-1}, \theta), \qquad (9.8)$$

where

$$P(Y_i \mid \gamma_{i-1}, \theta) = \int_{X_i \in \Omega_X} P(Y_i, X_i \mid \gamma_{i-1}, \theta) dX_i,$$

and where Ω_X is the domain for the state variables X. The maximum likelihood estimate of θ can be obtained by maximizing (9.8). However, for most state space models, the maximum likelihood estimate of θ cannot be determined in practical applications because the filtering algorithm must be applied many times. A self-organizing smoothing algorithm proposed by Kitagawa (1998) is recommended.

9.4 SELF-ORGANIZING ALGORITHM FOR STATE SPACE MODELING

To avoid complicated of notation when both subscript and superscript are required, we write $X(i)$ in place of X_i, and similarly $Y(i)$. Given the initial condition $X(0)$, which may be deterministic or stochastic with a known density $P(X(0))$, an algorithm based on Kitagawa (1998) consists of the following recursive steps:

1. Given θ^* and $X(i)$, $i = 1, \ldots, t_M$, generate n random samples of $X(i + 1)$ from $P(X(i + 1) \mid X(i), \theta^*)$. Denote the samples by $\{X^{(j)}(i + 1), j = 1, \ldots, n\}$.

2. Compute the importance factor $w_j = P(Y(i + 1) \mid X_i, X^{(j)}(i + 1), \theta^*)$ and $q_j = w_j/\Sigma w_j$, $j = 1, \ldots, n$, where $X_i = (X(0), \ldots, X(i))$.

3. Obtain n samples (resampling) from $\{X^{(j)}(i + 1), j = 1, \ldots, n\}$ with weight q_j. Denote these samples $X^*(i + 1)$.

4. Start with $i = 1$ and repeat steps 1 through 3 until $i = t_M$ to get random samples from $P(X \mid Y, \theta^*)$. Denote these samples by X^*.

5. Generate a sample of θ from $P(\theta \mid Y, X^*)$.

6. Use the average of the random samples from step 5 as the new θ^* in step 1 and repeat the process until convergence.

9.5 SOME EXAMPLES OF STATE SPACE MODELS

Instead of following the mathematical tradition of presenting the most general and rigorous formulation, three biologically motivated examples are presented in this section to illustrate the concept and procedure. Sufficient details are provided so that anyone familiar with modern sampling techniques would be able to use the procedure. It is believed that this easy-to- understand approach will contribute more to the risk assessment community than one with mathematical generality and rigorousness.

9.5.1 State space model for cell labeling

It is instructive to consider a simple problem of using labeling data to estimate cell birth (division) and death rates. The state space model for this problem involves some features of PBPK and BBDR models. The labeling index (LI), which is defined as the ratio of number of cells labeled (e.g., by [³H]-thymidine incorporation) and the total number of cells available for labeling at the time of observation, is often used as a proliferative marker for a cell population. The underlying assumption for using LI as a proliferative marker is that a cell can be labeled only when it is in the S-phase (onset of DNA replication) of a cell cycle, and a cell reaching the S-phase will always proceed to mitosis (cell division). It is also worthwhile to note, as will be discussed later, that the use of LI may result in a loss of valuable information.

Zheng (1997) pointed out that the procedure used to estimate the cell division rate using the experimental LI proposed by Moolgavkar and Luebeck (1992b) is not theoretically sound. The objective here is to use some of the concepts discussed in Zheng's paper to illustrate the unified modeling procedure by the state space model.

Let $U(t)$ and $W(t)$ be, respectively, the number of unlabeled and labeled cells observed at time t. At time $t = 0$, the entire cell population is unlabeled and is equal to $U(0)$. Let β and δ represent, respectively, the birth and death rates. Thus, by definition of being unlabeled (and alive), $U(t)$ is distributed as binomial with parameters $U(0)$ and $\exp[-(\beta + \delta)t]$, that is, $U(t) \sim \text{bin}(U(0), \exp[-(\beta + \delta)t])$. Based on the fact that $E(W)/E(N) = 1 - \exp(-\beta t)$, where $N(t) = U(t) + W(t)$, Moolgavkar and Luebeck (1992b) postulated that $W(t) \sim \text{bin}(N(t), 1 - \exp(-2\beta t))$. However, this may not be appropriate if U and W are not independent. One way to solve this problem is to consider it as a state space model. Under this framework, the state variables are $S(t) = (U(t), W(t))$, for $t = 0, \Delta t, \ldots, k\Delta t$. For ease of notation, we will take $\Delta t = 1$ so that $t = 0, 1, \ldots, k$, if there is no possibility of confusion. The use of $\Delta t = 1$ involves no loss of generality because one can always reduce the time scale. The observations are number of the observed unlabeled and labeled cells $(U(s), W(s))$, for $s = 1, \ldots, r$.

The problem can be solved by using the self-organizing algorithm described earlier. However, as will be seen, it can also be solved using Markov chain Monte Carlo (MCMC) methods (see Gilks *et al.*, 1996), and WinBUGS (Spiegelhalter *et al.*, 2003), a computer program for Bayesian data analysis. To keep track of the number of labeled cells at time t, $W(t)$, one needs to know what happens to the $W(t - 1)$ cells (i.e., $W(t - \Delta t)$) and the number of the newly labeled cells, $NW(t)$, in the interval $(t - \Delta t, t]$. During $(t - \Delta t, t]$, each of the $W(t - 1)$ cells has a growth rate $(\beta - \delta)\Delta t$, and each of the $U(t - 1)$ cells is labeled at rate $2\beta\Delta t$. Therefore, $W(t)$ can be considered as the sum of $W(t - 1)$ and two binomial random variables. The conditional expected value of $W(t)$ given $(U(t - 1), W(t - 1))$ is

$$E(W(t) \mid W(t - 1), U(t - 1)) = W(t - 1) + W(t - 1)$$
$$\times (\beta - \delta)\Delta t + U(t - 1) \times 2\beta\Delta t.$$

Similarly, each $U(t - 1)$ cell has a probability of $\exp[-(\beta + \delta)\Delta t$ of being alive and non-labeled during $(t - \Delta t, t]$. Thus, $U(t) \sim \text{bin}(U(t - 1), \exp[-(\beta + \delta)\Delta t])$.

An alternative way to write down the model for the state space variable $S(t) = (U(t), W(t))$ is as follows. Let $B_W(t)$ and $D_W(t)$ denote respectively the numbers of new births and deaths of labeled cells (W cells) during $(t, t + \Delta t]$; $L_U(t)$ and $D_U(t)$ the new labeled (thus, also new birth), and deaths of unlabeled cells (U cells) during $(t, t + \Delta t]$. Then given $W(t)$, $(B_W(t), D_W(t))$ are multinomial with probabilities $(\beta\Delta t, \delta\Delta t)$; and given $U(t)$, $(L_U(t), D_U(t))$ are multinomial with probabilities $(\beta\Delta t, \delta\Delta t)$. Hence, by the conservation law,

$$W(t + \Delta t) - W(t) = B_W(t) - D_W(t) + 2L_U(t)$$
$$= W(t)(\beta - \delta)\Delta t + 2\beta U(t)\Delta t + \varepsilon_W(t)\Delta t, \quad (9.9)$$

$$U(t + \Delta t) - U(t) = -L_U(t) - D_U(t) = -(\beta + \delta)U(t)\Delta t + \varepsilon_U(t)\Delta t, \quad (9.10)$$

where the random noises are given by

$$\varepsilon_W(t)\Delta t = [B_W(t) - W(t)\beta\Delta t] - [D_W(t) - W(t)\delta\Delta t] + 2[L_U(t) - \beta U(t)\Delta t],$$

$$\varepsilon_U(t)t = [\beta U(t)\Delta t - L_U(t)] - [D_U(t) - \delta U(t)\Delta t t].$$

By dividing both sides of equations (9.9) and (9.10) by Δt, we obtain a system of stochastic differential equations,

$$\frac{dW(t)}{dt} = (\beta - \delta)W(t) + 2\beta U(t) + \varepsilon_W,$$

$$\frac{dU(t)}{dt} = -(\beta + \delta)U(t) + \varepsilon_U.$$

This is just an alternat expression for the same state space model as discussed earlier. However, it offers an opportunity to consider an approximate method for analyzing the labeling data. Note that if the random noise terms are dropped, the above system of equations reduce to the deterministic equations proposed by Zheng (1997). It is easy to obtain an analytic solution for this deterministic system of equations:

$$U = \exp[-(\beta + \delta)t],$$
$$W = [1 - \exp(-2\beta t)] \exp[(\beta - \delta)t],$$

which results in $W/N = 1 - \exp(-2\beta t)$.

The problem with this approach is that both U and W are assumed to be deterministic. In this chapter, the differential equation form will be retained because it offers a simple yet realistic example of state space modeling under the Bayesian framework. Therefore, our presentation should be viewed in the broader context of state space modeling rather than of solving a simple differential equation. This model can be solved under the Bayesian statistic framework by using WBDiff, a differential equation solver in WinBUGS developed by Dave Lunn of Imperial College. Note that this approach can be considered only as approximation of the state space model because the actual densities for the system and the observation equations are not explicitly considered even under the Bayesian framework. A similar (Bayesian) approach for a PBPK model would have to be used if a population pharmacokinetic model in which parameters are assumed to have probability distributions is considered (see Bois, 2001).

On the basis of three percentage LI measurements (8.7, 17.3, and 31.3, respectively, at days 2, 7, and 14) and the least squares method, Zheng (1997) estimated $\beta = 0.02329$ by using the approximation LI $= 1 - \exp(-2\beta t)$, which was originally proposed by Moolgavkar and Luebeck (1992b). This formulation is independent of both original cell numbers, $U(0)$, and cell death rate, δ. In light of the Zheng's theoretical concern about the Moolgavkar and Luebeck method and the discussion above, it is of interest to compare different formulations relating LI and cell birth rate β along with other factors, $U(0)$ and δ. Two issues are of interest here. First, is there a loss of valuable information because $U(0)$ and δ are not incorporated in the Moolgavkar–Luebeck formulation LI $= 1 - \exp(-2\beta t)$? Second, how can β and δ be estimated from the original data U and W when a state space model is used? It is of interest to estimate the parameters β and δ because of their importance in a BBDR model. Furthermore, it seems reasonable to infer that if LI were indeed independent of $U(0)$ and δ, then the use of LI would lead to loss of some valuable information from the labeling data. The first issue can be addressed, as shown in Table 9.1, by comparing LI values for a given set of parameters. These LIs are calculated by using three approaches:

(i)   the state space model with exact distribution;

(ii) differential equation solved under Bayesian framework; and

(iii) the Moolgavkar–Luebeck method (last column) in which LI is approximated by $1 - \exp(-2\beta t)$.

Table 9.1 Posterior mean (and standard deviation) of LI calculated by three different methods. N is number of cells at $t = 0$; β and δ are, respectively, birth and death rates per cell per day. LI is approximated by $1 - \exp(-2\beta t)$, as proposed by Moolgavkar and Lubeck (1992b) and discussed in Zheng (1997). This method does not depend on the initial number of cells $U(0)$ and the death rate δ.

					Differential equation method	Moolgavkar–Luebeck method
			Exact distribution method			
t, days	$N = 50\,000$ $\beta = 0.023\,29$ $\delta = 0.001$	$N = 50\,000$ $\beta = 0.023\,29$ $\delta = 0.001$	$N = 50\,000$ $\beta = 0.023\,29$ $\delta = 0.02$	$N = 500\,000$ $\beta = 0.023\,29$ $\delta = 0.02$	$N = 50\,000$ $\beta = 0.023\,29$ $\delta = 0.001$	$\beta = 0.023\,29$ independent of N and δ
2	0.089 (8.15×10^{-4})	0.089 (8.18×10^{-4})	0.090 (8.33×10^{-4})	0.090 (2.54×10^{-4})	0.089 (2.06×10^{-3})	0.089
4	0.170 (1.26×10^{-3})	0.170 (1.26×10^{-3})	0.172 (1.33×10^{-3})	0.172 (4.10×10^{-4})	0.170 (1.73×10^{-3})	0.170
6	0.244 (1.48×10^{-3})	0.244 (1.46×10^{-3})	0.247 (1.50×10^{-3})	0.247 (4.81×10^{-4})	0.244 (1.46×10^{-3})	0.244
7	0.278 (1.52×10^{-3})	0.278 (1.51×10^{-3})	0.282 (1.54×10^{-3})	0.282 (4.92×10^{-4})	0.278 (1.39×10^{-3})	0.278
8	0.311 (1.56×10^{-3})	0.311 (1.55×10^{-3})	0.315 (1.60×10^{-3})	0.315 (5.08×10^{-4})	0.311 (1.40×10^{-3})	0.311
10	0.372 (1.59×10^{-3})	0.372 (1.59×10^{-3})	0.377 (1.64×10^{-3})	0.377 (5.12×10^{-4})	0.372 (1.23×10^{-3})	0.372
12	0.428 (1.58×10^{-3})	0.428 (1.58×10^{-3})	0.433 (1.65×10^{-3})	0.433 (5.07×10^{-4})	0.428 (1.33×10^{-3})	0.428
14	0.479 (1.55×10^{-3})	0.479 (1.57×10^{-3})	0.484 (1.63×10^{-3})	0.484 (5.09×10^{-4})	0.479 (1.37×10^{-3})	0.479

Three WinBUGS programs, which are provided in the Appendix, are used in these simulations. Except for the third and fourth columns under the exact distribution method, the results in Table 9.1 suggest that all three methods provide the same estimate of the mean but different standard deviations (in parentheses). The results in the third and fourth columns under the exact distribution method suggest, however, that mean LI can change with δ. For instance, at 10 days, LI increases from 0.372 to 0.377, and there is a 1.7 % increase in birth rate from 0.02326 to 0.02366 if the Moolgavkar–Luebeck formula is used to estimate birth rate from LI.

Although these differences seem numerically negligible, it does recall a heatedly discussed issue of Moolgavkar (1994) and Crump (1994). On the basis of animal bioassay data, Crump (1994) demonstrated that an increase of merely 1 % of cell birth rate can result in an explosive (10^5) increase in the excess risk when the two-stage carcinogenesis model is used. In his response to Crump's comment, Moolgavkar (1994), while acknowledging the problem, indicated the importance of considering the change in both birth and death rates simultaneously. Thus, the use of LI to estimate birth rate alone could result in a loss of valuable information and a misleading prediction of excess risk, even if the numerical differences in Table 9.1 are small.

Therefore, an appropriate approach is to use state space modeling on the basis of original data used to compute LI. Furthermore, as expected, the LI standard deviation decreases when $U(0)$ increases, suggesting the importance of taking into account the original cell number $U(0)$. Two WinBUGS programs based on the differential equation method are provided in the Appendix: one is used to simulate the data $U(t)$ and $W(t)$, $t = 1, 2, \ldots, 14$, using $U(0) = 50\,000$, $\beta = 0.02329$, and $\delta = 1 \times 10^{-3}$, and the other is used to optimize parameters β and δ using the simulated U and W as observed data. The simulated data are given as observed data in the optimization program in the Appendix. Based on these data, 10 000 burn-in iterations, and 40 000 additional iterations, the median estimate of β is practically identical to the 0.023 29 used to simulate the data, and the median for δ is 9.70×10^{-4}, also very close to the value 1×10^{-3} originally used to simulate the data.

Although it is possible to develop a similar optimization program under the exact distribution method using WinBUGS, it does not appear practical to carry out actual calculations because it was estimated, based on the first 1000 iterations, that it would take about five days to obtain convergence on a Pentium III PC with 256 MB RAM. It is possible to develop an alternative computing method using the Kitagawa algorithm.

9.5.2   State space model of carcinogenesis

Although it is possible to formulate the multistage model using deterministic differential equations (Chu, 1985), for instance, by considering each of the three cell populations in a two-stage model – normal (N), initiated (I), and malignant (M) – as three compartments in a PBPK model, the stochastic nature of each of the cell populations is no longer preserved. Tan and Chen (1998) provided a new modeling procedure using stochastic differential equations and showed that the two-stage model is a special case of this modeling procedure (see Theorem 1 on p. 62 in Tan and Chen, 1998). Let us here illustrate the state space approach with two examples: a three-stage model (Fig. 9.1), and a three-pathway model (Fig. 9.2), both of which are motivated by DeAngelo (1996) who postulated that liver carcinomas induced by dichloroacetic acid (DCA) arise from a multipathway carcinogenesis. DCA is a liver metabolite in animals (rats and mice), and perhaps also

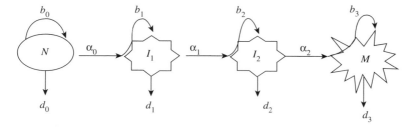

Figure 9.1   Three-stage model of carcinogenesis with transition rates α_i, $i = 0, 1, 2$; birth rate b_j and death rate d_j, $j = 0, 1, 2, 3$.

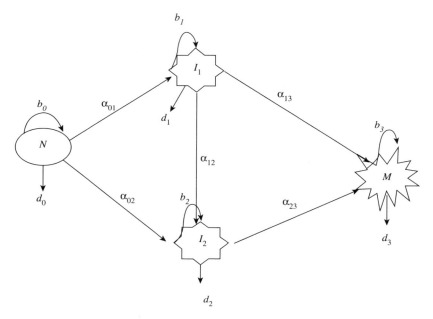

Figure 9.2 Three-pathway model of carcinogenesis with transition rates α_{ij}, $i = 0, 1, 2$, $j = 1, 2, 3$; birth and death rates b_i, d_i, respectively, $i = 0, 1, 2, 3$.

in humans, after exposure to trichloroethylene (TCE). DCA induces three types of liver tumors: hyperplastic nodules (HN), adenomas (AD), and carcinomas (CA). The normal cells, N, along with other tumor cell types, HN, AD, and CA, are denoted respectively as I_0(N), I_1(HN), I_2(AD), and I_3(CA) below.

9.5.2.1 A three-stage model of carcinogenesis

One three-stage model is the N–HN–AD–CA model where carcinomas are preceded by an adenoma, which in turn is preceded by a hyperplastic nodule, which originates from a normal stem cell (see Figure 9.1). Let α_i, $i = 0, 1, 2$ be the respective transition rate from I_i to I_{i+1}, $i = 0, 1, 2$ and b_j and d_j, $j = 0, 1, 2, 3$, cell division (birth) and differentiation (death) rates respectively for I_j, $j = 0, 1, 2, 3$. Let $X(t) = (I_0(t), I_1(t), I_2(t))$. As shown in Tan and Chen (1998), over a small time interval $(t, t + \Delta t)$, the transition from $X(t)$ to $X(t + \Delta t)$ is characterized by the following quantities:

$B_j(t) =$ number of new I_j cells during $(t, t + \Delta t]$ for $j = 0, 1, 2$,

$D_j(t) =$ number of dead I_j cells during $(t, t + \Delta t]$ for $j = 0, 1, 2$,

$M_j(t) =$ number of new I_j cells arising from I_{j-1} for $j = 1, 2, 3$, during $(t, t + \Delta t]$.

Note that $M_3(t)$ is the primary malignant cell occurring during the time interval $(t, t + \Delta t]$. Conditional on $X(t)$, to the order of $o(\Delta t)$, the above quantities are distributed as multinomial (Mult) and Poisson (Pois) variables:

$$\{B_j(t), D_j(t) \mid I_j(t)\} \sim \text{Mult}(I_j(t), b_j\Delta t, d_j\Delta t), \qquad \text{for} \quad j = 1, 2; \qquad (9.11)$$

$$\{M_j(t) \mid I_j(t)\} \sim \text{Pois}(I_j(t)\alpha_j\Delta t), \qquad \text{for} \quad j = 0, 1, 2. \qquad (9.12)$$

Expressions (9.11) and (9.12) are conditional probability functions that can be used for sampling. Because the conditioned variable I_j is a random variable, the actual implementation of (9.11) in a software package (such as WinBUGS) may require some modification. Now we have the following stochastic difference equations, for $N(t) = I_0(t)$, $I_1(t)$, and $I_2(t)$

$$N(t + \Delta t) = N(t) + B_0(t) - D_0(t),$$
$$I_1(t + \Delta t) = I_1(t) + M_1(t) + B_1(t) - D_1(t),$$
$$I_2(t + \Delta t) = I_2(t) + M_2(t) + B_2(t) - D_2(t).$$

By letting $\Delta t \to 0$, we have the stochastic differential equations,

$$\frac{dN(t)}{dt} = N(t)\gamma_0(t) + e_0(t), \qquad (9.13)$$

$$\frac{dI_1(t)}{dt} = N(t)\mu_0(t) + I_1(t)\gamma_1(t) + e_1(t), \qquad (9.14)$$

$$\frac{dI_2(t)}{dt} = I_1(t)\mu_1(t) + I_2(t)\gamma_2(t) + e_2(t). \qquad (9.15)$$

where

$$\gamma_j(t) = b_j(t) - d_j(t),$$
$$e_0(t)\Delta t = [B_0(t) - N(t)b_0(t)\Delta t] - [D_0(t) - N(t)d_0(t)\Delta t],$$

and, for $j = 1, 2$,

$$e_j(t)\Delta t = [M_j(t) - I_{j-1}(t)\alpha_{j-1}(t)\Delta t] + [B_j(t) - I_j(t)b_j(t)\Delta t] - [D_j(t) - I_j(t)d_j(t)\Delta t].$$

Denote $\Omega_j(t) = [B_j(t), D_j(t), M_{j+1}(t)]$, $j = 0, 1, 2$. The conditional probability of $\Omega_j(t)$, given $I_j(t)$, is a multinomial with parameters $\{I_j(t); \alpha_j(t)\Delta t, b_j(t)\Delta t, d_j(t)\Delta t\}$ to order $o(\Delta t)$ – that is,

$$\{\Omega_j(t) \mid I_j(t)\} \sim \text{Mult}[I_j(t); \alpha_j(t)\Delta t, b_j(t)\Delta t, d_j(t)\Delta t]. \qquad (9.16)$$

Given $X(t) = \{N(t), I_j(t), j = 1, 2\}$, the error terms e_i, $i = 0, 1, 2$, in (9.13)–(9.15) are uncorrelated and

$$E[e_i(t) \mid X(t)] = 0, \qquad \text{Var}[e_i(t) \mid X(t)] = I_{j-1}(t)\alpha_{j-1}(t)\Delta t + I_j(t)[b_j(t) + d_j(t)].$$

The system of equations (9.13)–(9.15), when combined with an observation equation that depends on the type of data available, can be used to estimate state variables and model parameters. It is instructive to provide an intuitive interpretation of (9.13)–(9.15), as the same concept can be easily applied to construct any model, no matter how complex Equation (9.13) says that the rate of change of the N-cells at time t is proportional to the number of N-cells at time t, with proportionality constant $\gamma_0(t) = \alpha_0(t) - \beta_0(t)$, the net difference of cell division and differentiation rates at time t, with a random error term e_0. Equation (9.14) says that the rate of change of the I_1 cells at time t equals the sum of newly formed I_1 cells from the normal cells and those from the net growth of the existing I_1 cells, with a random error term e_1. The interpretation of I_2 is similar to that of I_1, except that the role of N is now taken by I_1.

So far we have not considered malignant cells. Our interest in this aspect is the number of tumors (e.g., carcinomas) per animal and the incidence of malignant tumors (i.e., number of animals with the tumor). This is equally applicable to foci and benign tumors. Most of the existing two-stage models assume that a single malignant cell is equivalent to a tumor. This condition can be relaxed by assuming that a tumor develops solely from a primary malignant cell. For more discussion of this concept, see Yang and Chen (1991), and Chen et al. (1991).

Assume that a carcinoma becomes detectable when a clone originating from a primary malignant cell (i.e., I_3 or M-cell) contains at least n_M cells. According to Tan and Chen (1995), the probability of a clone originating from a primary malignant cell at time s and becoming detectable at time t, given it is non-extinct, is

$$P_M(s,t) = \frac{C_1(s,t)}{1 + C_2(s,t)} \left[\frac{C_2(s,t)}{1 + C_2(s,t)} \right]^{n_M - 1} \tag{9.17}$$

where

$$C_1(s,t) = \exp\left\{ \int_s^t (b(x) - d(x))dx, \qquad C_2(s,t) = \int_s^t b(x)C_1(x,t)dx. \right.$$

This probability function has a form proportional to a geometric distribution and thus can be interpreted intuitively as being the distribution for a random variable representing the number of Bernoulli trials until success. This is a generalization of the time homogeneous case investigated by Dewanji et al. (1989), and Chen et al. (1991).

Let $M(t)$ and $T(t)$ be, respectively, the number of malignant cells and number of tumors per animal at time t. By applying the same modeling principle as above, the number of malignant cells at time t, $M(t) = I_3(t)$, satisfies the differential equation

$$\frac{dM(t)}{dt} = I_2(t)\alpha_2(t) + e_M(t), \tag{9.18}$$

where e_M is the random noise for the three-event model, with

$$E(e_M(t) \mid I_2(t)) = 0, \qquad \mathrm{Var}(e_M(t) \mid I_2(t)) = I_2(t)\alpha_2(t).$$

To obtain the probability distribution of $T(t)$, let $M(s,t)$ be the total number of detectable tumors at time t arising from the primary M-cells during the time interval $(s, s + \Delta t)$. Then, to order $o(\Delta t)$, the probability distribution of $M(s,t)$, given $I_2(t)$ cells at time t, is a binomial variable with parameters $\{I_2(s), P_M(s,t)\}$. Therefore, the total number of observable tumors at time t is the sum of all $M(s,t)$, for $s \leq t$:

$$T(t) = \int_0^t I_2(s)\alpha_2(s)P_M(s,t)ds + e_M(t), \tag{9.19}$$

where the random noise e_M has expected value 0 and variance

$$\text{Var}[e_M(t)] = \int_0^t E[I_2(s)]\alpha_2(s)P_M(s,t)ds.$$

The probability distribution of observing a malignant tumor can be derived as

$$P(t) = 1 - \exp\left[-\int_0^t I_2(s)\alpha_2(s)P_M(s,t)ds\right].\tag{9.20}$$

These results, along with an observation equation that depends on the type of data at hand, can be used to form a state space model. It is interesting to note that the modeling procedure described here easily resolves the problem of computing the probability of observing tumor in animal bioassays discussed in Yang and Chen (1991), in which a theoretical formulation was developed but no practical computation approach was offered.

9.5.2.2 A multiple-pathway model

As discussed previously, the following three-pathway model was motivated by DCA-induced liver tumors: hyperplastic nodules, adenomas, and carcinomas. The model can be easily generalized to include additional pathways without unduly complicating the model formulation, although, the cost of computation would be increased.

Using the intuitive interpretation, the three-pathway model for the DCA can be readily written as follows:

$$\frac{dN(t)}{dt} = N(t)\gamma_0(t) + e_0(t),\tag{9.21}$$

$$\frac{dI_1(t)}{dt} = N(t)\alpha_{01}(t) + I_1(t)\gamma_1(t) + e_1(t),\tag{9.22}$$

$$\frac{dI_2(t)}{dt} = N(t)\alpha_{02}(t) + I_1(t)\alpha_{12}(t) + I_2(t)\gamma_2(t) + e_2(t),\tag{9.23}$$

where, as shown in Figure 9.2, $\alpha_{01}(t)$ and $\alpha_{02}(t)$ are the rates of transition from normal to I_1 and I_2 cells, α_{12} is the transition rate from I_1 to I_2, and $\gamma_i = b_i - d_i$, for $i = 0, 1, 2$. The number of malignant cell M at time t satisfies the equation

$$\frac{dM(t)}{dt} = I_1(t)\alpha_{21}(t) + I_2(t)\alpha_{22}(t) + e_M(t),\tag{9.24}$$

where α_{21} and α_{22} are, respectively, the transition rate from I_i, $i = 1, 2$, to M, and e_M is the sum of two random noises for the multiple-pathway model. The number of malignant tumors, $T(t)$, and the probability of observing a malignant tumor, $P(t)$, at time t can be similarly derived as in (9.19) and (9.20) above:

$$T(t) = \int_0^t [I_1(s)\alpha_{21}(s) + I_2(s)\alpha_{22}(s)]P_M(s,t)ds + e_M(t),\tag{9.25}$$

where the random noise e_M has expected value 0 and variance

$$\mathrm{Var}[e_M(t)] = \int_0^t \{E[I_1(s)]\alpha_{21}(s) + E[I_2(s)]\alpha_{22}(s)\}P(s,t)ds. \qquad (9.26)$$

The probability distribution of cancer incidence can be derived as

$$P(t) = 1 - \exp\left[-\int_0^t \{I_1(s)\alpha_{21}(s) + I_2(s)\alpha_{22}(s)\}P_M(s,t)ds\right]. \qquad (9.27)$$

9.6 A COMPUTING PROCEDURE FOR THE THREE-STAGE MODEL

There are at least two approaches to implementing the calculations for unknown state variables, X, and parameters, θ, in the three-stage model: using existing MCMC software for Bayesian statistical analysis such as WinBUGS and the probability distributions (9.7), (9.12), (9.16), (9.19), and (9.20), along with likelihood function, which depends on available data; or developing a program by using the algorithm based on the concepts of sampling and resampling by Smith and Gelfand (1992) and Kitagawa (1998).

The basic idea of both approaches is easy to understand if one considers an example of a classic problem of estimating an unknown θ given the observation Y. The main idea is to update the prior density, $P(\theta)$, to the posterior density, $P(\theta \mid Y)P(\theta)L(\theta \mid Y)$, through the medium of the likelihood function, $L(\theta \mid Y)$; that is, the likelihood function is acting as a resampling probability.

We will need the following notation to implement the self-organizing procedure: t_M, the maximum lifetime given in some time unit; $X(t) = (I_0(t), I_1(t), I_2(t))$, the state variables at time t; $X = \{X(1), \ldots, X(t_M)\}$, the collection of all values of X at each time point; $\Theta(t) = \{\alpha_i(t), i = 0, 1, 2; b_i(t), d_i(t), i = 0, 1, 2, 3\}$, the set of all parameters; and $\Omega(t) = \{M_0(t), M_1(t), B_i(t), D_i(t), i = 1, 2, 3\}$, the set of newly generated cells from transition, birth, and death processes. The observations are assumed to be $Y = \{y_{ij}, n_{ij}\}$, for n age groups indexed by $i = 1, \ldots, n$, and m exposure groups indexed by $j = 1, \ldots, m$; y_{ij} and n_{ij} are, respectively, the number of cancer cases and person years in the (i,j)th group from an epidemiological study.

The strategy for estimating the parameters θ and X is as follows:

1. For given state variables X and parameters θ, take a large sample from $P(\Omega \mid X, \theta)$ and resample by weight calculated from $P(Y \mid X, \theta)$. Denote the selected sample as Ω^*.

2. For given Ω^* and θ, take a large sample from $P(X \mid \Omega^*, \theta)$ and resample with weight calculated from $P(Y \mid X, \theta)$. Denote the selected sample as X^*.

3. Generate θ from $P(\theta \mid X^*, \Omega^*, Y)P(\theta)P(X^*, \Omega^*, Y \mid \theta)$, where $P(\theta)$ is the prior for θ.

4. Repeat steps 1–3 until convergence. Upon convergence, one can approximate the densities for X and θ by sampling, respectively, from $P(X \mid Y)$ and $P(\theta \mid Y)$.

To facilitate the procedure, various conditional densities are needed. Note that

$$P(X \mid \theta) = \prod_{t=1}^{t_M} \prod_{i=1}^{2} P[I_i(t) \mid I_{i-1}(t-1), I_i(t-1), \theta], \qquad (9.28)$$

where

$$P[I_i(t+1) \mid I_{i-1}(t), I_i(t), \theta] =$$

$$\sum_{j=0}^{I_i(t+1)-I_i(t)} p_i(j,t) \sum_{r=0}^{I_i(t)} C_r^{I_i(t)} C_{a_i(r,j;t)}^{I_i(t)-r} b_l^r(t) d_i^{a_i(r,j;t)} [1 - b_i(t) - d_i(t)]^{I_i(t+1)-2r-j\}},$$

$$(9.29)$$

in which C_r^n denotes the binomial combinatory coefficient, $a_i(r,j;t) = I_i(t) - I_i(t+1) + r + j$, for $i = 0, 1, 2$, and $p_i(j,t)$ is the density of a Poisson distribution with mean $\lambda_i = I_i(t)\alpha_i(t)$, for $i = 1, 2$. The conditional density of X and Ω, given $X(0)$ and Θ, is

$$P(X, \Omega \mid X(0), \theta) = \prod_{t=1}^{t_M} P(X(t) \mid X(t-1), \Omega(t-1), \theta)P(\Omega(t-1) \mid X(t-1), \theta),$$

$$(9.30)$$

where, on the basis of conditional distribution given by (9.11) and (9.12),

$$P(\Omega(t) \mid X(t), \theta) = \prod_{i=1}^{2} C_{B_i(t)}^{I_i(t)} p_{i-1}(M_{i-1}(t); t) b_i^{B_i(t)}(t)[1 - b_i(t)]^{I_i(t)-B_i(t)}, \qquad (9.31)$$

$$P(X(t) \mid X(t-1), \Omega(t-1)) = \prod_{1}^{2} C_{\eta_i(t-1)}^{I_i(t-1)} \left[\frac{d_i(t-1)}{1 - b_i(t-1)} \right]^{\eta_i(t-1)}$$

$$\cdot \left[1 - \frac{d_i(t-1)}{1 - b_i(t-1)} \right]^{\varsigma_i(t-1)}, \qquad (9.32)$$

with $\eta_i(t-1) = I_i(t-1) - I_i(t) + M_{i-1}(t-1) + B_i(t-1)$, $\varsigma_i(t-1) = I_i(t) - M_{i-1}(t-1) - 2B_i(t-1)$, for $i = 1, 2$.

The conditional distribution of Y_{ij}, given $I_2(i,j) = \{I_2(t;r,i,j), 0 \le t \le t_j, r = 1, \ldots, y_{ij}\}$, is binomial $Y_i(j) \sim \text{bin}(n_{ij}, P_{ij})$ This can be approximated by a Poisson distribution with expected value $\lambda_{ij} = n_{ij}P_{ij}$,

$$f_Y(y_{ij} \mid I_2(i,j)) = \frac{1}{y_{ij}!} \exp(-\lambda_{ij}) \lambda_{ij}^{y_{ij}}$$

$$= \frac{1}{y_{ij}!} \exp \left\{ y_{ij} \log(n_{ij}) - \sum_{r=1}^{y_{ij}} [X_r(t_{j-1}; i,j) \right.$$

$$\left. - \log(1 - \exp(-Z_r(i,j)] - \lambda_{ij} \right\}, \qquad (9.33)$$

where

$$X_r(t; i, j) = \sum_{l=1}^{t} I_2(l; r, i, j)\alpha_2(i, l), \qquad Z_r(i, j) = X_r(t; i, j) - X_r(t_{j-1}; i, j).$$

Thus, the joint distribution of $\{X, \Omega, Y\}$ conditional on θ is

$$P(X, \Omega, Y \mid \theta) = P(\Omega(0) \mid X(0)) \prod_{i=1}^{m} \prod_{j=1}^{n} f_Y(y_{ij} \mid I_2(i, j))$$

$$\cdot \prod_{l=t_{j-1}+1}^{t_j} P[X(i, l) \mid \Omega(i, l-1), X(i, l-1)] P(\Omega(i, l-1) \mid X(i, l)),$$

(9.34)

and the posterior distribution of θ, given (X, Ω, Y), is

$$P(\theta \mid X, \Omega, Y) \propto p(\theta) \prod_{i=1}^{m} p_i(\alpha_2(i)) \prod_{j=1}^{n} \prod_{s=1}^{2} \exp[-m_{s-1}(i, j)\alpha_{s-1}(i, j)]$$

$$\cdot [\alpha_{i-1}(i, j)]^{M_{s-1}(i,j)} [b_{s(i,j)}]^{B_s(i,j)} [d_s(i, j)]^{\eta_s(i,j)} [1 - b_s(i, j) - d_s(i, j)]^{\zeta_s(i,j)},$$

(9.35)

where

$$p_i(\alpha_2) = \exp\left\{ \sum_{j=1}^{n} \sum_{r=1}^{y_{ij}} [\alpha_2 X_r(t_{j-1} : i) - \log[1 - \exp(-\alpha_2 Z_r(j : i))]] - \right.$$

$$\left. \sum_{j=1}^{n} E\{\exp[\log(n_{ij}) - \alpha_2 X_r(t_{j-1} : i)][1 - \exp(-\alpha_2 Z(j : i))]\} \right\},$$

$$X_r(t : i) = \sum_{l=1}^{t} I_2(l : r, i, j),$$

$$Z_r(j : i) = X_r(t_j : i) - X_r(t_{j-1} : i),$$

$$X(t : i) = \sum_{l=1}^{t} I_2(l : i, j),$$

$$Z(j : i) = X(t_j : i) - X(t_{j-1} : i),$$

and where $I_2(l : i, j)$ is the number of individuals $I_2(l)$ in the (i, j)th group. The conditional distributions above can be used to implement the sampling procedure.

9.7   DISCUSSION

The modeling procedure used in this chapter was inspired by the desire to resolve a problem in Yang and Chen (1991) in which a stochastic model was developed to reflect more realistically the way in which tumors are counted in a laboratory: a primary solid tumor can only develop from a focus that originates from a primary initiated cell. However, the computational aspect of the model was a challenge. It turns out that the unified modeling procedure described in this chapter not only provides a solution to the problem in Yang and Chen (1991), but also is applicable to modeling other biological processes. This chapter demonstrates that it is possible to model dynamic events along the continuum from source of exposure to the disease endpoints using a single mathematical procedure that is conceptually similar to a conventional *deterministic* PBPK model but computationally more complicated when the events involved are *stochastic*. For risk assessors, the feature of being able to model this process as a PBPK model, at least conceptually, is highly desirable, because PBPK models have been routinely used in risk assessment practice and furthermore, because of the increasing use of population PBPK models which are also stochastic and computationally much more involved than conventional PBPK models. This argues for the need to further improve the procedure and to develop software to implement the computation more efficiently.

Although we have a far from complete understanding of the mechanism or mode of action of cancer and other diseases induced by exposure to a chemical, it becomes increasingly clear that we must attempt to exploit the exponential growth of information coming from current research activities. As envisioned by Strohman (2002), the dynamic system of phenotype generation involves the strategy used by dynamic protein networks that generate the phenotype from the genotype. Control of a global phenotype such as disease may be localized in a single regulatory system (metabolic, hormone signals, etc.) or distributed over many systems and levels. This type of information on cell signaling holds the promise of unraveling the cellular basis of a wide variety of adverse health effects, including cancers that may be related to chemical exposure. It also dictates the need to develop a flexible and easy-to-use mathematical tool that goes beyond the current modeling procedures, which are confined to the tissue-based PBPK model and the hard-to-modify BBDR model. With the advance of molecular biology, more biological information will become available and is expected to be incorporated into quantitative risk assessment. The importance of this emerging issue is underscored in US EPA (2003d).

It is desirable to develop a mathematical procedure which is easily applicable to construct a stochastic model that can incorporate biological information from source of exposure to activation of signaling pathways, to cellular response, and finally to disease endpoints. Such a procedure would be useful for assessing not only cancer, but also endocrine disrupters, just to mention two areas of keen interest in the risk assessment community. A unified modeling procedure to incorporate biological information from exposure to disease endpoints is proposed in this chapter. The procedure takes advantage of increasing computing power as well as the innovative statistical methods in sampling techniques such as the MCMC method, which has already been applied to extend a conventional PBPK model into a population model by using Bayesian statistics.

Although the theoretical foundation for the unified modeling procedure has mostly been resolved, the implementation of computation has yet to be accomplished.

It is possible to carry out some moderate modeling on desktop computers, but it often takes several days to obtain convergence. Part of the reason is that the existing software packages for MCMC are designed for general use for Bayesian statistical analysis. Even if one can trick the program into doing a task, it often cannot be computationally efficient because of its overhead for general usage. Clearly, a collective effort from the risk assessment community is needed if such a procedure is to become practical and user-friendly.

APPENDIX: SIMULATION PROGRAMS

Three WinBUGS computer programs that are used to carry out computations for the state space model for cell labeling are given in this Appendix. Simulation program I (exact distribution method) is used to simulate LI values in columns 2 to 5 in Table 9.1. Simulation program II (differential equation method) is used to simulate LI values in column 6 in Table 9.1. The data, $X(t)$ and $Y(t)$, for $t = 1, \ldots, 14$, are used as observations to test the optimization program. We conclude with an optimization program (differential equation method) for estimating parameters using simulated data.

Simulation program I

```
model
  { b<-0.02329
    d<-0.00100
    tb<-2*b
      br<-(b-d)
      bd<-exp(-(b+d))
    #Bugs does not allow index to start at 0=1
  x[1] <-48840 #actual simulated (observed) value
    y[1] <-2362 #actual simulated (observed) value
      for (i in 2:n.grid) {
    x[i] ~dbin( bd, x[i-1] )
  y1[i] ~dbin(br, y[i-1] )
  y2[i] ~dbin(tb, x[i-1] )
  y[i] <-y1[i] +y2[i] +y[i-1]
  LI[i] <-y[i] / (x[i] +y[i] )
    }
    }
DATA
list(
n.grid = 14
)
```

Simulation program II

```
model {
    solution[ 1:n.grid, 1:dim] <- ode(init[ 1:dim] , grid[ 1:n.grid] , D(C[ 1:dim] , t),
    origin, tol)
    D(C[X] , t) <- -g0 * C[X]
    D(C[Y] , t) <- g1* C[Y] +2* beta* C[ X]
    g0<-beta+delta
    g1<-beta-delta
    N<-C[1] +C[2]
# Initial conditions:
    init[X] <- 50000; init[Y] <- 0
# Stochastic model:
    for (i in 1:n.grid) {
        datay[i] ~dnorm(solution[i, Y] , tau) I(0,)
        datax[i] ~dnorm(solution[i, X] , tau) I(0,)
    LI[i] <-datay[ i] / (datax[i] +datay[i] )
    }
    tau ~ dunif(0, 0.001)
    }
DATA
list(
X = 1, Y = 2, beta=0.02329, delta=0.0010,
n.grid = 14,
dim = 2,
origin = 0,
tol = 1.000000E-3,
grid = c(1,2,3,4,5,6,7,8,9,10,11,12,13,14)
)
INITS
list( datax=c(100,100,100,100,100,100,100,100,100,100,100,100,100,100),
datay=c(100,100,100,100,100,100,100,100,100,100,100,100,100,100)
)
```

Optimization program

This model uses simulated data *x* and *y* as observations to optimize parameters.

```
model {
    solution[1:n.grid, 1:dim] <- LIModel(init[1:dim] , grid[1:n.grid] , theta[1:n.par] , origin, tol)
    theta[1] <- beta; theta[2] <- delta;
# Initial conditions:
    init[xx] <-50000; init[ yy] <- 0;
# Stochastic model:
    for (i in 1:n.grid) {
```

```
        datay[i] ~ dnorm(solution[ i,yy] , tau)
        datax[i] ~dnorm(solution[ i, xx] , tau)
        LI[ i] <-datay[ i] / (datax[ i] +datay[ i] )
    }
        beta ~ dnorm(data.beta, param.prec) I (0, 1)
    delta ~ dnorm(data.delta, param.prec) I (0, beta)
    tau ~ dunif (0, 0.001)
}
DATA
list ( xx = 1, yy = 2,
n.grid = 14,
dim = 2,
origin = 0,
tol = 1.0E-3,
grid = c ( 1, 2,3,4,5,6,7,8,9,10,11, 12, 13,14),
datax = c (
48840.00 47614.92, 46504.89, 45327.59, 44294.50, 43244.63, 42157.73, 41130.48,
40174.67, 39251.35, 38272.30, 37387.06, 36487.22, 35615.84),
datay = c (
2362.62, 4639.18, 6914.03, 9279.32, 11616.87, 13922.08,16269.94, 18499.90,
20926.26, 23199.02, 25649.21, 28032.79, 30402.31, 32768.56),
data.beta=0.05, data.delta=0.02,
n.par = 2,
param.prec=0.01
)
Initial values:
list(beta= 0.35, delta=0.022)
```

The above optimization program depends on the compiled program MODULE WBDiffLIModel:

```
    IMPORT
      GraphNodes,
      WBDiffODE,
      Math;

    TYPE
      Equations = POINTER TO RECORD (WBDiffODE.Equations) END;
      Factory = POINTER TO RECORD (GraphNodes.Factory) END;

    CONST
      nEq = 2;

      bb = 0; dd = 1;
      xx = 0; yy = 1;

      VAR
```

```
      fact-: GraphNodes.Factory;
PROCEDURE (e: Equations) Derivatives (IN theta, C: ARRAY OF REAL; n: INTEGER; t: REAL;   OUT
dCdt: ARRAY OF REAL);
      VAR
        i: INTEGER;
        beta, delta: REAL;
      K: ARRAY 2 OF REAL;

      BEGIN
        i: = 0;
        WHILE i < 2 DO;
          K[i] : = theta[ bb + i] ;


            INC(i);
        END;
        dCdt[xx] : = - (K[0] +K[1] ) * C[xx] ;
        dCdt[yy] : = (K[0] -K[1] ) * C[yy] + 2*K[0]*C[xx] ;
      END Derivatives;


      PROCEDURE (equations: Equations) SecondDerivatives (IN theta, x:
ARRAY OF REAL;
                      numEq: INTEGER; t: REAL;
                      OUT d2xdt2: ARRAY OF REAL);
      BEGIN
        HALT(126)
      END SecondDerivatives;


      PROCEDURE (equations: Equations) Jacobian (IN theta, x: ARRAY OF REAL;
                  numEq: INTEGER; t: REAL;
                  OUT jacob: ARRAY OF ARRAY OF REAL);
      BEGIN
        HALT(126)
      END Jacobian;


      PROCEDURE (f: Factory) New (option: INTEGER): GraphNodes.Node;
      VAR
        equations: Equations;
        node: GraphNodes.Node;
      BEGIN
        NEW(equations);
        node: = WBDiffODE.NewNode(equations, nEq);
        RETURN node
      END New;
```

```
    PROCEDURE Install*;
    BEGIN
      WBDiffODE.Install(fact)
    END Install;

    PROCEDURE Init;
    VAR
      f: Factory;
    BEGIN
      NEW(f); fact: = f
    END Init;

BEGIN
    Init
END WBDiffLIMod
```

CHAPTER 10

Modeling Lung Cancer Screening

Marek Kimmel
Rice University

Olga Y. Gorlova
MD Anderson Cancer Center

Claudia I. Henschke
Weill Medical College of Cornell University

10.1 INTRODUCTION

Screening for lung cancer remains a contentious issue. The reason is that, while chest X-ray (CXR) and sputum cytology increased detection rates for small isolated tumors, which have all the histological features of lung cancer, these findings were not translated into statistically significant differences in deaths due to lung cancer in randomized controlled trials. This, in turn, caused many experts to suggest that the increase in detection is merely overdiagnosis – discovery of non-progressing 'pseudo-cancers'. The controversy that followed is not limited to lung cancer screening. Similar doubts regarding efficacy of screening were expressed in the context of breast, prostate and colon cancer, to mention only the most important organ sites. With reference to lung cancer, the acuteness of this problem has increased as CT scanning for lung cancer is already well established in everyday diagnostic routine, generating findings that must be addressed by physicians.

One of the tools to elucidate this issue is mathematical modeling. It enables us to tie together the outcomes of screening studies, with and without control groups, as well as data from cancer registries. In addition, it makes it possible to determine the

Recent Advances in Quantitative Methods in Cancer and Human Health Risk Assessment
Edited by L. Edler and C. Kitsos   © 2005 John Wiley & Sons, Ltd

statistical power of randomized controlled trials planned as well as to predict the outcomes of long-term mass-screening programs.

This chapter starts with a review of past and current lung cancer screening studies. Then, we outline the principles of modeling of screening and treatment, by following the natural history of the disease and accounting for statistical effects such as length-biased sampling and lead-time bias. We review the existing modeling approaches, including issues such as model building, estimation of parameters, prediction of reduction of mortality from lung cancer, and cost-efficiency analysis. Finally, we explore the design issues, using as an example the current National Lung Screening Trial (NLST).

10.2   SCREENING AND OTHER RELEVANT STUDIES

10.2.1   Czechoslovak study

This randomized controlled trial of screening for lung cancer included males aged 40–64 years; all were current smokers. After removing 19 lung cancer cases detected at the prevalence screen, the participants were randomized into an intervention arm (3171 individuals) and a control arm (3174 individuals). The intervention group received a total of six CXR and sputum examinations at 6-month intervals. The control arm received a single examination by the same two modalities 3 years after the prevalence screen. After that a CXR examination was performed every year in both the intervention and control arms for 3 years (i.e., three more times).

10.2.2   Memorial Sloan-Kettering Cancer Center (MSKCC) and Johns Hopkins Medical Institution (JHMI) studies

These studies recruited male smokers (who had smoked at least one pack per day), were more than 45 years of age, with an estimated survival of no less than 5 years, no evidence of lung cancer on an initial evaluation, and sufficient lung function to tolerate lobectomy. The design was identical in both studies. Participants were randomized to either CXR alone or CXR and sputum cytology examination. CXR was performed annually and sputum cytology examination was performed every 4 months. The MSKCC trial had 4968 participants examined with both modalities and 5072 individuals receiving CXRs only. The JHMI trial enrolled 5226 individuals screened with both CXR and sputum examinations and 5161 individuals who got annual CXRs only.

10.2.3   Mayo Lung Project (MLP)

Like the MSKCC and JHMI studies, this study recruited males who smoked at least one pack per day, were older than 45, and had an estimated survival of no less than 5 years, no evidence of lung cancer on an initial evaluation, and sufficient lung function to tolerate lobectomy. Out of 10 933 subjects enrolled, 91 prevalence cases were excluded and the rest randomized into the screening or control group. The screened group had CXRs and sputum cytology examination every 4 months for 6 years; the control group received a recommendation to get yearly CXR and sputum examinations. Subjects were then followed up for between 1 and 5.5 years. By the end of the study the compliance fell to 75 % and more than a half of the control group also underwent CXR during the study period.

10.2.4 MD Anderson case–control study

This is an ongoing hospital-based case–control study. As of March 2004, almost 4000 cases and controls have been enrolled. The cases were accrued from the University of Texas M.D. Anderson Cancer Center, Houston, Texas. Patients were newly diagnosed, previously untreated with either chemotherapy or radiotherapy, and histologically confirmed. The controls were recruited on a volunteer basis from a large multi-specialty physician group with a network of 23 clinics in the Houston metropolitan area. The controls did not have a previous diagnosis of any cancer (except non-melanoma cancer of the skin). The identification and recruitment of the case and control study subjects is described in detail elsewhere (Hudmon *et al.*, 1997). This study includes more than 1700 cases and controls who are former smokers and more than 600 never smokers. The majority of cases and controls were also administered tests of mutagen sensitivity and DNA repair capacity (DRC), to determine the association of these indices with lung cancer. Molecular epidemiological studies have shown that sensitivity to mutagens and suboptimal DRC are independent risk factors for developing lung cancer (Wu *et al.*, 1998; Wei *et al.*, 2000). These assays use a chemical or physical mutagen challenge (such as the mutagen sensitivity assay), or measure cellular ability to remove adducts from plasmids transfected into lymphocyte cultures *in vitro* by expression of damaged reporter genes (host cell reactivation assay). This latter assay is a direct measure of repair kinetics, unlike the cytogenetic assays that only indirectly infer DRC from cellular damage remaining after mutagenic exposure and recovery (Berwick and Vineis, 2000), and as such likely reflect general and non-specific impairment of the DNA repair machinery.

10.2.5 Early Lung Cancer Action Project

The Early Lung Cancer Action Project (ELCAP) is a prospective study which enrolled a cohort of 1000 smokers and former smokers in New York City at two medical centers, Weill Medical College of Cornell University and New York University Medical Center. Baseline enrollment started in 1993 and continued to 1998; annual repeat screening was started in 1993 and continued to 2004. Those enrolled were volunteers who at baseline screening were at least 60 years of age, had a history of at least 10 pack-years of cigarette smoking and no prior diagnosis of cancer. At baseline, their median age was 67 years and the median number of pack-years of smoking was 45. The regimen of screening was defined by a protocol; the definition of a positive result of the initial low-dose CT and subsequent work-up was different on baseline and annual repeat screening. Baseline results are reported by Henschke *et al.* (1999) and annual repeat results by Henschke *et al.* (2001).

10.2.6 New York Early Lung Cancer Action Project

The New York ELCAP (www.NYELCAP.org) was started in 2001 because of the considerable interest in CT screening for lung cancer sparked by the ELCAP results and because it was recognized that expansion especially of the repeat screening experience was needed. It has recruited 6318 subjects for baseline screening and a single annual repeat screening using the same indications for screening and design as the original ELCAP. This design makes a sharp distinction between screening *per se* – the pursuit of early diagnosis – and the interventions that may result from this (Henschke *et al.*, 2003a, 2004a). The focus of NY-ELCAP was on evaluating the usefulness of a particular regimen of CT screening for lung cancer in terms of its diagnostic productivity. The entry criteria were the same as for ELCAP. Volunteers were recruited at 12 institutions throughout New York State and the screenings and management were performed at each of the participating sites with the Coordinating Center at Weill Medical College of Cornell University. At baseline, their median age was 66 years and the median number of pack-years of smoking was 40. The regimen of screening was defined by an updated protocol as new CT scanners were available which could obtain much thinner sections (Henschke *et al.*, 2002a, 2002b, 2005) and knowledge had been gained from the previous ELCAP study. As a result the definition of a positive result of the initial low-dose CT and subsequent work-up had to be updated and it was different on baseline and annual repeat screening. (Henschke *et al.*, 2002b).

10.2.7 International Early Lung Cancer Action Program

A third study, the International (I-)ELCAP (www.IELCAP.org) was started to perform 30 000 baseline and repeat screenings at institutions throughout the world with the goal of addressing the issue of overdiagnosis and curative effectiveness of the early interventions that the regimen's application provides for (Henschke *et al.*, 2003b). It was started in 2001 and left each institution free to set its own indication for screening as long as the same protocol for the screening regimen was used (www.IELCAP.org). It has accrued more than 25 000 baseline and repeat screenings. The data from the participating institutions can be pooled because an identical regimen in the pursuit of early diagnosis is being used and because the focus is not on the frequency of diagnosed cases of malignancy but on topics independent of the screening's indication, the proportion of those overdiagnosed among the unresected cases and the curability of the resected cases (Henschke *et al.*, 2003b).

10.2.8 National Lung Screening Trial (NLST)

This is a recently launched randomized controlled trial comparing CT scan versus CXR as two alternative modalities in screening for lung cancer. The participants are being enrolled by about 30 collaborating medical institutions. Eligible participants are 55–74 years old, smokers, either current or who quit within the past 5 years. The study will enroll 50 000 individuals, randomized into an experimental arm and a control arm. The experimental arm participants will receive a baseline screen and two annual repeats using the low-dose helical CT, with an additional 6–8 years of follow-up. The control arm participants will receive a baseline screen and two annual repeats using the postero-anterior (PA) CXR, followed, in the event of positive findings, by CT scan. In addition, periodic examinations of sputum, urine and blood specimens will be carried out, and a quality of life questionnaire will be administered. The endpoints recorded include overall and lung cancer death, clinical stage at detection and quality of life indicators. Accrual for this trial started in 2002 and has been concluded. Initial review of results (closed) is likely to take place in 2005.

10.3 PRINCIPLES OF MODELING OF LUNG CANCER SCREENING

10.3.1 Natural history of disease

The most natural way to model screening and therapeutic intervention in chronic disease is arguably to follow life histories of individuals drawn from defined populations at risk (Figure 10.1). This can be carried out using mathematical tools or, sometimes much more simply, by computer simulation. In this approach, it is assumed that the individuals at risk contract disease as a chance event at some age

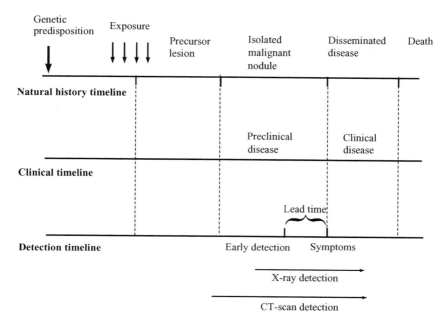

Figure 10.1 Timelines related to natural history and detection of cancer.

and then proceed through a succession of stages of random durations. These stages can be arranged in sequences (not necessarily a single sequence) with increasing detection probability and decreasing cure probability if detected. Ordinarily, the initial stage (sometimes called pre-clinical) includes small isolated nodules, visible only using early detection tools, but localized and potentially curable. At the other end of the spectrum, there will be advanced stages (sometimes called clinical), easily detectable because of the large size of the primary or because of presence of metastasis, but essentially incurable. Transitions between these stages can be modeled either by assigning random durations or, preferably, by defining a random path in the tumor size, nodal metastasis and distant metastasis (TNM) space. The relationship between these two modes of description of tumor progression is complicated (see Kimmel and Flehinger, 1991).

Once the model of disease natural history is developed, screening detection can be superimposed by assuming a schedule of examinations, which may be specific for a given individual, as well as a model of the detection process, in the simplest case a specification of the probability of detection given the stage of the disease. Finally, a model of treatment should be provided, in the simplest case a specification of cure probability given the stage of the disease.

Individual-based modeling provides a proper framework for understanding biases typical of the screening process. *Lead-time bias* arises when the cancer is detected early in its natural history. Then, even if this early detection does not alter the probability of cure, the interval from diagnosis to death is inflated. Consequently, survival curves based on screening-detected cases will be shifted to the right, even if early detection does not extent the patient's life length. *Length bias* arises from the distribution of durations of pre-clinical disease in different patients. The screening procedure, positioned at a given point in time, will preferentially detect longer-lasting cases. This will further inflate survivals of screening-detected cases. *Stage shift* is defined as appearance of an excess of early-stage cases, with an accompanying eventual decrease in the number of advanced cases, expected under screening, compared to usual clinical practice. *Overdiagnosis bias* is an extreme form of length bias, in which a fraction of screen-detected cases progresses so slowly that whether they are detected early, late, or not detected, is irrelevant for the patient. The above biases are naturally incorporated in the probabilistic individual-based model of lung cancer and no further 'corrections' for these biases are needed.

At the other extreme, some tumors may be detected small, but already metastasized. This can not be accurately modeled if the stage transitions are represented by their durations only, without reference to growth and increase in heterogeneity being driving forces. As far as we know, all existing models of lung cancer have this deficiency. Let us note that this phenomenon is not easily reconcilable with overdiagnosis (Strauss and Dominioni, 2000).

10.3.2   Critical parameters

Susceptibility is the probability that an individual at risk ever contracts lung cancer in his/her lifetime. It varies widely depending on the definition of the risk group. In the case of lung cancer, susceptibilities depend on behavioral factors such as cigarette smoking, or environmental factors such as exposure to asbestos, and on other host factors such as mutagen sensitivity and DRC. *Tumor growth rate* is the scale parameter of the exponential function approximating a given phase of tumor growth (Gorlova *et al.*, 2005). It is highly variable, and its estimates suffer from a serious ascertainment bias, which arises through a mechanism analogous to that responsible for the length bias. *Progression of disease* cannot be uniquely expressed in terms of primary tumor size. There is a complicated dependence between disease progression (appearance of nodal and distant metastasis) and tumor size. Transition through stages is a simplified mode of description of progression. In such description, the crucial parameters are those of the distribution of the random time spent in early and advanced stages, in particular, the *mean time* spent in a given stage. *Detection sensitivity* is the probability that a tumor is detected by the screening procedure, provided the tumor is present. The process of detection has a high random component; however, detection sensitivity increases with tumor size and stage (Gorlova *et al.*, 2005). *Cure rate* can be operationally defined as the probability of surviving indefinitely due to cancer cure, given the absence of other, competing, risks. It is also equal to the asymptotic value of the survival curve and as such is not affected by the shift caused by lead-time bias. Cure rate decreases with tumor size and stage.

10.3.3   Mortality versus case fatality versus survival

At the center of the discussions regarding modeling screening and screening itself, there is the question of the correct measure of the population effect of screening. As indicated above, survival can be inflated, in the sense of survival curves shifted to the right, as a result of lead-time and length biases. On the other hand, the asymptotic values of survival curves, if attained, measure the *probability of cure*, understood as the proportion of cases who do not die of lung cancer, in the absence of competing risks. A related concept is the *fatality rate*, which is equal to 1 minus the probability of cure, that is, it is the percentage of cases who eventually die of lung cancer in the absence of competing risk. However, the most objective statistic is the lung cancer *mortality*, that is, the fraction of population who die of lung cancer. Mortality rate is independent of the mode of detection of cancer and of the biases spelled out above. Therefore, it will differ between the screened and unscreened arms of a study only if the treatment of the earlier detected cases is more successful than the treatment of symptomatic cases. Of course, early detection by itself, not followed by an effective treatment, does not bring mortality reduction. Under stationary conditions, the conversion factor between fatality rate and mortality rate is the incidence of lung cancer in a given population. The incidence depends on the detection mode.

Mathematical modeling is the only means by which it is possible to relate these various measures of lung cancer death in non-stationary setups, for example, when a population of smokers enters a screening program. Therefore, it also provides the unique tool to project results of a limited trial to a larger population.

10.4   REVIEW OF MODELING APPROACHES

10.4.1   Statistical model of lung cancer progression, detection and treatment

The analytical model of Flehinger and Kimmel (1987) is based on the individual natural histories of lung cancer. It is assumed that the development of the disease is a stochastic process with two stages, early and advanced, characterized by mean durations, probabilities of detection, and cure probabilities. A screening program consists of periodic examinations intended to detect the cancer. Only a subgroup of the participants of the screening program will develop the disease, and the probability that an individual belongs to this subgroup is ρ. For a susceptible individual, the age of onset of the early stage is a random variable with a trapezoidal distribution. The durations of the early and advanced stages are independent random variables with exponential distribution and means μ_1 and μ_2, respectively. Given the presence of early (advanced asymptomatic) cancer, a single examination detects it with probability p_1 (p_2). Detection of successive examinations is independent. When a cancer is detected, screening is aborted and the patient is treated. The probability of cure for early stage is c_1 and it is set to zero for the advanced stage. Cure is defined pragmatically in terms of survival after detection: if cured, the survival is the same as if the patient had never had cancer; if not cured, the survival is the same as if the cancer had not been detected by screening. The participants in the screening program are also characterized by the distribution of age at enrollment and the distribution of age at death from other causes. These distributions were estimated directly from the screening data. In this model compliance with the screening schedule is assumed perfect and a possible change in detection probability within stage due to increase in tumor size is disregarded. The parameters of the model were estimated using the data on 10 040 participants in the Memorial Sloan-Kettering Lung Trial. The estimates that were obtained showed that CXR screening had poor sensitivity (probability of early stage detection no higher than 18 %). The mean time in early stage was at least 4 years, while the duration of the advanced asymptomatic stage was estimated as close to 2 years. The probability of susceptible group membership was estimated around 10 % (this is for adeno-carcinoma only). The estimate of early-stage cure probability was negatively correlated with the estimate of mean duration of early stage μ_1, close to 50 % when μ_1 was close to 4 years and close to zero when μ_1 was greater than 9 years. The authors concluded that only a limited mortality reduction of up to 18 % could be expected as a result of long-term annual screening of smokers, and that a short-term reduction would be impossible to detect in a CRX randomized controlled trial.

10.4.2   Simulation modeling of the Mayo Lung Project

Flehinger *et al.* (1993) describe what is in fact a simulation-based implementation of the model described in Section 10.4.1. This simulation study was designed to estimate the parameters of the model from the data collected by Mayo Lung Project. The basic assumptions of the model are the same as above, except that a special parameter λ is introduced, so that if a cancer were present and not detected at the first examination, then the next examination would detect it with probability λp. This parameter was assumed to be less than 1, since a small cancer missed on one examination because of its location in the chest is likely to escape detection again at the next examination. The duration of the screening trial and the frequency of examinations were assumed as in the MLP: 6 years of screening (followed by 1 year of follow-up) after the prevalence screen at which all participants with pre-existing cancer were removed from the sample. Assuming the most favorable set of the parameters consistent with the data, the long-term population reduction in mortality was estimated around 10 %.

10.4.3 Modeling of the long-term follow-up of Mayo Lung Project participants

Gorlova *et al.* (2001) extend the previous model to simulate the extended follow-up of the MLP participants. Data on mortality and survival for a follow-up period extended to a median of 20.5 years was published by Marcus *et al.* (2000). Again, no mortality difference was found between the study and control groups. However, some difference was observed in survival between the study and control subjects diagnosed with lung cancer. Marcus *et al.* (2000) concluded that screening provided no benefit, difference in survival being attributable to 'clinically irrelevant lesions found in screening'. When applying their model to this data, Gorlova *et al.* (2001) observed that the model not only fitted the results of 6 years of screening and 1 year of follow-up but also predicted, with the same set of parameters, the results of extended follow-up, which provided a long-term validation for the model. The results of this study strongly suggest that long-term screening with CXR does result in a reduction in lung carcinoma mortality. The limited extent of this benefit is the result of the low sensitivity of CXR as a screening tool. As a result, the MLP trial had low power, and extended follow-up did not make it more powerful.

10.4.4 Modeling the outcome of the Czechoslovak screening study

The model constructed by Walter *et al.* (1992) allows joint estimation of the distribution of the duration of the pre-clinical state of the disease and screening sensitivity from the data on the observed prevalence of disease at a screen and on the incidence of disease during intervals between screens (Walter and Day, 1983). Crucial parameters of the model are: incidence I, false negative rate of a screening examination β, and expected duration of the detectable preclinical stage $1/\lambda$. The authors applied this model to analyze the results of a randomized controlled trial of screening for lung cancer in Czechoslovakia (Walter *et al.*, 1992). They estimated the parameters of the natural history of lung cancer to show that the preclinical stage detectable by CXR screening is very short (6–8 months). They also concluded that this stage was detected by CXR with probability close to 1. This suggests that the preclinical detectable stage in their model corresponds to the advanced asymptomatic stage in the previous model, where this stage is also detected with perfect sensitivity. Its duration was estimated by Flehinger *et al.* (1993) as 2 years, compared to 6–8 months in this model. This may result from the difference in the type of CXR examination used.

10.4.5   Upper bound on reduction in cancer mortality due to periodic screening, based on observational data

The paper by Baker *et al.* (2003) can be considered a non-parametric counterpart of the model of Flehinger and Kimmel (1987). It is mathematically very elegant. The general idea is to balance incidences of cases detected, in the absence of screening, by screening (first or subsequent), and in the intervals between screenings. This allows the comparison of corresponding cancer mortalities under scenario *N*, no screening in an age interval followed by a single screen, with those under scenario *P*, periodic screening covering the age interval. The following Assumption 1 plays a key role: Lung tumor, once detectable on one screen, always remains detectable by screening. Under Assumption 1, the same numbers of cases are detected under scenarios *N* and *P*. If Assumption 1 violated, the incidence balance does not close and only provides and upper bound on *N* versus *P* mortality reduction. It is further assumed that mortality of interval cases is higher than mortality of cases detected in the absence of screening $(m_I > m_A)$. The paper concludes with a review of the application of the method to several screening studies. For MLP data, this leads to estimated upper bounds on reduction of mortality, due to a mass-screening program of the order of 100 deaths, in 10 000 study subjects, over 24 years.

10.4.6   Markov model of helical CT-screened and non-screened cohort

Mahadevia *et al.* (2003) present an example of a model which does not consider individual life histories of individuals, but only groups of cases, which, however, are not cohorts in the strict sense of this word. These groups follow a discrete Markov chain, involving stratifications with respect to some relevant variables, but not all. Non-screened smokers progress to either no disease, or lung cancer and death, or death from other causes. Annual transition rates (age-group and gender specific) as well as survivals are based on Surveillance, Epidemiology and End Results Registry (SEER) data. Screening-detected cases differ by stage shift, existence of over-diagnosis (understood as an intrinsic feature of a case and not as a dynamic artifact), and lead time (the latter specified separately from the stage shift; it is unclear how these two can be disentangled). All groups have quality of life and cost-effectiveness indices evaluated. The results concern a simulation of 100 000 non-screened and 100 000 annually CT-screened subjects, followed for a 20-year period.

A 50 % stage shift and 200 % overdiagnosis and length bias are assumed among screen-detected cases. The authors obtain 13 % mortality reduction in the screened group. However, the quality-of-life and cost-efficiency considerations do not seem to favor screening.

10.4.7   Cost-effectiveness study of baseline low-dose CT screening for lung cancer

To evaluate the cost-effectiveness of a single baseline low-dose CT for lung cancer screening in high-risk individuals, Wisnivesky *et al.* (2003) incorporated data from ELCAP into a decision analysis model comparing low-dose CT screening of high-risk individuals (60 years and older with at least 10 pack-years of cigarette smoking and no other malignancies) to observation without screening. Cost-effectiveness was expressed as the incremental cost per year of life saved. The analysis adopted a societal perspective. The probability of the different outcomes following the decision either to screen or not to screen an individual at risk was based on data from ELCAP, and SEER or published data, respectively. The cost of screening and treatment of lung cancer was established based on data from the New York Presbyterian Hospital's financial system. The base-case analysis was conducted under the assumption of similar aggressiveness of screen-detected and incidentally discovered lung cancers and then followed by multiple sensitivity analyses to relax these assumptions. Only when the likelihood of overdiagnosis was over 50 % did the cost-effectiveness ratio exceed $50 000 per year of life saved. The cost-effectiveness ratios were also relatively insensitive to estimates of the potential lead-time bias. They found that the incremental cost-effectiveness ratio of a single baseline low-dose CT was $2500 per year of life saved. They concluded that a baseline low-dose CT for lung cancer screening is potentially highly cost-effective, and compares favorably to cost-effectiveness ratios of other screening programs.

10.5   MODELING THE IMPACT OF NEW SCREENING MODALITIES ON REDUCTION OF MORTALITY FROM LUNG CANCER

10.5.1   Modeling the NLST trial

CT screening for lung cancer provides earlier diagnosis of lung cancer than chest radiography. Further evaluation using randomized controlled trials (RCTs) has been suggested to determine the mortality reduction under CT screening. Our aim is to understand how long and how large such a study would need to be to obtain a definitive answer. Using a previously validated mathematical model of screening for lung cancer, we determined the power of the RCT to detect a clinically significant mortality reduction when comparing CT screening with 'usual care' or CXR

Table 10.1 Power of RCT of 50,000 subjects (25,000 screenees vs. 25,000 controls) for evaluation of annual CT-scan screening versus chest X-ray (CXR) screening under (a) low CXR sensitivity and curability and (b) increased CXR sensitivity and curability, and a range of compliance levels. Abbreviations: a – compliance in both arms, p_{CT}, p_{CXR} – sensitivity of detection by CT and CXR, respectively, c_{CT}, c_{CXR} – curability following detection by CT and CXR, respectively.

(a)

Number of annual screens plus number of years of follow-up	Power under $p_{CT} = 0.6$, $p_{CXR} = 0.245$, $c_{CT} = 0.5$, $c_{CXR} = 0.35$		
	$a = 1.0$	$a = 0.75$	$a = 0.5$
$1 + 8 + 0$	0.951	0.886	0.829
$1 + 2 + 6$	0.795	0.681	0.538
$1 + 2 + 1$	0.299	0.243	0.207

(b)

Number of annual screens plus number of years of follow-up	Power under $p_{CT} = 0.6$, $p_{CXR} = 0.4$, $c_{CT} = 0.5$, $c_{CXR} = 0.4$		
	$a = 1.0$	$a = 0.75$	$a = 0.5$
$1 + 8 + 0$	0.684	0.584	0.444
$1 + 2 + 6$	0.450	0.406	0.284
$1 + 2 + 1$	0.180	0.167	0.122

screening under realistic scenarios of protocol non-adherence. In addition, we modeled the long-term impact of CT scan mass-screening on mortality reduction in a high-risk population (see Table 10.1(a)). The results indicate two trends. First, an increase in the length of follow-up after three screenings increases the power, but not sufficiently to bring it up to 80–90 %. This latter is achieved by an increase in the number of screenings. Second, non-compliance and higher than expected sensitivity of CXR (in the control arm) may seriously reduce the power.

10.5.2 Modeling the effects of long-term mass screening by CT scan

We also demonstrate, in the mass screening setup, that once screening is discontinued, the annual mortality rates gradually approach those of the unscreened population. Modeling of mass-screening programs suggests that, in the long run, CT-scan detection of early lung cancer followed by treatment leads to considerable reduction in lung cancer mortality (Figure 10.2). At the same time, RCTs for evaluation of screening require many participants who are screened annually for a sufficiently

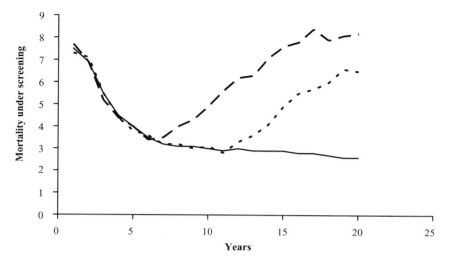

Figure 10.2   Annual number of lung cancer deaths under annual CT screening and follow-up. Screening performed for 5 years (dashed line), for 10 years (dotted line), and for 20 years (continuous line). Numbers of deaths expressed per 5000 participants per year.

long period to achieve a reasonable power in detecting a mortality reduction in the presence of realistic protocol non-adherence (Table 10.1(b)).

10.6   COMPARISON OF MODELS AND CONCLUDING REMARKS

The model of Baker *et al.* (2003) leads to conclusions concerning mortality reductions expected as a consequence of a screening trial, which are not contradictory to the conclusions based on the model developed in Flehinger and Kimmel (1987) and Flehinger *et al.* (1993). In particular, Baker *et al.* (2003) predict an upper bound of 100 individuals on reduction in the number of cancer deaths following a 24-year mass screening program, based on MLP data. From Figure 5g of Gorlova *et al.* (2001), the corresponding expected reduction is equal to about 30 individuals. Consistency is reached despite different technical assumptions of the models.

The model of Walter *et al.* (1992) is based on the data from the Czechoslovak study carried out in the 1970s. The quality of CXR films used is difficult to evaluate. The estimates obtained in the modeling study – detection probability close to 100 % and average duration of the detectable preclinical stage of 6–8 months – are not far from the estimates obtained by Flehinger and Kimmel (1987) for the asymptomatic advanced stage. This might reconcile the results of the two studies.

Mahadevia *et al.* (2003) obtained rather low expected reductions in mortality (13 %) following a CT-scan mass screening program based on SEER data and a discrete Markov chain model, not based on individual histories. Their estimate is comparable to that obtained by Gorlova *et al.* (2001) for CXR detection. However, Mahadevia *et al.* (2003) seem to assume arbitrary and difficult-to-evaluate values of stage shift (50 %) and overdiagnosis and length bias (200 %).

Modeling can be also used to evaluate efficacy of screening programs, if they are applied to differently defined high-risk groups. For example, it has been shown that lung cancer cases consistently exhibit higher mutagen induced chromosomal break scores as measured by a mutagen sensitivity assay and poorer DRC using the host-cell reactivation assay than age- and ethnicity-matched controls (Wu *et al.*, 1998, Wei *et al.*, 2000). Therefore, individuals with elevated mutagen sensitivity and/or reduced DRC constitute a natural subgroup of smokers to undergo screening. Gorlova *et al.* (2003) demonstrate, using the modeling approach of Flehinger *et al.* (1993), that, whereas annual CT screening of all smokers for 20 years can reduce mortality by 30 %, screening only individuals with elevated mutagen sensitivity and reduced DRC (12.5 % of all smokers) can reduce the overall mortality by 7 %.

A general remark based on modeling of short-term screening trials and long-term mass screening programs is that potentially considerable long-term reductions in mortality might not be detected by screening studies, even with an extended follow-up. Examples can be found in Gorlova *et al.* (2001) and in the modeling study of the ongoing NLST trial (Table 10.1 and Figure 10.2).

Application of the modeling allows several questions to be answered, concerning (a) the impact of behavioral and genetic factors underlying lung cancer and past lung cancer detection and treatment interventions on observed national trends in incidence and/or mortality, and (b) the population impact of hypothetical future mass screening and intervention programs. Processes of carcinogenesis and cancer progression are inherently stochastic and their pathways widely vary from one individual to another. This is the reason why any statements made about the course of the disease involve uncertainty. This interpopulation variability also lies at the root of biases of estimates of parameters of cancer progression derived from different observational studies (such as lead-time and length biases in screening studies and distortions of tumor growth rates in retrospective examinations of tumor size). To automatically take into account biases of this nature, modeling has to involve stochasticity. Consequently, model predictions have a probabilistic character, that is, they provide ranges of possible outcomes with their respective probabilities. The degree of uncertainty is influenced by limited data samples and interpopulation variability.

The principal challenge is constituted by the estimation of distributions and parameters and calibration/validation. Data on disease progression can be obtained indirectly from case repositories (e.g., SEER, hospital records) or from early detection programs (e.g., NCI 1967–1982 trials, ELCAP trials). These data cover intervals of the individual's lifetime, which are depicted in the clinical and detection timelines in Figure 10.1. Due to the recent introduction of the CT scan as a detection tool, some fraction of precursor lesions might be visualized and followed. On the other hand, genetic case–control studies and tobacco exposure studies provide estimates of risk of disease, which use the clinical disease as an endpoint. Mathematical modeling will enable all these data to be integrated and to be used to optimize future health care policies.

CHAPTER 11

Optimal Regimens of Cancer Screening

Leonid G. Hanin

University of Rochester

Lyudmila V. Pavlova

St. Petersburg State Polytechnical University

11.1 OPTIMAL SCREENING

Screening of large populations for breast, prostate, lung, and colon cancer as well as for some other cancer types has in recent decades become a widely used means of early cancer detection. Large-scale randomized trials were conducted to ascertain the survival benefits of screening and thus reduce the risks associated with late detection of the disease. The results of such trials were reported in numerous publications; see, for example, Flehinger *et al.* (1988), van Oortmarssen (1995) and van den Akker-van Marle *et al.* (1997). Some of them, such as the Cochrane report of Olsen and Gotzsche (2001) on trials that involved mammographic screening of at-risk women for breast cancer, led to highly controversial conclusions. It has been well documented by previous research that the efficacy of screening depends critically on the timing of medical exams. Because of this the use of conventional (typically, periodic) screening schedules may present a confounding source of uncertainty in the analysis of biomedical effects of screening. Such effects can be ascribed not only to the natural course of the disease, sensitivity of cancer detection technology, and curative treatment but also to the suboptimality of screening schedules. This makes constructing optimal screening schedules an indispensable step in methodologically sound evaluation of the benefits of screening, design of its improved schedules, and assessment of cancer related risks. Additionally, utilizing

Recent Advances in Quantitative Methods in Cancer and Human Health Risk Assessment
Edited by L. Edler and C. Kitsos © 2005 John Wiley & Sons, Ltd

optimal screening regimens leads to the possibility of increasing statistical power of randomized trials without increasing their sample size.

The goal of the present work is to study methodological, mathematical, and computational aspects of optimization procedures for screening regimens and discuss their biomedical significance with application to early detection of breast cancer. Optimization of cancer screening has been a matter of extensive investigation. Table 11.1 gives an overview of some of the most important work on cancer screening and its mathematical modeling since 1969. The problem becomes tractable only within the framework of a certain mathematical model of the disease progression. The modeling approaches used in most of the previous work were confined to the temporal aspects of the natural history of cancer (see references 1–36 in Table 11.1). By contrast, the present work is based on a comprehensive mechanistic model of cancer natural history that brings tumor size at detection (which implicitly incorporates the time dimension) to bear on the optimal design of screening schedules.

Tumor size is by far the most important single clinical covariate available at the time of diagnosis that largely determines the rate (or probability) of cancer detection and is at the same time highly predictive of long-term outcomes of the disease (cure, recurrence or cancer-related death). A methodological foundation for tumor size based models of cancer natural history that will be used in this study was laid in Hanin *et al.* (2001) and Bartoszyński *et al.* (2001). Some preliminary results related to optimal screening schedules in a somewhat simpler setting were obtained in Hanin *et al.* (2001). Incorporation of other clinical covariates from (and beyond) clinical tumor classification into the natural history of cancer requires a substantial additional modeling effort (Hanin and Yakovlev, 2004).

The problem of optimal screening design is set up as a search for optimal schedules of medical exams subject to certain constraints on their number and timing. Solving such a problem presupposes selection of a pertinent screening efficiency criterion. The most widely used efficiency functionals to be minimized are the expected total cost of screening, including both the cost of medical exams and somewhat elusive cost of late detection (see references 2, 6, 11, 16, 17, 19–25 and 29 in Table 11.1), and the expected difference between the times of cancer detection without and with screening (references 27, 29 in Table 11.1). For a detailed discussion of the merits and shortcomings of these approaches, see Hanin *et al.* (2001).

In a follow-up of this earlier paper, we will be dealing in this chapter with a biologically appealing screening efficiency functional defined as the expected difference between tumor sizes at detection in the absence and presence of screening. It is assumed that in the absence of screening a tumor can be detected spontaneously (i.e. by symptomatic surfacing of the disease typically followed by appropriate medical exams, or asymptomatically as a result of unrelated medical tests) and that the same mechanism is in place also in the presence of screening. Thus, our screening efficiency functional characterizes the net effect of screening and is, in principle, completely determined by the natural history of tumor development from the birth of a patient to the time of the last exam in the screening

Table 11.1 Chronological overview of literature on cancer screening and its mathematical modeling since 1969.

No.	Year of publication	Authors	Journal/Series
1	1969	Zelen and Feinleib	Biometrika
2	1974	Kirch and Klein	Management Science
3	1976	Prorok	Adv. Appl. Prob. (Parts I and II)
4	1976	Blumenson	Math. Biosci.
5	1977	Blumenson	Math. Biosci.
6	1977	Shahani and Crease	Adv. Appl. Prob.
7	1978	Albert *et al.*	Math. Biosci. (Parts I and II)
8	1978	Louis *et al.*	Math. Biosci.
9	1978a	Schwartz	Operations Research
10	1978b	Schwartz	Cancer
11	1983	Eddy	Medical Decision Making
12	1983	Walter and Day	Amer. J. Epidem.
13	1984	Day and Walter	Biometrics
14	1987	Brookmeyer and Day	Biometrics
15	1987	Flehinger and Kimmel	Biometrics
16	1991	Tsodikov and Yakovlev	Math. Biosci.
17	1991	Tsodikov *et al.*	Statistique des Processus en Milieu Médical
18	1991	Flehinger and Kimmel	Mathematical Population Dynamics
19	1991	Parmigiani	Biometric Bulletin
20	1992	Parmigiani	ISDS Duke University
21	1992	Tsodikov	Syst. Anal. Model. Simul.
22	1993	Parmigiani	J. Amer. Statist. Assoc.
23	1993	Parmigiani and Kamlet	Bayesian Statistics in Science and Technology: Case Studies
24	1993	Yakovlev *et al.*	Biométrie et Analyse de Données Spatio-temporelles
25	1993	Zelen	Biometrika
26	1995	Duffy *et al.*	Statistics in Medicine
27	1995	Tsodikov *et al.*	Biometrics
28	1996	H. H. Chen *et al.*	The Statistician
29	1996	Yakovlev and Tsodikov	Stochastic Models of Tumor Latency and their Biostatistical Applications
30	1997	Hu and Zelen	Biometrika
31	1997	Parmigiani	Biometrika
32	1998	Cronin *et al.*	Statistics in Medicine
33	1998	Lee and Zelen	J. Amer. Statist. Assoc.
34	1999	Shen and Zelen	Biometrika
35	2001	Pinsky	Biometrics
36	2001	Shen and Zelen	Journal of Clinical Oncology
37	2001	Hanin *et al.*	Mathematical and Computer Modelling
38	2004	Hanin and Yakovlev	Statistical Methods in Medical Research

schedule. The functional coincides with the Kantorovich distance (Kantorovich and Akilov, 1982) between tumor sizes at detection with and without screening.

One might, of course, adopt a more far-reaching approach by relating the screening efficiency to distant and clinically important outcomes such as cancer-specific mortality and survival. This approach, however, would require developing an overarching mathematical model of cancer natural history that includes not only tumor latency, progression and detection but also cancer treatment, recurrence and survival. The mathematical challenges associated with such a model are daunting. An additional statistical challenge consists of extrapolating model parameters reflective of the effects of cancer treatment, recurrence and survival to a general population to be screened. That is why in the present work we have adopted a simpler approach. This has distinct advantages: the approach is mathematically tractable and the clinical covariates (age and tumor size), requisite for estimation of model parameters, are readily available at the time of tumor detection.

The structure of the chapter is as follows. In Section 11.2 we describe a comprehensive mathematical model of cancer natural history including tumor latency, growth, and detection. An explicit computationally feasible formula for the screening efficiency functional is derived in Section 11.3. Data that resulted from Canadian randomized trials of mammographic breast cancer screening are described briefly in Section 11.4 (for more details, the reader is referred to Hanin *et al.*, 2004). This section also contains estimates of the parameters of our model of cancer natural history from these data. Optimal screening schedules based on these parameters are computed in Section 11.5. Finally, the discussion of our findings is relegated to Section 11.6.

11.2 A COMPREHENSIVE MODEL OF CANCER NATURAL HISTORY

According to a widely accepted classification, cancer progresses through the following stages:

1. *Tumor latency*, ranging from the birth of an individual to the appearance of the first clonogenic tumor cell (or to the time when a tumor reaches a minimal detectable size, as determined by the resolution of relevant detection technology). Such an event is called the onset of the disease. In the case of induced carcinogenesis, tumor latency is counted from the start of exposure to a carcinogen.

2. Once a tumor emerges (or becomes detectable), it enters the *preclinical stage* which lasts until the moment of tumor detection. The detection occurs either spontaneously or in the course of a pre-scheduled medical exam that might detect the lesion in the absense of clinical symptoms.

Let T be the duration of the stage of tumor latency measured from the birth of an individual, and let W be the sojourn time in the preclinical stage, that is, the time to tumor detection from onset of the disease. Durations T and W are thought of as random variables which are assumed to be absolutely continuous with probability density functions (p.d.fs) f_T and f_W, respectively.

11.2.1   Tumor latency

Elaborate mechanistic models of carcinogenesis are available to describe the time to onset of the disease. A widely accepted model of tumor latency is referred to as the Moolgavkar–Venzon–Knudson (MVK) model or alternatively the two-stage model of clonal expansion (TSCE) (Moolgavkar and Venzon, 1979; Moolgavkar and Knudson, 1981). Its most commonly used stationary version allows for an explicit formula for the distribution of the tumor latency time T (Kopp-Schneider *et al.*, 1994; Zheng, 1994). The simplest parametric form of this distribution is given by

$$\bar{F}_T(t) := \Pr(T > t) = \left[\frac{(A+B)e^{At}}{B + Ae^{(A+B)t}} \right]^{\rho}, \qquad t \geq 0; \qquad (11.1)$$

see Hanin *et al.* (2001) and Bartoszyński *et al.* (2001). Here A, B, $\rho > 0$ are identifiable parameters of the model (Heidenreich, 1996; Hanin and Yakovlev, 1996; Hanin, 2002), $\bar{F}_T := 1 - F_T$ is the survivor function of T, and F_T is its cdf.

11.2.2   Tumor growth

The following general functional form is assumed for the tumor size (the number of cells in a tumor) S :

$$S(w) = f(w), \qquad (11.2)$$

where w is the time from onset of the disease. The function f may depend on a parameter θ which may be scalar- or vector-valued, deterministic or random. It is assumed that, for each θ, the function f is strictly increasing, absolutely continuous, and that $f(0) = 1$. Note that the latter assumption is merely a matter of convenience, and that any given minimum detectable tumor size can be assumed without any significant change to the model. Denote by g the inverse function for f, and set

$$\Psi(w) := \int_0^w f(u)du.$$

Specific laws of tumor growth of primary interest are the following:

1. Deterministic exponential growth; in this case, $f(w) = e^{\lambda w}$, where $\lambda > 0$ is a constant growth rate. The problem of optimization of screening schedules for exponentially growing tumors was explored in Hanin *et al.* (2001).

2. Exponential growth with random growth rate λ that reflects individual variability of tumor growth rates. We will assume that the quantity $1/\lambda$ (which is proportional to the tumor doubling time) follows a gamma distribution with shape and scale parameters a and b, respectively. Other laws of tumor growth,

such as the Gompertz law, can easily be accommodated; see Bartoszyński *et al.* (2001).

11.2.3   Screening schedules

A sequence $\tau = \{\tau_1 < \tau_2 < \cdots < \tau_n\}$ of times of medical exams for a specific cancer counted from the birth of a patient will be called a *screening schedule*. Screening schedules may be subject to certain restrictions such as prescribing the number n of exams, setting up a lower bound for the time between any two successive exams, or imposing an upper bound on the age at the last exam. For the sake of convenience, we set $\tau_0 := 0$ and $\tau_{n+1} := \infty$.

11.2.4   Tumor detection

As it was pointed out in Section 11.1, we distinguish between *spontaneous* and *screen-based* tumor detection. The first occurs in the absence of or concurrently with screening and is thought of as a continuous process. By contrast, screen-based detection is an instantaneous event that may occur only at the moments of pre-scheduled medical exams and is therefore a discrete process.

Numerous attempts have been made to relate the probability of detecting a tumor to its size (Atkinson *et al.*, 1983, 1987; Brown *et al.*, 1984; Bartoszyński, 1987; Klein and Bartoszyński, 1991). Following Brown *et al.* (1984), we will assume that the hazard rate r_0 of the time to spontaneous tumor detection is proportional to the current tumor size,

$$r_0 = \alpha_0 S, \tag{11.3}$$

where α_0 is a positive constant.

Let the random variables W_0 and W_1 denote the times of spontaneous and screen-based detections counted from cancer onset, respectively. Then for the time W of combined detection, when both detection mechanisms are in place, we have $W = \min(W_0, W_1)$. Denote by

$$N_0 = f(W_0) \quad \text{and} \quad N = f(W) \tag{11.4}$$

the corresponding tumor sizes at spontaneous and combined detection.

If the parameter θ of the tumor growth function f is non-random, we derive from (11.3) that

$$\bar{F}_{W_0}(w) = e^{-\int_0^w r_0(u)du} = e^{-\alpha_0 \int_0^w f(u)du} = e^{-\alpha_0 \Psi(w)}.$$

Therefore, we obtain

$$\bar{F}_{N_0}(n) = \bar{F}_{W_0}(g(n)) = e^{-\alpha_0 \Psi(g(n))} \tag{11.5}$$

(recall that g is the inverse of f), and hence

$$\mathbb{E}N_0 = 1 + \int_1^\infty \bar{F}_{N_0}(n)dn = 1 + \int_1^\infty e^{-\alpha_0 \Psi(g(n))}dn = 1 + \int_0^\infty e^{-\alpha_0 \Psi(u)} f'(u)du,$$

where $\mathbb{E}$ stands for the expectation. In particular, for non-random exponential tumor growth with rate λ, we have

$$\bar{F}_{W_0}(w) = e^{-\frac{\alpha_0}{\lambda}(e^{\lambda w}-1)}, \qquad w \geq 0, \tag{11.6}$$

$$\bar{F}_{N_0}(n) = e^{-\frac{\alpha_0}{\lambda}(n-1)}, \qquad n \geq 1, \tag{11.7}$$

and

$$\mathbb{E}\,N_0 = 1 + \frac{\lambda}{\alpha_0}. \tag{11.8}$$

Equation (11.7) suggests that in this case tumor size at spontaneous detection N_0 follows a translated exponential distribution with parameter α_0/λ.

If the parameter θ is a random variable then an additional integration with respect to the distribution of θ is required. In the case where λ is a random variable such that $1/\lambda$ is gamma-distributed with parameters a, b, we derive from (11.8) that

$$\mathbb{E}\,N_0 = 1 + \frac{b}{\alpha_0(a-1)} \tag{11.9}$$

if $a > 1$ and $\mathbb{E}\,N_0 = \infty$ if $0 < a \leq 1$. As shown in Bartoszyński *et al.* (2001), N_0 in this case follows a translated Pareto distribution with p.d.f.

$$f_{N_0}(n) = \frac{\alpha_0 a}{b}\left[1 + \frac{\alpha_0}{b}(n-1)\right]^{-(a+1)}, \qquad n \geq 1.$$

We now specify, for any given screening schedule τ, the distribution of W_1. It suffices to define, for every $t \geq 0$, the conditional distribution of W_1 given $T = t$. Let $\tau_i \leq t < \tau_{i+1}$, $0 \leq i \leq n$. Let us introduce a discrete analog of the conditional hazard rate for the time of screen-based detection by

$$\mu_t = \sum_{k=i+1}^{n} r_t(k)\delta_{\tau_k-t}, \tag{11.10}$$

where $r_t(k)$ is the conditional detection intensity of the kth screen, $1 \leq k \leq n$, given the onset time $T = t$, δ_x stands for the Dirac measure at x, and the sum over the empty set of indices is set, as usual, to zero. By definition, the discrete measure μ_t is related to the conditional survival function of W_1 given that $T = t$ through the equation

$$\bar{F}_{W_1|T=t}(w) = e^{-\int_0^w d\mu_t(u)}, \qquad w \geq 0. \tag{11.11}$$

A relation between the conditional detection intensities $r_t(k)$ and conditional probabilities $p_t(k) := \Pr(W_1 = \tau_k - t | T = t)$ of tumor detection at kth screen given cancer onset at time t, $i+1 \leq k \leq n$, was obtained in Hanin *et al.* (2001).

Similar to (11.3), we are assuming that the discrete rate of screen-based detection is proportional to the current tumor size:

$$r_t(k) = \alpha S(\tau_k - t), \qquad i+1 \leq k \leq n, \tag{11.12}$$

for some constant $\alpha > 0$. Combining (11.11), (11.10) and (11.12) with (11.2), we find that, given any t such that $\tau_i \le t < \tau_{i+1}$, $0 \le i \le n - 1$,

$$\bar{F}_{W_1|T=t}(w) = e^{-\alpha \sum_{k=i+1}^{j} f(\tau_k - t)}, \qquad \tau_j - t \le w < \tau_{j+1} - t, \quad i + 1 \le j \le n. \tag{11.13}$$

11.3 FORMULA FOR THE SCREENING EFFICIENCY FUNCTIONAL

We proceed from the following two biologically natural assumptions.

1. The random variables W_0 and T are independent.

2. For every $t \ge 0$, W_1 and W_0 are conditionally independent given $T = t$.

For an in-depth discussion of these assumptions, see Hanin *et al.* (2001) and Bartoszyński *et al.* (2001). Let τ be any screening schedule. Assuming temporarily that the parameter vector θ that determines the law of tumor growth is non-random, we define the efficiency functional $\varphi(\tau; \theta)$ as the Kantorovich distance $d_K(N_0, N)$ between tumor sizes N_0 and N at spontaneous and combined detection. It is well known (Kantorovich and Akilov, 1982; Vallander, 1973) that

$$d_K(N, N_0) = \int_1^{\infty} |\bar{F}_{N_0}(n) - \bar{F}_N(n)| \, dn. \tag{11.14}$$

It follows from (11.4), the inequality $W_0 \ge W$, and monotonicity of the function f that N_0 stochastically dominates $N : \bar{F}_{N_0} \ge \bar{F}_N$. In the case where $\mathbb{E} N_0 < \infty$, this leads to the following alternative expression for the efficiency functional:

$$\varphi(\tau; \theta) = d_K(N, N_0) = \int_1^{\infty} \bar{F}_{N_0}(n) dn - \int_1^{\infty} \bar{F}_N(n) dn = \mathbb{E} N_0 - \mathbb{E} N. \tag{11.15}$$

We set $n = f(w)$ and condition upon T in (11.14) to obtain

$$\varphi(\tau; \theta) = \int_0^{\infty} |\bar{F}_{W_0}(w) - \bar{F}_W(w)| f'(w) dw$$

$$= \int_0^{\infty} \int_0^{\infty} |\bar{F}_{W_0}(w) - \bar{F}_{W|T=t}(w)| f'(w) dw f_T(t) dt,$$

where $\bar{F}_{W|T=t}$ is the conditional survivor function of W given that $T = t$, and f_T is the p.d.f. of the tumor latency time T. Since $W = \min(W_0, W_1)$, it follows from our Assumptions 1 and 2 that

$$\bar{F}_{W_0} - \bar{F}_{W|T=t} = \bar{F}_{W_0} - \bar{F}_{W_0}\bar{F}_{W_1|T=t} = \bar{F}_{W_0}F_{W_1|T=t}.$$

Therefore,

$$\varphi(\tau; \theta) = \int_0^{\infty} \int_0^{\infty} F_{W_1|T=t}(w)\bar{F}_{W_0}(w) f'(w) dw f_T(t) dt. \tag{11.16}$$

Observe that if $T = t$, where $\tau_i \leq t < \tau_{i+1}$, $0 \leq i \leq n$, then the only admissible values of W_1 are $\tau_{i+1} - t, \ldots, \tau_{n+1} - t$. More specifically,

$$W_1 = \begin{cases} \tau_j - t, \ i+1 \leq j \leq n, & \text{if } j\text{th exam detected a tumor,} \\ \tau_{n+1} - t = \infty, & \text{if the tumor was not detected by screening.} \end{cases}$$

Therefore, if $t \geq \tau_n$ or $\tau_i \leq t < \tau_{i+1}$, $0 \leq i \leq n - 1$, and $0 \leq w < \tau_{i+1} - t$, then $F_{W_1|T=t}(w) = 0$. This allows us to rewrite (11.16) as

$$\varphi(\tau; \theta) = \sum_{i=0}^{n-1} \int_{\tau_i}^{\tau_{i+1}} \sum_{j=i+1}^{n} \int_{\tau_j - t}^{\tau_{j+1} - t} F_{W_1|T=t}(w) \bar{F}_{W_0}(w) f'(w) dw f_T(t) dt.$$

Now, recall expression (11.13) for $\bar{F}_{W_1|T=t}$, and denote

$$G(x) := \int_x^{\infty} \bar{F}_{W_0}(w) f'(w) dw, \qquad x \geq 0.$$

Then we obtain

$$\varphi(\tau; \theta) = \sum_{i=0}^{n-1} \int_{\tau_i}^{\tau_{i+1}} \sum_{j=i+1}^{n} \left[1 - e^{-\alpha \sum_{k=i+1}^{j} f(\tau_k - t)} \right] [G(\tau_j - t) - G(\tau_{j+1} - t)] f_T(t) dt$$

$$= \sum_{i=0}^{n-1} \int_{\tau_i}^{\tau_{i+1}} \sum_{j=i+1}^{n} e^{-\alpha \sum_{k=i+1}^{j-1} f(\tau_k - t)} [1 - e^{-\alpha f(\tau_j - t)}] G(\tau_j - t) f_T(t) dt.$$

$$(11.17)$$

If, in particular, $f(w) = e^{\lambda w}$ with a constant rate λ, invoking (11.6) yields

$$G(x) = \frac{\lambda}{\alpha_0} e^{-\frac{\alpha_0}{\lambda}(e^{\lambda x} - 1)}, \qquad x \geq 0.$$

In this case the efficiency functional (11.17) takes on the form

$$\varphi(\tau; \lambda) = \frac{\lambda}{\alpha_0} \sum_{i=0}^{n-1} \int_{\tau_i}^{\tau_{i+1}} \sum_{j=i+1}^{n} e^{-\alpha \sum_{k=i+1}^{j-1} e^{\lambda(\tau_k - t)}} [1 - e^{-\alpha e^{\lambda(\tau_j - t)}}] e^{-\frac{\alpha_0}{\lambda}(e^{\lambda(\tau_j - t)} - 1)} f_T(t) dt.$$

$$(11.18)$$

If the parameter θ is random, the efficiency functional (11.17) has to be integrated additionally with respect to the distribution of θ. Let, in particular, $\theta = \lambda$ and $1/\lambda$ follow the gamma distribution $\Gamma(a, b)$. Then the efficiency functional $\varphi(\tau)$ has the form

$$\varphi(\tau) = \frac{b^a}{\Gamma(a)} \int_0^{\infty} \varphi(\tau, \theta^{-1}) \theta^{a-1} e^{-b\theta} d\theta = \frac{1}{\Gamma(a)} \int_0^{\infty} \varphi(\tau, bu^{-1}) u^{a-1} e^{-u} du,$$

$$(11.19)$$

where $\varphi(\tau; \lambda)$ is given by (11.18). Observe also that according to (11.15) in the case of deterministic tumor growth we have $\mathbb{E}N = \mathbb{E}N_0 - \varphi(\tau, \theta)$, while in the case of random tumor growth $\mathbb{E}N = \mathbb{E}N_0 - \varphi(\tau)$ holds, where the expected tumor size $\mathbb{E}N_0$ at spontaneous detection is assumed to be finite. These formulas allow for an explicit computation of the expected tumor size at combined detection.

11.4 THE DATA AND PARAMETER ESTIMATION

The above methodology was applied to optimal scheduling of breast cancer screening. Parameters of the comprehensive model of cancer development described in Section 11.2 were estimated from the data amassed in the Canadian National Breast Screening Studies (CNBSS). The CNBSS data set contains individual data on age and tumor size at detection generated in 1980–1996 for a population of about 90 000 women. The structure of the data resulting from CNBSS, modeling approaches, and parameter estimation techniques are discussed at length in Hanin et al. (2004). The data revealed a marked birth cohort effect on cancer incidence. To incorporate this effect into the model of tumor latency, the parameter ρ of the distribution (11.1) of tumor latency time T was assumed to be birth cohort dependent while other model parameters, including the parameters A and B of the MVK model, were assumed to be the same for all birth cohorts. Recall that ρ is the rate of proliferation of initiated cells divided by the rate of initiation; see Hanin and Yakovlev (1996).

The resulting maximum likelihood estimates for parameters of tumor latency distribution from the CNBSS data on cancer incidence are as follows: $\hat{A} = 8.3333 \times 10^{-6}$ month^{-1}, $\hat{B} = 1.0025 \times 10^{-2}$ month^{-1}, $\hat{\rho}_1 = 0.0691$, $\hat{\rho}_2 = 0.0737$, $\hat{\rho}_3 = 0.0985$, and $\hat{\rho}_4 = 0.1055$, where the indices 1–4 of the parameter ρ correspond to birth cohorts of the years 1921–1925, 1926–1930, 1931–1935, and 1936–1940, respectively. Assuming that the reciprocal tumor growth rate $1/\lambda$ is gamma-distributed with parameters a, b, the estimate for the expected value $\mu = a/b$ of $1/\lambda$ was obtained as $\hat{\mu} = 6.311$ months.

To account for the differences in breast cancer incidence between the CNBSS and the general American population, the estimates of the remaining model parameters obtained from CNBSS data were calibrated on the data on tumor-size-specific age-adjusted breast cancer incidence for the US female population accumulated by the Surveillance, Epidemiology and End Results program of the National Cancer Institute (for a detailed description of the calibration procedure, the reader is referred to Hanin et al., 2004). These calibrated parameters were a (the shape parameter of the gamma distribution assumed for $1/\lambda$), the rate α_0 of spontaneous detection, and the discrete detection rate α for mammography combined with physical exam. The calibrated estimates for these parameters were $\hat{a} = 0.7681$, $\hat{\alpha}_0 = 3.7367 \times 10^{-11}$ month^{-1}, and $\hat{\alpha} = 8.3000 \times 10^{-7}$. Therefore, $\hat{b} = \hat{a}/\hat{\mu} = 0.1217$ month^{-1}, and the estimate of the standard deviation, σ, of $1/\lambda$ is $\hat{\sigma} = \sqrt{\hat{a}}/\hat{b} = 7.201$ months.

11.5 NUMERICAL EXPERIMENTS

In numerical experiments we computed the maximum screening efficiencies and the corresponding optimal screening schedules for the case of $n = 10$ exams separated by at least one year. The time of the last exam τ_{10} was restricted to $\tau_{10} \leq 1200$ months. Results for the randomized model of tumor natural history described in Section 11.2 in which $1/\lambda$ was assumed to follow a gamma distribution $\Gamma(a, b)$ were compared with those for a non-randomized version of the model where tumor growth is exponential with a fixed rate λ_0 such that $1/\lambda_0$ coincides with the expected value $\mu = a/b$ of $1/\lambda$. The optimal efficiencies and screening schedules in the non-randomized model were computed for the four groups of birth cohorts specified in Section 11.4. Since the patterns of optimal screening schedules for all groups of birth cohorts appeared to be very similar, and the value of the screening efficiency functional was the highest for the fourth group of birth cohorts (see Table 11.2), the computation in the randomized model was conducted for the fourth group of birth cohorts only (i.e., for $\rho = \rho_4$). The values of all other relevant parameters of both models (A, B, a, b, α_0, α for the randomized model and A, B, $\lambda_0 = b/a$, α_0, α for the non-randomized model) were kept the same at their maximum likelihood values given in Section 11.4.

Table 11.2 Optimal screening schedules $\tau_1, \tau_2, \ldots, \tau_{10}$ and optimal screening efficiencies $\varphi(\tau)$ for the non-randomized and randomized models. Screening ages are given in months. The values of common parameters of both models are as follows: $A = 8.3333 \times 10^{-6}\,\mathrm{month}^{-1}$, $B = 1.0025 \times 10^{-2}\,\mathrm{month}^{-1}$, $\alpha_0 = 3.7367 \times 10^{-11}\,\mathrm{month}^{-1}$, $\alpha = 8.3000 \times 10^{-7}$.

	Non-randomized model				Randomized model
	$\lambda_0 = 0.1584\,\mathrm{month}^{-1}$				$a = 0.7681$
	$V_{\mathrm{spont}} = 4.24\,\mathrm{cm}^3$, $D_{\mathrm{spont}} = 2.01\,\mathrm{cm}$				$b = 0.1217\,\mathrm{month}^{-1}$
	$\rho_1 = 0.0691$	$\rho_2 = 0.0737$	$\rho_3 = 0.0985$	$\rho_4 = 0.1055$	$\rho = \rho_4$
τ_1	743	742	740	740	845
τ_2	800	800	798	797	872
τ_3	854	853	851	850	899
τ_4	905	904	902	902	926
τ_5	955	955	952	952	954
τ_6	1004	1004	1002	1002	981
τ_7	1053	1053	1051	1051	1008
τ_8	1102	1102	1100	1100	1035
τ_9	1151	1151	1150	1150	1100
τ_{10}	1200	1200	1200	1200	1200
$\varphi(\tau)$	8.9020×10^8	9.4017×10^8	1.1922×10^9	1.2583×10^9	1.2261×10^9
V_{scrin}	$3.35\,\mathrm{cm}^3$	$3.30\,\mathrm{cm}^3$	$3.05\,\mathrm{cm}^3$	$2.98\,\mathrm{cm}^3$	
D_{scrin}	$1.86\,\mathrm{cm}$	$1.85\,\mathrm{cm}$	$1.80\,\mathrm{cm}$	$1.79\,\mathrm{cm}$	

Optimal screening times $\tau_1, \tau_2, \ldots, \tau_n$ (in months) for $n = 10$ and the corresponding values $\varphi(\tau)$ of the efficiency functional (expressed as the number of tumor cells) for both models were computed using MATLAB proceeding from formulas (11.18) and (11.19); see Table 11.2. Additionally, in the case of the non-randomized model, Table 11.2 contains the values V_{spont} and V_{scrin} of the expected tumor volumes at spontaneous and combined detection, respectively, as well as the corresponding tumor diameter D_{scrin} assuming that tumors have a spherical shape. The conversion between tumor size, expressed in number of cells, and volume, expressed in cubic centimeters, is based on the fact that $1\,\text{cm}^3$ of solid tumor contains about 10^9 cells (Klein and Bartoszyński, 1991). Note that the distribution (11.5) of tumor size at spontaneous detection is time-independent and hence the same for all birth cohorts. Observe also that for the data at hand $\hat{a} < 1$ so that the expected tumor size at spontaneous detection (and therefore for combined detection as well) is infinite in the randomized model (see (11.9)).

The optimality of all screening schedules was carefully ascertained. Specifically, in all computations the same value of the efficiency functional and the same optimal schedule resulted from a large variety of initial approximations. This included periodic schedules as well as schedules that are skewed toward young ages, and those involving old ages only. Fixing $n - 1$ exam times at their optimum value and letting

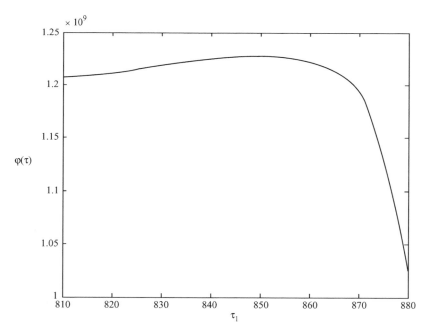

Figure 11.1 Profiles of the efficiency functional for the randomized model as functions of (a) τ_1, (b) τ_5 and (c) τ_9. Parameter values are as follows: $n = 10$, $A = 8.3333 \times 10^{-6}\,\text{month}^{-1}$, $B = 1.0025 \times 10^{-2}\,\text{month}^{-1}$, $\rho = \rho_4 = 0.1055$, $a = 0.7681$, $b = 0.1217\,\text{month}^{-1}$, $\alpha_0 = 3.7367 \times 10^{-11}\,\text{month}^{-1}$, $\alpha = 8.3000 \times 10^{-7}$.

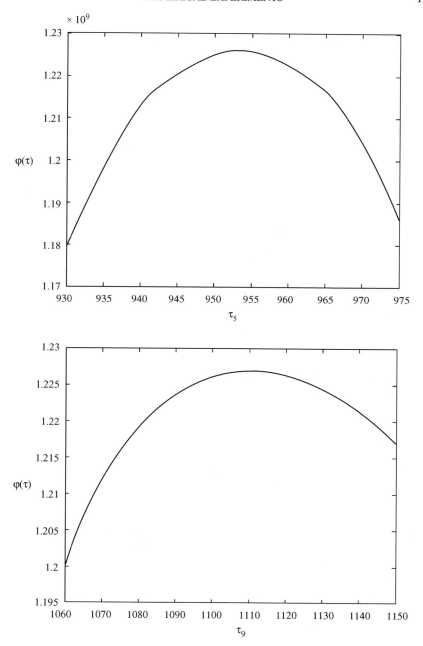

Figure 11.1   (*Continued*)

the remaining time range between the two neighboring optimal times, we constructed profile functions. All of them, except for the profile for τ_{10}, displayed a pronounced maximum at the point of extremum for the variable screening time (see Figure 11.1, where the plots of profile functions for τ_1, τ_5 and τ_9 in the randomized model case are displayed).

11.6 DISCUSSION

The results presented in Table 11.2 show that optimal screening schedules for all four birth cohorts in the non-randomized model of tumor natural history are very close to a periodic screening with a period of about 50 months. The age at the first exam is scheduled for about 740 months. It is reasonable to expect that optimal screening times follow the hazard of tumor detection. For spontaneous detection of exponentially growing tumors with non-random growth rate λ, the hazard function of the time to tumor detection is $h_0(w) = \alpha_0 e^{\lambda w}$ (see (11.6)). Accordingly, for screen-based detection, the hazard is close to $h(w) = \alpha e^{\lambda w}$, that is, increasing in time. This observation may serve as a heuristic justification for introducing the restriction $\tau_{10} \leq 1200$ months as well as an explanation for the following two related findings: that the ages of the last exam in all cases reach the allowed maximum of 1200 months; and that the profile function for τ_{10} is increasing in the neighborhood of 1200 months.

The effect of screening manifests itself in the reduction of tumor size at detection. The computed reduction of tumor size, as determined by the value of the efficiency functional and compared with the tumor volume at spontaneous detection, is $0.89\,\text{cm}^3$ (21 %), $0.94\,\text{cm}^3$ (22 %), $1.19\,\text{cm}^3$ (28 %), and $1.26\,\text{cm}^3$ (30 %) for 1–4 birth cohorts, respectively. The same effect, expressed in terms of tumor diameter at detection, is $0.15\,\text{cm}$ (7.5 %), $0.16\,\text{cm}$ (8.0 %), $0.21\,\text{cm}$ (10.4 %) and $0.22\,\text{cm}$ (10.9 %), respectively. These data suggest that, by contrast to optimal screening schedules, the optimal gain in tumor size is quite sensitive to the value of parameter ρ of the MVK model and increases with the growth of ρ.

The most striking finding of this study, though, is a significant difference in the pattern of optimal screening schedules for the randomized model and its non-randomized counterpart. The difference is observed in spite of the fact that both models share the values of all common parameters (A, B, ρ, α_0, α), and, additionally, the tumor growth rate λ_0 in the non-randomized model coincides with the corresponding expected value in the randomized model. Specifically, the starting age of screening in the randomized model is 845 months (as compared to 740 months in the non-randomized model), and the screening times $\tau_1, \tau_2, \ldots, \tau_8$ are essentially periodic with a period of 27 months versus about 50 months in the non-randomized model. Also, at the end of the screening regimen in the randomized model the periodic pattern deteriorates (see Table 11.2). The gain in tumor volume due to screening in the randomized model ($1.23\,\text{cm}^3$) is only slightly less than that for the non-randomized model with the same value of parameter ρ. This leads to the conclusion that, while the reduction of tumor size at detection due to optimal screening is relatively stable under variation of tumor growth rate in the screened population, the pattern of optimal screening ages is more sensitive to the variability of this critical parameter of tumor kinetics.

ACKNOWLEDGEMENT

This work was supported by Collaborative Linkage Grant PST CLG #979045 of the NATO Science Programme and by National Institutes of Health/National Cancer Institute grant U01 CA88177-01 (CISNET). A substantial portion of this work was completed in fall 2002 when Dr Pavlova visited with Dr Hanin at Idaho State University with the support of Yamagiwa-Yoshida Cancer Study Grant awarded by the International Union Against Cancer.

PART IV

STATISTICAL APPROACHES FOR CARCINOGENESIS STUDIES

Introductory remarks

Lutz Edler and Christos P. Kitsos

Ignoring the apparently never-ending controversy between 'frequentists' and 'Bayesians', methods from both camps are included in this book simply for pragmatic reasons of applicability. It is the practitioner's prerogative to apply any method which provides a useful answer. We are aware that different risk assessors may have different understandings of what probability is: a measure of belief in a proposition (Bayesian) or the long-term frequency of an event (frequentist). Such 'personal beliefs' may be essential to the way risk assessors or risk managers think about probability, and may influence the way information is extracted from experimental data and study results obtained from complicated statistical analyses. Sometimes, there is also confusion over the notions of measurement error, variability, (population) heterogeneity, and uncertainty in general. We felt that this text would not be the place to discuss such basic questions of the foundations of statistics, even if the discussion could contribute towards a better understanding the role of statistics in risk assessment. Our contribution to this discussion is to present in this part a number of papers which try to resolve parts of this controversy and misunderstandings simply by addressing topical statistical modeling problems of risk assessment.

Statistical analysis methods for survival data have penetrated almost all areas of clinical trials and epidemiology. This is particularly a consequence of the availability of robust and flexible non-parametric statistical methods, for example

Recent Advances in Quantitative Methods in Cancer and Human Health Risk Assessment
Edited by L. Edler and C. Kitsos   © 2005 John Wiley & Sons, Ltd

the Kaplan–Meier estimate of the survival curve, the log-rank test for parallel group testing, and proportional hazards regression for the identification of prognostic factors. Whenever time-to-event (time-to-occurrence) data are observed, survival time (failure time) analysis has become the state-of-the-art method. Since risk assessment studies often have a time component it is wise to watch out for options to define time points and lengths of duration in order to apply survival analysis methods. It has to be remarked that the term 'hazard' has an unequivocal definition in survival analysis as the instantaneous failure rate $\lambda(t) = \lim_{\Delta t \to 0} P(t < T \leq t + \Delta t | T > t)$, the probability of failure shortly (Δt) after time t given no failure has occurred by time t. Formally, this is an infinitesimal feature of the failure process at the time point t. The survival probability is a direct function of the hazard, namely, $S(t) = \int_0^t \exp(-\lambda(t))dt$. Statistical methods have been discussed in a number of texts, among them the breakthrough book of Kalbfleisch and Prentice (1980). Beyond the descriptive analysis and the parallel group testing of survival data, it was the introduction of regression models that revolutionized the use of statistical modeling in life sciences, starting with Cox (1972), one of the most often cited papers in statistics. His proportional hazards model is today surely the most frequently used method for the identification of prognostic factors in clinical studies as well as of risk factors in studies relevant to risk assessment. Chapter 12 considers possible extensions beyond the classical proportional hazards model which could be too idealized in a number of applications.

Methodologies for the extrapolation from effects observed under one set of conditions in one population to the whole human population were the focus of early work in risk assessment, known as low-dose extrapolation. Brown and Koziol (1983) summarize developments before 1980. As emphasized in the introductory remarks to Part I, traditionally obtained limits (reference doses), were based on the NOAEL derived from animal bioassay data. The NOAEL has been critically reviewed in Edler et al. (2002) and contrasted with the benchmark dose approach. We refer to this paper also for the use of uncertainty factors in risk assessment. Notice, that a reference dose is obtained by dividing a point of departure for the low-dose extrapolation (e.g. the NOAEL) by an uncertainty factor. This approach was first used by Lehman and Fitzhugh (1954), who proposed the uncertainty factor of 100, which later become a standard part of low-dose extrapolation.

In the 1970s, low-dose extrapolation used the logit and the one-hit model and fitted parametric models to (binomial) response data of lifetime tumor incidence. The logit model has also been used, in the tradition of the earlier used probit model developed for the estimation of the lethal dose 50 % (LD$_{50}$) value. Their use for the extrapolation to low doses was a recent development. The one-hit model is mathematically linear when approaching zero dose, in contrast to the logit model which has a highly non-linear shape and zero slope at dose zero. The tolerance distribution model was introduced independently by Gaddum (1933) in a report of the Britsh Medical Research Council and by Bliss (1934) in the journal *Science*. They considered simply the probability $P(d)$ that an individual will develop a particular disease characteristic during an experiment when exposed to the dose level d. A large class of dose-response models, namely the cumulative probability distributions, was obtained by assuming that the proportion of responders is monotone non-decreasing with dose exhibiting a sigmoidal shape, already considered by Fechner (1860). The probit model (without background risk) got its name because of the use of the Gaussian normal distribution as transformation.

In the 1980s these models were replaced by the more flexible linearized multi-stage model (US Environmental Protection Agency, 1986b). This model had some mechanistic basis, using the cell kinetic model approach of multistage car-cinogenesis modeling. At the same time, the type of response data changed from the lifetime tumor incidence data analyzed through rates and proportions to disease-specific time-to-occurrence data analyzed by survival methods; see Olin *et al.* (1995), who consider in detail the low-dose extrapolation and multistage models.

The Kaplan–Meier estimator of survival curves, the log-rank test or Mantel–Cox statistic, and other non-parametric methods have been used with overwhelming success in medical as well as in industrial applications. The availability of statistical packages is one of the reasons for today's widespread use of statistical methods. This is not the case when one wishes to perform risk assessment. Standard statistical software packages rarely provide the computational methods for risk assessment. Risk analysis software is rather buried in specialized research centers or embedded in expensive commercial software. The US EPA has started to provide special software packages, for example for the benchmark dose method. What is really lacking, however, is open source software for researchers. An overview of dose-response modeling is given in Chapter 13, which also introduces and defines the notion of point of departure for that dose within the experimental dose range from which a low-dose extrapolation can start, when one is unable to fit a dose-response model down to zero dose. Section 13.4.4 provides the link to Chapter 14 where the most prominent method to determine a point of departure, namely the benchmark dose approach, is presented in detail and with examples by Parham and Portier.

The analysis of uncertainty has become an integral part of practical risk assess-ment. Bois and Diack give a general introduction to the Bayesian approach to uncertainty analysis in Chapter 15. For the 'uncertainty in action' the reader may consult the references given in that paper. We particularly recommend the papers by Bois (2000a, 2000b) on the risk assessment of trichloroethylene in a special issue of *Environmental Health Perspectives*. This issues contains a number of other papers on this chemical, and demonstrates very impressively the crucial role that uncertainty analysis can play in a specific risk assessment problem.

The use of Bayesian methods seems to be quite natural since they allow a formal framework to define 'uncertainty' distributions for interesting model characteristics. For general remarks on sources of uncertainty in dose-response models and epi-demiological data, see also Stayner *et al.* (1999) who distinguish five sources: study design issue; choice of data sets; choice of dose-response model; choice of dosi-metry and errors in exposure estimates; and variability in susceptibility.

It is clear that statistical modeling is strongly related to the correct selection of data sets and statistical sampling. Both an appropriate statistical model and an optimal statistical plan for collecting the data are the two vital prerequisites of a valid statistical analysis. The theory of experimental design has a long history in the development of statistical methodology by R. A. Fisher since the 1930s. With its successful applications in agricultural sciences by Fisher and his contemporaries as well as all later generations, experimental design is one of the major research areas of mathematical and of applied statistics. Surprisingly, the impact on life sciences has been much less impressive, with the exception of clinical trials and their special demands on statistical planning. Non-plant biological sciences seem to have to account for more (but less understood) experimental factors and the linear model, which proved successful for agriculture, can rarely be applied to the usual non-linear processes observed in life sciences. Therefore, the application of optimal design principles has been rather rare in biological experiments and in assays performed for risk assessment. An exception has been the work invested by the US National Toxicology Program in standardizing their animal bioassays. Both theoretical and pragmatic considerations led them to a standard sample size of $n=50$ per dose group and a standard number of three or four dose groups and one control group.

It is important to note that there are many issues, practical, ethical and financial, which make it difficult to estimate risk parameters with sufficient precision. Both for economic and, increasingly often, ethical reasons only a restricted number of experiments can be performed. Therefore, an optimal design approach is needed. A review and recommendations are given in Chapter 16 in this part and in Chapter 21 in Part VI. Chapter 16 addresses experimental designs for bioassays by linking the biological question with the statistical theory and by addressing a non-linear dose-response relationship. The use of sequential designs is still in its infancy in risk assessment, compared with therapeutic research where it has become obligatory for the planning of a study, at least in humans. When adopting sequential methods one has to balance statistical optimality with biological practicability.

CHAPTER 12

Analysis of Survival Data with Non-proportional Hazards and Crossings of Survival Functions

Vilijandas B. Bagdonavičius

University of Vilnius

Mikhail S. Nikuline

*Victor Segalen University and
Steklov Mathematical Institute*

12.1 INTRODUCTION

The most popular and most widely applied survival regression model is the proportional hazards or Cox model, introduced by Cox (1972). The popularity of this model is based on the fact that there exist simple semiparametric estimation procedures which can be used when the form of the survival distribution function is not specified. On the other hand, the Cox model is rather restrictive and is not applicable when ratios of hazard rates under different fixed covariates are not constant in time. For example, if survival of patients with different perfomance status is analyzed, the hazard rates under different values of the covariate do not intersect but the ratios of hazard rates are monotone; see the survival data of 137 lung cancer patients given in Kalbfleisch and Prentice (1980).

When analyzing survival data from clinical trials, crossing of survival functions is sometimes observed. A classical example are the well-known data of the

Recent Advances in Quantitative Methods in Cancer and Human Health Risk Assessment
Edited by L. Edler and C. Kitsos © 2005 John Wiley & Sons, Ltd

Gastrointestinal Tumor Study Group, concerning effects of chemotherapy and radiotherapy on the survival times of gastric cancer patients (Stablein and Koutrouvelis 1985; Klein and Moeschberger 1997).

Piantadosi (1997, pages 483–488) gives data concerning the survival times of lung cancer patients. There were 164 patients divided in two groups who received radiotherapy (sample size of 86) or radiotherapy plus CAP (sample size of 78). The Kaplan–Meier estimators tend to cross twice: at a time around 7 months and around 33 months.

We present here several models and estimation procedures for data with non-proportional hazards with no, one or two crossings of the survival functions. Generalization to the case of more than two crossings is straightforward; see also Hsieh (2001) and Wu (2002, 2004). We also give three goodness-of-fit tests for the Cox model against different alternatives and apply those methods to lung and gastric cancer patient data.

12.2 MODELS

Let $S_x(t)$ and $\lambda_x(t)$ be the survival and the hazard rate functions under an m-dimensional, possibly time-dependent, explanatory variable $x = x(\cdot) = (x_1(\cdot), \ldots, x_m(\cdot))^{\mathrm{T}} \in E$, where E is the set of all admissible covariates, $x : [0, \infty) \to \mathbb{R}^m$. Denote by

$$\Lambda_x(t) = -\ln\{S_x(t)\}, \qquad x \in E,$$

the cumulative hazard under x and consider the following models: the *generalized proportional hazards* (GPH) *model* (with monotone ratios of hazard rates),

$$\lambda_{x(\cdot)}(t) = e^{\beta^{\mathrm{T}} x(t)} (1 + \Lambda_{x(\cdot)}(t))^{-\gamma+1} \lambda(t); \qquad (12.1)$$

the *simple cross-effects* (SCE) *model*,

$$\lambda_{x(\cdot)}(t) = e^{\beta^{\mathrm{T}} x(t)} \{1 + \Lambda_{x(\cdot)}(t)\}^{1 - e^{\gamma^{\mathrm{T}} x(t)}} \lambda(t); \qquad (12.2)$$

and the *multiple cross-effects* (MCE) *model*,

$$\lambda_{x(\cdot)}(t) = e^{\beta^{\mathrm{T}} x(t)} \left(1 + \gamma^{\mathrm{T}} x(t) \Lambda(t) + \delta^{\mathrm{T}} x(t) \Lambda^2(t)\right) \lambda(t), \qquad (12.3)$$

where $\beta^{\mathrm{T}} x(t)$ is the scalar product of vectors β and $x(t)$, $\lambda(t)$ the baseline hazard rate and

$$\Lambda(t) = \int_0^t \lambda(u) du$$

the baseline cumulative hazard. The parameter γ is one-dimensional for the GPH model and m-dimensional for the SCE model, the parameter δ is m-dimensional. In the case $\gamma = 0$ (or $\delta = \gamma = 0$) all the models coincide with the prortional hazards (Cox) model. The models have the following properties:

- *GPH model.* Under different constant covariates the ratios of the hazard rates increase, decrease or are constant, the hazard rates and the survival function do not intersect in the interval $(0, \infty)$.

- *SCE model.* Under different constant covariates the ratios of the hazard rates increase, decrease or are constant, the hazard rates and the survival function intersect at most once in the interval $(0, \infty)$.

- *MCE model.* Under different constant covariates the ratios of the hazard rates increase, decrease or are constant, the hazard rates and the survival function intersect at most twice in the interval $(0, \infty)$.

12.3 PARAMETRIC AND SEMIPARAMETRIC ESTIMATION

12.3.1 Parametric estimation

Let us consider for simplicity right-censored survival regression data, which are rather typical in survival analysis and constant in time covariates:

$$(X_1, \delta_1, x_1), \ldots, (X_n, \delta_n, x_n),$$

where

$$X_i = T_i \wedge C_i, \quad \delta_i = \mathbf{1}_{\{T_i \leq C_i\}} \quad (i = 1, \ldots, n),$$

T_i and C_i and are the failure and censoring times, $x_i = x_i(\cdot)$ the m-dimensional covariate corresponding to the ith object, $x_i(\cdot) = (x_{i1}(\cdot), \ldots, x_{im}(\cdot))^{\mathrm{T}} \in E$, $a \wedge b = \min(a, b)$, and $\mathbf{1}_A$ is the indicator of the event A. Equivalently, right-censored data can be presented in terms of the counting processes

$$(N_1(t), Y_1(t), x_1(t), t \geq 0), \ldots, (N_n(t), Y_n(t), x_n(t), t \geq 0),$$

where, for any $n = 1, 2, \ldots, n$,

$$N_i(t) = \mathbf{1}_{\{X_i \leq t, \delta_i = 1\}}, \quad Y_i(t) = \mathbf{1}_{\{X_i \geq t\}}, \quad x_i(t) = (x_{i1}(t), \ldots, x_{im}(t))^{\mathrm{T}}.$$

In this case for $t > 0$,

$$N(t) = \sum_{i=1}^{n} N_i(t) \quad \text{and} \quad Y(t) = \sum_{i=1}^{n} Y_i(t)$$

are the number of observed failures of all objects in the interval $[0, t]$ and the number of objects at risk just before the moment t, respectively. More on applications of counting processes for the analysis of censored data can be found in Andersen *et al.* (1993) and Bagdonavičius and Nikulin (2000).

Suppose that survival distributions of all n objects given $x_i(\cdot), x_i(\cdot) \in E$, are absolutely continuous with the survival functions $S_i(t, \theta)$ and the hazard rates

$\alpha_i(t, \theta)$, specified by a common parameter $\theta \in \Theta \subset \mathbb{R}^s$. Denote by G_i the survival function of the censoring time C_i. We suppose that G_i does not depend on θ. Suppose that the multiplicative intensities model is verified. In this case the compensators of the counting processes N_i with respect to the history of the observed processes are

$$\int Y_i(u)\lambda_i(u, \theta)du;$$

see Andersen *et al.* (1993). The likelihood function for θ estimation is

$$L(\theta) = \prod_{i=1}^{n} \lambda_i^{\delta_i}(X_i, \theta)\, S_i(X_i, \theta)$$

$$= \prod_{i=1}^{n} \left(\int_0^\infty \lambda_i(u, \theta)\, dN_i(u) \right)^{\delta_i} \exp\left\{ -\int_0^\infty Y_i(u)\lambda_i(u, \theta)\, du \right\}.$$

The maximum likelihood estimator $\hat{\theta}$ of the parameter θ satisfies the equation

$$U(\hat{\theta}) = 0,$$

where U is the score function

$$U(\theta) = \frac{\partial}{\partial \theta} \ln L(\theta) = \sum_{i=1}^{n} \int_0^\infty \frac{\partial}{\partial \theta} \ln \lambda_i(u, \theta)\{dN_i(u) - Y_i(u)\lambda_i(u, \theta)du\}. \quad (12.4)$$

The form of the hazard rates λ_i for the GPH, SCE, and MCE models is given by (12.1)–(12.3). The parameter θ contains the regression parameter β, the complementary parameters γ (or γ and δ), and the parameters of the baseline hazard λ, which is taken from some parametric family.

12.3.2   Semiparametric estimation

Let us consider a general approach (Bagdonavičius and Nikulin, 1997, 2002) to semiparametric estimation when the baseline hazard λ is supposed to be unknown. Note that for all the models considered above the expression $\lambda_i(t, \theta)dt$ in the parametric score function (12.4) has the form $g(x_i, \Lambda(t), \theta)\, d\Lambda(t)$: for the GPH model,

$$g(x, \Lambda(t), \theta) = e^{\beta^{\mathrm{T}}x}(1 + \gamma e^{\beta^{\mathrm{T}}x}\Lambda(t))^{1/\gamma - 1};$$

for the SCE model,

$$g(x, \Lambda(t), \theta) = e^{\beta^{\mathrm{T}}x}\{1 + e^{(\beta + \gamma)^{\mathrm{T}}x}\Lambda(t)\}^{e^{-\gamma^{\mathrm{T}}x} - 1};$$

for the MCE model,

$$g(x, \Lambda(t), \theta) = e^{\beta^{\mathrm{T}}x(t)}\left(1 + \gamma^{\mathrm{T}}x\Lambda(t) + \delta^{\mathrm{T}}x\Lambda^2(t)\right).$$

The martingale property of the difference

$$N_i(t) - \int_0^t Y_i(u)\lambda_i(u,\theta)du$$

implies the recursively defined 'estimator'

$$\tilde{\Lambda}(t,\theta) = \int_0^t \frac{dN(u)}{S^{(0)}(u,\tilde{\Lambda},\theta)}, \tag{12.5}$$

where ($u-$ denoting the left limit)

$$S^{(0)}(u,\tilde{\Lambda},\theta) = \sum_{j=1}^n Y_j(u)g(x_j,\tilde{\Lambda}(u-),\theta).$$

For all the models considered above the expression $\frac{\partial}{\partial\theta}\ln\lambda_i(t,\theta)$ in the parametric score function (4) is a function of x_i, $\Lambda(t)$ and θ:

$$\frac{\partial}{\partial\theta}\ln\lambda_i(t,\theta) = h(x_i,\Lambda(t),\theta).$$

So the modified score function is obtained replacing Λ by its consistent estimator $\tilde{\Lambda}$ in the parametric score function (12.4):

$$\tilde{U}(\theta) = \sum_{i=1}^n \int_0^\infty \{h(x_i,\tilde{\Lambda}(u),\theta) - E(u,\tilde{\Lambda},\theta)\}dN_i(u), \tag{12.6}$$

where

$$E(u,\Lambda,\theta) = \frac{S^{(1)}(u,\Lambda,\theta)}{S^{(0)}(u,\Lambda,\theta)},$$

$$S^{(1)}(u,\tilde{\Lambda},\theta) = \sum_{j=1}^n Y_j(u)\, g(x_j,\tilde{\Lambda}(u-),\theta)\, h(x_j,\tilde{\Lambda}(u-),\theta).$$

For the GPH model, $h(x,\tilde{\Lambda}(t),\theta) = (h_\beta(x,\tilde{\Lambda}(t),\theta), h_\gamma(x,\tilde{\Lambda}(t),\theta))$, where

$$h_\beta(x,\tilde{\Lambda}(t),\theta)) = x\,\frac{1+e^{\beta^\mathrm{T}x}\Lambda(t)}{1+\gamma e^{\beta^\mathrm{T}x}\Lambda(t)},$$

$$h_\gamma(x,\tilde{\Lambda}(t),\theta) = \frac{1}{\gamma}\left\{-\frac{1}{\gamma}\ln(1+\gamma e^{\beta^\mathrm{T}x}\Lambda(t)) + \frac{(1-\gamma)e^{\beta^\mathrm{T}x}\Lambda(t)}{1+\gamma e^{\beta^\mathrm{T}x}\Lambda(t)}\right\}.$$

For the SCE model, $h(x,\tilde{\Lambda}(t),\theta) = (h_\beta(x,\tilde{\Lambda}(t),\theta), h_\gamma(x,\tilde{\Lambda}(t),\theta))$, where

$$h_\beta(x,\tilde{\Lambda}(t),\theta)) = x\,\frac{1+e^{\beta^\mathrm{T}x}\Lambda(t)}{1+e^{(\beta+\gamma)^\mathrm{T}x}\Lambda(t)},$$

$$h_\gamma(x,\tilde{\Lambda}(t),\theta) = x\left\{-e^{-\gamma^\mathrm{T}x}\ln(1+e^{(\beta+\gamma)^\mathrm{T}x}\Lambda(t)) + \frac{(e^{\beta^\mathrm{T}x}-e^{(\beta+\gamma)^\mathrm{T}x})\Lambda(t)}{1+e^{(\beta+\gamma)^\mathrm{T}x}\Lambda(t)}\right\}.$$

For the MCE model, $h(x, \tilde{\Lambda}(t), \theta) = (h_\beta(x, \tilde{\Lambda}(t), \theta), h_\gamma(x, \tilde{\Lambda}(t), \theta), h_\delta(x, \tilde{\Lambda}(t), \theta))$, where

$$h_\beta(x, \tilde{\Lambda}(t), \theta)) = x,$$

$$h_\gamma(x, \tilde{\Lambda}(t), \theta) = \frac{x\tilde{\Lambda}(t, \theta)}{1 + \gamma^{\mathrm{T}} x \tilde{\Lambda}(t, \theta) + \delta^{\mathrm{T}} x \tilde{\Lambda}^2(t, \theta)},$$

$$\tilde{h}_\delta(x, \tilde{\Lambda}(t), \theta) = \frac{x\tilde{\Lambda}^2(t, \theta)}{1 + \gamma^{\mathrm{T}} x \tilde{\Lambda}(t, \theta) + \delta^{\mathrm{T}} x \tilde{\Lambda}^2(t, \theta)}.$$

12.3.3 Modified partial likelihood estimator

To estimate the unknown parameter θ we shall apply the so-called modified partial likelihood approach (Bagdonavičius and Nikulin, 1999b). According to this approach the modified maximum likelihood estimator $\hat{\theta}$ is the solution of the system of equations $\tilde{U}(\theta) = 0$.

Computing the modified likelihood estimators is very simple. This is due to the remarkable fact that these estimators can be obtained in another way: write the partial likelihood function

$$L_P(\theta) = \prod_{i=1}^{n} \left[\int_0^\infty \frac{g\{x_i, \Lambda(v), 0 \le v \le u, \theta\}}{\sum_{j=1}^{n} Y_j(u) g\{x_j, \Lambda(v), 0 \le v \le u, \theta\}} \, dN_i(u) \right]^{\delta_i}, \qquad (12.7)$$

and replace Λ in the score function by $\tilde{\Lambda}$. We obtain the same modified score function (12.5) as we obtained going from the full likelihood! So when computing the estimator $\hat{\theta}$ the score equation is not necessary. Better maximize the modified partial likelihood function which is obtained from the partial likelihood function (12.7) replacing Λ by $\tilde{\Lambda}$. The general quasi-Newton optimization algorithm (given in S-Plus) which seeks the value of θ which maximizes this modified function works very well (Bagdonavičius et al., 2002a).

For fixed θ the 'estimator' $\tilde{\Lambda}$ can be found recursively. Let $T_1^* < \cdots < T_r^*$ be observed and ordered distinct failure times, $r \le n$. Denote by d_i the number of failures at time T_i. Then

$$\tilde{\Lambda}(0; \theta) = 0, \qquad \tilde{\Lambda}(T_1^*; \theta) = \frac{d_1}{S^{(0)}(0, \tilde{\Lambda}, \theta)},$$

$$\tilde{\Lambda}(T_{j+1}^*; \theta) = \tilde{\Lambda}(T_j^*; \theta) + \frac{d_{j+1}}{S^{(0)}(T_j^*, \tilde{\Lambda}, \theta)}, \qquad (j = 1, \ldots, r - 1).$$

Given the consistency of $\tilde{\Lambda}$, the asymptotic covariance matrix of $\sqrt{n}(\hat{\theta} - \theta)$ is obtained by standard methods using the functional delta method and the central limit theorem for martingales. For consistency proofs of estimators, given by equations of type (12.5), see Ceci and Mazliak (2002).

The baseline cumulative hazard Λ and the survival function S_x for any value $x \in E$ of the covariate are estimated by

$$\hat{\Lambda}(t) = \tilde{\Lambda}(t, \hat{\theta}), \qquad \hat{S}_x(t) = e^{-\hat{\Lambda}_x(t)},$$

where

$$\hat{\Lambda}_x(t) = \int_0^T g(x, \tilde{\Lambda}(u), \hat{\theta}) d\tilde{\Lambda}(u, \hat{\theta}).$$

12.4 GOODNESS-OF-FIT FOR THE COX MODEL AGAINST THE CROSS-EFFECTS MODELS

Let us consider tests for checking the adequacy of the Cox model

$$H_0 \; : \; \lambda_x(t) = e^{\beta^T x} \lambda(t)$$

versus the alternatives (12.1), (12.2) and (12.3) with $\gamma \neq 0$ (GPH and SCE) or $(\gamma, \delta) \neq (0, 0)$ (MCE).
Set

$$\begin{aligned}
\hat{U}_\rho &= \tilde{U}_\rho((\hat{\beta}^T, 1)^T), & \rho &= \beta, \gamma & \text{(GPH model)}, \\
\hat{U}_\rho &= \tilde{U}_\rho((\hat{\beta}^T, 0^T)^T), & \rho &= \beta, \gamma & \text{(SCE model)}, \\
\hat{U}_\rho &= U_\rho((\hat{\beta}^T, 0^T, 0^T)^T), & \rho &= \beta, \gamma, \delta & \text{(MCE model)},
\end{aligned}$$

where $\hat{\beta}$ is the partial likelihood estimator of the regression parameter β under the Cox model.

Note that under the Cox model $\hat{U}_\beta = 0$ (for any of the three alternatives). For $\rho = \gamma, \delta$,

$$\hat{U}_\rho = \sum_{i=1}^n \int_0^\infty (\hat{h}_\rho(x_i, \hat{\Lambda}(u), \hat{\beta}) - \hat{E}_\rho(u, \hat{\Lambda}(u), \hat{\beta})) dN_i(u),$$

where

$$\hat{h}_\gamma(x, \Lambda(t), \beta) = -\ln(1 + e^{\beta^T x} \Lambda(t)), -x \ln(1 + e^{\beta^T x} t \Lambda(t)), x \Lambda(t),$$

for the GPH, SCE, MCE models, respectively,

$$\hat{h}_\delta(x, \Lambda(t), \beta) = x \Lambda^2(t),$$

$\hat{\Lambda}$ is the Breslow estimator of Λ under the Cox model, and

$$\hat{E}_\rho(u, \Lambda(u), \beta) = \frac{\hat{S}_\rho^{(1)}(u, \Lambda(u), \beta)}{\hat{S}^{(0)}(u, \beta)}, \qquad \hat{S}^{(0)}(u, \beta) = \sum_{j=1}^{n} Y_j(u)e^{\beta^{\mathrm{T}} x_j},$$

$$\hat{S}_\rho^{(1)}(u, \Lambda(u), \beta) = \sum_{j=1}^{n} Y_j(u)e^{\beta^{\mathrm{T}} x_j}\hat{h}_\rho(x_j, \Lambda(u), \beta).$$

The test is based on the statistic $\hat{U}$, where

$$\hat{U} = \hat{U}_\gamma \qquad \text{(GPH and SCE models)},$$
$$\hat{U} = (\hat{U}_\gamma^{\mathrm{T}}, \hat{U}_\delta^{\mathrm{T}})^{\mathrm{T}} \qquad \text{(MCE model)}.$$

The asymptotic distribution of the statistic $\hat{U}$ for the GPH and SCE models is given in Bagdonavičius *et al.* (2004a, 2004b).

Let us consider the slightly more complicated case of the MCE model. For this model

$$\hat{U}_\gamma = \sum_{i=1}^{n} \int_0^\tau \hat{\Lambda}(u-)\Big(x_i - E(u, \hat{\beta})\Big)dN_i(u),$$

$$\hat{U}_\delta = \sum_{i=1}^{n} \int_0^\tau \hat{\Lambda}^2(u-)\Big(x_i - E(u, \hat{\beta})\Big)dN_i(u),$$

where

$$E(u, \beta) = \frac{S^{(1)}(u, \beta)}{S^{(0)}(u, \beta)}, \qquad S^{(0)}(u, \beta) = \sum_{j=1}^{n} Y_j(u)e^{\beta^{\mathrm{T}} x_j},$$

$$S^{(1)}(u, \beta) = \sum_{j=1}^{n} x_j Y_j(u)e^{\beta^{\mathrm{T}} x_j}.$$

Set

$$S^{(2)}(t, \beta) = \sum_{j=1}^{n} (x_j(t))^{\otimes 2} Y_j(t)\, e^{\beta^{\mathrm{T}} x_j},$$

where $a^{\otimes 2} = aa^{\mathrm{T}}$ for any vector $a = (a_1, \ldots, a_m)^{\mathrm{T}}$. Denote by β_0 the true value of β.
    Consider the following assumptions:

(a) There exist a neighborhood B of β_0 (the true value of β) and functions $s^{(i)}(v, \beta)$, continuous on B, uniformly in $t \in [0, \tau]$ and bounded on $B \times [0, \tau]$, such that $s^{(0)}(v, \beta_0) > 0$ for all $v \in [0, \tau]$, and

$$\sup_{\beta \in B, v \in [0, \tau]} \left\| \frac{1}{n}S^{(i)}(v, \beta) - s^{(i)}(v, \beta) \right\| \longrightarrow 0 \quad \text{as} \quad n \longrightarrow \infty.$$

(b)

$$\frac{\partial}{\partial \beta} s^{(0)}(t, \beta) = s^{(1)}(t, \beta) \quad \text{and} \quad \frac{\partial^2}{\partial \beta^2} s^{(0)}(t, \beta) = s^{(2)}(t, \beta).$$

(c)

$$\sup_{i,j} |x_j^{(i)}| < \infty.$$

(d)

$$\Lambda(\tau) < \infty.$$

(e) The matrix

$$\Sigma(\tau) = -\int_0^\tau \left\{ s^{(2)}(u, \beta_0) - e(u, \beta_0)(e(u, \beta_0))^{\mathrm{T}} s^{(0)}(u, \beta_0) \right\} d\Lambda(u)$$

is positive definite.

To construct a test we need the asymptotic distribution of $\hat{U}$ under the Cox model.

Theorem 12.1 *Under assumptions (a)–(e) and the Cox model,*

$$T = n^{-1} \hat{U}^{\mathrm{T}} \hat{D}^{-1} \hat{U} \xrightarrow{\mathcal{D}} \chi^2(2m),$$

where $\hat{D}$ is a consistent estimator of the limit covariance matrix of the random vector $n^{-1/2}\hat{U}$ (the expression for $\hat{D}$ is given in the proof).

The proof is given in the Appendix.

The critical region of the chi-square type test with approximate significance level α is

$$T > \chi^2_{1-\alpha}(2m),$$

where $\chi^2_{1-\alpha}(2m)$ is the $(1 - \alpha)$-quantile of the chi-square distribution with $2m$ degrees of freedom; see for example, Greenwood and Nikulin (1996).

Similarly, in the case of the SCE model

$$T = n^{-1} \hat{U}^{\mathrm{T}} \hat{D}^{-1} \hat{U} \xrightarrow{\mathcal{D}} \chi^2(m),$$

where $\hat{D}$ is a consistent estimator of the limit covariance matrix of the random vector $n^{-1/2}\hat{U}$; see Bagdonavičius *et al.* (2004a, 2004b).

In the case of the GPH model (cf. Bagdonavičius and Nikulin, 1997),

$$T = n^{-1} \hat{U}^2 \hat{D}^{-1} \xrightarrow{\mathcal{D}} \chi^2(1).$$

12.5 EXAMPLES

We present goodness-of-fit results for the Cox model for three examples with different types of data.

12.5.1 Lung cancer prognosis

The survival data for 137 lung cancer patients given in Kalbfleisch and Prentice (1980) show that the hazard rates under different values of the covariate (performance status) do not intersect, but the ratios of hazard rates are monotone. So we apply the test for the Cox model when the alternative is the GPH model. Performance status is determined by the Karnofsky index: 10–30 denotes completely hospitalized, 40–60 partial confinement, 70–90 able to care for self. Nine observations were censored, representing a proportion of 0.0657.

We used the following models for the analysis:

(a) continuous covariate *per* (performance status).

(b) covariate $1_{\{perf \leq 50\}}$ (performance status dichotomized).

The goodness-of-fit test for the Cox against the GPH model was used. For the two cases (a) and (b) the test statistic T is equal to 8.156 and 8.563, respectively; p-values are 0.004 31 and 0.003 43. The distribution of the test statistic is approximated by the chi-square distribution with one degree of freedom. Obviously, the Cox model is rejected. We dichotomized the covariate to see wether the GPH model explains the data better than the Cox model. In the dichotomous covariate case the estimators of the survival functions obtained using the GPH model are much closer to the Kaplan–Meier estimators then the estimators obtained using the Cox model (Bagdonavičius *et al.*, 2002a).

12.5.2 Gastric cancer

The survival data for 90 gastric cancer patients given in Stablein and Koutrouvelis (1985) concern effects of chemotherapy (sample size of 45) and chemotherapy plus radiotherapy (sample size of 45). The Kaplan–Meier estimators pertaining to the treatment groups cross once. So we apply the test for the Cox model when the alternative is the SCE model. Eight observations were censored, representing a proportion of 0.0889.

The distribution of the test statistic is approximated by the chi-square distribution with one degree of freedom, with a value $T = 13.131$; the p-value is 0.000 211 4, so the proportional hazards hypothesis is strongly rejected.

We applied the SCE model for estimation of the influence of covariates on survival. The modified partial likelihood estimator of $\theta = (\beta, \gamma)$ is (1.8945, 1.3844). The estimators of the survival functions of the two treatment arms cross at about $t_0 = 2.3$ years. The resulting inference indicates that the radiotherapy would initially be detrimental to a patient's survival but becomes beneficial later on. Unfortunately, only about 20 % of patients survive to time t_0.

12.5.3 Lung cancer radiotherapy

The survival data for 164 lung cancer patients given in Piantadosi (1997, pages 483–488) concern the effects of radiotherapy (sample size of 86) or radiotherapy plus CAP (sample size of 78). The Kaplan–Meier estimators pertaining to the two treatment groups cross twice: around 7 months and around 33 months. So we apply the test for the Cox model when the alternative is the MCE model.

The distribution of the test statistic is approximated by the chi-square distribution with two degrees of freedom and its value is $T = 9.804$; the p-value is 0.007 43, so the proportional hazards hypothesis is rejected.

12.6 CONCLUDING REMARKS

The three models considered work well in the situations when the proportional hazards (Cox) model is not applicable, that is, when ratios of hazard rates under different fixed covariates are not constant in time. These models may be used when the ratios are monotone and either do or do not intersect. Situations with inter-sections of survival functions can be also treated. The proposed goodness-of-fit tests strongly reject the Cox model in the case of data where non-applicability of this model is suspected.

APPENDIX: PROOF OF THEOREM 12.1

Set

$$M_i(t) = N_i(t) - \int_0^t Y_i(u)e^{\beta_0^T x_i} d\Lambda.$$

The Doob–Meier decomposition, delta method and the equality

$$n^{1/2}(\hat{\beta} - \beta_0) = \Sigma^{-1}(\tau) \sum_{i=1}^n \int_0^\tau \{x_i - E(u, \beta_0)\} dM_i(u) + o_p(1)$$

(see Andersen *et al.*, 1993) imply that

$$n^{-1/2}\hat{U}_\gamma(t) = n^{-1/2} \sum_{i=1}^n \int_0^t \{x_i - E(u, \hat{\beta})\}\hat{\Lambda}(u)dN_i(u)$$

$$= n^{-1/2} \sum_{i=1}^n \int_0^t \{x_i - E(u, \hat{\beta})\}\Lambda(u)dM_i(u) + n^{-1/2} \int_0^t \{E(u, \beta_0)$$

$$\quad - E(u, \hat{\beta})\}S^{(0)}(u, \beta_0)\hat{\Lambda}(u)d\Lambda(u)$$

$$= n^{-1/2} \sum_{i=1}^n \int_0^t \{x_i - E(u, \beta_0)\}\Lambda(u)dM_i(u)$$

$$\quad - n^{-1} \int_0^t \frac{\partial E(u, \beta_0)}{\partial \beta} \Lambda(u)S^{(0)}(u, \beta_0)d\Lambda(u) \, n^{1/2}(\hat{\beta} - \beta_0) + o_p(1)$$

$$= n^{-1/2} \sum_{i=1}^n \int_0^t \{x_i - E(u, \beta_0)\}\Lambda(u)dM_i(u)$$

$$\quad - \Sigma_\gamma^*(t)\Sigma^{-1}(\tau)n^{-1/2} \sum_{i=1}^n \int_0^\tau \{x_i - E(u, \beta_0)\}dM_i(u) + o_p(1),$$

where $\Sigma(t)$ and $\Sigma_\gamma^*(t)$ are respectively the limits in probability of the random matrices

$$\hat{\Sigma}(t) = n^{-1} \int_0^t V(u, \hat{\beta}) dN(u) \quad \text{and} \quad \hat{\Sigma}_\gamma^*(t) = n^{-1} \int_0^t V(u, \hat{\beta}) \hat{\Lambda}(u) dN(u),$$

with

$$V(u, \hat{\beta}) = \frac{S^{(2)}(u, \hat{\beta})}{S^{(0)}(u, \hat{\beta})} - \left(E(u, \hat{\beta}) \right)^{\otimes 2}.$$

So

$$\langle n^{-1/2} \hat{U}_\gamma \rangle(t) = n^{-1} \sum_{i=1}^n \int_0^t \{x_i - E(u, \beta_0)\}^{\otimes 2} \Lambda^2(u) e^{\beta_0^T x_i} Y_i(u) d\Lambda(u)$$

$$- 2\Sigma_\gamma^*(t) \Sigma^{-1}(\tau) n^{-1} \sum_{i=1}^n \int_0^t \{x_i - E(u, \beta_0)\}^{\otimes 2} e^{\beta_0^T x_i} \Lambda(u)$$

$$\times Y_i(u) d\Lambda(u) + \Sigma_\gamma^*(t) \Sigma^{-1}(\tau) n^{-1} \sum_{i=1}^n \int_0^\tau \{x_i - E(u, \beta_0)\}^{\otimes 2} e^{\beta_0^T x^{(i)}}$$

$$\times Y_i(u) d\Lambda(u) \Sigma^{-1}(\tau) (\Sigma_\gamma^*(t))^T + o_p(1)$$

$$= \Sigma_\gamma^{**}(t) - \Sigma_\gamma^*(t) \Sigma^{-1}(\tau) (\Sigma_\gamma^*(t))^T + o_p(1),$$

where $\Sigma_\gamma^{**}(t)$ is the limit in probability of

$$\hat{\Sigma}_\gamma^{**}(t) = n^{-1} \int_0^t V(u, \hat{\beta}) \hat{\Lambda}^2(u) dN(u).$$

Similarly, the Lindeberg conditions (see Andersen *et al.*, 1993) are verified: for any $\varepsilon > 0$,

$$n^{-1} \sum_{i=1}^n \int_0^\tau \{x_{ij} - E_j(u, \beta_0)\}^2 \Lambda^2(u) \mathbf{1}_{\{|\Lambda(u)(x_{ij} - E_j(u,\beta_0))| \geq \sqrt{n}\varepsilon\}} e^{\beta_0^T x^{(i)}} Y_i(u) d\Lambda(u) \xrightarrow{P} 0$$

and

$$n^{-1} \sum_{i=1}^n \int_0^\tau \{x_{ij} - E_j(u, \beta_0)\}^2 \mathbf{1}_{\{|x_{ij} - E_j(u,\beta_0)| \geq \sqrt{n}\varepsilon\}} e^{\beta_0^T x^{(i)}} Y_i(u) d\Lambda(u) \xrightarrow{P} 0;$$

here x_{ij} and E_j are the jth components of x_i and E, respectively.

Analogously,

$$\langle n^{-1/2} \hat{U}_\delta \rangle(t) = \Sigma_\delta^{**}(t) - \Sigma_\delta^*(t) \Sigma^{-1}(\tau) (\Sigma_\delta^*(t))^T + o_p(1),$$

where $\Sigma_\delta^*(t)$ and $\Sigma_\delta^{**}(t)$ are the limits in probability of

$$\hat{\Sigma}_\delta^*(t) = \hat{\Sigma}_\gamma^{**}(t), \qquad \hat{\Sigma}_\delta^{**}(t) = n^{-1} \int_0^t V(u, \hat{\beta}) \hat{\Lambda}^4(u) dN(u),$$

respectively, and

$$\langle n^{-1/2}\hat{U}_\gamma, n^{-1/2}\hat{U}_\delta\rangle(t) = \Sigma_{\gamma\delta}^{**}(t) - \Sigma_\gamma^*(t)\Sigma^{-1}(\tau)(\Sigma_\delta^*(t))^\mathrm{T} + o_p(1),$$

where $\Sigma_{\gamma\delta}^{**}(t)$ is the limit in probability of

$$\hat{\Sigma}_{\gamma\delta}^{**}(t) = n^{-1}\int_0^t V(u, \hat{\beta})\hat{\Lambda}^3(u)dN(u).$$

Similarly, the Lindeberg conditions are verified.

Hence, the stochastic process $n^{-1/2}\hat{U}$ converges in distribution to a zero-mean Gaussian process, in particular

$$T = n^{-1}\hat{U}^\mathrm{T}\hat{D}^{-1}\hat{U} \xrightarrow{\mathcal{D}} \chi^2(2m)$$

where

$$\hat{D} = \begin{pmatrix} \hat{D}_\gamma & \hat{D}_{\gamma\delta} \\ \hat{D}_{\gamma\delta} & \hat{D}_\delta \end{pmatrix},$$

$$\hat{D}_\gamma = \hat{\Sigma}_\gamma^{**}(\tau) - \hat{\Sigma}_\gamma^*(\tau)\hat{\Sigma}^{-1}(\tau)(\hat{\Sigma}_\gamma^*(\tau))^\mathrm{T}, \quad \hat{D}_\delta = \hat{\Sigma}_\delta^{**}(\tau) - \hat{\Sigma}_\delta^*(\tau)\hat{\Sigma}^{-1}(\tau)(\hat{\Sigma}_\delta^*(\tau))^\mathrm{T},$$

$$\hat{D}_{\gamma\delta} = \hat{\Sigma}_{\gamma\delta}^{**}(\tau) - \hat{\Sigma}_\gamma^*(\tau)\hat{\Sigma}^{-1}(\tau)(\hat{\Sigma}_\delta^*(t))^\mathrm{T}.$$

The proof is complete.

CHAPTER 13

Dose-Response Modeling

Lutz Edler and Annette Kopp-Schneider

German Cancer Research Center

Harald Heinzl

Medical University of Vienna

13.1 INTRODUCTION

Quantitative human health risk assessment aims at the estimation of the likelihood and severity of damage to humans from exposure to hazardous agents. A major component of risk assessment (RA) is the search for and the study of a dose-response relationship with the goal of estimating the risk at specified doses, in particular, at doses in the range of human exposure levels. The risk assessor is usually highly interested in ascertaining the exposure level above which a compound is definitively harmful as well as the dose level below which exposure is harmless to humans. Knowledge of such threshold-type dose levels would make RA easy to communicate and to implement in regulatory guidelines. Whether this is always achievable and how dose-response models (DRMs) can contribute to the scientifically sound solution of this challenging task is one of the main issues to be dealt with in this chapter.

Efforts to estimate so-called safe dose levels have dominated RA methodology for several decades. Risk managers pursued the ambitious goal calculating a safe dose from experimental data, mostly of animal origin, at which exposure would not result in any appreciable risk for humans. RA was thus reduced to a dichotomous decision between the absence and the presence of a risk. Tests of many compounds were performed at doses convenient to assess the presence of toxicity at some dose level, but they were often rather non-informative for effects to be expected at presumed human exposure levels. This left human RA weak and with poor scientific foundations. The rigorous approach of either banning or accepting a compound has been debated from the outset as being incompatible with scientific principles of

Recent Advances in Quantitative Methods in Cancer and Human Health Risk Assessment
Edited by L. Edler and C. Kitsos © 2005 John Wiley & Sons, Ltd

dose-dependent effects. More adequate for a realistic RA is a toxicologically based notion of estimating the dose-response relationship on the basis of all available biological knowledge using empirical data and applying statistical inference. This approach will be followed in this chapter, and mathematical modeling and statistical analysis methods for DRMs will be reviewed.

The RA of a specific substance, for example a pesticide residue or a member of the dioxin family, often shows harmful effects at high doses in animal experiments. At the same time, this substance may be present ubiquitously and for a long time at very low doses in the food and human environment. When no effects after exposure to such substances at low doses are observed, one is tempted to believe that threshold doses exist below which no effects would happen or could happen. The discussion on the existence of threshold doses and their determination has been about toxicology and RA almost from the beginning. Obviously one can not conclude toxicity over the whole dose region when a toxic response is only observed when the substance is administered at a sufficiently high dose. On the other hand, it has also been recognized empirically that a threshold concept suffers from a lack of biological plausibility. Furthermore, when experimental dose-response data are evaluated using the appropriate statistical methods, determinations of threshold doses often lacked statistical support (Schneiderman *et al.*, 1979; Crump *et al.*, 1976). Apparently, the ability to detect a biological effect depends not only on the sensitivity but also on the design of the assay and the statistical power.

Nevertheless, from its very beginnings quantitative RA has discussed the validity of the threshold versus the non-threshold approach. The threshold concept was pragmatically based on the observation or non-observation of effects at some dose levels and has led to the use by risk assessors of the non-observed adverse effect level (NOAEL) or the lowest observed adverse effect level (LOAEL) as quantitative parameter of a dose-response curve. The NOAEL is a parameter directly derived from the observed dose-response curve defined as the highest administered dose where the effect is still not significantly different from that at dose 0. All effects at dose levels below the NOAEL must therefore be insignificant, and if there is none, the NOAEL has to be set equal to dose 0. The LOAEL ($>$ NOAEL) is the smallest administered dose level where the effect is (the first time) significantly different from the effects at dose 0, and if there is none, it cannot defined properly. Apart from being based on a multiple test procedure along the dose-response curve (see Section 13.3.1 below; see also Edler *et al.*, 2002), both parameters lack further statistical properties in terms of unbiasedness and precision. NOAELs and LOAELs are preferably then used in RA when the data are insufficient to build a DRM. In a recent guidance paper on RA of low levels of chemical in food and diet, Kroes *et al.* (2004) made extensive use of point estimates of NOAELs of various classes of compounds to define structure-based thresholds of toxicological concern in those cases. However, NOAELs and LOAELs were also used as apparently deterministic parameters easy to calculate and easy to communicate, although each of them carries, beyond the problem of technical detection, statistical variability, which is difficult to quantify. The existence and non-existence of thresholds had also been related to the absence and presence of genotoxic mechanisms, respectively.

Although theoretically appealing, this concept was not unanimously supported by empirical evidence (Edler and Kopp-Schneider, 1998). On the other hand, the non-threshold approach was based on mechanistically modeling effects over the whole dose range – from zero dose to the largest dose applicable in a test system, for example the maximum tolerated dose defined by acute toxicity or lethality. Obviously, humans would rarely be exposed to such large doses.

Irrespective of whether RA focused on resolving the controversy between the existence and the non-existence of thresholds or on the description of the dose-response relationship, considerable emphasis has been put on the use of sound biological and statistical principles for the construction of DRMs. The analysis of dose-response in a dose range where effects are actually observed is now considered as a first step for low-dose extrapolation. The second step would then be the set-up of a method which determines the risk estimates in the low-dose region, or estimates doses to be designed as without harm to humans, so-called reference doses (RfDs). This second step would constitute the genuine low dose extrapolation procedure and it would use information from the experimental dose regions only in a comprised form, for example as a starting point for low-dose extrapolation as defined in Section 13.4.4 below. This two-step approach seems well suited to overcoming deficiencies of earlier concepts where the RfD was estimated more or less in one step from the empirical dose-response data, for example, using the NOAEL or LOAEL together with some default safety factors. The benchmark dose (BMD) method, earlier developed for non-cancer endpoints only but recently also used for cancer endpoints, emphasizes the application of this two step approach. The BMD approach restricts any model prediction to the range of observed dose-response data. As such, it clearly separates the regulatory task of setting an RfD from the scientific task of estimating a dose-response curve (US Environmental Protection Agency, 1996).

This chapter will summarize the present status of dose-response modeling in RA by distinguishing between qualitative and quantitative DRMs for tumor incidence, for other quantal data as well as for continuous data. Models using age/time-dependent tumor incidence data will be addressed among the continuous DRMs. As a special case, quantal dose-response models including threshold-type models and tolerance distribution models will be considered. The multistage model and the two-stage model of clonal expansion are presented as valuable DRMs accounting for biological mechanisms. Section 13.5 considers aspects of the dose-response modeling of 2,3,7,8-tetrachlorodibenzo-*p*-dioxin (TCDD) as an example.

13.2   ELEMENTS OF DOSE-RESPONSE ASSESSMENT

Dose-response assessment in quantitative risk assessment evaluates the potential risks to humans at exposure levels of interest (Chapter 1, this volume; US EPA 1999). In order to put the assessment of the relationship of dose to response on a scientifically sound basis it is necessary to define both exposure and response in such a way as to be unequivocally suitable and implementable for the specific RA task. In this section we discuss some aspects of defining exposure, dose and risk response quantitatively.

13.2.1 Exposure and dose

Exposure describes the contact of the agent with the 'outer boundary' of the individual and has to account for all aspects of the individual's contact with the exogenous agent. Therefore, exposure is characterized by qualitative and quantitative elements. In contrast, dose data are quantitative in nature and describe the amount or concentration of an agent in the individual after that contact has occurred. Consequently, dose is a exact numerical quantity describing the amount of the agent entering the organism and acting at the target site. An agent can enter an organism at various instances (environmentally, accidentally, on purpose during medical treatment, etc.) and through various routes (inhalation, dermal, oral, etc.). Furthermore, on its way through the organism the agent passes various sites of the organism before being deposited at a final site of action or before being excreted. During this journey the parent agent can unleash its toxic action in various organs (targets). Most agents decay into sub-products, are metabolized into 'follow-up' compounds or induce in the organism the production of substances which may have a hazardous potential of their own. Those daughter substances may then interact with the organism in a similar manner to the parent compound. As a consequence, in most dose-response studies it is an oversimplification to concentrate on one exposure scenario of one dose. A more adequate course is to examine the complete route and cascade of the agent. This results in several notions of dose. One distinguishes between the *applied dose*, the amount presented for absorption; the *internal dose*, the amount crossing the absorption border; and the *delivered dose* (target dose), the amount available at the organ of the toxic interaction. The US EPA (1999) recommended that one check:

- whether dose is expressed as environmental concentration, applied dose, or delivered dose to the target organ;

- whether dose is expressed in terms of a parent compound, one or more metabolites, or both;

- whether the impact of dose patterns and timing are significant;

- the conversion from animal to human doses, when animal data are used;

- the conversion metric between routes of exposure.

In practical RA one may not be able to measure the target organ dose even if that would be most relevant. Reasons could be that data are available from animal experiments only and not from studies on humans, that no dose information is available for susceptible subgroups, that exposure data do not correspond to the type of exposure to be regulated, or that no measurement is possible at the target due to the complexity of the biological organism. Interspecies and intraspecies adjustment of dose, route-to-route extrapolation, and toxicokinetic analyses using physiologically based models have been developed to calculate at least approximately a dose parameter for the DRM. When exposure lasts over the individual's entire lifetime, individual dose averaging methods (e.g. using the AUC over the time course of the dose) have been proposed.

13.2.2 Response

Response data characterize the toxic endpoints. Because of the multiplicity of adverse effects and ambiguities as to what is a primary and what is a secondary endpoint, one should in principle account for multivariate response data $(Y_1, \ldots, Y_p)$. In addition to tumor incidence at various organ sites, immunological and neurological adverse events may be observed. In practice, DRMs have almost exclusively been analyzed as univariate DRMs, evaluating one variable Y_i at a time. A series of univariate evaluations has the advantage that its outcomes are much easier to interpret than the outcome of a multivariate response analysis because each component Y_j may be of very different quality.

13.2.2.1 Qualitative and quantitative tumor response data

Response data can be of a qualitative or of quantitative nature. In cancer risk assessment tumor incidence data and tumor-specific mortality data have been the basic response endpoints for the dose-response assessment. When considering lifetime tumor incidence, each individual is characterized by a dichotomous response variable Y with the two possible outcomes, 'tumor' or 'no tumor'. When the type of tumor is taken into account a multinomial response variable is recorded, for example when discriminating between different types of lung tumors such as adenomas and squamous cell carcinomas. A qualitative categorically ordered response variable is obtained when different grades of malignancy are determined. In contrast, the size of a tumor or the time to diagnosis of a tumor are quantitative response endpoints. The measurement scale of the response endpoint determines both the type of DRM and the type of error distribution of the data to be incorporated into the DRM.

13.2.2.2 Precursor lesions

Responses other than tumorigenicity may be considered when biological effects preceding the tumor development can be observed. Those effects could be DNA damage of cells of the target organ, hormonal or enzymatic changes, effects on cell growth and signal transduction, or physiological changes. If these effects can be traced down as having a direct effect on the tumor induction and tumor development one speaks of precursor lesions which were considered for dose-response in the context of the two-stage and the multistage hypothesis of tumor development (Chapters 5 and 8 this volume). A special case of precursor lesions are premalignant lesions in colon, prostate, endometrial, skin or liver (Chapter 4, this volume). Pre-malignant lesions occur with higher frequency than malignant tumors, may give rise to quantitative response and provide more information to build a

DRM (Kopp-Schneider, 2003). Skin and liver have been sites of carcinogenesis where the use of pre-malignant endpoints was most successful.

13.2.2.3 Premalignant lesions of the liver and the skin

The occurrence of foci of altered hepatocytes (FAH) has proven to be a valuable indicator of the ability of an experimental treatment to cause liver cancer (see Bannasch, 1996). Although the number of liver cancers induced in rodents by chemicals is orders of magnitude lower than that of FAH in the usual timeframe of these experiments, there is a clear correlation between the two. Consequently, the number of FAH has been considered as a sensitive surrogate marker of carcinogenic response and has been used as (surrogate) endpoint for the estimation of the carcinogenic potential of the agent. In addition, the finding that a compound alters the number of focal transections or the size distribution of the transections may give indications about the mechanism of action of the compound (Kopp-Schneider, 2003). Studies with FAH as endpoint can be evaluated quantitatively by determining the total area occupied by FAH in a liver section with a morphometric device. The carcinogenic potential of a treatment can be shown in an experiment treating less than 100 animals for only 3 months (Ittrich *et al.*, 2003), whereas studies with (qualitative) endpoint liver tumor incidence need to include several hundreds of animals for an observation period of 2 years. Therefore, the analysis of FAH has the potential to save time, cost, and animals in carcinogenesis testing.

Topical treatment of mouse skin has been widely used to study the mechanism and carcinogenic potential of chemicals. Skin papillomas are observed on the treated skin before skin carcinomas arise (Marks and Fürstenberger, 1987). These lesions can be observed repeatedly and it has been shown that some papillomas regress while others progress to carcinomas. The experimental two-stage mouse skin carcinogenesis model has played an important role in biological carcinogenesis theory. It led to the notion of initiation (conditioning of a normal cell) and promotion (cell proliferation with a growth advantage compared to normal cells). Further introduction of a second 'mutational' event describing the progression to carcinomas led to a very rich class of stochastic two-stage models which translated this theory into a class of mathematical models (see Kopp-Schneider 1997; Chapter 5, this volume).

Both experimental systems, liver and skin, have commonly been used to study dose-response relationships. Whether a dose-response relationship for the preneoplastic lesion can predict a dose-response relationship of the true carcinogenic endpoint has to be studied on a case-by-case basis. An example of the use of FAH and its predictivity of carcinogenicity of TCDD is provided below in Section 13.5.

13.2.3 Biomarkers

The notion of biomarkers was introduced in RA as a means to use more biologically realistic information and to make full use of all available biological measurements related both to exposure and to response. Biomarkers of exposure can be used as dose indicators, in contrast to biomarkers of effect which can be used to predict response and are useful as surrogate endpoints. A further class are the biomarkers of susceptibility useful for describing heterogeneity and effect modification, for example fast and slow metabolizers (see Chapter 3, this volume). Members of the cytochrome P450 isoenzyme family have been identified both as biomarkers of exposure and as biomarkers of response. The more biological information can be obtained about the investigated hazardous substance the easier it will be to define the role of a specific biomarker and to determine its function in a DRM either as a dependent or as independent variable.

13.3 DOSE-RESPONSE MODELS

The purpose of a DRM in quantitative RA is to find a relationship between the effect Y and the dose D which can be analyzed for the estimation of effects given specific dose levels as well as for the estimation of dose levels corresponding to specific effect levels. This first of all requires the DRM to be analytically tractable. Furthermore, sound and flexible statistical methods are essential to describe and explore experimental data by means of the DRM (curve fitting), to draw inferential conclusions on the nature of the dose-response, and to predict Y given dose D. A generic DRM has the form

$$f(D) : D \rightarrow Y(D), \tag{13.1}$$

where $f(D)$ represents the functional dependency of the effect Y on dose D. The effect could be a simple effect variable or a more complicated derived risk function. Construction and evaluation of $f(D)$ proceed in the following steps:

- Identify the type of data available on dose and response.
- Select the response and dose metric for assessment.
- Analyze the DRM using statistical methods.
- Explain the results of the dose-response assessment.

Statistical methods can be subdivided into two broad methodological approaches described below as qualitative and quantitative dose-response modeling. The type and extent of information available for the DRM and whether functional information on dose-response is available or not are determinants for choosing between the qualitative testing approach (Section 13.3.1) and the quantitative dose-response modeling approach (Section 13.3.2). In both cases we assume for a statistical analysis dose-response data of the form

$$(d_i, y_{ij}), \qquad j = 1, \ldots, n_i, i = 0, 1, \ldots, I, \tag{13.2}$$

where d_i is the ordered dose variable, say given I doses $0 < d_1 < d_2 < \ldots < d_I$. The control group is denoted by $d_0 = 0$. The design will assign n_i individuals to dose group d_i, respectively, and each of the n_i individuals exhibits its response value y_{ij} observed in the respective study.

Notice that throughout this section we will use 'dose', denoted by d, as a generic term for constructing and discussing mathematical dose-response models. In practical applications, dose metrics different from the administered dose are used, for example, the cumulative dose over lifetime in chronic toxicity experiments, or maximum given dose in acute toxicity experiments. For more evolved modeling of the dose and other dose metrics used in RA we refer to Chapter 7 (this volume).

13.3.1 Qualitative dose-response analysis

When no functional information on the dose-response relationship exists and consequently no function $f(D)$ is available, the dose-response data (13.2) can be analyzed qualitatively by testing for the presence of dose-response effects using statistical hypothesis testing. This is achieved by multiple testing procedures which allow conclusions on the presence or absence of a dose-response effect within the framework of error probabilities of hypothesis testing. In the simplest case, one tests the null hypothesis

$$H_0 : F_0 = F_1 = \cdots = F_I, \qquad (13.3)$$

where '$F_i = F_j$' describes the fact that the two groups treated with doses d_i and d_j do not differ in their outcome, versus an alternative H_1: (13.3) does not hold because at least one dose pair differs. If the symbol F is chosen to denote the cumulative distribution function of the stochastic outcome variable Y, then (13.3) will stand for the simultaneous equality of all $I + 1$ distribution functions characterizing the dose-response experiment.

More interesting then the alternative '(13.3) does not hold' is an alternative of increasing trend

$$H_1 : F_0 \,'\leq'\, F_1 \,'\leq'\, \cdots \,'\leq'\, F_I, \qquad (13.4)$$

where $F_i \,'\leq'\, F_j$ describes the fact that the response at dose d_j is larger than at dose d_i. Notice the symbolic use of '$\leq$' in (13.4). When calculating with cumulative distributions the '$\leq$' relationship in $F_i \,'\leq'\, F_j$ is correctly written mathematically as $F_i(y) \geq F_j(y)$, $y \geq 0$, y varying on the response scale.

If one assumes at each dose level d_i a normally distributed response $Y_{ij} \sim N(\mu_i, \sigma_i^2)$, with mean μ_i and variance σ_i^2, the alternative of a monotone increasing trend can be formulated in terms of the means of that normal distribution as

$$H_1 = \mu_0 \leq \mu_1 \leq \cdots \leq \mu_I, \qquad (13.5)$$

with $\mu_0 < \mu_I$. This test problem has been widely investigated in statistical literature (see Hothorn and Lehmacher, 1991).

If responses at doses d_i are proportions p_i, for example, the proportion of animals developing a tumor, the alternative

$$H_1 : p_0 \leq p_1 \leq \cdots \leq p_I \qquad (13.6)$$

with $p_0 < p_I$ can be tested using the Cochran–Armitage test for (linear) trend which is powerful for assessing monotone trends when response data follow a binomial or Poisson distribution. We refer to Piegorsch and Bailer (1997, Chapter 6) for more details of the statistical analysis of trend tests and for methods suitable for over-dispersed data, as well as for implementations in SAS software. Distribution-free rank-based methods are indicated in particular when instead of the monotone alternative (13.4)–(13.6) a downturn of the dose-response relationship is possible, for example the so-called umbrella alternative

$$H_0 : \mu_0 \leq \mu_1 \leq \ldots \mu_{i^*} \geq \mu_{i^*+1} \geq \ldots \geq \mu_I, \tag{13.7}$$

where i^* denotes the umbrella's turning point. This type of dose-response analysis has been intensively studied for the evaluation of mutagenicity data (Edler, 1992).

13.3.2 Quantitative dose-response analysis

When functional information is available a statistical analysis of a DRM can be performed such that one obtains estimates of specific parameters of the DRM as well as estimates of the dose-response curve as a whole to be used for the prediction of the response at a given dose. Furthermore, an inversion of the predicted DRM will allow the determination of the specific dose D_{y*} which is associated with a particular level of response y^*. Depending on the type of the response outcome, one distinguishes between continuous response models (Sections 13.3.2.1 and 13.3.2.2) and discrete response models (Section 13.3.2.3).

13.3.2.1 Continuous response models

The adverse effect of a toxic compound can give rise to continuous data $Y(d)$, such as tumor volume. A general DRM could be the regression model

$$Y(d) = \mu(d) + \varepsilon, \tag{13.8}$$

where μ denotes a predictor which may be nonlinear in d, and $\varepsilon \sim N(0, \sigma^2)$ the (residual) error term.

Notice that in practical applications a risk function is defined through normalization of the DRM (13.8). This could be achieved through subtraction of the background effect,

$$R(d) = Y(d) - \mu(0) \tag{13.9}$$

or through subtraction and additional scaling with the background effect $\mu(0)$,

$$R(d) = \frac{Y(d) - \mu(0)}{\mu(0)}. \tag{13.10}$$

Another type of normalization in the continuous response model is obtained by considering the probability that the standardized response $(Y(d) - \mu(0))/\sigma$ exceeds some boundary value δ when mapping the response Y onto the bounded 'risk interval' [0,1]:

$$Q(d) = P\left(\frac{Y(d) - \mu(0)}{\sigma} \leq \delta\right). \tag{13.11}$$

We refer to Kodell and West (1993) for an extended discussion of modeling of continuous response. The simplest form of a continuous model (13.8) is the linear regression

$$\mu(d) = \beta_0 + \beta_1 d \tag{13.12}$$

where the primary model parameter β_1 describes the slope of the DRM. Non-linear regression extends this concept by considering $\mu(d) = g(d, \beta)$ with a non-linear function g and parameter vector β. A large number of classes of non-linear functions g were discussed in Edler (1992) for modeling mutagenic response depending on dose.

A class of nonlinear hyperbolic functions has been used for modeling the amount or concentration of biomarkers, for example, the amount of specific enzymes of the P450 family. Most prominent has been the Michaelis–Menten (MM) equation

$$\mu(d) = \frac{V_{\max}d}{K_m + d} \tag{13.13}$$

where the role of the substrate concentration of the MM kinetic is taken over by the dose parameter and the MM reaction 'velocity' represents the response. The two model parameters have the well-known interpretation of maximum velocity $(V_{\max})$ and half-maximum dose (K_m). The MM model (13.13) has been generalized to the Hill equation

$$\mu(d) = \frac{V_{\max}d^n}{K_m + d^n} \tag{13.14}$$

where the additional parameter n, originally denoting the number of binding sites, describes the shape of the dose-response curve, sometimes interpreted as potency of the substance.

We refer to Kodell and West (1993) for an extended discussion of the modeling of continuous response.

13.3.2.2 Modeling age-dependent incidence

The risk of developing diagnosable cancer increases with the age of the individual not only because exposure may accumulate over time but also because cancer development is assumed to be slow and the latency from the first malignant cell to development of an overt tumor may last many years. Obviously cancer RA is much more realistic when not only the crude lifetime incidence is studied but also the development of the disease is examined over time. Age-dependent incidence data contain much more information and are more powerful for detecting differences between dose groups.

The simplest measurable quantity next to lifetime tumor incidence is the time from birth or start of exposure until the occurrence of an overt tumor. This time-to-occurrence (also called time-to-tumor) variable is a non-negative survival time which is possibly right-censored (in those individuals for whom the tumor had not occurred by the time of examination). In cases where the tumor is only observable through specific screening and the implementation of an inspection scheme, this survival time may even be interval-censored. Mechanistic stochastic modeling has mainly focused on this type of statistical data.

Statistical time-to-event models

Let us consider in this section the age-dependent incidence function $P(t, d)$ denoting the probability of occurrence of a tumor by age t if exposed to an agent at dose d by that time. Both parametric and semiparametric functions have been used to describe $P(t, d)$. Below are listed some parametric DRMs obtained by incorporating time (or age) of the individual straightforward into well-known tolerance distribution models or related models:

$$\text{Probit} \quad P(t,d) = p + (1-p) \cdot \Phi(a + bd + c \log t); \tag{13.15}$$

$$\text{Logit} \quad P(t,d) = p + (1-p) \cdot [1 + \exp(-(a + bd + c \log t))]^{-1}; \tag{13.16}$$

$$\text{Weibull} \quad P(t,d) = p + (1-p) \cdot (1 - \exp(-bd^m t^K)); \tag{13.17}$$

$$\text{Multi-hit} \quad P(t,d) = p + (1-p) \cdot \int_0^{d \cdot t} [b^n u^{n-1}/\Gamma(n)] \exp(-bu) du; \tag{13.18}$$

$$\text{Multistage} \quad P(t,d) = p + (1-p) \cdot \left\{ 1 - \exp\left[- \left(\sum_{i=0}^{K} a_i d^i \right) \cdot bt^K \right] \right\}. \tag{13.19}$$

Here p denotes the background risk $P(0,0)$ and a, b, c, K, m, n, and $\{a_i\}$ are model parameters. K denotes the number of stages in the multistage model. More generally, an age-dependent tumor incidence model can be defined using a non-parametric hazard function $\lambda^T(t, d)$ of the time-to-tumor T. The practical estimation of $\lambda^T(t, d)$ from carcinogenesis bioassay data requires statistical methodology for censored survival times. Methods of survival analysis (Kalbfleisch and Prentice, 1980) can be applied straightforwardly to analyze time-to-occurrence data, if the occurrence of the tumor can be observed. Notice, however, that one often will not be able to observe the tumor directly (occult tumor) but only through autopsy of the animal after natural death or sacrifice. Specific methods have been proposed to deal with this problem (Gart *et al.*, 1986). For the use of relative risk regression models based on the hazard function concept in RA we refer to Moolgavkar and Luebeck (2002).

When the distribution of time-to-death from a tumor is parameterized through quantiles of its distribution one can define a relationship between the dose and the quantiles. Druckrey (1967) investigated such a relationship for the median time-to-death with tumor (t_{50}),

$$t_{50}^n \cdot d = \text{const.}, \tag{13.20}$$

and considered it as a 'universal law' of carcinogenesis, where the power coefficient n was attributed a role of measuring carcinogenic potency (Druckrey index). In a similar vein, Sawyer et al. (1984) introduced the TD_{50} measure of carcinogenic potency for the long-term animal experiment accounting for occult tumors and serial/terminal sacrifice. TD_{50} is the dose, in units of mg/(kg body weight)/day, which, if administered chronically for the standard lifespan of the animal species, will halve the probability of remaining tumor-free throughout the standard lifespan. Denote the standard lifespan by T^* and the tumor incidence survival function by $S(t, d)$ describing the percentage of animals surviving time t without tumor given a dose d. Then TD_{50} is defined by

$$S(T^*, TD_{50}) = 0.5\, S(T^*, 0). \tag{13.21}$$

The hazard function $\lambda^T(t, d)$ for the tumor incidence, corresponding to $S(t, d)$, can only be estimated for observable tumors. For occult tumors it can be approximated by $\lambda^{DT}(t, d)$, the hazard function of time-to-death with tumor. Assuming the Cox proportional hazard model for λ^{DT} (i.e. $\lambda^{DT}(t, d) = \lambda_0(t) \exp(\beta \cdot d)$),

$$TD_{50} = \log\left[1 + \ln\frac{0.5}{\ln S_0(T^*)}\right]/\beta \tag{13.22}$$

where $S_0(T^*) = \exp(-\int_0^{T^*} \lambda_0(u)\, du)$ has to be estimated as baseline survivor function.

Stochastic models

A number of stochastic models have been suggested to describe the process of carcinogenesis and to analyze tumor incidence data. Generally it can be stated that the more realistic a model is, the more it becomes computationally complicated and therefore likely to be intractable for analytic calculations. A classification of carcinogenesis models with respect to their intended use, level of biological detail and analytic methods has been given by Kopp-Schneider (1997). These models describe the distribution to the time when the first detectable tumor occurs, the distribution of the number of tumors, the size distribution of the tumor, the probability of metastasis, etc. Taken by themselves all these models are primarily constructed to describe the natural course of the disease or the course of the disease under a specific condition. For their use as the basis for a DRM one has to introduce the dependency on the dose. This is most easily achieved through the use of dose-dependent model parameters. Take as an example the multistage carcinogenesis model of Armitage and Doll (1954); for a comprehensive explanation, see Whittemore and Keller (1978). The basic model parameters, transition rates μ_i between stage $i - 1$ and stage i, have been used to model a linear dose dependency as $\mu_i = a_i + b_i d$. Then one can calculate the probability of the occurrence of a tumor by time (age) t as

$$P(t, d) = 1 - \exp\left[-ct^K \left(\prod_{i=1}^{K}(a_i + b_i d)\right)\right], \tag{13.23}$$

with parameters $a_i \geq 0$, $b_i \geq 0$, and a global constant c, equivalent to (13.19). Given age t is fixed, for example at the length of the experiment or at the average lifespan of the individual, one obtains the multistage DRM in a polynomial form

$$P(d) = 1 - \exp[q_0 + q_1 d + q_2 d^2 + \cdots + q_K d^K] \tag{13.24}$$

with parameters $q_i \geq 0$, $0 \leq i \leq K$, (see also Chapter 5, this volume.)

The most prominent example in cancer RA has long been the multistage carcinogenesis model as described above. When the attempt was made to include more biological information in the construction of a carcinogenesis model, for example knowledge of cell proliferation and cell death, a second generation of multistage models, the so-called two-stage model of clonal expansion (TSCE model), emerged; see Chapter 5 (this volume). Within that model one can express the birth rates β_i, the death rates δ_i, or the mutation rates μ_i as a function of dose. In the absence of better mechanistic biological information a linear function of dose has usually been assumed. For alternatives and extensions, see Kopp-Schneider *et al.* (2002).

Research on the most realistic shape of the dose function and how it translates to the risk function $P(t, d)$ is still a challenge. Portier (1987) showed that additive treatment effects proportionate to dose will result in low-dose linear behavior. Another issue is model misspecification. Portier and Hoel (1983) investigated how the fit of the wrong dose-response relationship in the class of multistage models would affect dose estimates. Fitting a quadratic model to a true linear relationship results in an overestimation and, conversely, fitting a linear model to a true quadratic relationship results in an underestimation by 2–3 orders of magnitude. Even if the type of the model was determined by the data, this bias remained since the estimated model has a non-negligible chance of being misspecified and one may not be able to decide on the basis of the data whether the true model is purely linear, purely quadratic, or linear and quadratic in the dose.

13.3.2.3 Discrete response models

A variety of regression approaches exist in the statistical literature for other than continuous endpoints. It is convenient to distinguish between count data and dichotomous response data which describe the presence or absence of an event. Count data have been analyzed using log-linear regression models of the form $EY_i = \mu_i = g(d_i, \beta)$, where the dependent variable Y_i counts a property, for example number of defective cells in an individual dosed at level d_i. A common choice is the log-linear model $\mu_i = \exp(\beta_0 + \beta_1 d_i)$, equivalently $\log \mu_i = \beta_0 + \beta_1 d_i$ which is a special case of a generalized linear model; see Piegorsch and Bailer (1997) and Moolgavkar and Luebeck (2002).

Dichotomous response data have long been the standard form of data for cancer RA, obtained in particular from animal experiments. The notion of quantal data and quantal DRM was used to describe models for the risk $P(d)$ defined as the probability of the occurrence of the event (e.g. tumor). In cancer RA, lifelong duration of exposure at constant rate and lifelong observation usually constituted the standard experimental design when risk indices and reference dose levels were calculated. e.g., the allowable daily intake ADI.

When a DRM has been established risk estimation proceeds in two directions: forward estimation of the risk $P(d^*)$ for a given dose d^*; and backward estimation of the risk-specific dose RSD(r^*) for a given risk limit r^*.

It is convenient to allow a background response level, for example, due to some endogenous exposure or due to background exposure from other agents when both act on the same target as the investigated agent. If that contribution occurs independently from the administered exposure, one obtains an *independent background DRM*,

$$P(d) = p + (1 - p) f(d), \qquad (13.25)$$

where p denotes the background response at dose 0. If the agent adds its effect to a preexisting mechanism an *additive background DRM* of the form

$$P(d) = f(a + \varphi(d)) \qquad (13.26)$$

is more adequate where the function φ within the risk function f describes the way in which the agent's dose transmits its effect. In the next section we will discuss approaches to defining the risk function f. It is natural to separate the determination of the dose-risk function $f(g(d, \beta))$ into two steps: definition of $f(.)$, and definition of $g(d, \beta)$, with parameter vector β. Natural first choices for g are the linear function $g(d, \beta) = a + bd$, a polynomial $g(d, \beta) = \sum_{k=0}^{K} \beta_k d^k$ or a multiple regression $g(d, \beta) = \beta_0 + \sum_{k=1}^{K} \beta_k X_k$ where the dependency on the dose is subsumed in a general design X, which may involve further factors of the study.

Tolerance distribution models

The 'tolerance dose distribution' concept (Morgan, 1992) provided a class of dose functions $f(.)$ with some sort of biological interpretation based on the sensitivity or resistance of the individual. A toxic effect is considered to occur at dose d if the individual's resistance to the substance is broken at that dose. The risk $f(d)$ is then modeled as the probability that the tolerance dose of an individual is less than or equal to d:

$$\mathrm{pr}(\text{Tolerance} \leq d) = f(d), \qquad (13.27)$$

where $f(d)$ may be any monotone increasing function with values between 0 and 1. The right-hand side of (13.27) can be parameterized further as $f(g(d, \beta))$ using a parameterized dose function $g(d, \beta)$.

The tolerance distribution models relate the effect measure to the dose using a convenient mathematical parameterization. In statistical literature this approach was considered as a first attempt to model risk mechanistically. From a biological application point of view, however, the model is too simplistic; the model parameters are not directly informative so that usually functions of the model parameters are used to describe the result for the risk manager. The two classes of quantal DRMs (13.25) and (13.26) above, thus become

$$P(d) = p + (1 - p) f(g(d, \beta)) \tag{13.28}$$
$$P(d) = f(a + g(d, \beta)) \tag{13.29}$$

where the 'internal' dose function $g(d, \beta)$ can be taken from a flexible class of transformations parameterized by β. The probit, logit, Weibull and gamma models have been the most famous statistical models derived within the tolerance distribution concept. These are respectively written

$$P(d) = p + (1 - p) \cdot \Phi(a + bd), \tag{13.30}$$
$$P(d) = p + (1 - p) \cdot [1 + \exp(-(a + bd))]^{-1}, \tag{13.31}$$
$$P(d) = p + (1 - p) \cdot (1 - \exp(-bd^k)), \tag{13.32}$$
$$P(d) = p + (1 - p) \cdot \int_0^d [b^n t^{n-1} / \Gamma(n)] \cdot \exp(-bt) dt, \tag{13.33}$$

where Φ stands for the Gaussian distribution and Γ for the gamma function. These risk functions are obtained as special cases of the time/age-dependent functions (13.15)–(13.18) above when fixing the time at some point.

The Scientific Committee of the Food Safety Council (1978) released guidelines for quantitative risk assessment which proposed the use of these DRMs. The Committee considered in its guidance also the one-hit model as a special case of the Weibull model and the multistage model. At that time, the gamma-multihit model was recommended for estimating responses at low doses and RA was based on the virtually safe dose concept of Mantel and Bryan (1961); see also Brown and Koziol (1983).

Quantal dose-response model for d > 0

All models described above use dose d on its original scale. In many applications toxicologists prefer the use of a dose metric on a logarithmic scale since they feel that this scale will more often provide DRMs of linear shape which are easier to interpret than non-linear shaped curves. As long as the DRM does not include a control group $d_0 = 0$ one can use either dose d or the logarithm $\log(d)$ of the original dose d as the dose metric in the DRM. In the framework of quantal DRMs one therefore considers the generic model

$$P(d) = p + (1 - p) f(g(\log d, \beta)) \tag{13.34}$$

This model assumes, however, that data of a control group with dose $d = 0$ cannot be included in the model fit and that the fit of the DRM is restricted to the dose range $d > 0$.

By introducing a background incidence p as in (13.27)–(13.30) one can overcome this restriction at least for some quantal DRMs. The probit model (13.30) with logarithmic dose $\log(d)$,

$$P(d) = p + (1 - p) \cdot \Phi(a + b\log(d)),$$

is defined for $d = 0$ since at the limit $d \to 0$ and $\log(d) \to -\infty$ the limit of the Gaussian function $\Phi(a + b\log(d))$ is zero and therefore $P(d) = p$. The same argument holds for the logit and Weibull models.

Reparameterization and effective dose 50 %

Consider the simplest form of a quantal DRM without background:

$$P(d) = f(d). \tag{13.35}$$

One may parametrize f as distribution by its mean μ and its variance σ^2 to obtain

$$P(d) = f\left(\frac{\log d - \mu}{\sigma}\right) \tag{13.36}$$

From the identity

$$\log\left[\frac{d}{\exp(\mu)}\right]^{\frac{1}{\sigma}} = \frac{\log d - \mu}{\sigma} = a + b\log d = \log[\exp(a) \cdot d^b] \tag{13.37}$$

it follows that $a = -\mu/\sigma$ and $b = 1/\sigma$ and that $\exp(\mu)$ is a scale factor. The factor $b = 1/\sigma$ determines the shape of the dose-response curve. Obviously this relationship holds for any regular risk function, for example, the probit, logit and Weibull DRM.

Contrariwise, in the case of the simple one-hit model $P(d) = 1 - \exp(-bd)$ the effective dose 50 % ED_{50} is a direct function of the slope parameter b:

$$\mathrm{ED}_{50} = \frac{\log 2}{b}. \tag{13.38}$$

This definition can easily be extended for the background DRM $P(d) = p + (1 - p)f(d)$:

$$\frac{P(\mathrm{ED}_{50}) - p}{1 - p} = 0.5, \tag{13.39}$$

denoting that dose which would lead to 50 % tumor incidence over background. More generally, the effective dose p^* percent (ED_{p*}) is defined through $p^* = p_0 + (1 - p_0)f(g(\mathrm{ED}_{p*}, \beta))$. If $p_0 = 0$ and $g(d, \beta) = a + b\log d$,

$$\mathrm{ED}_{p*} = \exp\left(\frac{f_*^{-1}(p^*) - a}{b}\right). \tag{13.40}$$

13.3.2.4 Epidemiological models for human studies

Age- and cause-specific mortality data are usually collected in epidemiological studies. The age-dependent cause-specific incidence rate estimated in human studies is nothing more than the hazard function $\lambda(t, d)$ which corresponds to a survival function $S(t, d)$ of the occurrence of an event by age t if exposed at dose d, $P(t, d)$. The methodology of epidemiological data analysis is quite well developed. However, the major difficulty lies in the estimation of human exposure dose (Van den Brandt *et al.*, 2002). Lifetime average daily dose has been used as a reasonable dose metric for human studies.

The proportional hazard model $\lambda(t, d) = \lambda_0(t) \exp(\beta d))$ has been proposed for analyzing human data. Others have proposed an additive risk model $\lambda(t, d) = \lambda_0(t) + \beta d$ or a multiplicative risk model $\lambda(t, d) = \lambda_0(t)(1 + \beta d)$.

13.3.3 Threshold-type dose-response models

The existence and determination of threshold values for the dose have been intensively discussed in toxicology and also in carcinogenic RA. Given the existence of a threshold, $d^* > 0$, the threshold model is formally given by

$$P(d) = \begin{cases} p & \text{if } d \leq d^*, \\ p + (1 - p) \cdot f(d, d^*) & \text{if } d > d^*, \end{cases} \tag{13.41}$$

where p is the independent background response and $f(d, d^*)$ denotes a continuous, usually monotone increasing function with values between 0 and 1, for $d > d^*$. The threshold dose d^* is an additional parameter to be estimated from the data. The threshold model is therefore always more complex than the corresponding model without threshold and inclusion of this additional complexity requires justification. For specific types of threshold models see Edler and Kopp-Schneider (1998), and for a discussion of the limitations of this model in RA we refer to Slob (1999). Erroneous postulation of threshold behavior may be caused by logarithmic dose scale. Edler *et al.* (1994) pointed out the danger of using logarithmic scale transformations when they considered the Michaelis–Menten model for relating the effect concentration c_m to the substrate concentration c_x of a xenobiotic. Plotted as a function of c_x, a curve proportional to dose in the low-dose region is obtained which saturates to a maximal response in the higher doses. However, if unwisely plotted (half-logarithmically), this curve appears to be sigmoidal and its shape would suggest the presence of a non-linear response in the low-dose region. In essence, a model can be linear on the arithmetic dose scale that appears to have a threshold when presented on a log scale.

13.4 DOSE-RESPONSE MODELS IN RISK ASSESSMENT

The construction of a DRM and the estimation of its model parameters have in a RA framework the primary purpose of estimation of risk-specific quantities. This could be a risk-specific dose or a reference dose to be used as regulatory advice, as with the allowable daily intake in the case of food contaminants. In this section, we will discuss how the methods described above fit in with this purpose of RA and what has to be considered in their application. Model search and low-dose extrapolation will be discussed.

13.4.1 Model search

When specifying a DRM during the process of RA one may chose between two basic approaches: selection of an empirical model $f(g(d, \beta))$ and its fit to the data (curve fitting); and construction of a model based on biological and toxicological knowledge (mechanism-based model).

When biological knowledge is unavailable, insufficient or too imprecise to construct a DRM that reflects biological processes of carcinogenesis or the genesis of health effects, one searches for a dose-response function from the large class of quantal DRMs, which fits the observed dose-response data (empirical data) sufficiently well. These so-called curve-fitting or empirical models can be simple mathematical functions of the dose that adequately describe the pattern of response for a particular data set and provide means for hypothesis testing and interpolation between data points. They hardly provide qualitative insight into underlying mechanisms. Curve fitting has been the traditional dose-response modeling approach and has to be confined to the observed dose range. Quantal response data elicited the use of quantal DRMs, for example the family of tolerance distribution models described above. Longitudinal tumor incidence and tumor mortality data led to the application of failure-time data models. The nature of the data available, the presence of elaborate statistical procedures for their use, and the availability of evaluation software determine the success of their application. Extrapolation to low doses was recognized as a serious problem when the empirical modeling began to be used for RA (see Krewski and van Ryzin, 1981). Low-dose estimates differing by orders of magnitude, although their fit in the observed dose ranges was indistinguishable, has raised doubts as to the adequacy of the extrapolation of empirical models.

On the other hand, biologically based modeling as described above is a powerful tool for understanding and combining information on complex biological systems. Use of a truly mechanism-based approach can in theory enable reliable and scientifically sound extrapolations to the low-dose range and between species. US EPA (2003a) has encouraged the use of biologically based models when the mode of action of the agent is sufficiently known and a mechanistic mathematical model of the carcinogenic process can be built. The knowledge of the mode of action should include quantitative information on model parameters. This information should be obtained from experiments independent of those used for dose-response modeling. Otherwise, when the same data sources are used (a) to determine one subset of model parameters a priori and (b) to determine the rest of the model parameters by fitting that model to the data, an honest model validation would be impossible. When a model has been established new data must be generated to support the model as biologically valid or at least biologically plausible. Those data must be specific enough for the agent and the toxic process such that model parameters are identifiable.

13.4.2 Low-dose extrapolation

Risk assessment requires in almost all applications the extrapolation to doses which are lower and in most cases much lower than the doses used for the analysis of a DRM. Since the experimental data obtained in animal experiments are in almost all cases obtained at doses which are orders of magnitude larger than the doses to be assessed for the RA, and since dose-response data from human exposure are rare or also obtained at higher dose ranges (e.g. in chemical accidents or at occupational exposure) RA has to bridge the gaps by extrapolation both from high to low doses and from extrapolation from animals to humans. There exists no simple algorithm for such an extrapolation step of the dose-response assessment, and any extrapolation should use relevant information about biological processes which occur at that intermediate dose interval, or which can explain interspecies differences. One approach to filling the gap between high and low doses was to estimate using biological knowledge the type of shape of the DRM between the low-dose region and the region of the empirical model fit. The simplest classification was the first- and second-order curvature of the dose-response curve which is either the distinction between linear and non-linear or the distinction between linear, sublinear (convex) and supralinear (concave); see Edler and Kopp-Schneider (1998).

Some classifications used the presence or absence of the genotoxicity of a compound to decide on the most realistic shape of the DRM for RA. A threshold-type approach is used to deal with non-genotoxic carcinogens. An estimate of the 'threshold' is obtained and safety factors are applied for the extrapolation to low doses. In contrast, genotoxic carcinogens are assumed to follow a non-threshold dose-response relationship and a mathematical dose-response model is used for low dose extrapolation. In the past, linear extrapolation was used for DNA reactive agents including, for example, ionizing radiation and genotoxic compounds, as well as for compounds whose effects enhance effects of preexisting endogenous compounds. However, empirical support for those assumptions has not always been strongly convincing. Differences between countries using those approaches have been described by Cogliano et al. (1999a).

13.4.3 Linear versus nonlinear low-dose extrapolation

When investigating differences between linear and nonlinear DRMs for low-dose extrapolation, the slope of the dose response curve $P(d)$ at $d = 0$ is the basic mathematical feature. A substance has been denoted as low-dose linear in the case of a positive slope, irrespective whether the curve was a straight line or showed some curvature in the low-dose region. The slope can be used to describe risk increments in the low-dose region. Risk is then the product of the slope and anticipated exposure.

A zero or even negative slope at $d = 0$ would be called low-dose nonlinear and in that case no risk increments can be determined. The mode of action discussed in this context has often been based on a threshold-type argument. This aspect has been approached by the concept of hormesis. Its consequences for RA are discussed in detail by Amaral Mendes and Pluygers (Chapter 6, this volume). A default assumption of nonlinearity is appropriate when there is no evidence for linearity and sufficient evidence to support an assumption of nonlinearity.

13.4.4 Point of departure

According to the discussion above it is the exception rather than the rule that one DRM model or one dose-response function can be used for RA. In practice, one has dose-response information for a particular dose region $d^* \leq d \leq d^{**}$ and no information for $0 \leq d \leq d^*$, but wants to estimate the risk in a region $0 \leq d \leq d_1$, where d_1 could be some orders of magnitude lower than d^*. Low-dose extrapolation (see above) has to bridge the latter gap. However, the extrapolated risk measures would almost exclusively depend on the model chosen for this extrapolation since a large family of models could be fitted sufficiently well in the dose region $d^* \leq d \leq d^{**}$ of the observable data but their risk estimates in the region $0 \leq d \leq d_1$ would be different and there would be no further information to discriminate between those models.

Both the NOAEL approach and the benchmark approach of RA recognize this problem and advise that one investigate DRM in the first region $d^* \leq d \leq d^{**}$ and apply a low-dose extrapolation procedure in a separate step. Both define within the interval $d^* \leq d \leq d^{**}$ a lowest dose level from which the extrapolation can be started. This dose level has been named the point of departure (PoD) for low-dose extrapolation which then can also be performed using the safety factor approach (see Edler *et al.*, 2002).

Whereas the NOAEL approach tries to estimate some sort of approximation of a threshold dose using a portion of the available dose-response data, the benchmark dose method is better designed to make use of the full dose-response information. The BMD applies a DRM which has to be selected from a class of models as described above. The PoD ranges usually near the lower end of the $d^* \leq d \leq d^{**}$ region. In most practical cases the PoD has been a dose corresponding to a small portion of $1–10\,\%$ of adverse responses, that is between ED_{01} and ED_{10}. The LED_{10} (the 95 % lower confidence limit of the dose ED_{10} associated with an extra risk over background of 10 %) was proposed by US EPA (1999) for use as PoD. What then matters for low-dose extrapolation is not the finding of the best estimate of the dose-response curve in the observed range but the finding of the best PoD, that is, the least biased and most precise estimate of PoD on the DRM.

Some data could support extrapolation of the fitted model beyond the PoD when there are indications that the same mechanism is still active in the extrapolation region $d_1 \leq d \leq d^*$ as it had been in the region $d^* \leq d \leq d^{**}$ of the model fit. However, it may become difficult to estimate those estimates' precision and uncertainty.

Usage of the NOAEL as PoD is not without problems. The definition of an NOAEL as the experimental dose level immediately below the lowest dose that produces a (statistically significant) increase in the rate of adverse effects (e.g. tumor rate) over controls, allows some arbitrariness. It depends on the definition of the significance level, statistical variation is not accounted for, no efficient use is made of dose-response information, and the estimation of the NOAEL is highly dependent on the spacing of experimental doses. Furthermore, the power to detect an NOAEL at some dose level is directly dependent on the sample sizes chosen at those dose levels and therefore in most cases very small (Gaylor, 1989).

13.5   DOSE-RESPONSE MODELING OF 2,3,7,8-TETRACHLORODIBENZO-*p*-DIOXIN

2,3,7,8-tetrachlorodibenzo-*p*-dioxin (TCDD) is the most potent toxic member of a group of persistent environmental chemicals consisting of polychlorinated dibenzodioxins (PCDDs) and polychlorinated dibenzofurans (PCDFs). Environmental contamination is caused by emissions from various sources, for example waste incineration or production of pesticides. 'Hotspot' exposure situations have resulted from accidents in the chemical industry (e.g., in 1976 at the chemical plant in Seveso, Italy) and the use of defoliants during the Vietnam War. Adverse health effects of TCDD can be very serious and include dermal toxicity, immunotoxicity, reproductive effects and teratogenicity, endocrine disruption, and carcinogenicity. Today, human exposure to TCDD is estimated at about 90 % from environmental (background) exposure through the diet, where food of animal origin is the predominant source. Data from countries which started to implement measures to reduce dioxin emissions (e.g. by controlling waste incineration) in the late 1980s show decreasing PCDD/PCDF and polychlorinated biphenyl (PCB) levels in food and consequently significantly lower dietary intake. Due to the long half-life of TCDD and most of its congeners there is still great concern about dioxin-induced human cancer and health risks. Detailed reviews and risk assessments have been presented by the International Agency for Research on Cancer and US EPA.

Whereas the IARC finalized an RA for dioxins in 1997 (IARC, 1997) the EPA is still in the process of updating its RA from 1985 (US EPA, 1985) and two draft documents from 1994 and 2000 (US EPA 1994, 2000a) have been circulated via the EPA Internet site (www.epa.gov/ncea/). Meanwhile, under the auspices of the World Health Organization (WHO), the WHO-ECEH and the IPCS have issued a document on the health risk of dioxins which can also be consulted for the most recent status of dioxin RA (Anonymous, 2000). In this section we wish to address some of the basic features and outcomes of dose-response modeling for dioxin RA, referring to the above-cited documents for details. Because of the wealth of information on its mechanism and low-dose behavior TCDD can serve as prototype for exploring the use of mechanistic DRMs to improve RA.

13.5.1 Biological basis and mechanisms of action

A broad variety of data on TCDD has shown the importance of the aryl hydrocarbon receptor (AhR) in mediating the biological effects of dioxin. Pharmacological structure activity and mouse genetic studies using AhR deficient animals and cells have demonstrated the key role of the AhR. A number of genes encoding drug-metabolizing enzymes, such as the cytochrome P450 members CYP1A1 and CYP1A2, are part of the target gene battery for the AhR. After translocation of the receptor–ligand complex to the nucleus and binding to transcriptionally active recognition sites, the so-called dioxin responsive elements, changes of hepatic CYP1A1 and CYP1A2 (through transcriptional activation and alterations in gene mRNA products) and modulation of the estrogen receptor (ER) and the epidermal growth factor receptor (EGFR) have been examined as biomarkers of TCDD action describing intermediate effects after exposure; see Lucier et al. (1993).

Activation of the AhR by a ligand such as TCDD can trigger a still not fully explored cascade of further events which eventually lead to endocrine and paracrine disturbances and alterations in cell functions, including growth and differentiation. The high affinity binding of TCDD to AhR is likely to be linear at low concentrations. Some of these effects have been observed both in humans and animals, suggesting the existence of a common mechanism of action in both species. Overall it is believed that carcinogenic and human health effects due to exposure to dioxins are receptor-mediated effects and that the induction of members of the cytochrome P450 family such as CYP1A1 and CYP1A2 constitutes one possible pharmacodynamic pathway from exposure to cancer incidence.

13.5.2 Toxicokinetic dose-response models

Data on TCDD allow dose-response modeling between exposure and target tissue concentration (dosimetry), between target tissue concentration and gene products and cellular level endpoints (biomarker induction), and between cellular action levels and toxicity endpoints. Several PBTK models have been used to describe the kinetic behavior of TCDD and have contributed to the understanding of the fate of TCDD in the organism; see Edler and Portier (1992).

The model of Leung et al. (1990) included a TCDD binding component in the liver and it modeled the CYP1A1 and CYP1A2 concentrations as biomarkers of response using the Michaelis–Menten type relationship (13.13). The model adequately predicted tissue concentrations in one animal experiment. In another animal experiment, however, the model underpredicted them in the low-dose range and overpredicted them in the high-dose range. Portier et al. (1993) modeled CYP1A1, CYP1A2 and EGFR concentrations both as biomarkers of dose and as biomarkers of response dependent on the tissue concentration in rats using the Hill equation (13.14). Basal expression of these proteins was included as further model parameter. This allowed them to model the effect of the TCDD in two different ways, either acting independent of the endogenous induction of the biomarker or adding to its endogenous induction. Whereas both the independent and the additive model fitted the data equally well, the risk extrapolation differed in the low-dose range by several orders of magnitude. Andersen *et al.* (1993) modified the Leung *et al.* (1990) model to predict CYP1A2 in a steady state model and CYP1A1 as a time-dependent process. They correlated tumor promotion with induction of CYP1A1 and investigated low-dose non-linearity. An extensive model of the biochemistry of TCDD including all the above-mentioned enzymes and receptor concentration was presented by Kohn *et al.* (1993) to describe the effects of TCDD in the organism on the physiological and the cellular level.

13.5.3 Laboratory animal responses

TCDD has been shown in several chronic studies to be carcinogenic at multiple sites in multiple species in both sexes. The lowest observed adverse effect of TCDD was the development of hepatic adenomas in rats. TCDD also causes thyroid tumors in male rats. Among the most sensitive non-carcinogenic effects are: endometriosis, developmental neurobehavioral (cognitive) effects, developmental reproductive effects (sperm counts, female urogenital malformations), and immunotoxic effects. The most sensitive biochemical effects are CYP1A1 and CYP1A2 induction, EGFR down-regulation and oxidative stress.

TCDD does not bind covalently to DNA and no direct DNA-damaging (i.e. genotoxic) effects have been observed as such, providing support for the assumption that TCDD is not acting as an initiator of carcinogenesis. Data from initiation–promotion experiments with diethylnitrosamine (Pitot *et al.*, 1980) classified TCDD as a promoter. Studies on mouse skin support a lack of initiating activity and an ability to promote the growth of previously initiated lesions indicative of TCDD being a promoting agent. This is in agreement with the involvement of the AhR as a mediator of toxic effects. The ability of TCDD to enhance proliferation and inhibit apoptotic processes in focal hepatic lesions further supports an indirect mechanism of carcinogenicity.

Thorslund (1987) applied the two-stage model of clonal expansion (TSCE model) to investigate promotional activity. The birth rate of the intermediate (initiated) cells was modeled as a function of dose and fitted to rat tumor incidence data. The TSCE model was later used by Portier *et al.* (1996) to fit both tumor incidence data and the number and size of foci of altered hepatocytes (FAHs, specifically PGST positive hepatic focal lesions) from two independent experiments on rats. The area under the CPP1A2 concentration curve was estimated using the nonlinear Hill model (see Sections 13.3.2.1 and 13.5.2 above) and it served as a dose surrogate for mutational effects in another Hill model for the effect of TCDD on the rate of transformation form the normal state to the intermediate state. Tentatively, an added risk from exposure to TCDD was approximated for the low-dose region as $P(d) = 0.24d$ when fitting the animal tumor incidence data. Uncertainties are located in the choice of the dose surrogates, the choice of the dose-model parameter relationships and in the assumptions leading to the model. Moolgavkar and Luebeck (2002) describe the use of the TSCE to analyze distributions of the number and the size of enzyme altered hepatocytes (FAHs), yet with data from another TCDD experiment.

They obtained similar qualitative results on a proliferative effect of TCDD and saw also an effect on the initiation rate.

In its most recent analysis of animal data the US EPA in 2000 fitted the multistage Armitage–Doll model (13.23)–(13.24) to tumor incidence data (both for rats and mice) by either a linear dose response function βd or various non-linear functions of a power of dose βd^k. Eight out of 13 studies were best fitted by a linear model although the data may be described by a non-linear model as well. The ED_{01} was determined as PoD in units of ng/kg of a steady-state body burden of TCDD. In addition, there was an attempt to employ a mechanistic model to predict the incidence of liver tumors in female Sprague Dawley rats. The model assumed that dioxin exposure induced increased cellular proliferation and indirectly led to an increase in mutation rate due to induction of hepatic enzymes leading to oxidative stress. The hypothesis of no mutational effect was tested and could not be rejected for this model. The ultimate best-fitting linear model led to an estimate of the ED_{01}. Modeling of 45 non-cancer studies in rodents demonstrated that 21 were best fitted by a near-linear model, while 24 demonstrated non-linearity. The dose-response relationships for biochemical endpoints were mainly linear; but most of the relationships for clearly adverse endpoints showed non-linear behavior. When the ED_{01} for the biochemical endpoints was compared with the LOAEL, the ED_{01} was often higher than the measured response. In some studies, estimation of the maximum response was problematic and the biological plausibility of the curve fits was unclear, underlining the need for mechanistic models for non-cancer endpoints; for details see US EPA (2000a).

13.5.4 Human response

Epidemiological studies suggested effects of dioxins in human reproduction, neurotoxicity, diabetes, and cancer. The most informative studies for the evaluation of the carcinogenicity of TCDD are four cohort studies from herbicide production (one each in the United States, The Netherlands, and two in Germany), one from the Seveso area, Italy, contaminated after an industrial accident in 1976, and a comprehensive international study performed by IARC; see US EPA (1994), Kogevinas *et al.* (1997), and Anonymous (2000). Increased risks for all cancer types combined were seen in the occupational cohort studies, with the magnitude of the increase generally low. Increase in site-specific tumor incidence or cause-specific mortality was much more difficult to evaluate, both in occupational and in epidemiological cohort studies of the general population. The follow-up for the Seveso cohort is shorter than for the occupational cohorts, and further evaluations have to be awaited before cancer mortality can be assessed with more confidence.

Standard epidemiological analysis compared cancer disease-specific mortality indices such as the standardized mortality ratio (SMR) when the cohort was compared to national mortality figures or risk ratios (RRs) when compared to a control group. Mortality for all cancer combined was increased in the US study of the NIOSH cohort investigated by Fingerhut *et al.* (1991), in the German Boehringer

Hamburg cohort study of Manz *et al.* (1990), and in a highly exposed subgroup of the German BASF cohort study of Zober *et. al.* (1990).

Later on, it became possible to estimate the apparent elimination half-life of TCDD and to derive measures of internal TCDD exposure and target tissue concentrations to be used as dose measures in a DRM. On the basis of working records and measurement and estimation of internal TCDD exposure, individual dose metrics were obtained, in particular using back-calculation of the TCDD serum levels measured between the mid-1980s and mid-1990s when serum concentration measurements of TCDD became possible. For a dose-response analysis the cohorts were subdivided into a few exposure groups and for each exposure group an average TCDD exposure level was estimated. Then the SMRs or RRs were regressed on the dose estimate. Aylward *et al.* (1996) used three dose metrics – the area under the dioxin concentration curve (AUC), the peak serum lipid concentration, and the mean serum lipid concentration (AUC/age at time of observation) – and found an excess risk for lung cancer. In a series of papers (see, for example, Becher *et al.*, 1998) the investigators of the Boehringer Hamburg cohort used various statistical modeling techniques including the Cox proportional hazard model to test for a positive trend of the dose-response relationship. A similar analysis was applied by Ott and Zober (1996) on SMRs and standardized incidence ratios (SIRs) for the BASF cohort.

The US EPA (1994) draft analysis used the models of Section 13.3.2.3 to estimate the parameter β, and a lifetime incremental cancer risk per ppt/kg and daily intake (unit risk). The epidemiological evidence from the most highly TCDD-exposed cohorts studied produced the strongest evidence of increased risks for all cancers combined, along with less strong evidence of increased risks for cancers at particular sites, for example respiratory tract in males.

In its most recent analysis of animal data the US EPA (2000a) estimated a slope parameter from which ED_{01} was estimated such as to maintain a steady-state body burden associated with a 1 % excess risk over a lifetime. In order to compare risks between humans and animals, the body burden is a metric of choice. It is important to note that predictions of body burden based on lipid concentrations at high exposures may underestimate the total body burden and over- or underestimate specific tissue concentrations because of the hepatic sequestration. Use of PBTK models readily allows for conversion of body burden with tissue concentrations, as well as with daily dose. Less complicated models such as steady state/body burden models using first-order kinetics will give approximately the same results at exposures in the environmental range. Knowledge of the time-dependent free concentration in the target tissue would be the most appropriate dosimetry to use to equate risk across species, but this is difficult with the modeling techniques and data at present available.

Non-cancer endpoints in humans were evaluated in a variety of exposure scenarios. Among children exposed *in utero* to background levels, effects include subtle development delays and subtle thyroid hormone alterations. Multiple, persistent effects occurred among highly exposed children who had transplacental exposure, however, it is not clear to what extent dioxin-like and/or non-dioxin-like compounds are contributing to these effects when considering the complex mixtures that human individuals are exposed to. In children in Seveso who were highly exposed to TCDD, small, transient increases in hepatic enzymes, total lymphocyte counts and subsets, complement activity, and non-permanent chloracne were observed. Also an alteration of the sex ratio (more females than males) was observed in children born to parents highly exposed to TCDD; for details see US EPA (1994, 2000a). Of the many non-cancer effects evaluated in exposed adults many were transient, disappearing after the end of exposure. Non-cancer effects observed in adult male workers occupationally exposed to high levels of TCDD and, to a lesser extent, higher chlorinated PCDDs included changes in serum lipids, elevated serum gammaGT, increased incidence of cardiovascular disease and diabetes, and, last but not least, chloracne.

13.5.5   Further aspects

In the course of evaluating the adverse effects of dioxins at low doses, the usefulness of toxicokinetic and dose-effects modeling to calculate a benchmark, namely ED_{01}, for comparison in the assessment was explored by WHO-ECEH and IPCS (Anonymous, 2000). It was noted that the outcome of using this type of model would strongly depend on the assumptions used, and there are still a number of uncertainties in the interpretation of the results. Therefore, more traditional approaches using simple body burden calculations and simple empirical parameters such as the NOAEL or the LOAEL, have been used in the evaluation of WHO-ECEH and IPCS.

Estimation of a Tolerable Daily Intake (TDI) value for dioxin and related compounds would require that either a reliable NOAEL or a reliable LOAEL be identified for the most sensitive and relevant adverse response, which may serve as surrogate for all other adverse responses that might be expected. The consultation by WHO-ECEH and IPCS emphasized that the TDI represents a tolerable daily intake for lifetime exposure and that occasional short-term excursions above the TDI would have no health consequences provided that the averaged intake over long periods is not exceeded. Finally, breast-fed infants are exposed to higher intakes of these compounds on a body weight basis, although for a small proportion of their lifespan. However, the consultation by WHO-ECEH and IPCS noted that in studies of infants, breast-feeding was associated with beneficial effects, in spite of the contaminants present.

13.6   CONCLUDING REMARKS

The term dose-response analysis or dose-response modeling stands for a variety of mathematical, statistical and even more general methodological approaches all with the aim of deriving from ordered dose-response data a quantitative estimate usable for RA, the estimate of a risk at some dose point d or the estimate of a dose limit such that the risk dose not exceed a given barrier. The paradigm of postulating and subsequently estimating the 'true' biological dose-response relationship through an adequate DRM prevailing for some decades since the 1950s has recently been more and more abandoned in favor of either more complex biologically based mechanistic modeling or pragmatic approaches to find an optimal dose estimate given practical restrictions. Therefore the role of mathematical DRMs has changed; whereas in the first, methodologically often very challenging, path to RA a single mathematical model had to give way to complex systems usually no more amenable to analytical solutions and requiring extended use of computational methods, mathematical models now in the second path play much more the role of support methods in a more complex stepwise procedure.

In this chapter we have adopted a two-step approach. First, the relationship of dose to response in the dose range of observations in experiments and human studies has been evaluated. This evaluation was followed by an extrapolation to estimate response at lower environmental exposure levels. Examples were given of the use of the benchmark dose method and of the NOAEL as points of departure. Although the later parameter may suffer from serious statistical deficiencies it may in some instances constitute the only rational approach to starting a RA. The example of the ongoing RA for dioxins demonstrates this 'open' approach for RA forced to rescue itself in using a plurality of methods in order to reach for quantitative estimates.

CHAPTER 14

Benchmark Dose Approach

Fred Parham and Christopher Portier

National Institute of Environmental Health Sciences

14.1 INTRODUCTION

In order to achieve the statistical power to detect adverse health effects in animal experiments, it has generally been necessary to administer doses of possibly harmful chemicals at amounts much higher than would normally be encountered in the environment. Since the risk of cancer from environmental exposures is the quantity of interest, it is therefore necessary to extrapolate from the experimentally observed risks to risks at actually encountered levels.

In the absence of a mechanistic description of risk at low doses, the traditional method of extrapolation for regulatory purposes has been to either assume that low-dose risk is linear and to extrapolate from a low experimental dose or to derive a presumably safe level by dividing some experimentally determined dose by 'safety factors' or 'uncertainty factors'. The dose used as the upper end of the linear extrapolation or as the dose to be divided by the safety factor is generally referred to as the 'point of departure' (POD).

Historically, the method most commonly used for finding the POD involved applying multiple statistical tests to data and using biological insights to determine the no observed adverse effects level (NOAEL). The NOAEL is defined as the largest experimental dose that causes no statistically or biologically significant increase in adverse health effects. In the case of cancer, this would be the dose causing no statistically significant increase in tumor incidence. If all doses cause significant effects, the lowest dose causing adverse effects, the lowest observed acute effect level (LOAEL) can be used, but generally with larger uncertainty factors.

Crump (1984) suggested an alternative to the NOAEL – the benchmark dose (BMD). The BMD is defined as

Recent Advances in Quantitative Methods in Cancer and Human Health Risk Assessment
Edited by L. Edler and C. Kitsos © 2005 John Wiley & Sons, Ltd

a lower statistical confidence limit for the dose corresponding to a specified increase in level of health effect over the background level. The increased level of effect upon which the [benchmark dose] is based would be near the lower limit of the experimental range; i.e., near the lower limit of increases in health effects which can be measured with reasonable accuracy in toxicological studies. This value is estimated to be something on the order of a 10 % change from background at typical sample sizes.

The benchmark dose is obtained in three steps:

1. fitting a curve to the risk data;

2. finding the dose corresponding to the chosen increased level of risk on the curve;

3. finding a statistical lower confidence limit on the dose. This dose would be used as the POD for low-dose extrapolation.

As Murrell *et al.* (1998) point out, the BMD approach is a step between the simple empirical NOAEL method and full mechanistic modeling.

A note on terminology: the terminology used in the literature is not entirely consistent. This chapter will use the terminology used in the US Environmental Protection Agency (EPA) draft Benchmark Dose Technical Guidance Document (US EPA Risk Assessment Forum, 2000). BMD (or BMC, for benchmark concentration when that terminology is more appropriate) will refer to the dose found in step 2 above and BMDL (or BMCL) will refer to the lower confidence limit. The dose corresponding to a specific increased risk level of $X\%$ will be referred to as BMD_X or $BMDL_X$. For example, $BMDL_{05}$ is the lower confidence limit on the dose giving 5 % increased risk. BMD will be used as a general term for the benchmark dose approach to risk assessment. Finally, BMR refers to the benchmark response; for example, a BMD_{05} has a BMR of 5 %.

Crump (1984) pointed out several advantages of the BMD approach over the NOAEL approach. The NOAEL, by definition, can only be one of the experimental doses. The BMD need not be the NOAEL, and can even be used when every dose has a significant effect (i.e., when there is no NOAEL). The curve fitting uses all of the experimental data, while the NOAEL approach uses only the lowest significant increase in risk. Because an increase in study size will increase the power of the study to detect low risks, larger studies will make it more likely that significant effects will be found at low doses. Thus they will lower the NOAEL and result in more stringent regulatory guidelines. Since this stringency results from better ability to detect a low risk and not from the actual value of the detected risk, it may be unnecessary. This is one of the weaknesses in the use of the NOAEL as a POD. The BMD approach, however, behaves exactly how you would wish it to behave;

larger sample sizes result in less potential for bias and smaller confidence intervals. For the regulated industry tasked with doing an animal study to support safety, studies with larger sample sizes are then likely to yield more precise PODs and would more likely be supported than they would be for the NOAEL-based approach. If the chosen BMR is in the range of the data (interpolated BMD), the BMD should be less dependent upon the choice of regression model than if the BMR is outside of the range of the data (extrapolated BMD). Finally, the BMD approach provides the slope of the dose-response curve at the BMR. This can provide clues about the behavior of the risk at lower doses. For example, a steep slope means that the risk is decreasing rapidly and suggests that there may be threshold-like behavior (Barnes *et al.*, 1995).

14.2 USE BY REGULATORY AGENCIES

The US EPA has used the BMD approach to set exposure standards for non-cancer health effects. In this situation, it is often assumed that there are exposures below which no additional risk exists, making linear extrapolation from the BMD or BMDL to zero exposure, zero extra risk inappropriate; instead, a BMD/BMDL with an uncertainty factor approach is used. The EPA has also used BMDs to rank the toxicity (cancer and noncancer) of air pollutants (Barnes *et al.*, 1995).

Only recently has the EPA begun formal procedures to replace its traditional cancer risk assessment methods with a BMD-based approach. The traditional approach for cancer risk has been to use the linearized multistage model (Crump *et al.*, 1976) to extrapolate observable risk data to lower doses for which differences in risk could never be detected in a reasonably sized experiment. The linearized multistage approach posed several problems for the EPA that could easily be remedied by the use of a BMD-based approach. First, recent improvements in the mechanistic understanding of carcinogenesis could not readily be incorporated into the linearized multistage model approach, whereas this knowledge naturally fitted into the BMD-based methods. Secondly, there was strong desire to have a unified approach to risk assessment for both cancer and noncancer endpoints that again could not easily encompass the linearized multistage modeling approach but could utilize the BMD-based approaches. In draft documents on guidelines for cancer risk assessment, the most recent of which was issued in 2003 (US EPA, 2003c), the EPA recommends the use of the BMD approach for cancer.

The BMD approach has also been used by other agencies. For example, Health Canada uses a BMD-based approach for both cancer and noncancer data (Meek, 1999; Liteplo and Meek, 2001) for substances on the Priority Substances List. The World Health Organization and International Program on Chemical Safety (IPCS) have sporadically used the BMD approach to analyze data and are currently evaluating the use of this method as a general procedure in determining guidance values (IPCS, 2002).

14.3   CALCULATION METHODS

14.3.1   Types of models

BMD-based methods can be generally applied to any type of data for which a regression model could be used. As a general rule, regression methods involve two separate sets of assumptions: statistical assumptions regarding the variation resulting in different responses for replicate data points, and mathematical assumptions regarding the average behavior of the risk as a function of dose (Murrell *et al.*, 1998). For example, tumor incidence data are dichotomous data where animals either have a tumor or do not have a tumor. In this case, the general assumptions made in the analysis of the data are that animals in the same experimental group are independently drawn replicates from a Bernoulli distribution (statistical assumption) where the probability of tumor is some specified function of exposure (mathematical assumption). The discussion here will focus on the application of BMD methods to tumor incidence data (otherwise known as quantal data) as described in the example above. It is also possible to use BMD methods with continuous data such as data on the effects of chemical agents on DNA damage, exposure-driven changes in cellular replication rates, or alterations in maternal body weight as a function of exposure. Some of the mathematical and computational concepts will be illustrated by reference to studies using noncancer health data.

There are several mathematical functions that can be used to estimate the probability of tumor for tumor incidence data. The ones used in the US EPA Benchmark Dose Software (BMDS; see US EPA, 2003c) are listed in Table 14.1. All of the functions describe the probability (risk) of getting cancer as a function, $p(d)$, of the exposure being studied (d). The exposure may be the administered dose (in mg/kg body weight/day, for example) or an exposure derived from more complex modeling – the possibilities are endless, so only a few are discussed below.

Each function has several parameters (given as lower-case Greek letters in the table) which can be adjusted. The ultimate goal of most regression methods is to estimate values for the model parameters so that the dose-response curve described by the function is as close as possible to the dose-response observed experimentally. The data must include, at least, as many dose groups (including the control) as there are parameters for the model to fit with a unique set of parameters (Chernoff, 1953). In some cases, the parameters will be restricted to certain values in order to avoid biologically impossible behaviors. For example, for certain models and certain types of tumors, the dose-response curves have infinite slope at zero dose, which both is unrealistic and can lead to problems in the estimation of the benchmark dose.

It is also possible to use models with thresholds, that is, dose levels below which the probability of a tumor is the same as for controls. Including thresholds in models is problematic. For example, the threshold may have a confidence interval so wide as to include 0. In many cases, the presence or absence of a threshold in the model may not make a significant difference in fit of the model to the data (Barnes *et al.*, 1995), suggesting an overparameterization of the model. In other cases – for

Table 14.1 Dose-response functions used in benchmark dose analysis.

Name of model	Formula for risk p or extra risk F	Restrictions	Notes
General form	$p(d) = \gamma + (1 - \gamma)F(d)$	γ is the risk at zero dose; $0 \leq \gamma \leq 1$	$p(d)$ is risk of tumor at dose d. $F(d)$ is extra risk at dose d
Gamma	$F(d) = G(\beta d; \alpha)$	$\alpha \geq 1$ to avoid infinite slope at dose 0	G is the incomplete gamma function
Multistage	$F(d) = 1 - \exp\left(\sum_{j=1}^{N} -\beta_j d^j\right)$	All $\beta \geq 0$ to keep dose-response curve monotonic	N (the degree of the model) can be any positive integer. This is a generalization of a mechanistic model.
Weibull	$F(d) = 1 - \exp(-\beta d^\alpha)$	$\alpha \geq 1$ to avoid infinite slope at dose 0	
Quantal linear	As Weibull, with α fixed at 1		Identical to multistage model with degree 1
Quantal quadratic	As Weibull, with α fixed at 2		
Logistic	$p(d) = \dfrac{1}{1 + \exp(-\alpha - \beta d)}$		
Log-logistic	$F(d) = \dfrac{1}{1 + \exp(-\alpha - \beta \ln(d))}$	$\beta \geq 1$ to avoid infinite slope at dose 0	
Probit	$p(d) = \Phi(\alpha + \beta d)$		Φ is normal cumulative distribution function
Log-probit	$F(d) = \Phi(\alpha + \beta \ln(d)),$	$\beta \geq 1$ to avoid infinite slope at dose 0	

instance, the Haber *et al.* (1998) study of noncancer health risks from exposure to nickel compounds – including thresholds may be necessary to get a satisfactory fit to the data. It should be noted that the necessity for a threshold or the lack of need for a threshold in a model implies little about the presence or absence of a true biological threshold due to the crudeness of these data. The EPA guidelines (US EPA Risk Assessment Forum, 2000) recommend that thresholds not be used, but allow them if they are necessary to fit the data. The BMDS program does not include an option allowing for the use of thresholds.

14.3.2   Fitting to data

The recommended procedure for parameter estimation includes the use of an objective function, such as the statistical likelihood, and an optimization algorithm, such as the Davidon–Fletcher–Powell algorithm, to find the maximum or minimum of the objective function. Suppose there are M dose groups (including the control) with doses $d_1, \ldots, d_M$, with N_i individuals in the ith dose group and R_i individuals with tumors in the ith dose group. The distribution of R_i drives the estimation procedure in this case. For example, in cancer studies, it is generally assumed that R_i follows a binomial distribution with probability $p_i = p(d_i)$, where $p(d)$ is the estimated response for dose d from the chosen dose-response function. In this situation the log-likelihood function is then given by

$$\ln(L) = \sum_{i=1}^{M} [R_i \ln(p_i) + (N_i - R_i) \ln(1 - p_i) + \text{constant}].$$

In many cases, the objective function, like the log-likelihood, can also be used to assess model fit, calculate confidence intervals and test hypotheses (see below).

Algorithms for maximizing the log-likelihood, such as the Broyden–Fletcher–Goldfarb–Shanno algorithm, work by starting with an initial guess for the values of the parameters and then adjusting the parameters iteratively until a solution, that is, a set of parameter values for which the likelihood is a maximum, is found. In some cases, the procedure will converge to different solutions (local maxima of the likelihood function) when given different initial guesses. In such cases, the one with the highest likelihood is the true best solution.

14.3.3   Goodness of fit

Once the best set of model parameters has been chosen, it is necessary to measure the goodness of fit of the model to the data, since the best possible fit of a given functional form may still not be very good. The goodness of fit may be measured with a chi-squared test. To perform the test, compute the quantity

$$\chi^2 = \sum_{i=1}^{M} \frac{(R_i - p_i N_i)^2}{N_i p_i (1 - p_i)}$$

with p_i equal to the risk at dose level i computed using the optimized parameter values. This is the chi-squared (χ^2) goodness-of-fit statistic. The p-value for the chi-squared test is determined by comparing the test statistic to the chi-squared distribution with degrees of freedom equal to M, the number of adjustable parameters in the function. It is typical to reject the fit (i.e., assume the function does not fit the data well enough) if the p-value is less than a critical value of 0.05; the EPA draft benchmark dose guidance document recommends that a more stringent cutoff of 0.1 be used instead (US EPA Risk Assessment Forum, 2000).

It is also a good idea to plot the fitted curve versus the data, since the chi-squared test measures an overall goodness of fit and it is possible to fit the data at the highest doses but have a poor fit at the lowest dose levels, which are the ones of most interest (since they are near the POD). It may also be that the fitted curve is consistently above or below the data. Examination of the scaled residuals

$$(R_i - p_i N_i)/\sqrt{N_i p_i (1 - p_i)}$$

may also be helpful; if a residual's absolute value is greater than 2, there may be a problem. To summarize, nonrejection under the chi-squared test does not prove the adequacy of the model; examining the actual fitted curve is important.

In some cases, a model may not fit the data adequately, but it may be possible to fit the data if high dose groups are eliminated. Examples of this in the literature include modeling liver angiosarcoma resulting from vinyl chloride exposure (Storm and Rozman, 1997); modeling hepatic carcinogenicity due to N-nitrosodimethylamine in drinking water (Liteplo and Meek, 2001); and modeling developmental effects from exposure to halogenated compounds (Sand *et al.*, 2002). This is acceptable when the response at the highest dose is judged to be not relevant to low dose-response; for example, if carcinogenicity at high doses is due to toxic effects separate from the carcinogenic effects operating at low doses.

If there are several models that have acceptable goodness of fit, it is necessary to choose which one is best. A difference between the goodness-of-fit statistics for several models is not a sufficient criterion for choosing between models. One statistic that can be used to compare models is Akaike's information criterion (AIC), defined as $-2 \times$ (log-likelihood) $+ 2 \times$ (number of adjustable parameters). Generally speaking, a model with a lower AIC is better. The likelihood ratio test may be used to compare models which are members of the same family of models (e.g., the multistage model with increasing degrees of the polynomial, or the Weibull model vs. its special cases, the quantal linear and quantal quadratic models).

Once the model has been fitted to the data, it is necessary to compute the BMD. The BMD can be based on either extra risk or additional risk. For extra risk, the BMD is given by

$$\text{BMR} = \frac{p(\text{BMD}) - p(0)}{1 - p(0)}.$$

For instance, if the desired benchmark response is 10 % and the tumor risk for controls is $p(0) = 5$ %, the BMD is the dose which will cause, on average, 10 % of the rest of the population to develop tumors, that is,

$$0.1 = \frac{p(\text{BMD}) - 0.05}{0.95},$$

which implies that for this case $p(\text{BMD}) = 0.1495$. The BMD would thus be the dose which gives a value of $p = 0.1495$ in the model being used. With the additional risk model, the BMD is defined by $\text{BMR} = p(\text{BMD}) - p(0)$. For most of the models listed in Table 14.1, it is possible get an explicit formula for the BMD given the BMR.

14.3.4 Lower confidence limit

After the BMD has been computed, it is desirable to compute confidence bounds for the BMD. Of special interest to many agencies is the lower bound on the BMD, the

BMDL. The usual approach is to use the fact that the likelihood ratio has an asymptotic chi-squared distribution. The first step is to rewrite the risk function so that the BMD appears as a parameter. Details can be found in the EPA BMDS help manual (US EPA, 2001). For example, suppose the quantal linear model is being used. The extra risk function for that model is (see Table 14.1)

$$F(d) = 1 - \exp(-\beta d) \tag{14.1}$$

which implies that

$$BMR = 1 - \exp(-\beta \times BMD). \tag{14.2}$$

This can be rewritten as

$$\beta \times BMD = -\ln(1 - BMR), \tag{14.3}$$

which implies that

$$\beta = \frac{-\ln(1 - BMR)}{BMD}. \tag{14.4}$$

Finding the best fit of the model to the data gives a best value for β (call it β_B) and a log-likelihood for the best fit (call it L_B). Specifying the BMR and using (14.3) gives the BMD in terms of BMR and β_B; call this BMD value BMD_B. Substituting (14.4) into the extra risk function (14.1) gives

$$F(d) = 1 - \exp\left(\frac{d \ln(1 - BMR)}{BMD}\right).$$

This can be treated as a model function with one variable parameter, BMD. Using BMD_B, the value of BMD derived from the best fit to the data, will give the best fit of this new model function to the data, with the same log-likelihood, L_B. Using a different value for BMD will give a worse fit and therefore a lower value for the log-likelihood.

Suppose you want to find the $100(1 - \alpha)\%$ confidence limit. To do this, find the value of the BMD such that, when the other parameters are optimized, the log-likelihood is less than the log-likelihood for the best fit by the amount $\frac{1}{2}\chi^2_{1,1-2\alpha}$, where $\chi^2_{1,1-2\alpha}$ is the value of the $100(1 - 2\alpha)$ th percentile of the cumulative distribution of the chi-squared distribution with one degree of freedom. In the example using the quantal linear model, the value of BMR is a constant and so the only other parameter is the γ in the risk formula (see the first entry in Table 14.1). Specifying any particular value for BMD and finding the γ giving the best fit to the data will give a log-likelihood depending on the specified BMD; call it $L(BMD)$. To calculate a 95 % lower confidence limit, set α to 0.05 (so $1 - 2\alpha = 0.9$). The value of BMD for which $L_B - L(BMD) = \frac{1}{2}\chi^2_{1,0.9}$ is the BMDL.

Using the 95 % confidence limit is the standard. When comparing the BMDLs from different models, the EPA guidance document recommends that BMDLs within a factor of 3 be considered indistinguishable, with the one corresponding to the model with the lowest AIC being the one actually used. If they are not within a factor of 3, the document recommends using the lowest to be conservative

(US EPA, 2000b). When reporting results, both the BMD and the BMDL should be given.

14.3.5 Experimental design, dose selection and response metrics

When designing experiments to produce data for use with benchmark dose modeling, both the dose levels and the size of each dosing group must be considered. Several authors have addressed optimal experimental designs for obtaining BMDs.

Kavlock *et al.* (1996) simulated a developmental toxicity study with two variations in the sizes of the dose groups. One set of study designs had 80 litters divided among 4–8 dose groups; the other set had the number of dose groups fixed at 4 or 5, with 10–20 litters per group. Different dose spacings were tested. Toxicity data were randomly generated using a known log-logistic probability function, and the same function was used to fit the data. The best designs for estimating the BMD (minimum bias in the estimate) were from the studies with at least two dose groups having a significant positive (i.e., greater than control) response, with at least one of the responses near the true BMD. For those studies, increasing the size of the dose groups from 10 to 20 litters had little effect on the BMD. Adding more dose groups also had little effect. Next best were the studies with one positive dose group near the true BMD. In those studies, increasing the size of each dosing group had a noticeable effect of shrinking the size of the confidence limit, that is, raising the BMDL. The BMDLs were lower (more conservative) than in the case with two positive dose groups with one near the true BMD. Studies with no positive dose groups near the true BMD had highly variable estimates of the BMD and generally had low (conservative) BMDLs.

Woutersen *et al.* (2001) performed simulations with data from a study of several continuous biological endpoints in a study of rhodorsil silane toxicity in rats. The study had seven dose levels (including control) with 10 animals in each dose group. BMDs were computed for the full data set and for two reduced data sets, one with only five animals (selected randomly) per dose group and one with only four of the seven dose groups. The BMDs estimated from the data set with five animals/dose groups were generally closer to those from the full study than were the ones from the data set with only four dose groups.

Gephart *et al.* (2001) performed a study with simulated data in five patterns: (a) seven dose groups of 10 subjects each, with five having response over control level; (b) the same conditions as for (a), but with 5 subjects per group and half as many (rounded up) responding; (c) and (d) the same conditions as for (a) and (b), but with larger responses (a higher response at the lowest positive dose); (e) six dose groups, with 10 subjects per group and a positive response only at the highest dose level. Eliminating up to three of the high dose groups (not the dose group nearest the BMD) had little effect on the BMD or BMDL for the first four data sets. Eliminating nonresponding dose groups in the fifth data set could make very large changes in the BMDL, depending on which dose groups were eliminated.

Weller *et al.* (1995) examined experimental design using resampling from a large study on herbicides and prenatal death. They found that the variance of the BMD estimate increased somewhat as the number of dose groups increased, but the bias greatly decreased.

When designing experiments for benchmark dose calculation, then, studies with more dose groups are generally better. It is also important to have a range of responses. When the only responses are either at the control level or near the maximum level observed, there will also be problems with fitting the model and finding the BMD.

14.3.5.1   Dose metrics

It is also necessary to decide how to measure dose for modeling purposes. The simplest dose measure is an administered dose, such as a concentration in feed or a gavage dose. The draft EPA guidelines (US EPA, 2003c) have administered dose (an average daily dose or something similar) as the default dose metric, but prefer a measure of the amount of dose delivered to the organ where the tumor of interest is located. Physiologically based pharmacokinetic (PBPK) modeling can be used to compute such a dose.

Kim *et al.* (2002) used BMD methods with data on several continuous endpoints in dioxin studies. The BMDs were calculated using two dose metrics. One was the average daily dose (from gavage studies); the other was a body burden, computed via a PBPK model using the dosing information. The BMD average daily doses were then converted to equivalent body burdens using a simple kinetic model and compared to the BMD body burdens computed with the PBPK-derived dose metric. The BMD values from the two methods were generally within a factor of 5 of one another, with most within a factor of 2. In most cases the BMDs derived from the simple kinetic model were higher than those derived from the PBPK model.

PBPK modeling can also be used for intraspecies extrapolation. Bogdanffy *et al.* (1999) studied nasal tumors due to inhalation of vinyl acetate in rats. A PBPK model was used to predict levels of vinyl acetate and its metabolites in the nasal cavity for both rats and humans. A BMD exposure concentration was calculated from the rat data. Various measures of tissue dose corresponding to the BMD were calculated using the PBPK model for the rat, and the human BMD was calculated by using a human PBPK model to predict the vinyl acetate exposure concentration that would result in equivalent tissue doses.

14.3.5.2   Response selection

The BMR used to compute the BMD must not be either too low or too high. Using too low a BMR can lead to problems if calculation of the BMD requires extensive extrapolation below or above the observed levels of response; the point of using the BMD method is that the extrapolation to low dose levels (and therefore low response levels) is uncertain. Using too high a BMR can fail to take into account the shape of the observed dose-response curve at low doses.

Murrell *et al.* (1998) point out that the choice of the BMR affects the region where the model has to make a prediction. If the BMD is in the region where the response is nearly linear, the BMD will depend mainly on the response at the two nearest dose levels.

14.4 LITERATURE SURVEY

Several studies have been performed to compare ways of calculating the BMD. Haag-Gronlund *et al.* (1995) used a multistage model with a threshold to compute BMDLs for data from studies on trichloroethylene toxicity in rats and mice. The calculations were done for BMRs of 1 %, 5 %, and 10 %. They examined 31 quantal data sets, 12 of which were tumor data. Six of those data sets could not be fitted adequately by the model (i.e., they failed the goodness-of-fit test). This was generally because all noncontrol doses had a maximum or near-maximum response, resulting in a 'plateau' in the dose-response curve which could not be fitted by the model. In the six tumor studies for which a NOAEL was available, all of the NOAELs were greater than the $BMDL_{01}$, four were greater than the $BMDL_{05}$, and one was greater than the $BMDL_{10}$. Similar results, with many $NOAELS > BMDL_{10}$, were observed for nontumor data and for the continuous data sets also analyzed in the paper. The results suggest that the true extra risk at the NOAEL may be in the range of 10 %.

Liteplo and Meek (2001) used BMD methods to study data on hepatic carcinogenicity from a study of N-nitrosodimethylamine administered to rats in drinking water. The study had 16 dose groups, which is a very large number when compared to other toxicity studies. A multistage model was used to calculate BMD_{05}s and $BMDL_{05}$s. Several adjustments were made to the data. Some high-dose groups demonstrated a downturn in the dose-response curve, that is, a decrease in risk with increasing exposure. These groups (a different number for each sex–tumor combination) were eliminated as being not relevant to the response near the BMR. (The downturn was thought to be possibly related to animals' dying of other causes before having a chance to develop tumors; other authors have noted that this problem can be avoided by using survival-adjusted data. That is, the total number of animals in a dose group (N_i in the formulas above) is adjusted to reflect the number of animals which survived the full length of the experiment.) After this adjustment, the multistage model with a polynomial of degree greater than 2 still had problems fitting the data, so the number of dose groups was reduced by combining dose groups: the tumor count and total animals for adjacent similar dose groups were added together, and the dose level of the groups was averaged. This reduced the number of groups to 10 or less. If the multistage model still failed to fit, high-dose groups were dropped off one at a time until the goodness-of-fit criterion was satisfied.

Fowles *et al.* (1999) used log-probit and Weibull models to fit 117 acute inhalation lethality data sets from studies of 40 chemicals in six species of animals. Seventeen of the studies did not have acceptable goodness of fit when the log-probit model was used. Of the remaining 100 studies, seven did not have acceptable goodness of fit with the Weibull model. The log-probit model generally provided a better fit to the data (higher p-value from the goodness-of-fit test, smaller confidence intervals, and more models with acceptable goodness of fit). BMDLs were calculated for BMRs of 1 %, 5 %, and 10 %. The log-probit model gave higher BMDL values than the Weibull model, but the difference was usually small. The difference between the results of the two models increased as the BMR decreased.

Sand *et al.* (2002) used several models to fit data on cleft palate and hydronephrosis from developmental toxicity studies of several halogenated compounds (dioxins, furans, and biphenyls). They used the BMDS software with the logistic, log-logistic, probit, log-probit, Weibull, gamma, and multistage models. They used BMRs of 1 %, 2.5 %, 5 %, and 10 % and computed 90 %, 95 %, and 99 % lower confidence limits (BMDLs). The AIC was used to compare models. If none of the models could fit the data, dose groups were dropped, starting with the highest-dose group, until the goodness-of-fit criteria were satisfied for at least one model. Each model could fit 11 of the 12 cleft palate data sets; 10 of the 12 data sets could be fitted by all of the models. For seven of the 12 data sets, the multistage model had the best AIC. The log-logistic model could fit nine of the 10 hydronephrosis data sets, and the log-probit could fit eight of the 10; the other models could fit five or fewer.

BMDLs (95 % confidence limits) were presented for two cleft palate data sets both from studies of 2,3,7,8-tetrachlorodibenzodioxin. For any given model, the BMDLs were generally similar for the two studies. However, the best model (by AIC) was the log-probit for one study and the multistage for the other study. Comparing the BMDLs corresponding to the best models for each study shows larger differences, with the log-probit giving noticeably higher BMDLs at low BMRs. Examining the BMDLs for all BMRs and all three confidence limit sizes across all cleft palate data sets showed that the differences between models (as measured by the ratio of highest to lowest BMDL) increased as BMR decreased and the size of the confidence interval increased. For models other than the multistage, though, changing the confidence limit size from 90 % to 99 % made little difference in the size of the BMDL.

The differences in the AIC between models for the cleft palate data were generally due to the $2p$ term (twice the number of parameters) in the definition of the AIC. In many cases, estimated parameters for the multistage model were on the edge of the constrained parameter range. In those cases, BMDS regards the parameter as a constant when calculating the AIC, that is, it decreases the effective number of parameters. If this adjustment is not made, the multistage model is no longer the best model for several of the data sets. Adjusting the effective number of parameters also affects the degrees of freedom in the chi-squared test for goodness of fit, but the adjustment did not change whether the test rejected the fit.

Filipsson and Victorin (2003) compared the performance of BMDS and two other pieces of benchmark dose software – a commercially available program, THRESH, and the program QUAN (Kalliomaa *et al.*, 1998) – as applied to data from trichloroethylene studies. The other two software tools used the multistage model for quantal data, with a threshold included. The software was applied to 32 sets of dichotomous data, 13 of which were tumor data. The EPA BMDS using the log-logistic, multistage (with degree selected by finding the degree giving the highest p-value), or quantal linear model could fit 29 of the 32 data sets (12 of the 13 tumor data sets). Other models from the EPA BMDS (logistic, probit, log-probit, quantal quadratic) could fit from 16 to 23 of the data sets. The gamma model could fit 28 of the 32. The authors state that the Weibull model could fit 28 of the 32. Note, however, that the quantal linear, which could fit 29, is a special case of the Weibull model. This means that any functional form produced by the quantal linear can also be produced by the Weibull. However, the Weibull model has one more parameter, so the chi-squared goodness-of-fit test has one less degree of freedom. This means that some data fits that are accepted by the test under the quantal linear model will be rejected under the Weibull. For 16 of the 32 data sets, the log-logistic model had the lowest AIC value; for 10 of the 32, the multistage model had the lowest.

The other two software packages, THRESH and QUAN, used the multistage model with threshold and fitted 22 and 24 of the data sets, respectively. As with the EPA multistage model, the degree with the best p-value was used. Both of these used the multistage model. Each could fit 12 of the 13 tumor data sets. The authors speculate that the difference in the number of acceptable fits to these data sets may be due to using different starting values for the parameter values in the optimization algorithm; this points out the importance of changing the starting values if an initial try does not fit. In most cases, $BMDL_{10}$s for tumor data were similar when calculated with the multistage model using the three different software packages. For 10 out of 12 of the data sets that the models could fit, BMDS and THRESH gave identical results for $BMDL_{10}$ and the QUAN gave somewhat higher results. There is no explanation as to the reason for the differences between models.

14.5   SOFTWARE AND CALCULATION EXAMPLE

This section presents an example of BMD and BMDL calculation using the BMDS. (US EPA, 2003c). The data used for the calculation are given in Table 14.2. The version of the software used is 1.3.2, available on the web at http://cfpub.epa.gov/ncea. The BMR used for the calculation was 0.1, based on extra risk (using additional risk is an option in the software). A 95 % lower confidence limit was used for the BMDL. The restrictions listed for the individual models in Table 14.1 are options in the BMDS; for this example, all of the optional restrictions were used. As

Table 14.2 Data used for the benchmark dose calculation example.

Dose	Number of animals with tumors	Number of animals/dose group
0	3	50
25	8	50
50	25	50
75	45	50
100	50	50

Table 14.3 Goodness-of-fit data and benchmark doses from the benchmark dose calculation example.

Model	χ^2	p-value	AIC	BMD_{10}	$BMDL_{10}$
Multistage degree 3	0.43	0.8073	175.157	25.8125	15.7589
Weibull	0.52	0.7730	175.175	27.7054	20.7536
Logistic	3.18	0.3649	176.35	20.8072	16.7189
Probit	3.78	0.2861	176.459	18.5347	14.9449
Gamma	2.19	0.3342	177.138	32.1631	22.7937
Log-probit	2.97	0.2262	177.933	36.6226	26.0857
Log-logistic	3.10	0.2126	178.357	36.3597	27.0637
Multistage degree 2	5.70	0.1270	179.853	17.5445	14.5097
Multistage degree 1	30.08	<0.0001	211.381	5.31512	4.50544

was pointed out in the Notes column of Table 14.1, the quantal linear model is identical to the multistage model with degree 1, so its results are not presented separately. For this data set, the restriction on the β values for the multistage model resulted in a value of $\beta_1 = 0$ for the multistage model with degree 2, which means that for this data set it is equivalent to the quantal quadratic model.

Table 14.3 shows results of the BMD calculations, with models ranked by their AIC values from lowest (best) to highest. There are several interesting things to notice about the table. All but one of the models (the multistage with degree 1) would pass even the stringent goodness-of-fit test (p-value > 0.1) recommended by the Benchmark Dose Technical Guidance Document. The two best-fitting models, the multistage with degree 3 and the Weibull, have very similar AICs. Examining the parameter estimates from the BMDS output gives the following functional forms for those models: for the multistage with degree 3,

$$p(d) = 0.0621 + 0.9379\left(1 - \exp\left(-6.168 \times 10^{-4}d - 5.2 \times 10^{-6}d^3\right)\right),$$

and for the Weibull,

$$p(d) = 0.0690 + 0.9310\left(1 - \exp\left(-3.683 \times 10^{-6}d^{3.089}\right)\right).$$

Note that $\beta_2 = 0$ for the multistage model in this case. So these two models give very similar results in this case.

Figure 14.1 plots the results produced by the BMDS for the multistage model with degree 3. Shown are the data points with 95 % confidence intervals, the fitted curve, and part of the 95 % lower confidence limit on the fitted curve, with marks at the $BMDL_{01}$, $BMDL_{05}$, $BMDL_{10}$, $BMDL_{20}$, and $BMDL_{30}$. For comparison, Figure 14.2 shows the multistage model with degree 2, which is the worst-fitting model with an acceptable goodness of fit and also the model with the lowest calculated BMD_{10} and $BMDL_{10}$. The fit of the model is noticeably worse at all data points. Figure 14.3 shows the log-logistic model, which has the highest $BMDL_{10}$ and the second-highest BMD_{10} of the models. It fits the high-dose

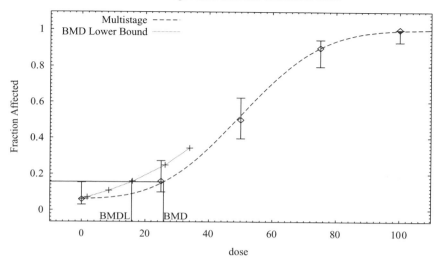

Figure 14.1 BMDS plot of results of the multistage model of degree 3 applied to the example data set. Diamonds: data points. Lines through data points: 95 % confidence intervals. Dashed line: the fitted curve. Dotted line: part of the 95 % lower confidence limit on the fitted curve, with marks at zero dose and at the $BMDL_{01}$, $BMDL_{05}$, $BMDL_{10}$, $BMDL_{20}$, and $BMDL_{30}$ (in that order, from lowest to highest value). The BMD_{10} and $BMDL_{10}$ are noted on the dose axis.

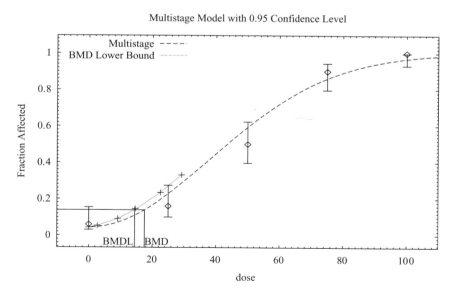

Figure 14.2 BMDS plot of results of the multistage model of degree 2 applied to the example data set; see Figure 14.1 for legend.

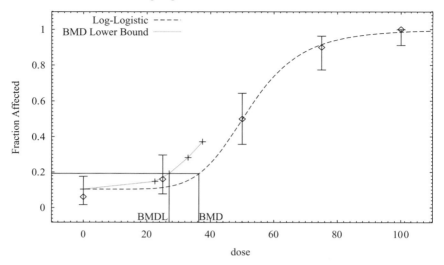

Figure 14.3 BMDS plot of results of the log-logistic model applied to the example data set; see Figure 14.1 for legend.

data well, but the curve is nearly flat at low doses, so the dose needed to achieve a 10 % extra risk is higher. The log-probit model, which also gives a high BMD, also is nearly flat at low doses. Despite the differences in fit, however, the lowest and highest $BMDL_{10}$ from the models that fit the data are within a factor of 2. In this case, there is little difference between the $BMDL_{10}$ from the model with the lowest AIC and the lowest of the calculated $BMDL_{10}$s (which would be the conservative choice).

CHAPTER 15

Uncertainty Analysis: The Bayesian Approach

Frédéric Y. Bois and Cheikh T. Diack

INERIS, Institut National de l'Environnement Industriel et des Risques

15.1 INTRODUCTION

Cancer models are idealised representations of the essential aspects of a set of complex biological phenomena. They can help with knowledge synthesis and scientific inference, by aggregating various sources of data in a unified framework. They can also be used to explore the logical consequences of postulated mechanisms, guiding further experiments to validate theoretical claims. Finally, they can also predict risks or make prognoses (risk assessment), and help design prevention and treatment strategies (risk management). All these activities fall under the heading of decision analysis: decisions about nature or decisions on how to act to acquire new knowledge or fight disease.

The current trend for mechanism-based quantitative risk assessment, and its focus on sensitive subgroups, relies on complex models to derive individual or population risks. Models are not perfect, however, and neither are data. Cancer is a very complex disease, and uncertainty is the permanent companion of knowledge in the area. Uncertainty, the inability to make precise and unbiased statements, results from a combination of imperfect knowledge of the biological phenomena, an inability to model them precisely and an inaccurate gathering of information. Cancer mechanisms are still far from clear. Even if they were, summing up in a model the massive amount of information required would in itself be a challenge. In addition, cancer bioassays or epidemiological studies are very costly and yield a limited amount of data, particularly on dose-response relationships. Risk assessment is inevitably carried out on the basis of incomplete scientific evidence, and risk estimates are therefore uncertain. On this basis, risk management has to make choices among alternatives actions with uncertain consequences. Any decision

Recent Advances in Quantitative Methods in Cancer and Human Health Risk Assessment
Edited by L. Edler and C. Kitsos   © 2005 John Wiley & Sons, Ltd

process aimed at minimising risk then becomes substantially more complicated. Questions arise such as: What action is likely to be the best? Does a single best choice exist? What is the loss (or cost) incurred from a (wrong) decision? How confident should one be in the efficacy of the decisions taken? Uncertainty in risk estimates or management goals leads to a range of options, most of which are wrong choices.

Uncertainty analysis aims at spanning this range, understanding, quantifying and devising ways to reduce uncertainties. It is therefore an essential step in decision-making. Rational decision-makers are willing to depart from simplistic models and default assumptions, but such an effort should clearly be justified by a gain in precision and accuracy of the risk estimates. This is what motivated, for example, the US Environmental Protection Agency and the Occupational Safety and Health Administration to request uncertainty analyses in the framework of their recent trichloroethylene and dichloromethane risk assessments (Bois, 1999, 2000a, 2000b). In those cases, at the interface between modelling and risk assessment, uncertainty analysis brought a clear reduction in uncertainty, while at the interface between assessment and management, it offered a perspective of the limited knowledge we had on what constitutes a good measure of effective dose.

The mechanics of inductive inference in the presence of uncertainty depend strongly on its representation and on the methodology used. Many approaches are available. This is briefly discussed in Section 15.2. Understanding uncertainty requires the identification of its causes. This is an integral part of uncertainty analysis and is discussed in Section 15.3, while the different types of uncertainty are analysed in Section 15.4. Sections 15.5 and 15.6 discuss methods to quantify and reduce uncertainty, respectively.

15.2 REPRESENTATIONS OF UNCERTAINTY

A firmly grounded uncertainty analysis requires a representation of the uncertainty surrounding the quantities of interest. A representation of uncertainty formalises incomplete information. Such a representation can be obtained by assuming that uncertain quantities or statements are known only to the extent that their values belong to a set (classes of models, ranges of parameter values, etc.). In the case of uncertain statements, standard Boolean logic can be used to build valued sets. Current approaches for representation of uncertainty include interval mathematics for handling imprecise measurements (Broadwater et al., 1994), Dempster–Shafer belief (or evidence) theory (Dempster, 1968; Shafer, 1976; Gordon and Shortliffe, 1990; Josang, 2001), fuzzy theory for the analysis of uncertainty due to vagueness rather than to the stochastic nature of some variables (Bonissone, 1990; Dubois and Prade, 1990; Klir and Yuan, 1995; Nestorov, 2001), and probabilistic analysis (Bedford and Cook, 2001; Coyle, 2003). Fuzzy theory was introduced in the 1960s by Zadeh to model the uncertainty of natural language. The theory is built to handle the concept of partial thruth. For example, the statement 'chemical x causes cancer' may be conceived as neither completely true nor completely false. The probabilistic approach is the most widely used to characterise uncertainty in physical systems. There is no universally best representation and the choice of one over the others should depend on the domain of application. In any case, the justification and mechanics of any inductive inference will depend on the representation adopted for uncertainty.

Clearly, any representation of uncertainty (in the current state of knowledge) takes into account current beliefs (assumptions). Such beliefs may change when an increase in knowledge is provided by data (observations of facts). The Bayesian theory provides a statistical framework that formalises the process of updating existing beliefs with the data at hand (O'Hagan, 1994; Gelman et al., 1995). In a Bayesian setting, all unknown quantities are considered as random variables. The probability distribution of an unknown parameter is interpreted in terms of degrees of belief about its possible values. Before analysing an experiment, a prior probability distribution, P, is constructed for each unknown to reflect current knowledge about it. The use of a probability distribution to represent prior knowledge offers a unified way to account for precise as well as vague information available before an experiment. When little knowledge is available on a particular parameter, a non-informative (i.e., flat-shaped) distribution can be used, although the representation of complete ignorance can be problematic. If stronger prior knowledge is at hand, the prior should represent that information as appropriately as possible.

Although the Bayesian method is convenient to analyse uncertainty, a solid alternative is provided by so-called classical statistics. Both theories have advantages and drawbacks. For the sake of conciseness, we focus in the following on the probabilistic representation of uncertainty within the Bayesian framework.

15.3   CAUSES OF UNCERTAINTY

Besides the reduction of uncertainty, the first aim of uncertainty analysis is the identification of its sources and elaboration of ways to quantify it. Uncertainty is often taken to be inherent in the physical system under consideration, but another view is that our limited knowledge is the sole source of uncertainty. For example, biological systems tend to produce responses that we cannot predict exactly, and we qualify such responses as uncertain. What is really uncertain are our predictions not the responses themselves, and the involvement of the modeller in any modelling process must be considered. Hence, the ultimate source of uncertainty is the imperfect knowledge of the causal relationships underlying observations. Yet we stumble, for three main reasons.

The first reason is inaccurate or incomplete gathering of data. Data are realisations of underlying stochastic processes. In a Bayesian context, the data values at hand are considered as fully known, and therefore certain. The data are the raw material of any statistical investigation since they do have some persistent relationship with the world from which they were drawn. Indeed, there is uncertainty about the underlying process by which data were obtained (coding and reading errors, systematic measurement errors, censored values, etc.), or about the value of future data. The whole purpose of modelling is precisely to provide a statistical distribution of the 'true state of the world' that data reflect. Deterministic models focus usually on the mean of the data and are supplemented with statistical models to specify distributions. Purely stochastic models directly provide full distributions.

The second reason for stumbling is variability and uncertainty. Our inability to describe a system precisely may be the result of not understanding it, or may come from its high variability. Here, variability refers not only to the heterogeneity (intra- and interindividual variability: gender, age, genetic variations, social status, sensitive sub-populations, etc.) almost always present in any data set, but also to the inherent imprecision of measurement systems. Variability is not uncertainty. In some cases it is possible to have full knowledge of the variability, for example by exhaustive enumeration, with no uncertainty attached. However, variability may be a source of uncertainty in predictions if we do not fully understand it and ascribe it to randomness. In that case, we cannot exactly predict the characteristics or responses of future items, experimental units, individuals, etc. In addition, describing variability through distributions (or by any other means) is a large source of modelling errors and model uncertainty (what is the correct distribution?). Note that while variability can be quantified by measurements, it is often irreducible and unavoidable, since it is a state of nature.

A final stumbling block is human subjectivity. This may be caused by limited knowledge. In this case, the world is not fully understood and therefore not modelled exactly. Summing up in a model a massive amount of information can in itself be a technical challenge. Assumptions have to be made to construct models or make decisions. Uncertainty is necessarily attached to them. Human subjectivity may also be caused by difficulty in rationalising preferences and being fully rational in a complex decision process.

15.4   TYPES OF UNCERTAINTY

Uncertainties can affect all components of the decision chain: models, parameters, future scenarios, predictions, decision rules and decisions. Figure 15.1 illustrates the information flow in a Bayesian modelling and decision problem. The analysis of data, conditionally on the model and prior parameter distributions, yields posterior parameter distributions. These can be used with the same model to make predictions for future scenarios. Using these predictions, decisions are made. Uncertainty affects every node of the graph, except the data node, which is a 'given'.

15.4.1   Model uncertainty

For practical use, statistical models need only to be sufficiently complex to capture interesting aspects of reality (i.e., those that matter for the inferences or decisions to be made). There is uncertainty in the definition of these 'interesting aspects' (this is discussed in Section 15.4.2). The source of uncertainty about model structure is

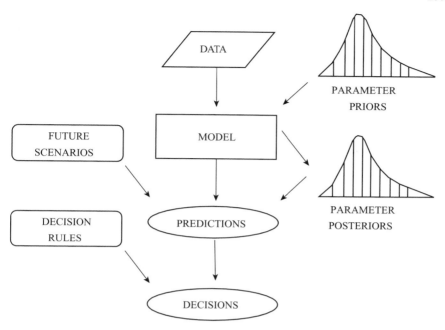

Figure 15.1   Information flow in a modelling and decision problem.

primarily a lack of theoretical knowledge to correctly describe the phenomenon of interest on all scales. For example, the number and sequence of limiting steps for the development of cancer of a given organ is still poorly known. It is therefore unclear if cancer is best described as a multistage or a multihit process (Kopp-Schneider, 1997). In those conditions, choosing a two-stage carcinogenesis model maybe sensible but is quite arbitrary, and we cannot be sure that the model will provide reasonable predictions of biological outcomes. Another source of model uncertainty stems from the assumptions made about structure of the stochastic processes eventually involved in carcinogenesis or about the probability distributions used to describe uncertainty itself. For example, assuming that the number of animals bearing tumours is binomially distributed is justified only if the probability of having a tumour is independent and identical for each individual in the cohort. Uncertainty is attached to such an assumption. In addition, there are usually several plausible models. Bernardo and Smith (1994) differentiate three cases. The M-closed case corresponds to believing that one of the models considered is 'true', without the explicit knowledge of which one it is. The M-complete case corresponds to acting as if the models considered are simply to be compared to some reference model (even if it cannot be said to be the true one). Finally, the M-open view requires comparison of the models in the absence of a reference. These three cases lead to different treatments of the problem of model choice and model comparison under uncertainty. We refer the reader to Bernardo and Smith (1994, Chapter 6) for further details.

15.4.2   Parameter uncertainty

Given a particular model structure, assumed to be correct, quantitative modelling requires the estimation of model parameter values, initial conditions, etc. These values may be obtained a priori, on the basis of the scientific literature or previous experiments, or a posteriori, via statistical model fitting (called 'calibration' in a Bayesian context). A Bayesian treatment of information allows prior information and data to be convolved to obtain 'posterior' distributions of the parameter estimates. The spread of that distribution reflects the degree of residual uncertainty after all information has been summarised by the model. Parametric uncertainty is often the easiest to assess and quantitative uncertainty analyses tend to focus on it.

15.4.3   Decision framework uncertainty

This uncertainty arises in the predictive or decision-making phase of modelling. Decision rule uncertainty is about whether the model settings (in input or output) represent the concerns of the decision-maker, given that those concerns might not be clearly expressed and might not be fully rational. In a decision-analytic framework this can be construed as uncertainty in the definition of 'utility' (Bedford and Cook, 2001). The apparent irrationality of some decision-maker is more difficult to describe, but is actively investigated in the areas of game theory and sociology (Fehr and Fischbacher, 2003). Here are some examples of questions falling in the realm of decision rule uncertainty:

- If future exposure scenarios are to be explored, how should they be defined?

- What is an acceptable level of risk?

- Should an 'average' person be considered for a risk estimate? What is an average person? Is the average defined in terms of exposure or in terms of susceptibility?

- Which are the sensitive subgroups? How precisely are they defined?

One can see that there is probably as much uncertainty attached to each of these questions as is attached to model choice. The decision-maker may not necessarily know a priori what trade-offs are involved. Fortunately, interactions of uncertainty analysts with planners and decision-makers are usually not a one-way approach. Presenting the results of an uncertainty analysis (and/or sensitivity analysis) will highlight new aspects of the problem and new questions will arise. This is critical in the area of risk analysis.

15.5   QUANTIFYING UNCERTAINTY

As mentioned above, almost every box or node in Figure 15.1 is affected by uncertainty. How it is quantified will depend on the type of item we are dealing with.

15.5.1 Parameter uncertainty

In probabilistic analysis, and in particular in a Bayesian framework, one starts by assigning statistical distributions to each model parameter. Assigning distributions to parameters is relatively easy when they are real numbers or integers, which is most often the case. Note that the shape of the distributions themselves may not be known and may therefore fall under the heading of model uncertainty. If we assume that the shape is known and that the model is correct (e.g., for theoretical reasons), the spread of those distributions provides a measure of uncertainty in the parameter values.

Bayesian updating of prior information with that contained in the data calls upon Bayes' theorem. The theorem states that the joint posterior (i.e., updated) parameter probability (or probability density in the case of continuous parameters) is simply proportional to the product of the prior parameter probability (density) and the likelihood function evaluated for the given data. More precisely,

$$P(\mathbf{\theta}, \mathbf{D}) = P(\mathbf{\theta}|\mathbf{D})P(\mathbf{D}) = P(\mathbf{D}|\mathbf{\theta})P(\mathbf{\theta}).$$

Therefore,

$$P(\mathbf{\theta}|\mathbf{D}) = \frac{P(\mathbf{D}|\mathbf{\theta})P(\mathbf{\theta})}{P(\mathbf{D})}$$

where $\mathbf{\theta}$ is the set of parameters to estimate, $\mathbf{D}$ the data, $P(\mathbf{D}|\mathbf{\theta})$ the likelihood function, $P(\mathbf{\theta})$ the prior probability, $P(\mathbf{\theta}|\mathbf{D})$ the posterior parameter probability and $P(\mathbf{D})$, a constant with respect to $\mathbf{\theta}$.

The likelihood function is the probability of observing the data for given parameter values. In simple cases, and when prior distribution shapes are carefully chosen to have special mathematical properties (conjugacy), the posterior parameter distributions can be obtained explicitly. This leads to statements of the type 'the posterior distribution of a is normal with mean 0.05 and variance 0.1'. With non-linear models and unconstrained choice of shape for the priors, the posterior distribution is not known explicitly and the current practice is to resort to Monte Carlo simulations to obtain a sample of parameter values from that distribution. If one can compute the prior probabilities and the likelihood function, several algorithms can be used, and in particular the so-called Markov chain Monte Carlo (MCMC) samplers (Smith and Roberts, 1993; Gelman and Rubin, 1996; Gilks *et al.*, 1996).

In summary, prior distributions can be used to quantify parameter uncertainty; but if data are available, the parameter posterior distributions should be used. Such posterior can generally be obtained using appropriate Monte Carlo sampling algorithms.

15.5.2 Model uncertainty

A general statistical approach to quantifying model uncertainty is to first evaluate the lack of accuracy of the models $(M_1, M_2, \ldots, M_k)$ considered when predicting some data sets. An underlying assumption is that the data are 'correct on average' and can be used to discriminate between models. Several loss functions can be used to quantify the distance between model predictions and data (Lehmann, 1986). The use of the likelihood as loss function has proved to be successful in great variety of problems in classical statistics. It is also consistent with Bayesian theory. The fact that complex models are more likely to fit the (eventually spurious) details of the data has led to attempts to penalise overparameterised models (e.g., using the Akaike criterion). With the Bayesian use of (proper) prior information, models should be assigned a prior probability of being correct (although it can be set equal for all models considered) and should be compared on the basis of their posterior probability (which can be estimated via MCMC simulations: Gilks *et al.*, 1996). The posterior probability, which automatically penalises larger models by a dilution effect of the posterior, when the dimension of the prior increases, is a criterion for model choice. In the M-closed case (see definition above), only a known set of models is entertained and the true model is part of the set, but we may not be able to designate it with certainty. The posterior probabilities of the models considered define a discrete distribution of the probability of being the 'true model', which correctly reflects model uncertainty. In the M-complete case the true model is not supposed to be in the set considered and models are just ranked on the basis of the loss function. The posterior model probabilities then do not fully reflect uncertainty because some possibly good models are left out of the picture. This, in our opinion, is problematic. Treatment of the M-open view is more challenging. In that case, the major problem when attempting to quantify uncertainty in the model structure is to define a measurable space for models. Bayesians will also want to be able to define meaningful prior distributions on that space. It is also necessary to be able to compute loss functions or posterior probabilities for any point of that space and sample from it efficiently. It may be possible to define a general class of models that contains the model(s) of interest. If that class is parametric (i.e., models have a common structure, but differ in parameter values) we are back in a situation of parameter uncertainty. In all three cases, it is possible to avoid choosing one particular model by doing 'model averaging': models and their parameter values can be Monte Carlo sampled following their posterior probabilities and used to make predictions. Each model is then represented with its own weight (Hoeting *et al.*, 1999).

However, simple averaging over a class of models that does not necessarily contain the true model, as suggested by Hoeting *et al.* (1999), is not safer than treating a single non-rejected model as correct. It is preferable to reflect the range of possibilities generated by model uncertainty. In any case, analyses of model uncertainty can be computationally costly. In addition, in the Bayesian framework, using posterior probabilities as a criterion for model choice, and performing goodness-of-fit tests, requires the use of prior model probabilities, which may be difficult to assign (and the use of arbitrary or non-informative priors is problematic in this context). In any case, posterior model probabilities will depend strongly on priors if the data are poor (but this may rather be seen as a problem with the data).

15.5.3   Decision framework uncertainty

Future scenarios and decision rules usually come only in input of the modelling/ prediction exercise. The challenge here also is to elicit a range (continuous or not) of options from the planners and decision-makers (see the literature on medical decision-making, e.g. Cancré *et al.*, 1999). Once this is achieved, it is possible to assess the impact of this uncertainty on model outputs or decisions to be made by exhaustive enumeration or Monte Carlo sampling (Cancré *et al.*, 1999; Greenland, 2001; see also Figure 15.1).

15.5.4   Sensitivity analysis

Understanding the major determinants of model output uncertainty is called sensitivity analysis. Sensitivity can be studied locally (in the parameter space) by computing the variation in outputs subsequently to a small perturbation of para-meter values (Iman and Helton, 1988). In our opinion, it is preferable to study it globally, via Monte Carlo sampling from distributions describing parameter uncertainty. A parameter may have a low impact on outputs when assessed locally (around its mean value, for example), but if its value is very uncertainty, it may have an overall large sensitivity. Global sensitivity analysis can be easily performed by simply studying, in a univariate or multivariate setting, the relationships between sampled parameter values or scenario definitions (what-if analysis) and outputs (Gelman *et al.*, 1996).

15.6   REDUCING UNCERTAINTY

Measuring uncertainty provides a range of possibilities. The goal of uncertainty analysis is to state and discuss this range, but also to point to ways to reduce it. To this end, we can benefit from recent developments in data mining and multilevel modelling.

15.6.1   Data preparation

Bringing all the data together under the umbrella of a common model and fitting them jointly might help to reduce uncertainty. However, when the volume of data increases, model complexity tends to increase too. When large amounts of data are available, the techniques of data mining may help reduce uncertainty. The process starts in particular by getting to know the data in order to understand how reliable the measurements are. This involves cleaning up the data by visualising them, checking for outliers or out-of-range values, replacing missing values (without obscuring the fact that they were missing), etc.

15.6.2   Accounting for variability to reduce uncertainty: multilevel modelling

Variability is almost always present in nature and is often an important source of uncertainty. Yet the two can be disentangled, therefore leading to a reduction in uncertainty, with statistical multilevel (or 'population') models (Gelman *et al.*, 1996; Wakefield, 1996; Bernillon and Bois, 2000; Greenland, 2000; Bois, 2001). The objective of multilevel models is to extract, from data on individuals units (e.g., subject, family, group), a quantitative description of the variability in given characteristics within a large population. The basic idea is that the same model can describe the data for each unit, and that the model parameters differ randomly between units, or between observations within the same unit, etc. Such randomness characterises variability *per se*, and is described by (multivariate) probability distributions. A parameter characterising individual susceptibility to cancer, for example, will be assumed to be normally distributed around a 'population mean', with a 'population variance' which measures variability in the population. Population means and variances (one for each parameter supposed to vary across units) are termed 'population' parameters. They are estimated during the model calibration process, together with the model parameters for each unit.

A typical multilevel model is presented in Figure 15.2. The hierarchical structure of the model is apparent, with two major components: the subject level and the population level. At the subject level, data (**y**) are measured in conditions specified by the design variables **X**. A set of individual characteristics (parameters **θ**) also condition the observations. Some of these characteristics may be known (e.g., sex, age, genotype), in which case they are considered as 'covariates', but usually some interesting characteristics are unknown and need to be estimated from the data. This estimation can be achieved by data fitting. At this level the model is made of two parts:

- A statistical model that links some 'predictable' aspects of the data (e.g., their expected values, or their variance) to the actual measurements (**y**). Deviations between measurements and their expected values may be due to limited assay precision, modelling error, or random intra-individual variability. Such deviations may, for example, be assumed to be independent normal random variables, with mean zero and variance σ^2. That variance can, if necessary, be estimated along with the other model parameters. The model chosen will specify the data likelihood.

- A pharmacokinetic or pharmacodynamic (e.g., cancer) model, f, links the 'predictable' aspects chosen to **X** and **θ**.

At the population level, interunit variability is described by considering that the individual parameters, **θ**, are randomly drawn from given statistical distributions, each with population mean **μ** and variance Σ^2, as described above. The population parameters are to be estimated together with the parameters **θ** and the residual variance σ^2.

In this setting, uncertainty enters the calibration process through the residual variance σ^2 (which typically includes limited assay precision, modelling error, and neglected levels of variability). It is possible to split σ^2 in order to identify separately its various components. For example, a further level can be defined to

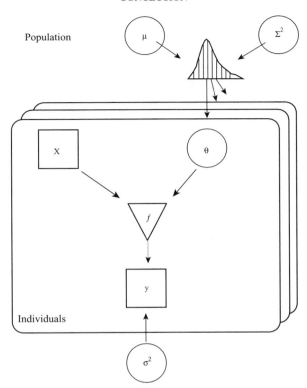

Figure 15.2 Graphical representation of a multilevel model. At the individual level, design (controlled) variables (**X**) and individual characteristics (parameters, **θ**) condition the observations (data, **y**). A model, f, describes the relationships between **X**, **θ** and **y**. Individual characteristics are randomly distributed in the population. Population means and variances (**μ** and Σ^2) describe the shape of that distribution. Measurement errors, modelling errors, and intra-individual variability are lumped in a common variance term σ^2. Unknown quantities are in circles, known quantities in squares.

deal with intraunit variability. However, some measurement and modelling errors are likely to remain, even with the best available data and models. A less obvious source of uncertainty, which affects the population parameters, is the finite size of the population sample. Even if the characteristics of each individual were perfectly known, the population parameter values inferred from a non-exhaustive sample would still be affected by uncertainty.

15.7   CONCLUSION

The goal of uncertainty analysis is to provide an evaluation of the limits of our knowledge. In that respect, it is likely that exploring limits will always be more difficult that simply going for a single reasonable model. Parameter uncertainty is now routinely analysed, thanks to the diffusion of Monte Carlo simulations techniques, for which several software tools are available (@Risk®, Crystal Ball®, etc.). Progress in the inclusion of evidence from data has been fostered by the development of MCMC simulation software for Bayesian updating (MCSim, BUGS, etc.). Such computations remain heavy when dealing with complex models, but progress in statistical modelling, numerical analysis, and computer science and technology, should help alleviate these difficulties. More challenging is the need to deal with model and decision rule uncertainties. A major difficulty seems to come from a split in modelling philosophy. A first approach, mostly entertained by statisticians, is to develop large classes of flexible models that 'let the data speak for themselves'. In that case, examining models individually is not feasible and sampling techniques are actively investigated. The second approach, exemplified by climate research or physiological modelling, proceeds from a mechanistic understanding of the process studied and tends to focus on a few complex models. It relies heavily on prior knowledge, and special statistical tools are required (Poole and Raftery, 2000). Given this split, unification of tools and wide availability of general software for model uncertainty analysis are probably a long way off. However, the question be addressed in health risk assessments as a matter of urgency. The realisation that cancer models can differ widely in their low-dose predictions (Zeise *et al.*, 1987) led, during the 1980s, to the default choice of a somewhat conservative multistage model. This can be construed as a precautionary move in the face of very large uncertainties. Yet we should try to reduce those uncertainties through a joint effort of modelling, data gathering, and statistical analysis.

But here may lie the paradox: uncertainty analysis itself cannot be precise! One has to choose, for example, between alternative methodologies (fuzzy theory, Bayesian or classical statistics, etc.). The robustness of analysis of uncertainty may therefore be questionable. One should not be mistaken, however, about the problem to tackle. A good analysis of uncertainty should help elucidate and focus on the uncertainties that matter most to the decision-maker. In that sense, uncertainty analysis goes hand in hand with sensitivity analysis. The ultimate goal of an uncertainty analysis is to tell us by how much we can be wrong and still be ok!

ACKNOWLEDGEMENTS

This work was funded by grant no. BCRD-AP2002-DRC-13 from the French Ministry of Ecology and Sustainable Development.

CHAPTER 16

Optimal Designs for Bioassays in Carcinogenesis

Christos P. Kitsos

Technological Educational Institute of Athens

16.1 INTRODUCTION

The aim of this paper is to bridge the theoretical insight obtained from an experimental design with its practical applications such that in the cancer risk assessment research field, the optimal experimental design theory finds more recognition than it has found in the past. Although other equally strong mathematical approaches have been widely used in carcinogenesis (Tan, 1991), experimental design theory has not been widely adopted for experimental carcinogenesis problems. As the statistical software becomes more user-friendly for experimentalists, we believe that the optimal design approach can eventually be adopted in the field of cancer risk assessment, as it has been applied successfully in other fields.

This chapter is organized as follows. Section 16.2 refers to the background of the optimal design theory, and various examples are provided for the discrete and continuous case. In Section 16.3 the theory is applied to the Michaelis–Menten model as an example of a continuous response model. In Section 16.4 the sequential design approach is adopted for the Weibull tolerance distribution model as a binary response model.

16.2 ON THE OPTIMAL DESIGN THEORY

Experimental design methods belong to one of the most important classes of statistical methods used for investigational processes in various technical and biological fields. Experimental designs can be considered as the most important statistical

Recent Advances in Quantitative Methods in Cancer and Human Health Risk Assessment
Edited by L. Edler and C. Kitsos © 2005 John Wiley & Sons, Ltd

procedures for investigating particular characteristics of a process by means of setting the appropriate optimal conditions. The design of a study defines the system of experimentation through a formal description of constraints, especially constrains on the allocation of subjects. We consider here an experiment as a task where the researcher controls the experimental conditions. For a general discussion on the design of experiments, see Atkinson and Bailey (2001). When we consider an experiment as a test, then a designed experiment is a series of planned tests, such that the researcher obtains information on the underlying link between the input variables and the output response or responses.

An optimal (experimental) design is one which gives the best possible parameter estimates, under a specified criterion. Such a criterion can be to minimize the variance of the estimators, to minimize the sum of variances of the estimators, etc.; see Ford *et al.* (1989) for a detailed review.

An experiment in which the presence of a chemical is quantified, by using living organisms, is known as bioassay. There exist different definitions of the term bioassay: 'An assay for determining the potency (or concentration) of a substance that causes a biological change in experimental animals' (www. epa.gov/isis/gloss8.htm), or 'Determination of the potency or concentration of a compound by its effect upon animals, isolated tissues, or microorganisms, as compared with an analysis of its chemical or physical properties' (www.jackorchard.org/2_glossary.asp).

For any experiment certain rules have to be followed. First, one has to define the k predictor variables (explanatory, input variables) denoted $x = (x_1, x_2, \ldots, x_k)$. The range of their values, usually a subset of the k-dimensional real space, is known as the experimental region, $X \subseteq \mathbb{R}^k$. Typical examples of explanatory variables are 'time' or 'concentration' in biological systems. Next, one has to define a structure on the experimental region. This is achieved by a measure ξ on the experimental region X. The pair (X, ξ) is known as the design space, with ξ being a design measure from a family of measures Ξ (Silvey, 1980; Ford *et al.*, 1989). Practically speaking, the design measure tells the experimenter what portion of observations to allocate at the optimal design points of the experiment.

Whereas the theory of optimal linear design has been well established in the second part of the past century by the theory of linear models, the theory of nonlinear designs is still in its infancy. On the other hand, most real-life applications, in particular, in risk assessment lead to nonlinear models. Two different problems arise for nonlinear optimal designs:

(i) The underlying model describing the physical phenomenon is nonlinear. The aim is then to estimate the involved parameters as well as possible.

(ii) A nonlinear function of the unknown parameter, known as the general nonlinear aspect, is to be estimated as well as possible.

Typical examples are presented below. We consider a response variable, *Y*, which is either discrete or continuous.

16.2.1 Binary outcome designs

The main aim of statistical modeling is to present a simplified and smooth representation of the underlying population separating systematic features (such as gender, age, height, weight, etc.) from random variation (error, noise). The systematic features are represented by a model function, while the random variation, unrelated to the input variables, is usually presented by a probability distribution, with one or two (mostly unknown) parameters. The analysis of the binary response problems leading to binomial data has been developed within the theory of generalized linear models; see McCullagh and Nelder (1989).

The first application of regression-like models with binomial data was done for bioassays with individual responses being success or failure, and with the proportions of 'successes' as the outcome variable. A typical example is the proportion of animals killed by a toxic substance at various doses; see, for example the classical models of quantal responses as developed by Finney (1947).

For a binary response, the outcome of n experiments is denoted by $Y_i = 0$ or 1, $i = 1, 2, \ldots, n$. The outcome is then linked with the covariate or input variable x from the design space Ξ and the parameter vector θ from the parameter space $\Theta \subseteq \mathbb{R}^p$, through a probability model PM. This model simply assigns a probability p to 'success':

$$p(x, \theta) = \text{PM}(x; \theta) = p(Y_i = 1 \mid x) = = 1 - p(Y_i = 0 \mid x). \tag{16.1}$$

It is assumed that the function PM is a 'smooth' (monotone and differentiable) function.

Example 16.1   Carcinogenesis bioassay models. Typical probability models for bioassays are the *logit, probit* and *exponential* models:

$$\text{PM}_\text{L}(x, \theta) = \log\{p(x; \theta)(1 - p(x; \theta))\},$$
$$\text{PM}_\text{P}(x, \theta) = \Phi^{-1}\{p(x; \theta)\},$$
$$\text{PM}_\text{E}(x, \theta) = \exp(-\theta x)$$

with Φ being the cumulative distribution function of the standard normal distribution. The probability $\text{PM} = p(x, \theta)$ denotes the individual success probability and its relation to the predictor variable x has to be modeled. In carcinogenesis bioassays the binary response describes 'tumor' or 'no tumor' and x is usually the dose or the logarithm of the dose. Notice that PM_E model is the one-hit model well known in carcinogenesis theory.

Example 16.2   The contingent response model (Zocchi and Atkinson, 1999). Let us now denote by x the log-dose and consider the following pairs of responses (Y_{1k}, Y_{2k}):

$Y_{1k} = 1$, the kth subject has a toxic response, $Y_{1k} = 0$, otherwise,
$Y_{2k} = 1$, the kth subject has a disease failure, $Y_{2k} = 0$, otherwise,

with $k = 1, 2 \ldots, n$. Let us concentrate on the following three possible outcomes: $\{Y_{1k} = 0, Y_{2k} = 0\}$ benefit and no harm; $\{Y_{1k} = 0, Y_{2k} = 1\}$ no harm, but no benefit; $\{Y_{1k} = 1\}$ harm and no statement on benefit.

A parametric location–scale model can be assumed to model this two-dimensional outcome. Using two logit models, we obtain a multinomial logistic model of the form

$$p(Y_{1k} = 0 \mid x) = F(a_1 + b_1 x)$$
$$p(Y_{2k} = 0 \mid Y_{1k} = 0\,x) = G(a_2 + b_2 x),$$

where both F and G denote the logistic function $1/(1 - e^s)$. Using the notation $F' = 1 - F$ and $G' = 1 - G$, the probability of toxicity is F' and the probability of disease failure is $F'G'$. Therefore $p(Y_{1k} = 0, Y_{2k} = 0 \mid x) = F'G$. The optimal dose level that maximizes $F'G$ can be evaluated by setting the derivatives of $F'G$, say $D(F'G)$, equal to zero: $0 = D(F'G) = F'D(G) + GD(F') = F'D(G) - GD(F)$. Obviously, this approach is not confined to F and G being only logistic functions and any model from a location–scale family can be also be used, although the derivates may be somewhat more complicated.

Example 16.3   Dose-finding in Phase I/II clinical trials (Thall and Russel, 1998). It is the very clearly expressed goal of a clinical trial to perform an experiment that satisfies specific safety and efficacy requirements. For ethical reasons, only doses which are both safe and efficacious should be administered to patients. This requires the estimation of the rates of the events at preset dose levels. Using as dose-response curve the logit model PM_L, the cumulative odds model can be used. So the underlying model describing the experiment is again a nonlinear model where a binary indicator describes the levels of toxicity. One has to impose a trial target to estimate that optimal level of dose among different candidate dose levels that satisfies both the efficacy and toxicity criteria.

Example 16.4   Subject allocation for the logistic model. Given the model $PM_L = \{1 + \exp[-\theta_1(x - \theta_2)]\}^{-1}$, the optimal design allocates half the observations ($\xi = 1/2$) at the optimal design points $(1.54 - \theta_1)/\theta_2, (-1.54 - \theta_1)/\theta_2$. For the *probit model* with mean θ_1 and variance θ_2 the optimal design points are $(1.14 - \theta_1)/\theta_2, (-1.14 - \theta_1)/\theta_2$, while for the *one-hit model* the optimal design point is $1.59/\theta$. That is, we allocate all the observations at one point only; see Kitsos (1986, 1999). Example 16.7 below considers this situation in more detail in a simulation study.

Notice, that the estimation of the model parameters using the maximum likelihood theory depends in its quality on the number of experimental units observed in a bioassay. When the sample size is small, the likelihood function might not provide a valid estimate of the model parameters. That occurs when a batch of only successes or only failures results as outcome, that is, the $Y_i s$ are all 1 or 0. Simulation results for the one-hit model (see Kitsos, 1999), provide evidence that, in practice, even if the sample size is $n = 50$ there may be two or three experiments, out of 1000 simulated ones, that do not provide a maximum likelihood estimate. Obviously, the situation gets worse with smaller sample sizes. Roughly speaking, the maximum likelihood method for the binary response problems can provide a valid estimate only when both successes and failures occur; for a detailed discussion see Kitsos (1999). For further theoretical and practical applications of the maximum likelihood approach we refer to Tan (1991), McCullagh and Nelder (1989) and Ewens and Grant (2002).

Notice from the above examples that the optimal design points depend on the unknown parameters we would like to estimate. To overcome this problem various techniques have been suggested: local optimum designs, optimum average designs, minimax designs, and sequential design; see Ford *et al.* (1989).

16.2.2   Continuous outcome designs

In a continuous regression model, the input variable x is linked with the model parameter θ through a (deterministic) function, $f(x, \theta)$ to describe the response (output) variable. In practice, the response is only observed with experimental error, say e. This results in a stochastic nonlinear regression model of the form

$$y_i = f(x_i, \theta) + e_i, \qquad i = 1, 2, \ldots, n, \tag{16.2}$$

where the function f is a smooth, intrinsically nonlinear regression function. Moreover, the errors are assumed to be independent and identically distributed random variables with mean $E(e_i) = 0$ and variance $V(e_i) = \sigma^2 > 0$. Denote the expected value of the binary response Y by η, i.e $E(Y) = \eta$.

Example 16.5   Circadian rhythms (Kitsos *et al.*, 1988). In the investigation of circadian rhythms one uses the so-called cosinor model to describe a parameter around which systematic oscillation occurs. This clinical parameter, known as a mesor, indicates the overall expiratory capacity when a circadian rhythm is measured. There is a second positive parameter which measures the degree of diurnal variation. Interest is focused on their ratio. This is, therefore, an example where a ratio of unknown parameters has to be estimated in a nonlinear model. Different optimality criteria can be discussed in relation to the geometry involved in this biological problem. For a list of regression kinetic models and their corresponding optimal design points, see Kitsos (1995). For the nonlinear regression problems the main estimation method is ordinary least squares; see Bates and Watts (1988) or Seber and Wild (1989). We will apply those methods below for the estimation of the parameters of Michaelis–Menten model.

16.2.3   Definition of the optimal design

In this section, we briefly discuss how an optimal nonlinear design can be defined. For a very valuable theoretical approach to the optimal design analysis see Chapter 21 in this volume. Let us start formally.

The variance–covariance matrix, C, for both models (16.1) and (16.2) is defined as

$$C(\hat{\theta}, \xi) = \sigma^2 [(\nabla\eta)^T (\nabla\eta)]^{-1} \qquad (16.3)$$

with $\eta = E(y)$ and $\nabla\eta$ being the vector of partial derivatives of η with respect to the parameter $\theta = (\theta_1, \ldots, \theta_p) \in \Theta$. The average per-observation information matrix $\mathbf{M}$ for the design measure ξ is defined as

$$M(\theta, \xi) = \frac{1}{n}(\nabla\eta)^T \nabla\eta = \frac{\sigma^2}{n} C^{-1}(\theta, \xi). \qquad (16.4)$$

The matrix $I(\theta, \xi) = nM(\theta, \xi)$ is also known as Fisher's information. A design measure $\xi \in \Xi$ is said to be optimal if it minimizes a (convex) functional of $M^{-1}(\theta, \xi)$ (Kitsos, 1986). An important example of a design criterion is the so-called D-optimality, which minimizes $\det M^{-1}(\theta, \xi)$. The D-optimality criterion will be adopted for the Michaelis–Menten model in the next section.

16.3   THE MICHAELIS–MENTEN MODEL

A general theory for enzyme kinetics was firstly developed by Michaelis and Menten (1913) in their pioneering work on the metabolism of an agent described by a reaction rate. The basic toxicokinetic model of metabolism, the so-called Michaelis–Menten (MM) model, applies when an enzyme, say E, binds reversibly with a substrate, say S, to form an enzyme–substrate complex, say ES, which can dissociate to the product, say P. The following stoichiometric scheme is assumed:

$$E + S \underset{k_2}{\overset{k_1}{\rightleftarrows}} ES \overset{k_3}{\longrightarrow} E + P$$

with k_1, k_2, k_3 the associated rate constants. Set

$$K_M = \frac{k_2 + k_3}{k_1}$$

(known as the MM constant) and

$$V_{max} = k_3 C_{TOT},$$

where C_{TOT} is the total enzyme concentration. A plot of the initial velocity of reaction u, against the concentration of substrate, C_S, will provide the MM rectangular hyperbola of the form

$$u = \frac{V_{max} C_S}{K_M + C_S}. \qquad (16.5)$$

With the modeling set up of (16.2), we have $\theta = (V_{max}, K_M)$, and $x = C_S$. The deterministic relation (16.2) is the functional relationship $f(x, \theta)$. Several different linear transformations have been suggested to estimate the model parameters depending on how the input variable C_S is curvilinearly related to the response u (see Currie, 1982). The most used forms are

$$n = V_{max} - K_M \frac{u}{C_S},$$

$$\frac{C_S}{u} = \frac{K_M}{V_{max}} + \frac{1}{V_{max}} C_S, \tag{16.6}$$

$$\frac{1}{u} = \frac{1}{V_{max}} + \frac{K_M}{V_{max}} \frac{1}{C_S}.$$

The third form, known as 'double reciprocal' transformation, is the most popular one. In this case estimates for K_M and V_{max} are obtained straightforwardly using linear regression. The second transformation has been shown in practice as the most efficient one, in terms of parameter estimation.

Endrenyi and Chan (1981) assumed that the error variance is proportional to the mean, Currie (1982) discussed the heteroscedasticity in the MM model, while Gilberg et al. (1999) provide an extensive discussion of the transform-both-sides model. To avoid heteroscedasticity problems in model (16.6), we consider the MM model in its original form (16.5) and search for an estimator solving the normal equations.

Example 16.6 Consider the data set of Seber and Wild (1989, p. 93) for enzyme velocity y and substrate concentration C_S:

C_S :	2.0	0.667	0.4	0.286	0.222	0.2
y :	0.0615	0.0334	0.0138	0.0129	0.0083	0.0219
	0.0527	0.0258	0.0258	0.0183	0.0169	0.0087

At each design point two experiments were performed and two responses were obtained. Suppose that the MM model is fitted to the data. Then the least-squares estimate of the vector of the unknown parameters is (0.105 79, 1.7077), provided (0.057, 0.6) is used as an initial guess. The MM model normal equations are

$$\sum_{i=1}^{n} \left(y_i - \frac{V_{max} C_{S,i}}{K_M + C_{S,i}} \right) \nabla u = 0, \tag{16.7}$$

with $u = (u_1, u_2, \ldots, u_n)$ and

$$\nabla u = \left(\frac{\partial u}{\partial V_{max}}, \frac{\partial u}{\partial K_M} \right)^T = \left(\frac{C_S}{K_M + C_S}, -\frac{V_{max} K_M C_S}{(K_M + C_S)^2} \right)^T. \tag{16.8}$$

For a single observation (u, C_S), Fisher's information is given as $(\nabla u)^T (\nabla u)$ and the average per-observation information matrix for n observations can be calculated as $\sigma^{-2} n \, M(\theta, \xi)$ (recall (16.4); see also Dette and Biedermann, (2003)). Therefore, asymptotically, the 2×2 variance–covariance matrix,

$$\mathbf{C} = \mathbf{C}(\hat{\theta}, \xi) = (n M(\hat{\theta}, \xi))^{-1}, \tag{16.9}$$

can be calculated and asymptotic approximate confidence intervals can be obtained for $\theta = (V_{\max}, K_{\mathrm{M}})$, as in the linear case. Another approach is to apply Beale's measure of nonlinearity (Kitsos, 1986, p. 81) which involves the curvature of the nonlinear model. This curvature is less than $1/2(F(\alpha, p, n - p))^{1/2}$, with F being the well known F distribution with parameters $(p, n - p)$, and α denoting the significance level. The supremum value of Beale's measure of nonlinearity reduces to

$$B = 1 + \frac{n}{n - 2}\frac{1}{\sqrt{F}}. \tag{16.10}$$

Therefore an approximate confidence region for the MM parameter vector $(V_{\max}, K_{\mathrm{M}})$ is given by

$$\left(\theta - \hat{\theta}\right)^{\mathrm{T}} I\left(\hat{\theta}, \xi\right)\left(\theta - \hat{\theta}\right) \leq Bps^2 F(a, p, n - p). \tag{16.11}$$

With $B = 1$, one obtains a linear approximation. A suitable estimator of σ^2 is

$$s^2 = \frac{1}{n - 2}\sum_{i=1}^{n} (y_i - \hat{y}_i)^2.$$

16.3.1   D-optimal design of the Michaelis–Menten model

There are two lines of thought in the search for an optimal design for the MM model. First, from a biological point of view, one may search for information on how enzymatically induced interactions influence the production of a carcinogen. This production has been described by biologists using the parameters K_{M} and $V_{\max}$. Secondly, one may take a statistical point of view and consider the MM model within the class of nonlinear models. In this section we try to bridge the two lines of thought, keeping a strong theoretical background and providing useful results for the experimentalist.

Designs for the MM kinetic were first discussed in Duggleby (1979). He constructed geometric designs with substrate concentrations set at the points rK_{M}, with $r = 0.25, 0.5, 1.0, 2.0, 4.0$ or $r = 0.5, 1.0, 2.0$. This design is optimum for estimating the ratio $V_{\max}/K_{\mathrm{M}}$ if the variance σ^2 is constant. Currie (1982) was working with geometric locally optimal designs where he could calculate efficiencies. A near-optimal design for estimating $V_{\max}$ and K_{M} with efficiency 70 % is the one at the design points $0.5K_{\mathrm{M}}, K_{\mathrm{M}}, 2K_{\mathrm{M}}$. Although there is a sequential flavor in these designs they are neither sequential (as there is not a sequential scheme which converges) nor optimal (as the design points are selected without adopting an optimality criterion, for example, to minimize the variance).

Endrenyi and Chan (1981) obtained D-optimal design points without minimization of the information matrix by a rather empirical approach. They worked out different designs claiming efficiencies from 95 % to 100 %. It is obvious that in enzyme kinetic studies with constant variance one design point should be at the highest possible concentration and another at the maximal feasible velocity.

Next, in a sequence of propositions, we work out locally D-optimal designs for the MM model.

Proposition 16.1 The D-optimal design for the MM model as in (16.5) does not depend on V_{max}.

Proof Indeed, from Kitsos (1986, p. 44),

$$\nabla u = \begin{pmatrix} 1 & 0 \\ 0 & V_{max} \end{pmatrix} \begin{pmatrix} C_S(K_M + C_S)^{-1} \\ -C_S(K_M + C_S)^{-2} \end{pmatrix} \tag{16.12}$$

with ∇u as in (16.8). It follows that the vector ∇u can be written as a product of a matrix with elements 0,1 and V_{max} and a vector which depends only on K_M. The model is partially nonlinear and so the parameter V_{max} does not influence the D-optimal design for estimating $\theta = (V_{max}, K_M)$.

Proposition 16.2 The D-optimal design for an extended MM model,

$$u = \frac{V_{max} C_S}{K_M + C_S} + \theta_0 C_S, \tag{16.13}$$

with parameter $\theta = (V_{max}, K_M, \theta_0)$ does not depend on V_{max} and θ_0.

Remark This means in practice that the D-optimal design points are not influenced when an extra linear term is introduced in the MM model. One then needs no more prior knowledge to perform the experiment. The experimenter needs only an initial guess for K_M, say K_0.

Proposition 16.3 Consider the MM model (16.5), with $C_S \in (0, U]$. The locally D-optimal (discrete) design at $K_M = K_0$ allocates half of the observations at points U and OptC$_S$, each, with

$$\text{Opt}C_S = \frac{K_0 U}{2K_0 + U} \tag{16.14}$$

and U denoting the maximum allowable substrate concentration.

Remark When C_S is within the left open, right closed interval (0,U] then the optimum C_S is at

$$\text{Opt}C_S = \frac{K_0 U}{2K_0 + (U - L)}, \qquad K_0 > 0, 0 < L < U. \tag{16.15}$$

Moreover, when the sample size n is odd, say $n = 2q + 1$, we can allocate q and $q + 1$ observations at the two optimum design points, U and OptC$_S$, in both permissible ways. The optimal design for the MM model is now a two-point design. There is no need to assign subjects at three or more design points.

Proposition 16.4   For the locally D-optimal design of Proposition 16.3 the determinant of the inverse average per-observation information matrix is given explicitly as:

$$d = \frac{V_{max}^2 U^6}{16 K_0^2 (K_0 + U)^6}. \tag{16.16}$$

Remark   This value can be compared with those of Endrenyi and Chan (1981). With Proposition 16.4 the experimenter has to calculate $\det \mathbf{M}^{-1}(\theta, \xi)$; recall (16.4) for the MM model. Notice that in (16.14) and (16.15) an initial guess for K_M is needed.

Proposition 16.5   If $U \gg K_0$ the locally D-optimal design ξ is

$$\xi^* = \left\{ \begin{array}{cc} U & K_0 \\ 0.5 & 0.5 \end{array} \right\}. \tag{16.17}$$

Remark   This design allocates one half observations at the maximum value U of the concentration of substrate and the other half at the initial guess K_0 for the MM constant. With Proposition 16.5 it is very simple to construct a D-optimal design.

Proposition 16.6   The D-optimal designs from Proposition 16.3 or 16.5 are also the D-optimal for estimating the ratio $\Phi = V_{max}/K_M$.

Remark   Proposition 16.6 informs the experimenter that the optimal two-point design for the MM model is needed to estimate the ratio of the parameters. This means that the optimal design for the estimation of the parameters of the MM model is at same time optimal for the estimation of their ratio. This is not generally true (see Kitsos *et al.*, 1988).

For the construction of *sequential optimal designs*, see Kitsos (1989, 2001). One problem is to find the initial guess K_0. We recommend devoting some observations for the estimation of the initial estimates and then to proceed with a two-stage procedure:

1. Devote a proportion p for n observations at first stage, that is, allocate $np/2$ observations at U and K_0, as in (16.17) or at U and $\text{Opt}C_S$ as in (16.15) or (16.14). Calculate the estimates. Use these estimates for the next step.

2. Use these estimates to perform static design.

The two-stage design is a compromise between a static design (devote all the observations once at the optimal design points) and a full sequential design (perform the experiment by devoting one observation per replication).

16.3.2   Applications of the D-optimal design

Let us consider now Example 16.6 in more detail. There are six design points within the closed range [0.2, 2.0] for C_S. There are 12 responses, obtained from a double replication of the experiment. An optimal design needs to be replicated at the optimal design points; see (16.14). One might think of obtaining estimates by performing the experiment at $U = 2.0$ and at $C_S = 0.4$, for an initial guess $\theta_0 = (V_{max}, K_M) = (0.057, 0.6)$ or at $C_S = 0.6$. Another approach could be to devote a portion of observations at these points: for example, allocate three observations at each optimal point, perform the experiment and then redesign it with the obtained estimate – that is, we devote half of the observations at each stage. If we devote two observations at each point, then a three-stage optimal design would be obtained.

Now consider the approximate confidence region (16.11) for the estimated vector $\widehat{\theta} = (\widehat{V}_{max}, \widehat{K}_M) = (0.105\,79, 1.7077)$. The matrix $\sigma^{-2} nM(\hat{\theta}, \xi)$ is evaluated with diagonal elements 0.8629, 0.011 69 and off-diagonal elements equal to -0.0314. An estimate of σ^2 is obtained from the data and the estimated vector $\hat{\theta}$ as $\widehat{\sigma}^2 = s^2 = 0.000\,02$. Hence with (16.4) we can evaluate Fisher's information matrix as

$$I(\hat{\theta}, \xi) = 12M(\hat{\theta}, \xi) = \begin{pmatrix} 43\,145 & -157.0 \\ -157.0 & 584.5 \end{pmatrix}.$$

The supremum value of Beale's measure of nonlinearity is $B = 1.049\,38$ using (16.10). From (16.11) the approximate confidence region is the ellipse

$$43.14V_{max}^2 + 0.58K_M^2 - 3.14V_{max}K_M - 82.92V_{max} - 0.92K_M + 1.50 \le 0.$$

If we apply the 'double reciprocal transformation' we obtain $(\widehat{V}_{max}, \widehat{K}_M) = (0.113\,636, 1.988\,63)$.

Notice that there is a difference compared with the values reported above even at the first decimal place, when using the nonlinear calculation. The fit is rather insufficient with $R^2 = 72.7\,\%$ due to calculating s^2, with the 'linear' approximation. The experimenter can obtain different values for the approximate values of Beale's measure of nonlinearity: with $\alpha = 0.05$, and sample sizes $n = 4, 6, 8, 10, 20, 30, 60$ the corresponding supremum values of Beale's measure of nonlinearity are respectively $B = 1.2294$, 1.5693, 1.5881, 1.5918, 1.5897, 1.5862, and 1.5828 after applying (16.10). It is therefore easy to get a more accurate confidence region with (16.11), than with $B = 1$.

16.4   DOSE EXTRAPOLATION DESIGNS

Early estimates of a virtually safe dose in carcinogenic risk assessment were based on confidence intervals using the class of multistage models of carcinogenesis (see Wosniok *et al.*, 1999). The essential differences between the candidate models heavily influence the extrapolation towards zero. The dose-response problem is also discussed in Chapter 13 of this volume.

Let us recall the tolerance distribution model of Section 16.2.1 above. Let X be the individual tolerance dose considered as a random variable, then the function $F(x) = P(X \le x)$, with x being the dose level administered, is of practical use. $F(\cdot)$ can be considered as a cumulative distribution function.

16.4.1   The Weibull model

A typical model in life testing is the Weibull model, which also belongs to the class of multistage models. It is of the form

$$F(x) = 1 - \exp(-\theta x^s), \tag{16.18}$$

where s is a shape parameter. If $s > 1$ the model is sublinear, if $s < 1$ it is supralinear, and if $s = 1$ the model coincides with the so-called one-hit model, the exponential. The one-hit model postulates that cancer is the result of a single cell, while the Weibull model introduces the shape parameter and has a different hazard function.

Suppose that we want to estimate the $L_p, p \in (0, 1)$, quantile for the Weibull model. This is equivalent to solving the equation $R(x) = F(x) - p = 0$. Assume that only observations of $y_i = R(x_i) + e_i$, $i = l_1, \ldots, n$, are available, with e_i being the error term with mean zero and variance σ^2.

Proposition 16.7   For the Weibull model the sequence of the $100p$ percentiles $L_{p,n}$

$$L_{p,n+1} = L_{p,n} - \left(n\theta(1-p)L_p^{s-1}\right)^{-1}(y_n - p), \qquad n = 1, 2, 3, \ldots, \tag{16.19}$$

converge (in mean square) to the real pth percentile point L_p and this design minimizes the variance, that is to say, is a D-optimal design.

Example 16.7   Simulation study for a sequential approach (Kitsos, 1999). The approach outlined above has been adopted for constructing an optimal sequential design for the calculation of percentiles in a simulation study. Binary response data $y_i = 1$ or 0, $i = 1, 2, \ldots, n$, were generated for the one-hit model. $\theta = 3.18$ was chosen as a true value of θ. For this model the D-optimum design point is $x = 1.59/\theta$. The simulation study was based on $N = 1000$ simulations and the following two strategies were considered:

(i) The case where the initial values were 'far' from the unknown true value (2.156 or 7.15). The iterative scheme devoting one observation per stage is the fully sequential design which is at the same time the stochastic approximation scheme. The results of the simulation study provide evidence that the sequence of estimates behaves very close to normal distribution, as the values of skewness and kurtosis are close to those of the normal distribution. Also, the calculated MSE(θ) is 'small' and the average estimated value of the unknown parameter is very close to the true value.

(ii) The iterative scheme (16.19) for 'small' values of p, near to zero, yields estimates of L_p, which have a minimum variance, as the iterative scheme provides D-optimal estimates, even with a small number of observations. The method works well also as far as the percentile estimates are concerned, providing estimates with small mean square error, and average values of the unknown percentile very close to the true one.

16.5 DISCUSSION

This chapter has discussed problems of optimally designing bioassays when the underlying mechanism to be modeled is nonlinear model, with special emphasis on the nonlinear Michaelis–Menten kinetic model which is still widely used in toxicology and in risk assessment applications. The optimal design approach can be adopted to resolve design problems with this kinetic. Even if it is difficult to evaluate the optimal design points in the laboratory, it is better to perform a nearly optimal design than just an experiment with no planning.

Various examples were presented where an optimal design approach can be adopted. The procedure applied above for the analysis of the MM model may serve as an example of how to proceed in similar situations. An important extension of the nonlinear MM model is the so-called Hill model,

$$u = \frac{V_{max} C_S^n}{K_M^n + C_S^n},$$

which has found much interest among risk assessors when enzyme concentrations are considered (see Toyoshiba *et al.*, 2002). Compared to the standard MM model (16.5), this model contains a third model parameter, the so-called Hill coefficient n, which has an intrinsic role in the shape of the concentration response curve. Future work is needed to defined optimal designs for the estimation all three parameters of this nonlinear kinetic.

ACKNOWLEDGEMENTS

Firstly, I would like to thank the NATO CCMS for the generous fellowship in pilot studies under the leadership of Prof. G. Zapponi (Rome) which introduced me to risk assessment. Secondly, I am grateful to the German Cancer Research Center (Heidelberg) for a travel grant to collaborate with Dr. Lutz Edler on cancer risk assessment.

PART V

SPECIFIC MODELING APPROACHES FOR HEALTH RISK ASSESSMENT

Introductory remarks

Lutz Edler and Christos P. Kitsos

The Belgian astronomer L. A. J. Quetelet (1796–1874) stated that all the mental and physical characteristics of human beings follow a consistent frequency distribution, the same distribution that Carl Friedrich Gauss (1777–1855) had already postulated from a completely different astronomical study. The curve, with its symmetrical shape, shows deviations from a central line, and therefore it often illustrates the errors of exact measurements. Quetelet's measurements of human characteristics included height, limb size, weight, head size and intelligence. It was about that time that the idea of 'a model' of human activities and characteristics was introduced. A pioneer of modeling was the English economist Thomas Malthus (1766–1834), who in 1798 had published his book on *An Assay on the Principle of Population* and who eventually proved that population growth follows an exponential model, thereby influencing Charles Darwin (1809–1892) and his theory of evolution. Since these times statistics has impacted the development of biology. The following three chapters are devoted to the link between statistical modeling and risk assessment.

In an optimal experiment, the parameters of interest are estimated as well as possible under the chosen optimality criterion and with a limited number of observations. Optimal experimental design as discussed in Chapter 16 provides the statistical framework for this estimation. The question of the best optimal

Recent Advances in Quantitative Methods in Cancer and Human Health Risk Assessment
Edited by L. Edler and C. Kitsos © 2005 John Wiley & Sons, Ltd

statistical design applies in particular when risks originating from chemical mixtures have to be evaluated. Mixtures of chemicals and their risk assessment have become extreme important since it is obvious that humans are always exposed to mixtures of hazardous substances and not to single agents, as holds for animals in the artificial set-up of a bioassay. The elaboration of designs for combining chemical agents is an urgent and extremely difficult task. Chapters 17 and 18 work with appropriate designs and present methods for assessing cumulative risks. It is obvious that more research efforts must be devoted to this topic in the future.

Parametric methods for survival data have played a minor role in medical applications although they were the first methods developed for the analysis of survival data. The Weibull, the extreme value and Gompertz distributions (Pike, 1966) were distributional models applied to animal assay data for hazard identification and hazard characterization. Lack of fit to an increasing number of bioassay data sets and weaknesses of biological motivations for a specific class of distributions for the time-to-tumor have prevented their use. However, parametric methods were more successfully used for complex stochastic modeling of failure time data. For example, according to Yakovlev and Tsodikov (1996), parametric models have the advantage of allowing the natural interpretation of parameters when having a biological meaning, the ability to predict risk forward in time, the possibility of estimation of the survivor fraction, the provision of the basis for the design of surveillance strategies, and the prevention of nonidentifiability. These authors also show how the risk of tumor recurrence (tumor latency) either spontaneously occurring, occurring under treatment or manifesting itself as novel tumor can be modeled through parametric stochastic models. They use the generic survival model $S(t) = \exp(-\int_0^t h(x)F(t-x)dx$, where h denotes the rate of formation of lesions and F the rate of their progression. This model has laid the basis for modeling the tumor size at detection assuming that a tumor becomes detectable when it attains a threshold size or a critical number of cells; see Chapter 11 in Part III as well as chapter 19 in this part, where the focus is on the natural history of breast cancer. This chapter in a sense bridges the modeling chapters and the case study chapters of our text, since besides its theoretical deduction it reports applications using data from the National Cancer Institute's Surveillance Epidemiology and End Results (SEER) program.

CHAPTER 17

Cancer Risk Assessment for Mixtures

Christos P. Kitsos

Technological Educational Institute of Athens

Lutz Edler

German Cancer Research Center

17.1 INTRODUCTION

Mixtures of chemicals are ubiquitous in the environment – in the air we breathe, in the food we eat, in the water we drink. Therefore, in our natural environment we are exposed to a large number of potentially hazardous agents. Exposure to a chemical mixture changes in terms of composition and intensity during a lifetime, and the hazardous potential of the mixture may also strongly depend on its components. Since exposure to mixtures is the rule rather than the exception any realistic risk assessment of humans has to address exposure to mixtures. Henschler *et al.* (1996) said that 'The potential adverse effects of realistic exposure levels to mixtures of chemicals should be a primary research topic of toxicologists for the near future, focusing on mechanisms of action and development of approaches to assess interaction data'. Considerable research effort has been devoted to mixture risk assessment including the need to develop efficient designs of studies, to analyze the data sufficiently and to interpret the results correctly (El-Masri *et al.*, 1997).

Statistical analysis methods need to be extended for a realistic analysis of human cancer and health risk due to exposure of mixtures. Obviously, risk characterization for a mixture is much more complicated than for a single chemical investigated under a standard experimentation regime and analysed using a standard statistical approach. This is because chemical mixtures add more and more complex

Recent Advances in Quantitative Methods in Cancer and Human Health Risk Assessment
Edited by L. Edler and C. Kitsos   © 2005 John Wiley & Sons, Ltd

information into a statistical analysis model. However, it is also clear that the mixture problem has to be distinguished from the problem of the best use of covariate information in a bioassay, as has been discussed by Kitsos (1998). The problem of mixtures in bioassays has attracted interest since the nineteenth century. In this chapter we will present the main aspects of the mixture theory for risk assessment. We try to bridge the biological point of view with the statistical approach.

The toxicological analysis of chemical mixtures and mixture bioassays has been investigated by many authors; see Hodgson and Levi (1987), Mumtaz *et al.* (1993), Mauderly (1993), Yang (1994a, 1994b) and World Health Organization (1987). The examination of multiple target organs was reported by Simmons (1995), while Yang and Rauckman (1987) provided tables for chemical mixtures and the dosages for toxicity studies. Groten *et al.* (1991) focused on oral toxicity of cadmium in rats. The chemical mixture of groundwater contaminants was discussed by R.S.H. Yang *et al.* (1989), while Dirven *et al.* (1990) studied effects in the liver and the serum of rats, as did Cassee *et al.* (1996) for the effect of mixtures of formaldehyde, acrolein and acetylaldehyde.

Unfortunately, there exist a variety of definitions and nomenclatures in the biological and statistical literature concerning not only mixture exposure and mixture effects. It is one aim of this work to introduce a uniform terminology, in order to improve communications between the statistical and biological lines of thought for a more efficient use for risk assessment.

Mumtaz *et al.* (1993) tried to resolve parts of the complexity of the mixture problem by structuring it and putting three aspects into the focus of research:

1. Which hazards result from a long-term and low-dose exposure through mixtures?

2. Which specific hazard-related toxicological endpoints can be assessed quantitatively?

3. Do there exist interactions between the components of the mixture, and how do they affect low-dose extrapolation?

Another approach to resolving the complexity of mixtures tried to first classify the combined effects of different agents and then to find the most suitable analysis method. This line of thinking started with the ground-breaking work on effect amplification and effect inhibition of Frei (1913) and Loewe (1928), two researchers who can be credited with the introduction of the notion of synergism and antagonism into the evaluation of mixtures. Another more instrumentally oriented line of thought was introduced later by the notion of additive and sub- or superadditive effects. This chapter aims to clarify the meaning and the definition of these modes of combined action of components of a mixture, and we will introduce experimental design methods which may be helpful to distinguish between modes of action.

We are aware of other approaches which classify mixture effects using pharmacological, chemical or physical properties of the components to take competition, cooperation, inhibition or induction of biological processes into account. These will not be addressed in this chapter. We should also mention that some pragmatic propositions have been made for mixture risk assessment: testing only a limited number of components, called top-ten testing, as proposed by Feron *et al.* (1997). It was also proposed to characterize the single components and derive from them the properties of the mixture in stepping from the margin to the kernel. These approaches may be very helpful in practical situations of risk assessment in case studies for the solution of an environmental risk problem. However, in their present formulation they seem too *ad hoc* to be useful in a formal quantitative methodology.

17.2 BASIC PRINCIPLES

A simple mixture may in practice consist of a very large number of very different chemicals, as in the case of cigarette smoke and automobile exhaust fumes. Practical analyses of chemical mixtures consider usually no more than 10 chemicals, but even then it becomes very difficult to separate the individual from the combined effects. An analysis of the interactions of individual effects is a tedious procedure and involves the qualitative and quantitative interplay of the chemicals involved. Even if sound and substantial knowledge from available chemical and biological experiments is available, not all important interactions may be sufficiently explored and the addition of one newly synthesized chemical may substantially change the quality and quantity of the response. A typical example is the composition of atmosphere, its changes due to the industrial development and the resulting effects.

When investigating the action of mixtures one has to combine two views. One view is concerned with the mode of action of the chemicals of the mixture, where one can distinguish between (a) the same mode of action and (b) different modes of action. Another view is concerned with effects induced in the exposed individual (animal or human), where one can distinguish between effects on the (i) the same target organs and (ii) different target organs.

Two basic conceptual lines of thought have been established in the scientific literature: that of *synergism and antagonism* and that of *potentiation*. If toxicity is greater than would be expected from the toxicities of the compounds administrated separately, one speaks usually of synergism; if it is less than expected, one speaks of antagonism. If the components in the mixture show qualitatively different toxicity when administered together than when administered alone, one speaks of potentiation, for example when one substance has an effect only in the presence of another.

Biostatistical theory has been concerned with the combination of experimental factors for a long time, since R.A. Fisher introduced for agricultural bioassays the term interaction in order to deal appropriately with the combination effects of two or more than two components. This approach does not however, fully address the complex problem of chemical mixtures outlined above and therefore other considerations are needed to adopt a uniform statistical methodology for the risk assessment of mixtures. Mumtaz *et al.* (1993) define toxicological interaction as a phenomenon 'in which exposure to two or more chemicals results in a qualitatively or quantitatively altered biological response relative to that predicted from the action of a single chemical', whereas Berenbaum (1977) pragmatically states that interaction is present if the observed effect in the mixture differs from what would be expected from the effects known from the components. In the following we will discuss these basic principles of joint action from the statistical modeling perspective, restricting ourselves to two components for simplicity of presentation.

17.2.1 Synergism

Discussions on the notion of synergism go back to the work of Fraser (1872); see the important work of Berenbaum (1977, 1981, 1985, 1990) for an excellent analysis of the problem. The combined action of two components S_1 and S_2 administered at doses (z_1, z_2) can be described by a dose-response surface $F(z_1, z_2)$ in a plane spanned by the two doses $z_1 \geq 0, z_2 \geq 0$. Notice that each of the two components can then be described alone by its own dose-response function $f_1(d) = F(d, 0)$ and $f_2(d) = F(0, d)$. Loewe and Muischnek (1926) introduced isoboles (from the Greek *bole*, meaning 'amplitude') in order to classify the surface F by so-called isobolograms. These are simply projections I_c of curves of the same effect on the surface onto the dose space, the non-negative plane $z_1 \geq 0, z_2 \geq 0$:

$$I_c = \{(z_1, z_2) : F(z_1, z_2) = c\}.$$

Isoboles hitting one of the axes – corresponding to a zero dose value for one component – define special effect levels, namely effect-equivalent single doses of component S_1 or S_2, respectively:

$$
\begin{aligned}
z_1^* &= f_1^{-1}(F(z_1, z_2)), \\
z_2^* &= f_2^{-1}(F(z_1, z_2)).
\end{aligned}
\tag{17.1}
$$

A biological interaction between two components takes place if the effect of one component changes – that is, is enhanced or inhibited – in the presence of the other. For a better understanding of those effect changes it is helpful to consider first a fixed combination of two doses (z_1, z_2) and when component S_2 acts on the effect of component S_1. This results in a local and asymmetrical definition of synergism: we say that the action of S_2 on S_1 in (z_1, z_2) is

$$
\begin{aligned}
synergistic \quad & \text{if } F(z_1, 0) < F(z_1, z_2), & (17.2a) \\
inert \quad & \text{if } F(z_1, 0) = F(z_1, z_2), & (17.2b) \\
antagonistic \quad & \text{if } F(z_1, 0) > F(z_1, z_2); & (17.2c)
\end{aligned}
$$

or equivalently

$$
\frac{z_1}{f_1^{-1}(F(z_1, z_2))}
\begin{cases}
< 1 \Leftrightarrow \text{synergistic,} \\
= 1 \Leftrightarrow \text{inert,} \\
> 1 \Leftrightarrow \text{antagonistic.}
\end{cases}
$$

Similarly, one defines local action of S_1 on S_2. The isoboles method has been extensively discussed by Cassee *et al.* (1998) in a review paper, which also provides an example of a 4-week oral toxicity study of the combination of different and well-known chemicals in rats. Yang and Rauckman (1987) considered a number of chemicals frequently detected in groundwater contaminants.

The definition of local synergism, inertism or antagonism can be extended to a global one if one postulates relationship (17.2) to hold for all dose combinations $z_1 \geq 0, z_2 \geq 0$. Notice, however, that a global occurrence of one of the three mechanisms over the entire dose space is very rare. In reality, the dose space would contain regions of different types of action. Notice also that so far the asymmetry of the action of S_2 on S_1 in (17.2) still prevails. More important than extending the definition of local synergism to a global synergism is to characterize a one of those actions symmetrically with respect to the two components S_1 and S_2 by requiring the respective equation (17.2a)–(17.2c) to hold both for S_2 on S_1 and for S_1 on S_2. Gobal symmetric action occurs if the respective equations of type (17.2a)–(17.2c) hold for all dose combinations $z_1 \geq 0, z_2 \geq 0$. Therefore two components exhibit global (symmetric) synergistic action if

$$\max[F(z_1, 0), F(0, z_2)] < F(z_1, z_2), \qquad \text{for all } z_1 \geq 0, z_2 \geq 0.$$

Notice that this definition can be generalized to more than two components immediately for synergistic action, but not for inertism or antagonism. As a consequence, an isobole which at one point (z_1, z_2) shows local (symmetric) synergism always has regions with other points (z_1', z_2') where there is local asymmetrical antagonism or synergism. This exhibits a logical difficulty of the definition of synergism and antagonisms (and inertism) in a dose region which is either not realized or which elicits attempts to find more appropriate definitions (see Unkelbach and Wolf, 1984, 1985). This may be one reason for the confused used of the term synergism in toxicology as was described by Berenbaum (1977): 'Synergy, however, is a topic on which confusion reigns. The relevant pharmacological literature is often obscure (some papers, indeed, are models of incomprehensibility) and is profusely littered with technical terms that are not always clearly defined. Several different terms are used to describe the same phenomenon and the same term means different things to different authors.' In practice, one therefore tends to rely more on a distinction between additive and non-additive action, than on synergism and antagonisms. Unfortunately, there has also been confusion over synergism and additivity. We will therefore define additivity explicitly in the next subsection.

17.2.2   Additivity

The notion of additivity is based on the observation that related chemical substances should be similar in their effects. Similar action of two substances is compared with the (self-)similar action of two samples obtained when one substance is subdivided into two aliquots and the combined effect of the two aliquots, at different doses, is examined (self-similarity). Notice that additivity in this sense automatically assumes the presence of global symmetric synergistic action of the two aliquots in the sense defined above. It is highly illuminating to investigate additivity for the case where one examines one substance as it is given and the other as a thinned (or thickened) version of that substance. Assume, for example, that component S_1 is identical to S_2 except that it is thinned by a factor f, $f < 1$ ($f > 1$ would correspond to thickening). One can then replace the dose z_1 of S_1 by an appropriate dose z_2 of S_2 namely fz_2, which has the same effect as dose z_1. This equivalence can be expressed in a formula

$$z_1(S_1) \leftrightarrow fz_2(S_2),$$

or

$$\frac{1}{f}z_1(S_1) \leftrightarrow z_2(S_2).$$

The effect of the combination (z_1, z_2) of S_1 and S_2 is therefore identical to that of $fz_1 + z_2$ of S_2, or $z_1 + (1/f)z_2$ of S_1; see Unkelbach and Wolf (1985). The factor f is called the relative potency of S_1 to S_2 and $\rho = 1/f$ is called the relative potency of S_2 to S_1. Notice the isobole through (z_1, z_2) hits then the single-dose axes of S_1 and S_2 at $(z_1^*, 0)$ and $(0, z_2^*)$, where

$$z_1^* = [z_1 + \frac{1}{f}z_2] = [z_1 + \rho z_2],$$

$$z_2^* = [f \cdot z_1 + z_2]$$

are the single doses of identical effect. This effect is then given as $F(z_1, z_2)$, i.e. the effect size at the combination dose (z_1, z_2). The concept of self-similarity and thinning was used to define additivity/non-additivity of different components S_1 and S_2. The combined effect of two components S_1 and S_2 $F(z_1, z_2)$ in (z_1, z_2) is

$$
\begin{aligned}
&\text{superadditive,} &&\text{if} \\
&\text{additive,} &&\text{if} && \frac{z_1}{z_1^*} + \frac{z_2}{z_2^*} = \frac{z_1}{f_1^{-1}(F(z_1,z_2))} + \frac{z_2}{f_2^{-1}(F(z_1,z_2))} &&\begin{cases} < 1, \\ = 1, \\ > 1, \end{cases} \\
&\text{subadditive,} &&\text{if}
\end{aligned}
$$

$$\text{(17.3)}$$

when z_i^* is defined by (17.1). The marginal points $(z_1^*, 0)$ and $(0, z_2^*)$ corresponding to the effect $F(z_1, z_2)$ in (z_1, z_2) then span a straight line which separates the region of super- and subadditive effects (Figure 17.1). In general, M components are additive in $(z_1, \ldots, z_M)$ if

$$\sum_{i=1}^{M} \frac{z_i}{z_i^*} = \frac{z_1}{z_1^*} + \frac{z_2}{z_2^*} + \cdots = 1.$$

If (17.3) holds for all doses (z_1, z_2) one speaks of global additivity. All isoboles are then straight lines with positive intercept. Koshinsky and Khachatourians (1992a,

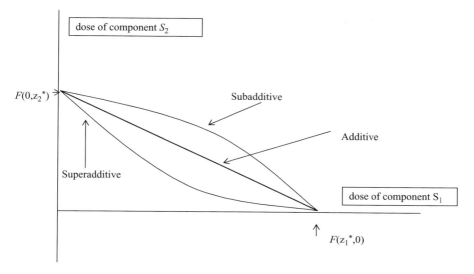

Figure 17.1 Isobols of additive effects. The straight line connects dose points of same effect and separates regions of super- and subadditivity.

1992b) discuss and apply the three notions of synergism, additivity and antagonism for bioassay data, while Svendsgaard and Hertzberg (1994) discuss the statistical methods relative to these fundamental ideas. We would like to emphasize again that synergy (as defined above) is not equivalent to an additive response; see Hastie and Tibshirani (1984) for details.

17.2.3 Modeling Additivity

Examination of additivity is performed in two steps. At first one define a parametric additive dose-response model, e.g., a probit model $F(z_1, z_2) = \Phi\left(\frac{1}{\sigma}\ln(z_1 e^{-\mu_1} + z_2 e^{-\mu_2})\right)$. Then one is going to examine $z_1/z_1^* + z_2/z_2^*$ for each dose combination (z_1, z_2) in the dose-response region. Gennings and Carter (1995) describe a mixture model based on a number of c solitary experiments performed on the individual components and one experiment performed on the combination and they apply therefore a generalized linear model.

A graphical method first described by Loewe (1953) has been widely used for analyzing mixture effects (Steel and Peckham, 1979; Cassee et al., 1998). One constructs pointwise a region of additivity around the isobole of a fixed effect using the dose-response curves of the single components. Monotone envelopes are then constructed from a deterministic variation principle which defines a region of tolerable deviation from additivity at which observed effects are compared (Edler, 1999).

17.2.4 Further concepts

The effect of the combination of S_1 and S_2 at doses (z_1, z_2) is called independent if

$$1 - F(z_1, z_2) = [1 - f_1(z_1)] \cdot [(1 - f_2(z_2)],$$

otherwise superindependent (if $<$ holds) or subindependent (if $>$ holds). The type of independent effects is equivalent to multiplicativity of effect rates. There is no direct relationship between this type of effect and additive effects. See the early work of Plackett and Hewlett (1948), as well as Wahrendorf et $al.$ (1980) and Elashoff et $al.$ (1987).

Two one-dimensional dose-response curves $f_i(d), i = 1, 2$, are called similar if they are related to each other such that one component is a thinning of the other. Then there exist two constants ρ_k , $k = 1, 2$, such that $f_1(\rho_1 d) = f_2(\rho_2 d)$ for all $d > 0$. The two components are called simple similar if an equivalent amount of both components generates the same effect. Simple similarity is equivalent to similarity and global additivity (see Unkelbach and Wolf, 1985, chapter 4.3.2). In the case of simple similar action the isoboles are straight lines with positive intercept. Statistical tests for similarity have been proposed by Giltinan et $al.$ (1988) and a generalized dose additive model for similar action has been given in Chen et $al.$ (1989).

Simple similar action has an important application in carcinogenic risk assessment when the combined exposure to strongly related compounds is investigated. Occupational exposure to polychlorinated dibenzo-p-dioxines (PCDDs), furanes (PCDFs) and biphenyls (PCBs) is such an example of exposure to components for which a simple similar action has been proposed. The components show extremely different toxic potency, from the extreme toxicity of the 2,3,7,8-tetrachlorodibenzo-p-dioxin (TCDD) to almost no toxicity of other congeners (Jung and Konietzko, 1994). So-called $toxicity$ $equivalent$ $factors$ (TEFs) were introduced to summarize combined exposure and to obtain a combined dose metric for the risk assessment of dioxins and furans (Van den Berg et $al.$,1998). The biological basis for a joint mechanism of action is the binding of all dioxins and furans at the Ah-receptor which initializes the subsequent cascade of toxicodynamic effects. Assuming a simple similar action of the combination effect of doses z_i, the individual components are combined to a combination dose CD as the weighted sum of the z_i and the factors TEF_i

$$CD = \sum_{i=1}^{K} TEF_i z_i;$$

see Portier et $al.$ (1999). It should be observed that the risk assessment of dioxins and furans depends on the assumption of simple similar action.

17.2.5 The additive model reconsidered

Let $P(z_i)$ denote the probability of a toxic response to concentration z_i of toxicant S_i such that $P(z_i) = F_i(z_i)$, for some given 'smooth' monotonic functions $F_i(i = 1, 2)$.

If we suppose that the one toxicant is a dilution of the other, then $z_1 = \rho z_2$, with ρ being the relative potency of toxicant 2 to toxicant 1. Then the joint probability of a toxic response to the combination of z_1 and z_2, assuming *concentration additivity*, can be evaluated as

$$P(z_1, z_2) = F_1(z_1 + \rho z_2) = F_2(z_1/\rho + z_2).$$

Now let z to be a mixture of the two chemical toxicants S_1 and S_2 in proportions π_1, and π_2, respectively; then the joint probability is

$$P(z_1, z_2) = F_1[(\pi_1 + \rho \pi_2)z] = F_2[\pi_1/\rho + \pi_2)z].$$

Moreover, the probability of a joint toxic response to the combination S_1 and S_2, assuming *response additivity*, is

$$\begin{aligned}
P(z_1, z_2) &= P(z_1) + [1 - P(z_1)]P(z_2) \\
&= P(z_2) + [1 - P(z_2)]P(z_1) \\
&= P(z_1) + P(z_2) - P(z_1)P(z_2) \\
&= F_1(x_1) + F_2(x_2) - F_1(x_1)F_2(x_2).
\end{aligned}$$

That is, the response to the second toxicant over and above that of the first is simply an added effect based on the proportion not responding to the first toxicant, and vice versa. This joint probability represents the union of two statistically independent events. Now the joint response for response additivity may be predicted from the regressions of the response on z_i by adopting scale-parameter models

$$P(z_1, z_2) = F_1(a + b_1 z_1) + F_2(a + b_2 z_2) - F_1(a + b_1 z_1)F_2(a + b_2 z_2).$$

The evaluation of a group of m chemicals, that is, evaluating $F(z_1, z_2, \ldots, z_m)$ is considered in Chapter 18 of this volume.

Example Consider the one-hit model of carcinogenesis with

$$P(z_1) = F_1(z_1) = 1 - \exp[-\vartheta_1 z_1],$$
$$P(z_2) = F_2(z_2) = 1 - \exp[-\vartheta_2 z_2].$$

In this case the concentration addition and response addition models are statistically indistinguishable. In practice, this means that their predicted joint responses are identical. Using a double logarithmic transformation, one obtains parallel lines with slope equal to 1. This enables the estimation of the parameters ϑ_1, ϑ_2 and thus the relative potency, $\rho = \vartheta_2/\vartheta_1$. Thus, under an assumed concentration-additive joint response,

$$\begin{aligned}
P(z_1, z_2) = F_1(z_1, z_2) &= 1 - \exp[-\vartheta_1(z_1 + \rho z_2)] \\
&= 1 - \exp[-\vartheta_1(x_1 + \vartheta_2/\vartheta_1 z_2)] \\
&= 1 - \exp[-(\vartheta_1 z_1 + \vartheta_2 z_2)].
\end{aligned}$$

Assuming a response-additive joint response, one obtains

$$
\begin{aligned}
P(z_1, z_2) &= F_1(z_1) + F_2(z_2) - F_1(z_1)F_2(z_2) \\
&= 1 - \exp[-\vartheta_1 z_1] + 1 - \exp[-\vartheta_2 z_2] - 1 + \exp[-\vartheta_1 z_1] + \exp[-\vartheta_2 z_2] \\
&\quad - \exp[-\vartheta_1 z_1]\exp[-\vartheta_2 z_2] \\
&= 1 - \exp[-(\vartheta_1 z_1 + \vartheta_2 z_2)].
\end{aligned}
$$

Now consider the case $f_1(z_1) = F(z_1, 0)$ and $f_2(z_2) = F(0, z_2)$ as already defined. The question is how we can evaluate $f_1(z_1)$ and $f_2(z_2)$ for given dose levels z_1 and z_2. Kelly and Rice (1990) suggested applying the theory of splines, particularly B-splines, working with one of the most famous bioassay data sets, namely that of Bliss (1939) on two series of trials on house flies sprayed with alcoholic solutions of rotenone, pyrethrins and a mixture of the two.

17.2.6 Probabilistic point of view

The National Research Council (1980) defined toxicological interaction, as a situation in which exposure to two or more chemicals results in a qualitatively or quantitatively altered biological response relative to that predicted from the actions of a single chemical. Consider two chemical components A and B in a mixture and denote by P_A, P_B and P_{AB} the probability of toxicity of A, B, and A or B (denoted as the union $A \cup B$), respectively. When there is no correlation between A and B the relation $P_{A \cup B} = P_A + P_B - P_A P_B$ holds. If $P_{A \cup B} = P_A + P_B$ a negative correlation holds; if $P_{A \cup B} = P_A$ or $P_{A \cup B} = P_B$ a strictly positive correlation holds. See also Section 17.4.

17.3   DESIGN OF MIXTURE EXPERIMENTS

An obvious problem with the investigation of mixtures is the overwhelming number of possible combinations to be examined as the number of chemicals to be tested for carcinogenicity increases. With several tens of thousands compounds, for example, on hazardous waste disposal sites, risk assessment is such a complex and difficult task that no more perfect approaches and protocols exist (Yang and Rauckman, 1987; R.S.H. Yang et al., 1989). Response surface methods and experimental design analysis have been mentioned by various authors, among them Cassee et al. (1998), El-Masri et al. (1997) and Gennings (1995). Mixture designs have been applied to food technology; see the early work of Hare (1974). Wahrendorf et al. (1981) proposed an optimal design to examine the effect of two carcinogens. The comparison of in vitro and in vivo studies is considered by Terse et al. (1993), and guidelines for the health risk assessment of chemical mixtures can be found in US EPA (1986a). Although the need for statistical support has been clearly expressed, no appropriate statistical software exists to assist the experimenter in the planning of mixture experiments. The problem is obvious when one looks at the number of possible combinations of compounds.

If all combinations of the components of a mixture are to be studied at different dose levels the number of experimental combination groups is impractically large. For a mixture consisting of 4, 5 or 6 chemicals one has to test $2^4 - 1 = 15$, $2^5 - 1 = 31$, $2^6 - 1 = 63$ treatment groups, respectively, even if there is only one dose group and a control group. If three chemicals are involved in a mixture, each to be tested at five different dose levels (a control and four non-zero dose levels), 125 treatment groups result, and if only five animals are assigned to each treatment group a total of 625 animals are needed. An experiment of this size would only be carried out in exceptional circumstances because of restrictions not only on laboratory space and finances, but also on research time. Furthermore, if one were to perform experiments with such a large number of groups, biases and experimental fallacies would increase due to large experimentation time and many more persons working for this bioassay. Thinking of a 25-chemical mixture with $2^{25} - 1 = 33\,554\,431$ combinations will make this handicap obvious. A systematic toxicity testing using the NTP subchronic study protocol in only one species would cost more than \$3 trillion (R.S.H. Yang *et al.*, 1989). Therefore, such studies are impossible from an economical, practical or even ethical point of view, and an appropriate design theory is needed.

Different types of optimal experimental designs have been proposed in the statistical literature to study the problem of mixtures. We close this chapter with an overview of these designs.

17.3.1 The 2^k factorial design

For a full 2^k factorial experiment all combinations of the two levels of the k input variables are realized in the experiment. The experimental design region is therefore a hypercube. For the 2^2 factorial, one usually examines the two-variable linear regression model

$$\eta = \beta_0 + \beta_1 x_1 + \beta_2 x_2 + \beta_{12} x_1 x_2, \tag{17.4}$$

where x_1 is the dose of chemical S_1 and x_2 is the dose of chemical S_2. The constant parameter β_0 is the unknown intercept and represents the overall mean response. β_1 is the slope parameter associated with chemical S_1, and β_2 is the slope parameter associated with chemical S_2. The term β_{12} is an unknown parameter associated with the interaction between chemicals S_1 and S_2, the most important term for analyzing mixtures. If $\beta_{12} = 0$ the model is called additive. For $\beta_{12} > 0$, a synergism can be claimed between chemical S_1 and chemical S_2, while for $\beta_{12} < 0$, an antagonism is claimed (see Figure 17.2).

Gennings (1995) analyzed a 2^5 experimental design, known as the '5 PAH mixture study', using the additive model. A 5^3 experimental design was used by Narotsky *et al.* (1995) to examine the toxicity of the mixture of trichloroethylene, di(2-ethylhexyl) phthalate and heptachlor. They were able to evaluate the two-way and three-way interactions in their model for synergism or antagonism of the agents. Factorial experiment designs have also been used in combination toxicity studies by Groten *et al.* (1996).

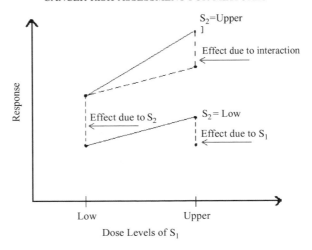

Figure 17.2 Parallel dose-response curves indicate additivity. Non-parallel curves indicate the presence of an interaction.

17.3.2 2^{k-q} fractional factorial experiment

A full factorial experiment using k input variables needs a very large number of experimental runs even in the case of a moderate value of k, therefore a proportion 2^{-q} of the 2^k experiments is needed and a 2^{k-q} fractional design is created. The fractional factorial confuses the higher-order effects with the main effects of interest. If it is assumed that the main effects are small enough, so that they can be ignored, this could become a useful design; see Haaland and O'Connell (1995) and Bisgaard (1994).

17.3.3 Rotatable designs

A response surface design is called rotatable when the standardized variance function $\frac{N}{\sigma^2} \mathrm{Var}(\hat{y}(x))$, where $\hat{y}(x)$ denotes the fitted response, is only a function of the distance of a design point from the design origin. The method has so far been applied mainly in industrial experiments; see Box and Draper (1987).

17.3.4 q-component mixture model: response surface analysis

Consider next a mixture experiment in which q factors or input variables generate the mixture. Denote the proportion of the ith component by x_i and assume

$$x_i \geq 0, \qquad i = 1, 2, \ldots, q,$$

$$\sum_{i=1}^{q} x_i = x_1 + x_2 + \cdots + x_q = 1.$$

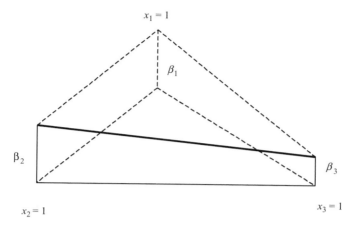

Figure 17.3 First-degree planar surface above the three-component triangle.

The input x_i represents the non-negative fractions of the mixture. Response surface methods provide are a convenient statistical relationship between the doses of each component and the response variable; see El- Masri *et al.*, (1997) and Cassee *et al.* (1998). We briefly describe this method in Figures 17.3–17.5. It is assumed that there exists a link function of the form $\varphi(x_1, \ldots, x_q)$ between the variables involved, with φ being a smooth function. The expected response is then given by

$$E(y) = \eta = \varphi(x_1, x_2, \ldots, x_q);$$

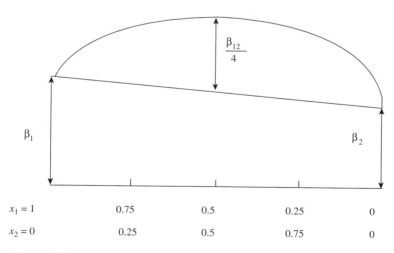

Figure 17.4 Quadratic blending with $\beta_{ij} > 0$, see model equation (17.5).

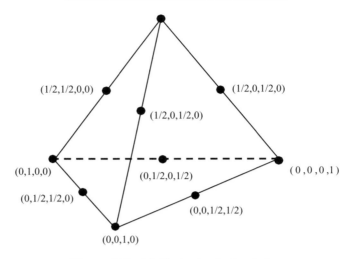

Figure 17.5 $\{4, 2\}$ simplex lattice design.

$\varphi(x_1, x_2, \ldots, x_q)$ should preferably be a low-degree polynomial. For n observations, the statistical model is

$$y_i = \eta_i + \varepsilon_i, \qquad 1 \leq i \leq n,$$

with additive experimental error term ε_i, uncorrelated and identically distributed with zero mean and common variance σ^2. The unknown model parameters are estimated using the least-squares method.

When $q = 2$ this reduces to a first-degree polynomial of the form

$$y_i = \beta_1 x_{1i} + \beta_2 x_{2i} + \varepsilon_i, \qquad i = 1, 2, \ldots, n.$$

Quadratic blending is illustrated in Figure 17.4. Notice that the quadratic term $\hat{\beta}_{12} x_1 x_2$ represents the excess response of the quadratic model over the linear model

$$E(y) = \beta_1 x_1 + \beta_2 x_2 + \beta_{12} x_1 x_2. \qquad (17.5)$$

Depending on the sign of β_{12}, the term $\beta_{12} x_1 x_2$ describes the interaction due to nonlinear blending. The linear term $\beta_1 x_1$ only contributes to the model when $x_1 > 0$; and the maximum contribution occurs at $x_1 = 1$, in which case the maximum effect contributed by x_1 is β_1 (see Figure 17.3). The quadratic term $\beta_1 x_1 x_2$ contributes to the model at every point in the simplex where $x_1 > 0$ and $x_2 > 0$. The maximum contribution occurs at the edge joining the vertices x_1 and x_2 at the point $x_1 = x_2 = 1/2$. The maximum contribution to the model is $\beta_{12}/4$ (see Figure 17.4).

For a three-compound mixture, the expected response is

$$\eta = \beta_0 + \beta_1 x_1 + \beta_2 x_2 + \beta_3 x_3 + \beta_{12} x_1 x_2 + \beta_{13} x_1 x_3 + \beta_{23} x_2 x_3 + \beta_{123} x_1 x_2 x_3,$$

where the last four terms display the interaction among the three different dose levels x_1, x_2, x_3. It is essential to realize that in mixture experiments the primary target may not be to investigate the main effects but to find out whether two or more chemicals can give rise to interaction effects.

17.3.5 Simplex lattice and simplex centroid designs

The simplex lattice design was introduced by Scheffé (1958) and describes a design where the experimental points are located at the vertices of a k-dimensional simplex. If q denotes the number of components and m the degree of the polynomial used to describe the mixture, this design is characterized by the parameter pair $\{q, m\}$. A trivial design is one where the points are positioned uniformly over the simplex factor space. The points in the simplex factor space take $m + 1$ equally spaced values $x_i = 0, 1/m, 2/m, \ldots, 1$ in the unit interval [0,1]. For example, if $q = 3$ the three components are the proportions $x_i = 0$, 1/2, and 1. If, furthermore, $m = 2$, the $\{3, 2\}$ simplex lattice consists of the six points on the boundary of the triangular factor space: $(1, 0, 0), (0, 1, 0), (0, 0, 1), (1/2, 1/2, 0)$, $(1/2, 0, 1/2), (0, 1/2, 1/2)$.

The three vertices (1,0,0), (0,1,0) and (0,0,1) represent individual components, while the points $(1/2, 1/2, 0), (1/2, 0, 1/2)$ and $(0, 1/2, 1/2)$ represent the binary blends or two-component mixtures. They are located at the midpoints of the three sides of the simplex, a triangle in this case. The $\{3, 2\}$, $\{3, 3\}$ and $\{4, 2\}$ simplex lattice designs are the most common designs; see Figure 17.5 for the $\{4, 2\}$ design. In general, the number of points in a $\{q, m\}$ simplex lattice design is given by

$$N = \frac{(q + m - 1)!}{m!(q - 1)!}.$$

The simplex centroid design was introduced by Scheffé (1963) and is characterized by one parameter q, which defines the number of design points, $2^q - 1$. These design points correspond to the q permutations of $(1, 0, 0, \ldots, 0)$, the $\binom{q}{2}$ permutations of $(1/2, 1/2, 0, 0, \ldots, 0)$, the $\binom{q}{3}$ permutations of $(1/3, 1/3, 1/3, 0, \ldots, 0), \ldots$, until the last centroid point $\left(\frac{1}{q}, \frac{1}{q}, \ldots, \frac{1}{q}\right)$. The design points are located at the centroid of the $(q - 1)$-dimensional simplex and at the centroids of all the lower-dimensional simplices contained within the $(q - 1)$-dimensional simplex. With $q = 3$ components one obtains a cubic polynomial.

17.3.6 Response trace plots

Response trace plots constitute a technique where the proportion of one single component is changed while the relative proportion of the other components are kept fixed (Cornell, 1990). Response trace plots have become useful when interactions between different drugs have to be interpreted; see Gershwin and Smith (1973). A typical example are toxic substances in drinking water; see Gennings *et al.* (1990). To study the combination of ethanol and chloralhydrate they adopted therefore the model (17.4) and estimated the response using the logit model for the proportion of animals responding. ED_{50} contours and the associated line of additivity were obtained.

17.4 DISCUSSION

An experiment is probably the most important way to collect information about a process under investigation. As we discussed above, a mixture experiment is a special type of experimental design, in which the factors are ingredients or compounds of the mixture and the response is a function of the proportion of each ingredient. Various methods have been discussed. For specific applications, the appropriate technique has to be chosen, mainly depending on the data. For example, the primary difference between standard regression polynomials and a mixture polynomial is that a special form of design is needed. The experimenter needs both biological and statistical points of view when a mixture problem is under consideration.

CHAPTER 18

Designs and Models for Mixtures: Assessing Cumulative Risk

James J. Chen and Ralph L. Kodell

National Center for Toxicological Research

Yi-Ju Chen

Pennsylvania State University

18.1 INTRODUCTION

Health risk assessment is used to derive acceptable exposure levels or to estimate the risks from exposure to chemicals that may exist as contaminants in food, drinking water, air, or the environment. Risk assessment is usually conducted on a single toxic agent through a single route of exposure. Although it is important to establish safe levels of exposure for humans for each toxic agent, people frequently are exposed to many chemicals simultaneously or in sequence by different routes. The exposures to multiple chemicals could cause unexpected cumulative potential effects through various media. The combined risk from exposures to multiple chemicals may be greater or less than what would be predicted from data on individual chemicals. Methods for risk assessment of chemical mixtures fall into two general categories: the whole-mixture approach and the component-based approach. The whole-mixture approach involves either direct evaluation of the mixture of concern or an assessment of the mixture of concern using data available on a sufficiently similar mixture. The mixture is evaluated as a single entity. The component-based approach considers the additive or interactive actions among the mixture components.

Recent Advances in Quantitative Methods in Cancer and Human Health Risk Assessment
Edited by L. Edler and C. Kitsos © 2005 John Wiley & Sons, Ltd

A principal objective in risk assessment of mixtures is to study the effects of individual component concentrations and their interactions in the mixture response. In the whole-mixture approach the desired data include the effects of the total mixture dose as well as of the component proportions. Experimental design is an important issue in studying mixtures. Traditional procedures for the assessment of joint toxicant effects fall into the general framework of response surface analysis using factorial designs. In a factorial experiment, the components represent different dose concentrations of the chemicals in the mixture. A complete factorial experiment can provide a great amount of toxicity information on the mixture as well as on the individual components. An important problem for implementing a complete factorial experiment is that it requires a great deal of resources. Moreover, a complete factorial experiment may not be useful in toxicological studies. For example, in animal carcinogenesis bioassays, if the maximum tolerated doses (MTDs) are used for each of the individual compounds, then the dosage administered at their respective MTDs together is likely to cause significant mortality. This chapter describes a design based on a proportion-concentration response model for mixture experiments.

The whole mixture of concern provides a direct approach to assessing the joint effects of mixtures. But in most practical situations, little information exists on the exposures to multiple chemicals. In the absence of whole-mixture toxicity testing data, risk assessments often are performed using the component-based approach assuming no interactions between the components in the mixture. The most widely used component-based methods are dose addition and response addition. Dose addition assumes that the chemicals act on similar biological systems and behave similarly in terms of the primary physiologic processes (absorption, metabolism, distribution, elimination), and elicit a common response (EPA, 2000b). Response addition assumes that the chemicals behave independently of one another, so that the body's response to the first chemical is the same whether or not the second chemical is present; in simplest terms, a response addition model is described by statistical independence.

One of the important problems in risk assessment of mixtures is how to cumulate the total risk from exposures to multiple chemicals with a common mechanism of toxicity (Mileson *et al.*, 1998; Wilkinson *et al.*, 2000). For example, organophosphate (OP) pesticides have been widely used in agriculture, home, garden, and veterinary practice. Many apparently share a common mechanism of cholinesterase inhibition and can cause similar symptoms. The US Environmental Protection Agency (US EPA, 2002) has been considering the cumulative risks of several common mechanism pesticides and other substrates. Toxicological assessment of exposures from combinations of cholinesterase inhibiting compounds has also been addressed by the UK Pesticides Safety Directorate (PSD, 1999).

The issue of a common mechanism of toxicity has recently been addressed by a working group of experts convened by the ILSI Risk Science Institute (Mileson *et al.*, 1998). The working group concluded that common mechanism determinations are difficult to establish because chemicals often exhibit a different spectrum of adverse effects in different organs and tissues. A feasible assumption for a common mechanism of toxicity is that the chemicals act on similar biological systems in eliciting a common effect and that the type of joint action which might occur will be additive (noninteractive) in nature (US EPA, 2002). Therefore, a dose addition model to estimate cumulative risk of multiple chemicals with a common mechanism of toxicity is reasonable (Wilkinson *et al.*, 2000; Code of Federal Regulations (CFR), 1998); it is consonant with US EPA policy that 'pesticide chemicals that cause related pharmacological effects will be regarded, in the absence of evidence to the contrary, as having an additive deleterious action' (CFR, 1998).

In this chapter we assume that common mechanism groups can be satisfactorily determined. In this context, a common mechanism group is defined as a group of pesticides determined to cause adverse effects by a common mechanism of toxicity. Such chemicals are said to occupy the same 'risk cup' (US EPA, 2002). Cumulative risk is the likelihood for the cumulation of a common toxic effect resulting from all routes of exposure to substances that share a common mechanism of toxicity. We present a component-based procedure to estimate cumulative risks from exposures to multiple chemicals via dose addition modeling. The dose-addition model for estimating the cumulative response for quantitative response data is described in the context of cholinesterase inhibition effects. The cumulative response is estimated by directly fitting the combined dose-response function for the chemicals with a common mechanism under dose addition.

18.2   EXPERIMENTAL DESIGNS AND MODELS FOR WHOLE MIXTURE

Two designs commonly used in response surface analysis are the factorial design and simplex-lattice design (Scheffé, 1958). In a factorial experiment, the components represent different dose concentrations of the chemicals in the mixture. For a binary mixture, if k_1 and k_2 are the numbers of nonzero doses of two chemicals C1 and C2, respectively, then a factorial design will have $(k_1 + 1) \times (k_2 + 1)$ dose combinations. The effect of components on the mixture response is modeled by a polynomial model such as a linear-quadratic model,

$$y = \beta_0 + \beta_1 c_1 + \beta_2 c_2 + \beta_{11} c_1^2 + \beta_{22} c_2^2 + \beta_{12} c_1 c_2 + e,$$

where c_1 and c_2 are concentrations of C1 and C2, respectively. The response is a function of concentrations of C1 and C2.

In many toxicology studies, the primary interest may be the effect of the relative proportions in the mixture rather than their absolute amounts. For example, individual components of air pollution vary from one area to another, and an important objective in the study of air quality is to investigate the effects of changes in proportions of individual components on endpoint responses. The effect of relative proportions can be analyzed by Scheffé's canonical polynomial (Scheffé, 1958). The Scheffé canonical model is not applicable to the study of dose-response assessment since it considers only one concentration. A proportion-concentration response model, a generalization of Scheffé's model that incorporates the concentration and its implied design for the mixture experiment, is described below.

Consider a mixture experiment containing m components with g total mixture concentrations. Let the proportion of the ith component in an m-component mixture be denoted by x_i ($i = 1, \ldots, m$), where $0 \le x_i \le 1$ and $x_1 + \cdots + x_m = 1$. Denote the kth total mixture concentration level as T_k ($k = 1, \ldots, g$). The joint response for a subject from the experimental group $\mathbf{x} = (x_1, \ldots, x_m)$ with concentration T_k can be modeled by the proportion-concentration model (Chen $et\ al.$, 1989)

$$Y = \boldsymbol{\beta}'_0 \mathbf{x} + \boldsymbol{\beta}'_1 \mathbf{x} T_k + \boldsymbol{\beta}'_2 \mathbf{x} T_k^2 + \cdots + \boldsymbol{\beta}'_r \mathbf{x} T_k^r + \cdots, \qquad (18.1)$$

where $\boldsymbol{\beta}'_r \mathbf{x}$ is the Scheffé (1958) canonical polynomial (proportion response model)

$$\boldsymbol{\beta}'_r \mathbf{x} = \sum_{i=1}^{m} \beta_{i,r} x_i + \sum_{i<j}^{m} \beta_{ij,r} x_i x_j + \sum_{i<j<l}^{m} \beta_{ijl,r} x_i x_j x_l + \cdots + \beta_{12\cdots m,r} x_1 x_2 \cdots x_m.$$

$$(18.2)$$

The total mixture concentration T is the sum of individual component concentrations $T = c_1 + c_2 + \cdots + c_m$, where $c_i = T x_i$ is the individual component concentration, $i = 1, \ldots, m$. The proportion-concentration approach models the mixture response as a function of the relative proportions of individual components $\mathbf{x} = (x_1, \ldots, x_m)$ and the total concentration T. The response surface approach (factorial design) models the mixture response as a function of individual component concentrations $\mathbf{c} = (c_1, \ldots, c_m)$.

The proportion-concentration model (18.1) consists of two components: the proportion component described by a Scheffé polynomial $\boldsymbol{\beta}'_r \mathbf{x}$ and the concentration component described by a polynomial function of T. There are several simpler models in terms of the two components. For example, a quadratic-proportion and quadratic-concentration model ($r = 2$) is

$$Y = \left(\sum_{i=1}^{m} \beta_{i,0} x_i + \sum_{i<j}^{m} \beta_{ij,0} x_i x_j \right) + \left(\sum_{i=1}^{m} \beta_{i,1} x_i + \sum_{i<j}^{m} \beta_{ij,1} x_i x_j \right) T$$

$$+ \left(\sum_{i=1}^{m} \beta_{i,2} x_i + \sum_{i<j}^{m} \beta_{ij,2} x_i x_j \right) T^2.$$

A quadratic-proportion and linear-concentration model ($r = 1$) is

$$Y = \left(\sum_{i=1}^{m} \beta_{i,0} x_i + \sum_{i<j}^{m} \beta_{ij,0} x_i x_j \right) + \left(\sum_{i=1}^{m} \beta_{i,1} x_i + \sum_{i<j}^{m} \beta_{ij,1} x_i x_j \right) T.$$

Similarly, a linear-proportion and quadratic-concentration model is

$$Y = \left(\sum_{i=1}^{m} \beta_{i,0} x_i \right) + \left(\sum_{i=1}^{m} \beta_{i,1} x_i \right) T + \left(\sum_{i=1}^{m} \beta_{i,2} x_i \right) T^2.$$

If there is only one concentration, the proportion-concentration response model is the proportion response model,

$$Y = \sum_{i=1}^{m} \beta_i x_i + \sum_{i<j}^{m} \beta_{ij} x_i x_j + \sum_{i<j<l}^{m} \beta_{ijl} x_i x_j x_l + \cdots + \beta_{12\cdots m} x_1 x_2 \cdots x_m.$$

The β_i represent the expected response from treatment group with component i only, and $\eta_1 = \sum_{i=}^{m} \beta_i x_i$ represents the linear component (effect) of the mixture. The quadratic terms $\beta_{ij} x_i x_j$, $i < j$, represent deviations from linearity. The higher-order terms are generally used for checking the adequacy of the quadratic polynomial. The likelihood ratio test under the Scheffé model is used to assess the significance of the coefficients. The model building process is based on the sequential model fitting approach beginning with the 'linear' model. The likelihood ratio test of the homogeneous linear model versus the heterogeneous linear model ($H_0 : \beta_1 = \cdots = \beta_m$) is computed by

$G = 2 \ln [\text{likelihood without the restriction/likelihood with the restriction}]$

$= \text{deviance with the restriction} - \text{deviance without restriction}.$

The deviances are given in, for example, McCullagh and Nelder (1989). Under the null hypothesis, the likelihood ratio statistic G asymptotically has a chi-square distribution with $m - 1$ degrees of freedom. Other hypotheses of interest or inferences on the coefficients of the proportion-concentration can be tested similarly.

Scheffé introduced the simplex-lattice design, corresponding to the canonical polynomial model, for mixture experiments with one concentration. In a simplex-lattice design, the components represent the relative proportions of the chemicals in the mixture for a fixed total concentration. A proportion–concentration mixture design contains many total concentrations, in which each concentration contains several proportions. Figure 18.1 is a proportion-concentration mixture design for two chemicals C1 and C2. Points on the X-axis correspond to a proportion 1:0 proportion mixture for C1:C2, and on the Y-axis correspond to the proportion 0:1 for C2:C1. Each line connected by the X- and Y-axis represents different combinations of proportions for the two chemicals having the same total concentration. Ray lines emanating form the origin represent combinations of different concentrations with a constant mixing proportion (Finney, 1971; Abdelbasit and Plackett, 1982).

The number of parameters provides guidance for the number of experimental groups. For $m = 2$, for example, the quadratic proportion and quadratic concentration model becomes

$$Y = (\beta_{1,0} x_1 + \beta_{2,0} x_2 + \beta_{12,0} x_1 x_2) + (\beta_{1,1} x_1 + \beta_{2,1} x_2 + \beta_{12,1} x_1 x_2) T$$
$$+ (\beta_{1,2} x_1 + \beta_{2,2} x_2 + \beta_{12,2} x_1 x_2) T^2.$$

This model contains nine parameters. The model requires at least three concentrations with three proportions for each concentration, such as the three proportions (1,0), (1/2,1/2), and (0,1), for a total of at least nine groups. Replication of the experimental groups makes the lack-of-fit test possible.

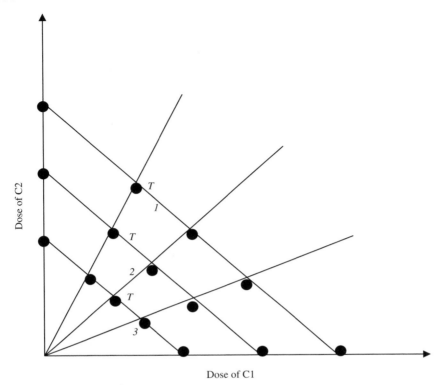

Figure 18.1 Proportion-concentration design. Coordinate axes represent concentrations of C1 and C2 of individual components. Points on the *X*-axis correspond to the proportion 1:0 mixture for C1:C2, and on the *Y*-axis correspond to the proportion 0:1 for C2:C1. Points on the line connecting the *X*- and *Y*-axes represent different combinations of the two chemicals having the same total concentration, T_k. Points on a ray emanating form the origin represent combinations of different concentrations with the same proportion.

The proportion-concentration response model described above is for modeling quantitative response data. Dose-response data for risk assessment often are quantal responses such as presence or absence of a particular adverse effect, such as, liver tumor. The probit, logistic, and multistage models are commonly used for quantal response data. For example, the quadratic-proportion and quadratic-concentration logistic model for a two-chemical mixture is

$$P(Y=1 \mid x_1, x_2, T)$$

$$= \frac{\exp\left[\beta_{1,0}x_1 + \beta_{2,0}x_2 + \beta_{12,0}x_1x_2 + \sum_{r=1}^{2}(\beta_{1,r}x_1 + \beta_{2,r}x_2 + \beta_{12,r}x_1x_2)T^r\right]}{1 + \exp\left[\beta_{1,0}x_1 + \beta_{2,0}x_2 + \beta_{12,0}x_1x_2 + \sum_{r=1}^{2}(\beta_{1,r}x_1 + \beta_{2,r}x_2 + \beta_{12,r}x_1x_2)T^r\right]}.$$

J. J. Chen *et al.* (1996b) used a logistic proportion model for the analysis of a dietary mixture experiment to study the effects of dietary fat, carbohydrate, and fiber calories on DMBA-induced mammary gland tumors. It should be noted that the same design configuration (e.g., the number of concentrations and the number of proportions) can be applied to the quantal or quantitative response data, except that the quantal response data generally require more subjects per group.

18.3   DOSE-RESPONSE MODELING FOR COMPONENT-BASED APPROACH

18.3.1   Relative potency factor method

Consider the hypothetical data set of six pesticide chemicals shown in Table 18.1. These data represent the cholinesterase activity levels in each dose group for the six chemicals. The common endpoints measured in cholinesterase bioassays are plasma, red blood cell, and brain cholinesterase levels. The activity levels given in Table 18.1 represent typical ranges measured in a cholinesterase bioassay. The data are control-normalized so that the mean of each control groups is 1 (control groups not shown). A natural logarithmic transformation is applied to stabilize the variances. The constant variance model for a given chemical appears to be adequate for the transformed data. The mean of the log-transformed data in the control group is 0. Assume that the dose-response function for an individual chemical is given by

$$m(d) = \alpha + \beta \log d, \qquad d > 0.$$

EPA (2000b) recommended using the relative potency factor (RPF) approach to normalize and combine the different toxic potencies among the chemicals for cumulative risk assessment. An initial step in the RPF approach is to identify a point of departure (POD). A POD is generally defined as a point estimate of the dose or exposure level that is used to depart from the observed range of empirical response (or incidence) data for the purpose of extrapolation (EPA, 2000b). In the case of a cumulative risk assessment, the POD is a dose reflecting a uniform response level for the common toxic effect for each chemical. The RPF can be estimated as the ratio of the POD of the index chemical (a well-studied chemical) to that of each other chemical in the group, $RPF_i = POD_{\text{index chemical}}/POD_i$. The exposure dose to each chemical is multiplied by the RPF to express all exposures in terms of the index chemical. The summation of these values provides a total combined exposure dose expressed in terms of the index chemical (index chemical equivalent dose) for prediction. That is,

index chemical equivalent dose $= \text{exposure}_1 \times RPF_1 + \text{exposure}_2 \times RPF_2 + \cdots$.

The index chemical equivalent dose is treated as the dose level of the index chemical to assess the cumulative risk of the m chemicals. For example, the cumulative dose can be divided by the uncertainty factors for the index chemical and compared with the reference dose (RfD) for assessment.

For the example data set, suppose we are interested in cumulative risk assessment at the exposure doses $d_1 = 0.030$, $d_2 = 0.035$, $d_3 = 0.200$, $d_4 = 0.200$, $d_5 = 0.030$,

Table 18.1 A hypothetical group of six chemicals.

Chem	Dose					
1	0.02	1.024	1.020	0.865	1.029	0.824
	2.3	0.500	0.603	0.444	0.400	0.059
	22.5	0.250	0.232	0.265	0.221	0.209
	213	0.147	0.144	0.124	0.129	0.126
2	0.017	1.139	1.113	1.246	0.861	0.869
	1.7	0.499	0.693	0.507	0.507	0.510
	17.0	0.220	0.212	0.229	0.214	0.203
	177	0.125	0.127	0.186	0.139	0.151
3	0.03	1.316	1.233	1.168	1.188	1.299
		1.253	1.243	1.270	1.319	1.286
	1.1	0.865	0.937	0.793	0.829	0.970
		0.803	0.862	0.852	0.875	0.977
	15.0	0.299	0.289	0.309	0.306	0.270
		0.293	0.306	0.247	0.276	0.286
	168	0.171	0.151	0.128	0.125	0.138
		0.168	0.148	0.155	0.132	0.148

Chem.	Dose					
4	0.05	1.147	1.027	1.075	1.123	1.023
	2.00	0.775	0.835	0.889	0.749	0.784
	19.0	0.216	0.204	0.222	0.189	0.198
	205	0.135	0.114	0.129	0.090	0.102
5	0.019	0.936	0.652	0.824	0.830	0.933
	1.3	0.546	0.546	0.630	0.593	0.749
	13.8	0.256	0.270	0.240	0.259	0.265
	189	0.078	0.097	0.109	0.086	0.117
6	0.01	0.631	0.651	0.504	0.740	0.824
	0.1	0.429	0.644	0.451	0.656	0.556
	10.8	0.273	0.218	0.256	0.204	0.211
	250	0.058	0.138	0.153	0.173	0.140

Table 18.2 Maximum likelihood estimates (standard errors) of the coefficients of the individual dose response model, exposure dose d, predicted response Pred(d), point of departure (POD) for a uniform response level of -0.05, total (RPF) exposure dose d_{RPF}, and predicted response at d_{RPF} for the six chemicals.

Chemical	α	β	σ	d	Pred(d)	POD	d_{RPF}	Pred(d_{RPF})
1	-0.774	-0.212	0.170	0.030	-0.0316	0.0327	0.1965	-0.4290
	(0.041)	(0.011)	(0.027)					
2	-0.768	-0.221	0.201	0.035	-0.0278	0.0387	0.2324	-0.4455
	(0.047)	(0.013)	(0.032)					
3	-0.548	-0.289	0.322	0.200	-0.0832	0.1782	1.0701	-0.5676
	(0.080)	(0.023)	(0.051)					
4	-0.483	-0.260	0.233	0.200	-0.0642	0.1894	1.1370	-0.5164
	(0.039)	(0.012)	(0.026)					
5	-0.853	-0.232	0.307	0.030	-0.0385	0.0315	0.1892	-0.4668
	(0.072)	(0.020)	(0.049)					
6	-1.104	-0.169	0.248	0.002	-0.0548	0.0019	0.0114	-0.3480
	(0.056)	(0.014)	(0.039)					
sum				0.1202	-0.3001			

and $d_6 = 0.002$ for the six chemicals. In the RPF approach, the linear dose-response function

$$m(d) = \alpha + \beta \log(d)$$

is first fitted to the log-transformed data for each chemical. Suppose that the estimated dose corresponding to the predicted mean response of -0.05 is defined to be the POD so that $\hat{\alpha} + \hat{\beta} \log(\text{POD}) = -0.05$. Note that -0.05 corresponds to a dose level near the low end of the dose-response range for all six chemicals. Table 18.2 contains estimates of dose-response parameters, POD, the index chemical equivalent dose, and the predicted response with each chemical as an index chemical. For example, the total equivalent dose with respect to the index chemical 1 is

$$d_{RPF} = 0.030(0.0327/0.0327) + 0.035(0.0327/0.0387) + 0.200(0.0327/0.1782)$$
$$+ 0.200(0.0327/0.1894) + 0.030(0.0327/0.0315) + 0.002(0.0327/0.0019)$$
$$= 0.1965.$$

The index chemical equivalent dose can be divided by an uncertainty factor for chemical 1 to obtain the RfD.

The predicted mean response associated with the index chemical equivalent dose d_{RPF} can be estimated by using the dose response model of index chemical 1,

$$\text{Pred}(d_{RPF}) = \hat{\alpha}_1 + \hat{\beta}_1 \log(d_{RPF})$$
$$= -0.774 + (-0.212) \times \log(0.1965) = -0.4290.$$

It can be seen that different index chemicals will result in different predicted values.

18.3.2 A dose addition model for mixtures

In Section 18.3.2.1 we describe an approach in which the predicted response does not depend on the index chemical if the chemicals are dose additive. Section 18.3.2.2 illustrates an application of the approach to the example data set in Table 18.1.

18.3.2.1 Dose addition for mixtures

A dose response function for binary response data, denoted by $P(d) = F$, relates the probability of response to the dose d, where F is a probability distribution function. The general model can be expressed as

$$P(d) = F(\alpha + \beta \log d), \qquad d > 0,$$

or

$$P(d) = F(\alpha + \beta d).$$

Two commonly used dose-response models are the probit model and the logistic model. The probit model expressed in terms of the log dose is

$$P(d) = c + (1 - c) \int_{-\infty}^{\alpha + \beta \log d} \frac{1}{\sqrt{2\pi}} \exp(-1/2t^2) dt,$$

and the logistic model is

$$P(d) = c + (1 - c) \frac{\exp(\alpha + \beta \log d)}{1 + \exp(\alpha + \beta \log d)},$$

where the parameter c represents background effect and $P(d)$ is defined to be c when $d = 0$. The parameters α and β are the intercept and slope of the dose-response model. The dose-response model in the dose scale has a similar expression. In the presentation that follows, dose-response models will be in terms of the log dose.

The response at a dose may be a continuous (quantitative) variable representing a magnitude of the adverse effect, such as cholinesterase inhibition. Denote the mean response from exposure to dose d as $m(d)$. For quantitative response data, the dose-response function is given by

$$m(d) = \alpha + \beta \log d, \qquad d > 0.$$

Note that the expected response at $d = 1$ is α. In the context of risk assessment, the response at $d = 0$ is normalized to either 1 or 0 depending on the measurement scale.

Consider only two chemicals. Denote the dose-response function for chemical 1 at dose d_1 as

$$F_1(d_1) = \alpha_1 + \beta_1 \log d_1,$$

and the dose response function for chemical 2 at dose d_2 as

$$F_2(d_2) = \alpha_2 + \beta_2 \log d_2.$$

If $F_1(d_1) = F_2(d_2)$, the ratio of the equally effective doses $\rho_{12} = d_1/d_2$ is called the relative potency of chemical 2 to chemical 1. Recently, Chen *et al.* (2001) showed that two chemicals have a constant relative potency if and only if the slopes of the (log) dose response functions are equal, that is, $\beta_1 = \beta_2$. Under dose addition, the response to the combination of d_1 and d_2 for chemical 1 and chemical 2 is $F_1(d_1 + \rho_{12}d_2) = F_2(d_1/\rho_{12} + d_2)$, where ρ is the relative potency of chemical 2 to chemical 1. The combined mean response can be derived through addition of doses of chemical 1 and chemical 2 based on the RPF. Briefly, under dose addition, if two chemicals have a constant relative potency and if the joint response is dose-additive, then the dose-response function from exposure to d_1 of chemical 1 and d_2 of chemical 2 is

$$
\begin{aligned}
F(d_1, d_2) &= F_1(d_1 + \rho_{12}\, d_2) \\
&= \alpha_1 + \beta_1 \log(d_1 + \rho_{12}\, d_2).
\end{aligned}
\tag{18.3}
$$

For a group of m chemicals in which the relative potency between any two chemicals is constant, the joint response of the m chemicals can be derived as

$$
\begin{aligned}
F(d_1, \ldots, d_m) &= F_1\left(d_1 + \sum_{t=2}^{m} \rho_t d_t\right) \\
&= \alpha_1 + \beta \log\left(d_1 + \sum_{t=2}^{m} \rho_t d_t\right),
\end{aligned}
\tag{18.4}
$$

where $\rho_t = \exp[(\alpha_t - \alpha_1)/\beta]$ is the relative potency of chemical t to index chemical 1, $t = 2, \ldots, m$. The joint response can also be expressed in term of any other chemical as an index chemical s,

$$
F(d_1, \ldots, d_m) = \alpha_s + \beta \log\left(d_s + \sum_{t \neq s}^{m} \rho'_t d_t\right),
\tag{18.5}
$$

where $\rho'_t = \exp[(\alpha_t - \alpha_s)/\beta]$. It can be seen that $\rho'_t = \rho_t/\rho_s$ for $t = 1, \ldots, m$, where $\rho_1 = 1$. The two models are equivalent, that is, the estimated risk at any doses does not depend on the choice of index chemical.

For a set of m chemicals, the chemicals can be clustered into several subclasses of constant relative potency $\{S_1, S_2, \ldots, S_s\}$, where each S_i consists of chemicals having constant relative potency. For example, the set $\{\{c_1, c_2, \ldots\}, \{c_q, c_{q+1}, \ldots\}, \ldots \{c_m\}\}$ represents the fact that the chemicals $c_1, c_2, \ldots$ in the first subclass have constant relative potency with respect to each other, as do the chemicals $c_q, c_{q+1}, \ldots$ in the second subclass; the relative potency factor between the last chemical c_m and the other chemicals is different at different response levels. Let m_i be the number of chemicals in the ith cluster $S_i, i = 1, \ldots, s, \sum_{i=1}^{s} m_i = m$. Under dose addition, the combined dose-response function for the cluster S_i is

$$F_i(d_1, \ldots, d_{m_i}) = F_i\left(d_1 + \sum_{t=2}^{m_i} \rho_{it} d_t\right)$$

$$= \alpha_i + \beta_i \log\left(d_1 + \sum_{t=2}^{m_i} \rho_{it} d_t\right). \quad (18.6)$$

Further, assume response addition for chemicals from different clusters, that is, the chemicals in the different clusters behave independently of one another. For binary response data, the combined risk for the m chemicals $\{S_1, S_2, \ldots, S_s\}$ is

$$F(d_1, \ldots, d_m) = \sum_{i=1}^{s} F_i(d_1, \ldots, d_{m_i}) - \sum_{i \neq j}^{s} F_i(d_1, \ldots, d_{m_i}) F_j(d_1, \ldots, d_{m_j}) + \cdots$$

$$(18.7)$$

For quantitative response data, the combined response is simply the sum of responses of individual subclasses,

$$F(d_1, \ldots, d_m) = \sum_{i=1}^{s} F_i(d_1, \ldots, d_{m_i}). \quad (18.8)$$

Chen *et al.* (2003) proposed two tree classification algorithms, top-down and bottom-up schemes, to cluster a set of m chemicals into subclasses such that the chemicals in the same subclass have a common slope (constant RPF). The top-down classification starts with the assumption that the slopes of the m chemicals are all different. At each step, the adjacent pair of chemicals with the most similar slope is grouped into one cluster based on a pre-specified significance level, say, $\alpha = 0.25$. The procedure continues to the next step until it fails to meet the latter grouping criterion. Note that the significance level of 0.25 is commonly used when accepting the null model (hypothesis) is of interest. The bottom-up classification starts with the assumption that the slopes of the m chemicals are equal. At each step, the adjacent pair of chemicals with the greatest slope difference is separated into two clusters based on a pre-specified significance level, say, $\alpha = 0.05$. Again, the procedure continues to the next step until it fails to meet the separation criterion. In both procedures, a (global) goodness-of-fit test is performed on the terminal tree against the two trivial trees $\{1, 2, \ldots, m\}$ and $\{\{1, 2, \ldots, m\}\}$.

The top-down classification forms the tree from the top. It assumes that the slopes of the chemicals are different. At each step, a chemical (or subclass of chemicals) is combined with another chemical (or subclass of chemicals) to form a new subclass. Therefore, the number of subclasses at each step is one less than at the previous step. On the other hand, the bottom-up algorithm forms a tree by division. It assumes that the slopes of the chemicals are equal. A new subclass is formed at each step. These two algorithms may result in different tree structures. The concept of dose addition between two chemicals is equivalent, operationally, to a common slope between the two dose-response functions. Under this premise, the top-down algorithm initially assumes that the chemicals in the group are not dose-additive, and at each step the classification algorithm determines if two chemicals (chemical clusters) are dose-additive to form several dose-additive subgroups; while the bottom-up algorithm initially assumes that the chemicals are dose-additive, and the classification algorithm separates the nonadditive chemicals into new groups.

Estimation of the parameters of dose-response coefficients can be obtained by the maximum likelihood method. Let y_{ijl} denote the control-adjusted response data for the lth observation at dose level d_{ij} from the ith chemical ($i = 1, \ldots, m, j = 1, \ldots, g_i$, and $l = 1, \ldots, n_{ij}$), where n_{ij} denotes the number of subjects in dose group j from chemical i, and g_i is the number of dose groups from chemical i. Suppose y_{ijl} is normally distributed with mean $m_i(d_{ij})$ and variance σ_i^2. The log-likelihood function for chemical i is

$$LL = -\frac{1}{2} \sum_{j=1}^{g_i} \sum_{l=1}^{n_{ij}} \left(\frac{[y_{ijl} - m_i(d_{ij})]^2}{\sigma_i^2} + \log 2\pi\sigma_i^2 \right),$$

where $m_i(d_{ij}) = \alpha_i + \beta_i \log d_{ij}$. The log-likelihood function for the m_i chemicals of constant relative potency in terms of chemical s (the index chemical) is

$$LL = -\frac{1}{2} \sum_{i=1}^{m_i} \sum_{j=1}^{g_i} \sum_{l=1}^{n_{ij}} \left(\frac{[y_{ijl} - m_s(D_{ij})]^2}{\sigma_i^2} + \log 2\pi\sigma_i^2 \right),$$

where $m_s(D_{ij}) = \alpha_s + \beta_s \log D_{ij}$ and $D_{ij} = d_{is} + \sum_{t \neq s}^{m_i} \rho_{st} d_{it}$.

18.3.2.2 Numerical illustration

For the hypothesis data set (Table 18.1), the six slope estimates are, in ascending order,

$$\hat{\beta}_3(-0.289) < \hat{\beta}_4(-0.260) < \hat{\beta}_5(-0.232) < \hat{\beta}_2(-0.221) < \hat{\beta}_1(-0.212)$$
$$< \hat{\beta}_6(-0.169).$$

Both the top-down and bottom-up algorithms show that the six chemicals can be grouped into three clusters $\{1, 2, 5\}, \{\{3, 4\}, \{6\}\}$ of constant relative potency. The data set of six chemicals can be fitted based on the three subclasses, for example,

$$m(d_1, d_2, d_5) = \alpha_1 + \beta_1 \log(d_1 + \rho_{12}d_2 + \rho_{15}d_5),$$
$$m(d_3, d_4) = \alpha_3 + \beta_3 \log(d_3 + \rho_{34}d_4),$$
$$m(d_6) = \alpha_6 + \beta_6 \log d_6.$$

The parameter estimates for the subclass $\{1, 2, 5\}$ and $\{3, 4\}$ using different index chemicals are given in Tables 18.3 and 18.4, respectively. For example, the total

Table 18.3 Maximum likelihood estimates (standard errors) of the coefficients of the combined dose-response function, total exposure dose D, and predicted response at d_{RPF} for chemicals 1, 2, and 5.

s	α	β	ρ_a	ρ_b	σ	D	Pred(D)
1	−0.760	−0.221	1.032	1.599	0.170	0.11413	−0.2796
	(0.054)	(0.010)	(0.347)	(0.538)	(0.027)		
2	−0.767	−0.221	0.968	1.550	0.200	0.11055	−0.2796
	(0.054)	(0.010)	(0.326)	(0.522)	(0.032)		
5	−0.864	−0.221	0.625	0.645	0.307	0.07133	−0.2796
	(0.053)	(0.010)	(0.210)	(0.217)	(0.048)		

Table 18.4 Maximum likelihood estimates (standard errors) of the coefficients of the combined dose-response function, total exposure dose D, and predicted response at d_{RPF} for chemicals 3 and 4.

s	α	β	ρ	σ	D	Pred(D)
3	−0.576	−0.269	0.680	0.322	0.33599	−0.2833
	(0.062)	(0.011)	(0.187)	(0.051)		
4	−0.473	−0.269	1.471	0.232	0.49415	−0.2833
	(0.044)	(0.011)	(1.405)	(0.026)		

exposure dose for the subclass $\{1, 2, 5\}$ is $D = 0.030 + 1.031 \times 0.035 + 1.599 \times 0.020 = 0.1141$ with chemical 1 as index chemical. The predicted response is -0.2796. Similarly, the mixture dose for the subclass $\{3, 4\}$ is $D = 0.3360$ (chemical 3 as index chemical) with the predicted response -0.2833, and the predicted response for chemical 6 is -0.0548. The combined response is the sum of the responses of the three subclasses $(-0.2796) + (-0.2833) + (-0.0548) = -0.6177$.

18.4 COMPONENT-BASED RISK ASSESSMENT FOR QUANTITATIVE RESPONSE DATA

Risk is customarily defined as the statistical probability of the occurrence of an adverse effect at a given level of exposure. Dose-response models for adverse quantal response data are well defined since an adverse effect is self-evident, that is, the occurrence of an adverse effect is observed on individual subjects empirically. By contrast, a clear-cut adverse effect for continuous quantitative responses is difficult both to define and to observe unequivocally. The characterization of risk for continuous quantitative responses in terms of probability of occurrence does not naturally follow. Methods for risk estimation of continuous quantitative response data for a single toxin have been proposed by many authors (Crump, 1984; Chen and Gaylor, 1992; Kodell and West, 1993; J. J. Chen *et al.*, 1996a). This section describes an approach to estimating the cumulative risk of an adverse continuous quantitative effect under dose addition.

Let $y(d)$ be a control-adjusted response variable of an individual exposed to a chemical at dose d. Assume that $y(d)$ has a normal distribution with mean $E(y(d)) = m(d)$ and variance σ^2. Note that we assume a constant variance across dose groups of a chemical. Without loss of generality, suppose c^* is a critical value for an abnormally low level of response, a level below which a response is considered to be atypical. For example, c^* may be a certain threshold such as a 3 standard deviation reduction (difference) from the control mean or 20% reduction relative to the control mean. Under the difference scale, c^* can alternatively be expressed as $c^* = -k\sigma$, where k is appropriately chosen to yield a specific low percentage point of the distribution of unexposed individuals. For exposure to a given dose d, the proportion of the individuals with response $y(d)$ below the critical value $c^* = -k\sigma$ is given by

$$P(d) = P[y(d) \leq c^*] = P[y(d) \leq -k\sigma] = \Phi\left[-k - \frac{m(d)}{\sigma}\right], \qquad (18.9)$$

where Φ is the standard normal cumulative distribution function. Under the ratio scale, c^* can be expressed as $c^* = 1 - k\sigma$. The probability of adverse effect at dose d becomes

$$P(d) = \Phi\left[-k - \frac{m(d) - 1}{\sigma}\right]. \qquad (18.10)$$

Note that in either case $P(0) = \Phi(-k)$. The dose d^* corresponding to the critical level $y(d^*) = c^*$ is regarded as a safe dose. The risk is the probability that $y(d)$ is less than or equal to the critical value c. By expressing c in terms of k and σ the probability of adverse effect can be calculated. Since the risk estimate depends on the standard deviation estimate, different index chemicals will predict different total risk estimates, even for chemicals in the same subclass (Tables 18.3 and 18.4). One approach is to assume a constant variance model for the chemicals in the same subclass. For a given critical value c, denote $\hat{m}_i(D)$ as the predicted response for the ith subclass of a constant RPF. The total risk estimate measured on the difference scale is

$$\hat{P}_i(D) = \Phi\left[-k_i - \frac{\hat{m}_i(D)}{\hat{\sigma}_i}\right], \qquad (18.11)$$

where $c = -k_i\sigma_i$ and $\hat{\sigma}_i$ is the common variance estimate for the ith subclass.

For the example data set, with $k = 3$, the cumulative risk is the probability of the control-adjusted response less than or equal to three standard deviation units. Table 18.5 (column 3) contains the risk estimate at the exposure dose d for $k = 3$. The sum of individual risk estimates is 0.0155. Using the RPF method with chemical 1 as the index chemical, three standard deviations below the control

Table 18.5 The estimated cumulative risk from the individual model, RPF method and the dose addition model for the six chemicals.

Chemical	Individual model		RPF method	Dose addition model	
	d	$\hat{P}(d)$	$\hat{P}(d_{RPF})$	$\hat{P}(D)$	$\hat{P}^a(D)$
1	0.030	0.0024	0.3169	0.0320	0.3209
2	0.035	0.0021	0.2166	0.0320	0.3209
5	0.030	0.0020	0.0695	0.0320	0.3209
3	0.200	0.0031	0.1079	0.0242	0.2230
4	0.200	0.0032	0.2166	0.0242	0.2230
6	0.002	0.0027	0.0552	0.0027	0.3053
Sum		0.0155		0.0580	

mean is $0.171 \times 3 = 0.513$; this value corresponds to $\exp(-0.513) = 0.600$ in terms of the original measurement. Therefore, the critical value can be interpreted as a 40 % reduction from the control mean. The estimated cumulative risk for six chemicals using the dose response model of index chemical 1 is

$$P(D) = \Phi\left[-3 - \frac{\hat{\mu}_1(D)}{\hat{\sigma}_1}\right] = \Phi\left[-3 - \frac{-0.4290}{0.171}\right] = 0.3169.$$

Column 4 contains the cumulative risk estimates using the RPF method.

Under a constant variance model, the standard deviation estimate for the subclass $\{1, 2, 5\}$ is 0.2437. The estimated cumulative risk for the three chemicals is

$$P(D) = \Phi\left[-3 - \frac{\hat{\mu}_1(D)}{\hat{\sigma}_1}\right] = \Phi\left[-3 - \frac{-0.2796}{0.2437}\right] = 0.0320.$$

The standard deviation estimate for the subclass $\{3, 4\}$ is 0.2760. The estimated cumulative risk for the two chemicals is 0.0242. The risk for chemical 6 is 0.0027. The cumulative risk for the six chemicals using equation (18.7) is 0.0580. Alternatively, the cumulative risk can be computed based on the predicted cumulative response -0.6177 under response addition. The cumulative risk in terms of chemical class $\{1, 2, 5\}$ is

$$P^a(D) = \Phi\left[-3 - \frac{-0.6177}{0.2437}\right] = 0.3209.$$

Under the alternative approach, the estimated cumulative risk of the joint response depends on the standard deviation of the index chemical class. The cumulative risks for the two methods are shown in columns 5 and 6. It can been that the estimated risk based on simply summing the individual probabilities heavily understates the risk as compared to the estimates from the RPF method or dose-addition model.

18.5 DISCUSSION

The dose-addition model described above assumes a constant relative potency between two chemicals. If the relative potency factor between chemical 1 and chemical 2 is different for different response levels, the joint response from exposure to d_1 of chemical 1 and d_2 of chemical 2 in terms of chemical 1 is

$$F(d_1, d_2) = \alpha_1 + \beta_1 \log(d_1 + \rho_{12} d_2^{w_{12}}),$$

where $w_{12} = \beta_2/\beta_1$, and $\rho_{12} = \exp[(\alpha_2 - \alpha_1)/\beta_1]$. The cumulative response from exposure to chemical 1 and chemical 2 can also be expressed in terms of chemical 2. However, if the relative potency is not constant, then the response predicted based on chemical 1 will differ from that predicted based on chemical 2. For m chemicals, the combined response in terms of, say, chemical s can be derived as

$$F(d_1, \ldots, d_m) = F_s\left(d_s + \sum_{t \neq s}^{m} \rho_{st} d_t^{w_{st}}\right)$$

$$= \alpha_s + \beta_s \log\left(d_s + \sum_{t \neq s}^{m} \rho_{st} d_t^{w_{st}}\right).$$

The $\rho_{st} = \exp[(\alpha_t - \alpha_s)/\beta_s]$ is a potency ratio of chemical t to the index chemical s, and $w_{st} = \beta_t/\beta_s$ is the slope ratio, $t = 1, \ldots, m$, and $t \neq s$. The predicted value will depend on the index chemical class (Chen *et al.*, 2001).

The dose unit d described in the previous sections is an administered (applied) dose in a general sense. Concern as to relating exposures to the actual dose that is delivered to the body, and finally to the target organ, has been raised from time to time. Ideally, estimation of the risk requires knowledge of the functional (dose-response) relationship between the biological (effective) target tissue dose and the probability of toxic response, and the functional relationship between the applied dose and the effective dose. It is preferable to model the dose-response function in terms of the effective dose. Depending on several factors, such as the chemical involved, the route of administration, and the target organ, the actual 'effective' toxic dose at the target organ may be an altered dose. The dose-response model used for risk assessment should be based on the 'transformed' target dose rather than the 'administered' dose. In general, the effective dose is assumed to be proportional to the applied dose since it is seldom known. It is possible, however, that the functional relationship between the applied dose and effective dose may be nonlinear due to a nonlinear pharmacokinetic transformation (Gehring *et al.*, 1978). The true dose-response relationship between the effective dose and response may be linear at low doses, but the relationship between the applied dose and the effective dose may be nonlinear.

Van Ryzin and Rai (1987) proposed a kinetic dose-response model where the applied dose is transformed in accordance with incoming and outgoing Michaelis–Menten nonlinear kinetic equations to a biologically 'effective' toxic dose concentration at the target organ. Denoting by D the effective dose at the target organ, they showed that in the steady state the functional relationship between D and d is

$$D = g(d) = \frac{r_1 d}{1 + r_2 d},$$

where the function g is the pharmacokinetic transformation with two parameters r_1 and r_2 operating on the applied dose d. The dose-response function for a chemical under the effective dose $D = g(d)$ is

$$P(g(d)) = P(D) = F(\alpha + \beta D).$$

The joint dose-response model for the mixture involving multiple chemical exposures can be derived similarly. Finally, we consider a log transformation of dose, $\log d$, because the logarithm of the dose has been commonly used in toxicology to model dose-response relationships. Nevertheless, the log transformation can be regarded as a functional relationship between the applied dose and the effective dose.

CHAPTER 19

Estimating the Natural History of Breast Cancer from Bivariate Data on Age and Tumor Size at Diagnosis

Alexander V. Zorin, Leonid G. Hanin and Andrej Y. Yakovlev
University of Rochester

Lutz Edler
German Cancer Research Center

19.1 INTRODUCTION

The natural history of cancer is represented by a set of biologically meaning-ful quantitative characteristics of the initiation, promotion and progression stages of tumor development, with the structure of the latter stage being dependent on a specific mechanism of cancer detection. This paper is con-cerned with statistical inference on unobservable characteristics of tumor latency from multivariate data on those quantities that may be observed at the time of tumor detection. The natural history of cancer is interrupted by the (random) event of detection and the question arises as to whether the clinical information available at the time of diagnosis can be utilized to estimate such characteristics.

The traditional approach to modeling of carcinogenesis and cancer detection tends to describe the process of tumor development in only one dimension, that is, in time. It is generally agreed that the period of tumor latency can conveniently be

Recent Advances in Quantitative Methods in Cancer and Human Health Risk Assessment
Edited by L. Edler and C. Kitsos © 2005 John Wiley & Sons, Ltd

divided into the following three stages:

- formation of initiated cells;
- promotion of initiated cells resulting in the first malignant clonogenic cell;
- subsequent tumor growth and progression until the event of detection occurs.

It should be noted that the third stage is also known as the preclinical stage, the term widely used in the literature on models of cancer screening. The length of each stage is treated as a random variable. The most popular two-stage models of carcinogenesis yield the distribution of the total duration of the first two stages. In theoretical exploration of such models as well as in numerous analyses of animal and human carcinogenesis, the period of tumor latency is interpreted as the sum of the two stages. It is not absolutely clear why an explicit description of the third stage, where cancer detection normally occurs, is typically obviated in stochastic models of carcinogenesis. Part of the explanation has to do with identifiability aspect of the problem.

The notion of identifiability is defined as follows. Let $g(t; \mathbf{z})$ be a probability density function with vector of unknown parameters $\mathbf{z}$. The model represented by $g(t; \mathbf{z})$ is said to be identifiable if the equality $g(t; \mathbf{z}_1) = g(t; \mathbf{z}_2)$ for all t implies $\mathbf{z}_1 = \mathbf{z}_2$. It is clear that a mathematical model whose parameters are not identifiable is of little utility in practical applications, because there may be (typically infinitely) many parameter combinations leading to the same probability density function. In terms of parameter estimation, non-identifiability manifests itself in the instability of estimation procedures.

In the context of stochastic models of carcinogenesis, let T be the time to the occurrence of the first malignant cell measured from the date of birth of an individual, and W the time to the event of tumor detection measured from the moment of tumor onset. In other words, T is the age at tumor onset, while $T + W$ is the age at tumor detection. Even assuming that T and W are independent, it is still a serious problem to find a practically useful and still realistic model incorporating both stages of the natural history of the disease. Indeed, to make sure that estimation of model parameters from time-to-tumor observations is feasible, one needs to answer the following question. Suppose $\mathcal{P}$ and $\mathcal{G}$ are two specific families of probability distributions on $[0, \infty)$ chosen for the random variables T and W. Assume, in addition, that T and W are independent and both families are identifiable. Is the family of convolutions $P * G$, where $P \in \mathcal{P}$ and $G \in \mathcal{G}$, identifiable? In other words, does $P_1 * G_1 = P_2 * G_2$, where $P_1, P_2 \in \mathcal{P}$ and $G_1, G_2 \in \mathcal{G}$, imply that $P_1 = P_2$ and $G_1 = G_2$?

It is sometimes not an easy task to check identifiability of a particular convolution. Bartoszyński *et al.* (2001) provide sufficient conditions that may be useful for this purpose. However, examples show that even for the most popular choices of $\mathcal{P}$ and $\mathcal{G}$ the above question remains unanswered. For example, suppose we specify the distribution of T using the Moolgavkar–Venzon–Knudson (MVK) model with constant (in time) parameters, properly reparameterized in terms of identifiable combinations of its basic parameters (Heidenreich, 1996; Hanin and Yakovlev, 1996; Heidenreich *et al.*, 1997), while choosing the Gompertz distribution for the random variable W as suggested by a quantal response model of cancer detection (see Section 19.2). These parametric families do not not satisfy the sufficient conditions given by Bartoszyński *et al.* (2001). This is not to say that the model represented by the convolution of the two distributions is necessarily non-identifiable, but the issue remains unresolved. Great care should be exercised when improving the structure of a specific model with the aim of achieving its identifiability. As discussed by Clayton and Schifflers (1987) in the context of the age–period–cohort model for cancer incidence, non-identifiability is not a purely methodological problem that needs only methodological advances in model building. All improvements in a given model should be biologically grounded and not just driven by the desire to overcome its non-identifiability.

An alternative idea is to invoke additional data relevant to the natural history of cancer. It is well known that increasing the dimension of the vector of observations may help overcome non-identifiability of a model by enriching the information to be analyzed. The process of tumor progression is multidimensional in nature (Zelen, 1968; Feldstein and Zelen, 1984) and cannot be reduced to a simple sequence of distinct stages. Therefore, it is possible to more efficiently extract the information on the natural history of cancer from the vector of clinical covariates recorded at the time of diagnosis if we are able to develop pertinent methods of statistical inference from such multivariate observations. In this chapter, we confine ourselves to just two important variables represented by tumor size and age of a patient at diagnosis. An analytic expression of the joint distribution of these stochastically dependent random variables can be derived (Bartoszyński *et al.*, 2001) within the framework of the so-called quantal response model that relates the rate of tumor detection to the current tumor size. The quantal response concept was introduced by Puri (1967, 1971; Puri and Senturia, 1972) as an alternative to threshold models of biological effects. This concept was developed further in the context of cancer detection by Bartoszyński and other authors (Atkinson *et al.*, 1983, 1987; Brown *et al.*, 1984; Bartoszyński, 1987; Klein and Bartoszyński, 1991); see also Bartoszyński *et al.* (2001) for further thoughts and results. The present chapter deals with statistical inference from bivariate data on tumor size and age at detection aimed at estimating the natural history of cancer. The focus of our study is to explore applied aspects of the proposed approach and illustrate its usefulness with an application to the relevant data on breast cancer available from the Utah Population Data Base linked to the Utah Cancer Registry.

19.2 THE MODEL

Let T be the age of an individual at tumor onset, and W the time of tumor detection measured from the onset time T. In the application reported in Section 19.3, use was made of the MVK model with constant parameters to specify the probability density function, $p_T(t)$, of the random variable T. The model is given by the following survival function

$$\bar{P}_T(t) := \Pr(T > t) = \left[\frac{(A + B)e^{At}}{B + Ae^{(A+B)t}}\right]^{\rho}, \qquad t \geq 0, \qquad (19.1)$$

from which the density $p_T(t)$ can be derived. In (19.1), ρ is the ratio of the initiation rate and the rate of proliferation of initiated cells, while A and B are parameters of the promotion time distribution. These parameters are identifiable from time-to-tumor observations. The MVK model has proven to provide a good fit to diverse data on animal and human carcinogenesis; see Gregori *et al.* (2001) for goodness-of-fit testing.

Introduce a random variable S to represent tumor size (the number of cells in a tumor) at detection. In practice, it is not the number of tumor cells S that is observable but the volume V in appropriate units, and one needs to change variables using the equality $S = V/c$, where c is the volume of a single tumor cell ($c \simeq 10^{-9}$ cm^3).

Suppose the law of tumor growth is described by a deterministic function f : $[0, \infty) \rightarrow [1, \infty)$ with $f(0) = 1$, so that $S = f(W)$. It is assumed, in addition, that

(1) random variables T and W are absolutely continuous and stochastically independent;

(2) function f is differentiable and $f' > 0$;

(3) the hazard rate for tumor detection is proportional to the current tumor size with coefficient $\alpha > 0$.

It follows from the above assumptions that

$$p_W(w) = \alpha f(w) e^{-\alpha \int_0^w f(u)du}, \qquad w \geq 0.$$

Therefore, we have

$$p_S(s) = \alpha s g'(s) e^{-\alpha \int_0^{g(s)} f(u)du}, \qquad s \geq 1,$$

where g stands for the inverse function for f : $g = f^{-1}$. In the case of deterministic exponential tumor growth with rate $\lambda > 0$ ($f(w) = e^{\lambda w}$) we obtain the following formulas:

$$p_S(s) = \frac{\alpha}{\lambda} e^{-\frac{\alpha}{\lambda}(s-1)}, \qquad s \geq 1, \qquad (19.2)$$

and

$$p_W(w) = \alpha e^{\lambda w - \frac{\alpha}{\lambda}(e^{\lambda w} - 1)}, \qquad w \geq 0. \qquad (19.3)$$

It is clear from (19.2) and (19.3) that, in this particular case, tumor size at detection S follows a translated exponential distribution with parameter α/λ, while the distribution of age at detection measured from the disease onset is a Gompertz distribution.

In a typical cohort study, we observe the random vector $\mathbf{Y} := (T + W, S)$ whose components are interpreted as age and tumor size at diagnosis, respectively. The probability density function of $\mathbf{Y}$ is given by

$$p_{\mathbf{Y}}(u, s) = p_T(u - g(s))p_S(s), \quad u \geq g(s), s \geq 1. \tag{19.4}$$

This distribution is known to be identifiable (Hanin, 2002). The above joint distribution specifies the structure of dependence between the random variables $U = T + W$ and S. In addition, it can be shown that U and S are positively correlated. Furthermore, the following lemma gives a lower bound for the covariance $\mathrm{cov}(U, S)$.

Lemma   The following lower bound for $\mathrm{cov}(U, S)$ holds true:

$$\mathrm{cov}(U, S) \geq C \, \mathrm{var}(W),$$

where $C := \inf\{f'(t) : t \geq 0\}$ is assumed to be a positive constant.

Proof   Notice that since the random variables T and W are assumed to be independent, the same is true for T and S. Hence we conclude that $\mathrm{cov}(T, S) = 0$. Therefore, $\mathrm{cov}(U, S) = \mathrm{cov}(W, S)$. Observe in addition that for any two random variables X and Y defined on the same probability space $(\Omega, \mathbb{P})$,

$$\mathrm{cov}(X, Y) = \mathbb{E}\{XY\} - \mathbb{E}\{X\}\mathbb{E}\{Y\}$$
$$= \frac{1}{2} \int_{\Omega \times \Omega} [X(\omega) - X(\omega')][Y(\omega) - Y(\omega')]d\mathbb{P}(\omega)d\mathbb{P}(\omega').$$

Therefore,

$$\mathrm{cov}(W, S) = \frac{1}{2} \int_{\Omega \times \Omega} [W(\omega) - W(\omega')][f(W)(\omega) - f(W)(\omega')]d\mathbb{P}(\omega)d\mathbb{P}(\omega').$$

By the mean value theorem in the case $W(\omega) \geq W(\omega')$, we have

$$f(W)(\omega) - f(W)(\omega') = f(W(\omega)) - f(W(\omega')) \geq C[W(\omega) - W(\omega')],$$

where $C = \inf\{f'(t) : t \geq 0\}$. This implies that, for all $\omega, \omega' \in \Omega$,

$$[W(\omega) - W(\omega')][f(W)(\omega) - f(W)(\omega')] \geq C[W(\omega) - W(\omega')]^2,$$

and consequently

$$\mathrm{cov}(U, S) \geq \frac{C}{2} \int_{\Omega \times \Omega} [W(\omega) - W(\omega')]^2 d\mathbb{P}(\omega)d\mathbb{P}(\omega') = C \, \mathrm{var}(W).$$

Suppose that tumor growth is exponential with (non-random) growth rate λ. Then it follows from (19.4) that the joint probability density $p_{\mathbf{Y}}(u, s)$ is of the form

$$p_{\mathbf{Y}}(u, s) = p_{U,S}(u, s) = \frac{\alpha}{\lambda} e^{-\frac{\alpha}{\lambda}(s-1)} p_T\left(u - \frac{\ln s}{\lambda}\right), \quad u \geq 0, 1 \leq s \leq e^{\lambda u}. \tag{19.5}$$

The model given by (19.5) can be generalized by assuming that some of its parameters are random. In particular, suppose $1/\lambda$ is gamma-distributed with parameters a and b. Then we have

$$p_{U,S}(u,s) = \frac{\alpha b^a}{(\ln s)^{a+1}\Gamma(a)} \int_0^u (u-x)^a \exp\left\{-\frac{b+\alpha(s-1)}{\ln s}(u-x)\right\}p_T(x)dx,$$

$$(19.6)$$

for $u \geq 0$, $s \geq 1$. In this case, the marginal distribution of tumor size is a Pareto distribution (Bartoszyński et al., 2001). Unfortunately, no theoretical results are available to check identifiability of the joint distribution (19.6) because the corresponding mathematical problem is very difficult to tackle. However, our simulation studies of the corresponding likelihood profiles have shown that the identifiability property established for the distribution (19.5) is preserved under the compounding procedure used to derive (19.6).

19.3   ESTIMATION OF MODEL PARAMETERS

The existing data sets on human cancers present with considerable amounts of censoring and missing tumor size information. Censoring is due to competing mortality and other random causes (such as the relocation of an individual) that preclude the event of cancer diagnosis from occurring during the follow-up period. Poor reporting procedures may result in missing tumor size information; in such cases we know the time of diagnosis, but the size of the detected tumor remains unknown. Let n be the sample size and denote by $\delta_i, i = 1, \ldots, n$, an indicator variable such that $\delta_i = 0$ if the ith observation is censored, $\delta_i = 1$ if the ith observation is exact, providing the information on (u_i, s_i), and $\delta_i = 2$ if the event of cancer detection at age u_i is recorded but the information on tumor size is missing. Based on the joint distribution (19.6) the likelihood function for the sample under consideration is of the form

$$L(\theta) = \prod_{i=1}^n p_{U,S}^{\delta_i(2-\delta_i)}(u_i, s_i \mid \theta)\, p_U^{\delta_i(\delta_i-1)/2}(u_i \mid \theta)\, \bar{P}_U^{(1-\delta_i)(2-\delta_i)/2}(u_i \mid \theta), \quad (19.7)$$

where $\bar{P}_U$ is the survival function for the marginal probability density p_U of age at detection, and $\theta = (\alpha, \rho, A, B, a, b)$ is the vector of unknown parameters.

Maximization of the likelihood given by (19.7) is a challenging problem because it involves many time-consuming computations. There may be many thousands of complicated double integrals representing the survival function $\bar{P}_U$ to be computed for all censored observations, for censoring is heavy in studies of this kind. Therefore, we resorted to simulations in order to estimate the contributions of censored data, rather than evaluating these integrals numerically. The simulation model generates individual histories of cancer development and detection in accordance with the postulates formulated in Section 19.2. The time of tumor onset was generated according to the distribution given by (19.1), while for the preclinical stage duration W the Gompertz distribution given by (19.3) was employed. The reciprocal of the growth rate was generated from a two-parameter gamma distribution. The survival function $\bar{P}_U$ and the probability density function p_U were estimated nonparametrically from the simulated data. The contributions of the exact pairs (u_i, s_i) were computed numerically in accordance with (19.6).

There is always a certain level of random noise in the simulated likelihood, calling for stochastic approximation methods to find a maximum of its expected value. Therefore, we used the Kiefer–Wolfowitz procedure (Pflug, 1996) to obtain maximum likelihood estimates. Unfortunately, when applied to the log-likelihood function the Kiefer–Wolfowitz procedure results in biased estimates and one needs to generate extremely large simulation samples to keep this bias to a minimum. For this reason, we provided 10^4 simulated samples when estimating $\bar{P}_U(u_i)$ and 10^6 samples when estimating $p(u_i)$ for each iteration of the Kiefer–Wolfowitz procedure employed in the application presented in the next section. In a separate set of simulation experiments, we assured ourselves that this sample size was sufficient for obtaining stable results.

An alternative method is a Monte Carlo EM (MCEM) algorithm, first proposed by Wei and Tanner (1990) (see also Chan and Ledolter, 1995; McLachlan and Krishnan, 1997). In the standard EM algorithm, the E step involves computing the conditional expectation of the log-likelihood for complete data given the observed data. In the MCEM algorithm, the conditional expectation of the log-likelihood is estimated by averaging the conditional log-likelihood functions of simulated sets of complete data. The MCEM algorithm does not possess the monotone convergence properties of the standard EM algorithm, but it has been shown by Chan and Ledolter (1995) that, under suitable regularity conditions, an MCEM sequence will, with high probability, get close to a maximizer of the likelihood of the observed data. We used the MCEM algorithm in addition to the Kiefer–Wolfowitz procedure applied to the simulated likelihood. Both methods resulted in very similar estimates. Therefore, we report only the results produced by the method of direct maximization of the (partially simulated) likelihood function given by (19.7).

19.4   DATA ANALYSIS

We obtained the data necessary for our analysis from the Utah Population Data Base (UPDB), which contains genealogical records that have been linked to cancer incidence and mortality data supplied by the Utah Cancer Registry (UCR). More than 1.3 million individuals are covered, all of whom were born, died, or married in Utah or *en route* to Utah during the nineteenth and twentieth centuries. Genealogy records are represented as families that have been linked across generations and, in some instances, the records encompass eight generations. The individuals in these records have been linked to other data sets, including cancer records, birth and death certificates, and Health Care Financing Administration records.

The Utah population differs little from most Caucasian populations, but it has generally had relatively low rates of breast cancer in comparison with the rest of the USA. The rates, about 15 % lower, are probably the result of reproductive factors such as large family sizes and early age at first pregnancy, or other lifestyle factors.

The UCR has been a component of the National Cancer Institute's Surveillance Epidemiology and End Results (SEER) program since its inception in 1973. Every incident cancer case diagnosed among residents of the state of Utah has been recorded in the UCR since 1966, and detailed extent-of-disease data are available from 1973 on. The UPDB has been successfully used to study familiality of cancer and the influence of reproductive factors on cancer risk. Pathologically confirmed and individually verified tumor size data has been a key part of the data collected by the SEER registries since the inception of the program. Since 1983, tumor diameter data have been available in millimeter units, with codes for missing data, no mass measurable, diffuse tumors, and tumors greater than 10 cm. The latest data (after 1987) provide the tumor diameter at diagnosis in millimeters, while older records give coarser intervals. To avoid computing additional integrals we decided to remove the data grouping by uniformly distributing the observations over each interval.

The study population consisted of people recorded in the UPDB who were born between 1918 and 1947 and for whom follow-up information is available that places them in Utah during the years of operation of the UCR. The analysis was performed on cohorts based on birth year. In particular, we looked at female breast cancer cases in five separate birth cohorts (B1, B2,...,B5) each encompassing a contiguous six-year period. More specifically, B1 is composed of the subpopulation of women whose birth date falls in the interval between 1918 and 1923, B2 includes all women born between 1924 and 1929, B3 covers the interval 1930–1935, B4 corresponds to the interval 1936–1941, and B5 to the interval 1942–1947. The relevant information on each birth cohort in the study population is given in Table 19.1.

Table 19.1 Data summary.

Birth cohort	Sample size	Number of exact observations	Primary tumors of unknown size
B1	16 677	960	368
B2	15 039	804	300
B3	12 884	576	185
B4	11 374	410	96
B5	13 437	333	79

In our analysis of the UPDB data, we proceeded from the distribution (19.6) assuming that the reciprocal of growth rate is gamma-distributed with mean $\mu = a/b$ and standard deviation $\sigma = \sqrt{a}/b$. As the UCR includes records since 1966, the likelihood (19.7) was modified in the usual way (Klein and Moeschberger, 1997) in order to incorporate left random truncation. Descriptive statistical analysis has shown a pronounced birth cohort effect manifesting itself in the behavior of breast cancer incidence in the population under study. If we allow the initiation rate ρ to vary among different birth cohorts, there will be five parameters ρ_1, ρ_2, ρ_3, ρ_4, ρ_5 forming the proportional hazards structure of the onset time distribution (see (19.1)). Therefore, we attributed the birth cohort effect to these parameters, as suggested by Boucher and Kerber (2001). The remaining parameters A, B, μ, σ and the sensitivity parameter α are common to all birth cohorts. Therefore, there are 10 parameters in total to be estimated from the data by the method of maximum likelihood. We obtained the following estimates: $\hat{\rho}_1 = 0.0384$, $\hat{\rho}_2 = 0.0472$, $\hat{\rho}_3 = 0.0552$, $\hat{\rho}_4 = 0.0584$, $\hat{\rho}_5 = 0.0613$, $\hat{A} = 7.5 \times 10^{-5}$, $\hat{B} = 0.1319$, $\hat{\mu} = 0.1422$, $\hat{\sigma} = 0.1291$, $\hat{\alpha} = 1.4570 \times 10^{-9}$. It is clear from these estimates that the birth cohort effect in terms of the parameter ρ is quite strong.

Since our analysis is limited to cases with known tumor sizes, the maximum likelihood estimates $\hat{\rho}_i$ cannot be used to model the total age-specific incidence: the model needs to be calibrated with respect to the parameter ρ to account for missing cases. The estimated values of all biologically meaningful parameters incorporated into the model give an exhaustive account of all components of the natural history of breast cancer, that is, the processes of initiation, promotion and preclinical development of the disease. Figure 19.1 displays the best-fit model in terms of the probability density function of tumor size and the hazard function of age at detection. Their nonparametric counterparts are also shown; it is clear that the model provides a very good fit to the histograms of tumor size and to the hazard functions estimated by (Epanechnikov) kernel smoothing techniques (Klein and Moeschberger, 1997) for all birth cohorts. Unfortunately, no theoretically based statistical tests are available to assess goodness of fit for the bivariate distribution given by (19.6), while parametric bootstrap techniques are computationally prohibitive with a model of such complexity.

A key assumption behind the model discussed in this chapter is that the random variables T and W are stochastically independent. At first glance it would seem that such an assumption is not plausible and the model could be generalized by making the growth rate (or the preclinical stage duration) dependent on the age of a patient at the time of tumor onset. However, if this were the case we would see variations in the distribution of tumor size at detection from one birth cohort to another. As is obvious from Figure 19.1, there is no tangible birth cohort effect on the nonparametrically estimated distribution of tumor size at detection. The Kruskal–Wallis test does not reject the global null hypothesis of no birth cohort effect as well. Therefore, the model does not call for any extension in this regard.

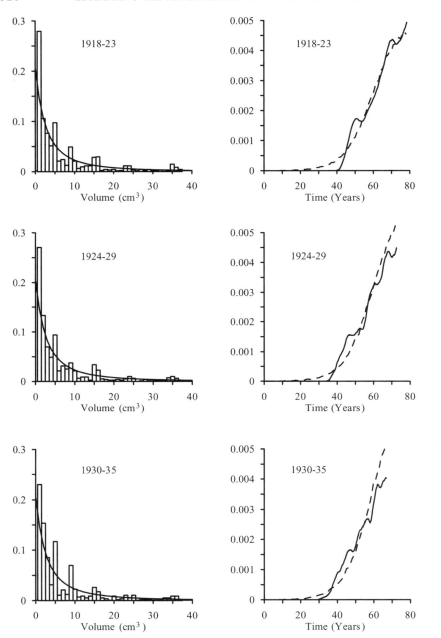

Figure 19.1 Parametric (left panels, solid lines; right panels, dashed lines) versus nonparametric estimates resulting from the analysis of five birth cohorts (B1, . . . ,B5). Left panels: probability distribution density of tumor size at diagnosis of breast cancer. Right panels: hazard function of age at diagnosis.

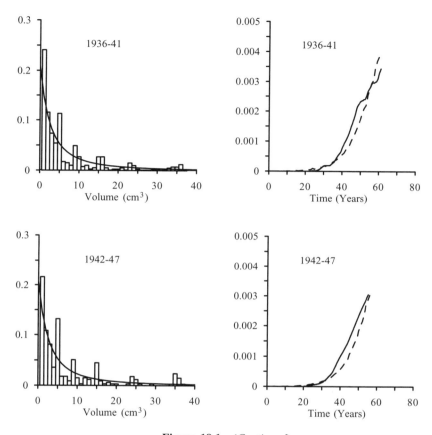

Figure 19.1   (*Continued*)

ACKNOWLEDGEMENTS

This paper was prepared when Dr. A. Yakovlev was visiting the Biostatistics Unit at the German Cancer Center (Heidelberg) with the support of the Alexander von Humboldt Foundation. The research was supported in part by NIH/NCI grant U01 CA88177-01 and Collaborative Linkage Grant NATO SA PST CLG 979045 under the NATO Science Programme. The analysis of epidemiological data was supported by the Utah Population Data Base and the Utah Cancer Registry funded by contract NO1-PC-67000 from the NCI with additional support from the Utah State Department of Health and the University of Utah.

PART VI

CASE STUDIES

Introductory remarks

Lutz Edler and Christos P. Kitsos

The beneficiaries of the use of mathematical modeling became clear for physics and engineering during the 19th century when the consequences of the industrial revolution were obvious and the need to find optimal solutions was recognized by the stakeholders of the related industries. In the mid-twentieth century it became clear that biology, economics, geography, sociology, medicine and psychology would also come to benefit from adopting mathematical modeling and statistical inference. The procedure for model solving can generally be organized into seven steps:

1. Formulate the model.

2. Define the assumptions for the model.

3. Describe the mathematical problem.

4. Solve the problem.

5. Interpret the solution.

6. Validate the model.

7. Use the model to explain, predict, and decide about the real phenomenon.

This procedure holds for a wide set of modeling approaches, deterministic as well as stochastic. In biology and medicine, deterministic modeling does not capture the real-life situation where the data are obscured by measurement errors. Therefore a statistical or a stochastic model is more appropriate than a solid deterministic mathematical solution function, but it is also more complex. Apart from modifications of the first three steps, stochastic modeling is to a large extent part of step 4 of the above procedure. It comprises the following steps:

Recent Advances in Quantitative Methods in Cancer and Human Health Risk Assessment
Edited by L. Edler and C. Kitsos © 2005 John Wiley & Sons, Ltd

4a. Construct the statistical model.

4b. Generate the experimental data.

4c. Fit the combined mathematical and statistical model to the data.

4d. Determine the parameter estimates and their uncertainty.

Part VI tries to bridge risk assessment methods with the analysis of real-life data. Most data arise from epidemiological studies where data analyses are obliged to develop new statistical strategies. We have included a small number of case studies covering a wide range of methods. This small selection may motivate practitioners to adopt other approaches, discussed here, for cancer risk assessment problems. Form the point of few of the data, the six case studies range from basic molecular data via clinical data on lung function and the neurophysiological system to cancer data on childhood leukemia, melanoma and thyroid carcinoma. From the methodological point of view, statistical methods for classification, discrimination and regression have always been among the most frequently used ones in the determination of risk factors. The method of logistic regression was already outlined earlier in Chapter 3 for the use in the assessment of lung cancer risk factors. Chapters 21 and 22 present more sophisticated applications of logistic regression and address the design problem as well as the question of unbiased estimation in the case of sparse data when asymptotics no longer prevail and therefore 'Exact' methods have to be applied.

The impact of radiation is an excellent example of the limitations of a study performed on a specific area population. Results for the area of Zaragoza (Spain) cannot be extrapolated to the population of Spain or of Europe as a whole, but still provide useful information for that area. For extrapolation to be considered, data are needed for other regions. The exposure to arsenic of a small but over time period highly contaminated area of Slovakia contrasts with the Spanish example by showing strong effects. On the other hand, this study demonstrates clearly the importance, and at the same time the intrinsic difficulties, of exposure measurement in epidemiological studies. Exposure can often only be measured indirectly, as in this example where the content of arsenic in the hair of a selected subpopulation served as sort of surrogate exposure value. A totally new development, which may impact all aspects of risk assessment, including the exposure assessment and factors influencing individual exposure, is that of the measurement of individual genomic data.

The Korean example of the search for a set of differentially expressed genes which are correlated with different colorectal tumor types gives an introduction to the forthcoming data analysis problems of the analysis of genomic data. Methodologically, the search for a predictive set of genes is not so far from the search for the best predictive covariates in the Polish example of standard clinical data on childhood leukemia, where classification, discrimination and regression were applied.

Finally, when statistical data analysis is used to predict risks and is eventually used to determine risk parameter estimates which may be used to set up regulatory standards, one should critically assess the statistical modeling approach as outlined in steps 4a–4d above. The following six questions provide a checklist which is helpful for an examination of the appropriateness and correctness of this statistical task:

1. Was the statistical techniques adequate for analyzing the data?
2. Was an optimal design approach adopted?
3. Was the model useful and the software appropriate?
4. Were rival models and situations considered and discussed?
5. Has the particular biological, medical, etc. case been sufficiently studied?
6. Were all data considered?

We would like to encourage the reader to check for him/herself how far the case studies of this part have complied with these requirements and to use this knowledge when he/she gets involved in quantitative risk assessment tasks in the future.

CHAPTER 20

Statistical Issues in the Search for Biomarkers of Colorectal Cancer Using Microarray Experiments

Byung-Soo Kim, Sunho Lee, Inyoung Kim, Sangcheol Kim, Sun Young Rha and Hyun Cheol Chung

Yonsei University

Sunho Lee

Sejong University

20.1 INTRODUCTION

DNA microarray technology has been established as a major tool for high-throughput analysis which measures the expression levels of thousands of genes simultaneously. The simultaneous monitoring of so many genes made it possible to characterize tissue specimens at the most basic level, namely, that of the genes. Its implications for cancer research are considerable. The results can be used to accurately diagnose and molecularly classify tumors (Golub *et al.*, 1999; Alizadeh *et al.*, 2000; Sørlie *et al.*, 2001; Yeoh *et al.*, 2002; Dyrskjot *et al.*, 2003), assess their risk of metastasis (van't Veer *et al.*, 2002), develop molecular prognostic predictors for survival (Rosenwald *et al.*, 2002; Vasselli *et al.*, 2003) and identify genes that correlate with sensitivity/resistance to anticancer drugs (Kihara *et al.*, 2001; Chang *et al.*, 2003). It is a new statistical challenge to analyze the data from microarray experiments, not simply because they involve large amount of data, but because they comprise a nonstandard statistical problem which is often referred to as a

Recent Advances in Quantitative Methods in Cancer and Human Health Risk Assessment
Edited by L. Edler and C. Kitsos © 2005 John Wiley & Sons, Ltd

'large p, small n' problem (West, 2003); we have p explanatory variables (genes), n sampling units, and $p \gg n$. Therefore, standard statistical methods do not handle these data effectively. For a tutorial on the microarray experiment, see Nguyen *et al.* (2002); for a recent review of statistical problems, Speed (2003) and Parmigiani *et al.* (2003) would be good references. A microarray movie (520 MB file) prepared by W. Huber, G. Sawitzki and H. Sültmann at the German Cancer Research Center is available for free download at www.dkfz-heidelberg.de/abt0840/whuber/.

One of the major aims of microarray experiments is to isolate a few genes that discriminate between cancer and normal tissues by searching for biomarkers of the specific cancer that can be used in population screening. Pepe *et al.* (2003) elegantly used the receiver operating characteristic curve to address this problem. The goal of cancer screening is to detect tumors sufficiently early that a successful treatment can be administered. A substance secreted by tumor tissue, not secreted by nontumor tissue, and easily detectable in serum or urine is an ideal biomarker. Furthermore, for the cancer screening the false positive probability should be maintained at a very low level, because even with a small false positive probability a large number of people are subject to unnecessary diagnostic procedures which involve psychological and physical stresses. The risk assessment will be a major issue in the final stage of population screening of colorectal cancer. However, at this stage of screening genes for biomarker development we will not deal with the risk assessment issue, but will provide necessary prerequisities for this future task. The aim of our study is to identify a set of differentially expressed (DE) genes in colorectal cancer, compared with normal colorectal tissues, to evaluate the predictivity of a new specimen and to rank genes for the development of biomarkers for population screening of colorectal cancer.

Colorectal cancer is one of the most common causes of cancer-related death in developed countries. Long-term decline in colorectal cancer incidence has been shown since mid-1990s. Early detection of precancerous colorectal polyps prevents progression to invasive cancer, which is considered one of the contributing factors of the long-term decline. Therefore, it is essential to discover lesions early in their neoplastic evolution. Characterization of gene expressions associated with colorectal cancer is crucial to understand the cellular and molecular process of colorectal cancer pathogenesis. Traditional studies showed that a number of genes, including *APC* (Powell *et al.*, 1992), *k-ras* (Forrester *et al.*, 1987), *p53* (Baker *et al.*, 1989), *HER-2/neu* (Kapitanovic *et al.*, 1997) and *Wnt-2* (Vider *et al.*, 1996), were involved in colorectal cancer carcinogenesis. However, it is important to monitor thousands of genes simultaneously, instead of a handful of genes one by one, to understand the common pathway of carcinogenesis and progression of colorectal cancer. Several high-throughput technologies, including serial analysis of gene expression (SAGE), array-based comparative genomic hybridization (CGH) and microarray gene expression, have been developed for this purpose. Of these, microarray gene expression technology is the most accurate and comprehensive way of simultaneously analyzing the mRNA expression of thousands of genes. Microarray technology was driven by the explosive proliferation of the microtechnology itself. The development of Affymetrix's GeneChip® contributed to the easy and wide availability of the microarray technology. A number of studies have already employed microarray gene expressions to investigate the molecular behavior of various cancers, including liver (Okabe *et al.*, 2001), breast (Perou *et al.*, 2000), stomach (Oien *et al.*, 2003), lung (Wikman *et al.*, 2002) and colorectal cancers (Zou *et al.*, 2002; Williams *et al.*, 2003).

In Section 20.2 we describe the experiment and the structure of our data, which consist of a set of paired observations and two independent sets of observations. We also raise statistical issues relevant to the data set. In Section 20.3 we compare three statistical procedures for detecting a set of DE genes from the training set and then we validate the chosen set of DE genes by using them for classifying the test set. In the context of detecting DE genes we propose a new method of using Hotelling's T^2 statistic. We also propose using a new statistic (t_3), based on the t statistic, as a means of detecting DE genes for data sets which are a mixture of paired observations and two independent sets of observations. A discussion concludes the chapter.

20.2 EXPERIMENTS, DATA AND STATISTICAL ISSUES

Cancer and normal tissues were obtained from 58 colorectal cancer patients who underwent surgery at Severance Hospital, Yonsei Cancer Center, Yonsei University College of Medicine, Seoul, Korea, from May to December 2002. Basic patients characteristics are shown in Table 20.1. The fresh samples were snap-frozen in liquid nitrogen right after resection and stored at $-70\,^{\circ}\mathrm{C}$ until required.

Table 20.1 Clinical characteristics of patients ($n = 58$).

Gender	Male: Female 32:26
Age (years)	Median (range) 65 (28–90)
20–29	1
30–39	3
40–49	4
50–59	12
60–69	26
70–79	11
≥ 80	1
Tumor location	
Colon	20
Rectum	29
Sigmoid	9
Dukes stage	
B	23
C	27
D	8

We originally attempted to extract total RNAs from tumor and normal tissues from all patients. From each of 20 patients we had RNA specimens both for tumor and normal tissues. However, from 16 patients RNA specimens for normal tissues only were available. From another 22 patients RNA specimens for tumor only were obtainable. Thus, we have a matched pair sample of size 20 and two independent samples of sizes 16 and 22. We conducted a cDNA microarray experiment using a common reference design with 17K human cDNA microarrays. We pooled 11 cancer cell lines from various origins and used this as our common reference. After total RNAs were extracted from fresh frozen tissues, the specimens were labeled and hybridized to cDNA microarrays based on the standard protocol established at the Cancer Metastasis Research Center (CMRC), Yonsei University College of Medicine. We used $M=\log_2(R/G)$ for the evaluation of relative intensity, where R and G represent the cy5 and cy3 fluorescent intensities, respectively. A laser scanner measures two fluorescent dye intensities by emitting excitation light of different wave lengths. A photo multiplier tube converts the emitted photon into electric current, and finally an analog to digital converter is used to convert the electrons into a sequence of digital signals of which the range is from 0 to $2^{16}-1$. Thus, both R and G may take integer values between 0 and 65 535. Quantitative real-time reverse transcription polymerase chain reaction (RT-PCR) assay was performed with six selected genes using a Rotor Gene 2072D real-time PCR machine (Corbett Research, Australia) following the manufacture's instructions. We used SYBR Green (Quiagen, CA, USA) for the labeling. The amplified fluorescence signal was measured and the level of transcript of each specimen was calculated based on the standard curve. The standard curve was drawn by plotting the measured threshold cycle versus the arbitrary unit of copies/reaction according to the amount of serially diluted standard RNA. The threshold cycle (Ct) value was determined as the cycle number at which the fluorescence exceeded the threshold value.

20.2.1 Preprocessing the data

We conducted two cDNA microarray experiments, firstly on the matched pair sample of size 20 and secondly on the two independent samples of sizes 16 and 22. One easy way of utilizing all the information in the matched pair data set and two independent data sets would be to use the matched pair sample for the training set for detecting DE genes and the two independent samples for the test set for validating the chosen DE genes. By detecting a set of DE genes in the training set of matched pairs we could control the between individual variation. The independence within and between the two samples of sizes 16 and 22 would make them the ideal test set. We define the no missing proportion (NMP) of a gene as the proportion of valid observations out of the total number of arrays. For example, if a gene has valid observations for 32 arrays out of 40, its NMP is 0.8. We preprocessed the data in the following order:

1. We normalized the log intensity ratio ($\log_2 R/G$) using within-print tip group, intensity-dependent normalization following Yang *et al.* (2002).

2. We used 0.8 and 0.7 as NMP cut points to delete genes from the training and the test sets, respectively. We used slightly different cut points to balance the number of genes at $\sim$13 500 both for the training and the test set. Genes were deleted simultaneously within the training set and also within the test set. However, due to different NMP values in the training set and the test set, genes were not deleted simultaneously in all three data sets.

3. We employed the k-nearest-neighbor ($k=10$) method for the imputation of missing values.

4. We averaged values for multiple spots. The numbers of duplicated, triplicated, and quadruplicated spots were 1329, 10, and 5, respectively.

5. We merged the training set and the test set. We ended up with a data set represented by a $12\,311 \times 78$ matrix, where 12 311 represents the number of genes and 78 stands for the number of microarrays. We investigated various box plots (not shown) after the (location parameter) normalization and concluded that it was not necessary to have the scale normalization either between blocks within an array or between arrays.

20.2.2 Data structure and notation

We define notation for the data and then clarify the structure of the data. For the 20 patients in the matched pair data set let $\{(X_i, Y_i)\}_{i=1}^{20}$ represent the data, where X_i and Y_i denote M-values for the common reference versus normal tissue hybridization and the common reference versus tumor hybridization, respectively, for the ith patient. For the 16 patients from whom RNA specimens for normal tissue only are available we observe M-values only for the common reference versus normal tissue hybridizations and this M-value is denoted by U, which has the same marginal distribution as X ($=X_1$). For the 22 patients from whom RNA specimens for tumor only are available we also have 22 M-values only for the common reference versus tumor hybridizations, which is represented by V. V has the same distribution as Y ($=Y_1$). Thus, we have three data types as shown in Table 20.2.

Table 20.2 Three data types of the experiment. X and Y represent log intensity ratios for common reference vs normal and common reference vs tumor hybridizations, respectively. U and V have the same distribution as X and Y, respectively.

Hybridization		
Common reference vs normal	Common reference vs tumor	Number of cases
X	Y	20 (n_1)
U	missing	16 (n_2)
missing	V	22 (n_3)

20.2.3 Statistical issues

As a means of utilizing the entire data sets we first use the matched pair data set as a training set from which we detect a set of DE genes between the normal tissue and the tumor. Then we use the pool of two independent data sets $\{U_i\}_{i=1}^{16}$ and $\{V_j\}_{j=1}^{22}$ as the test set for validating the chosen set of DE genes. We employ the following three procedures for detecting a set of DE genes from the matched pair sample of size 20:

    (i)   paired t test and Dudoit *et al.*'s max T procedure for controlling the family-wise error rate (FWER) (Dudoit *et al.*, 2002b; Ge *et al.*, 2003);

    (ii) Tusher *et al.*'s SAM procedure (Tusher *et al.*, 2001);

    (iii) Lönnstedt and Speed's empirical Bayes procedure using B statistics (Lönnstedt and Speed, 2002).

Dudoit *et al.* (2002b) employed the FWER to control the Type I error and used Westfall and Young's step-down procedure for calculating the adjusted p-value. We have 2^{20} sign change permutations for the paired t statistic for 20 patients from which we can derive the null distribution of the paired t statistic. We used, however, 100 000 bootstrap samples of size 20, due to computation limitations, to derive the null distribution of the paired t statistic. Tusher *et al.*'s SAM procedure is a permutation test with a modified t statistic. They adopted the false discovery rate (FDR: Benjamini and Hochberg, 1995) for controlling the Type I error, the FDR being defined as the number of false positive genes divided by the number of genes declared significant. The FDR is more sensitive in detecting significant genes (Ge *et al.*, 2003). We set $k=10$ when we use the k-nearest-neighbor method for imputing missing values and fix the number of permutations at 5000 in running the SAM program. Lönnstedt and Speed (2002) used the empirical Bayes method to derive a Bayes log posterior odds, B. The experimenter may take the top 100 genes in terms of B values in combination with experimental preference.

We can adopt and modify the standard methods as follows for the data set at hand. As an initial attempt at employing a multivariate method we propose using Hotelling's T^2 statistic for the detection of a set of DE genes. We propose a t-based statistic, say t_3, which combines three data types for the detection of DE genes.

20.3   RESULTS

We employed univariate procedures (i)–(iii) to detect DE genes in colorectal cancers compared with normal colorectal tissues based on the matched pair data set of size 20. We noted that these three procedures yielded more or less same set of DE genes. We classified the test set as a validation of the chosen set of DE genes and observed that only a few genes were required to achieve the 0 % test error. As an initial attempt at using a multivariate procedure we employed Hotelling's T^2

statistic by pairing two genes in all possible ways and found that the list of the top 25 pairs had less than 40 % overlap with the top 50 gene list of the univariate t statistic. Finally, we proposed a t-based statistic, t_3, as a means of combining the paired data set and two independent data sets of Table 20.2.

20.3.1 Detecting differentially expressed genes based on the matched pair data set

Even for the FWER of 0.01 using procedure (i) we were able to detect more than 700 genes for the differential expression, which far exceeds the number of candidate genes for the biomarker development for colorectal cancer screening. Using each of three procedures we were able to detect the top 100 genes. These three procedures coincide reasonably well with each other, as Figure 20.1 shows. From now on we rank the genes according to the significance of the p-values which are computed by procedure (i).

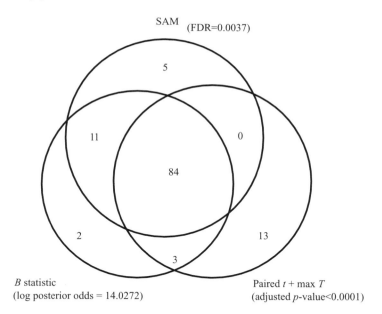

Figure 20.1   Overlap pattern of differentially expressed genes detected by three procedures: Dudoit *et al.*'s t test and max T procedure; Tusher *et al.*'s SAM; and Lönnstedt and Speed's B statistic. The number in each intersection indicates the number of genes jointly detected by two or three procedures.

20.3.2 Classifying the test set: validating the chosen set of differentially expressed genes

We restricted ourselves to the top 50 genes for the classification of the test set which comprised 16 normal and 22 tumor specimens. The experimenter thought that 50 was the maximum number of genes for which she could perform the confirmatory experiments. Using these 50 genes we employed diagonal quadratic discriminant analysis (DQDA) for the classification. We found that only the top 5 genes were required to achieve a 0 % test error.

Dudoit *et al.* (2002a) showed that diagonal linear discrimnant analysis (DLDA) yielded the lowest test error rate even with its simplicity when they compared several discriminant methods, including DQDA, using lymphoma, leukemia and NCI 60 data sets. We found in this colorectal cancer data set that DQDA needed only the top 5 genes to achieve 0 % test error, whereas DLDA required the top 7 genes. Our data set, which consists of tumors and normal tissues, is more heterogeneous than the data sets used by Dudoit *et al.* (2002a). This heterogeneity motivated us to use different variances for two groups in our DQDA, and it turned out to be more efficient than DLDA.

20.3.3 Hotelling's T^2 Statistic

We computed Hotelling's T^2 statistic by pairing two genes in all possible ways from the training set and obtained the top 25 pairs in order of magnitude. It is interesting to note that this list of 25 pairs has less than 40 % overlap with the top 50 gene list of the univariate t statistic. Hotelling's T^2 statistic (Anderson, 2003) for a pair of genes is a function of several parameters including the correlation coefficient (ρ). It takes a large value when at least one of two genes in a pair has a large t statistic and $|\rho|$ is large with $t_1 t_2 \rho < 0$, where t_1 and t_2 refer to t statistics for two genes in a pair. Therefore, the T^2 statistic can detect some of genes that are not detected by the univariate t test, such as gene 1' in Table 20.3, but has high correlation with a gene of a very large t value. We ranked gene pairs by T^2 statistic. We employed DQDA for classifying the test set based on the list of top 25 pairs and found that the top 3 pairs in Table 20.3 were sufficient to yield 0 % test error.

Table 20.3 Top 3 pairs of genes selected by Hotelling's T^2 statistic.

Gene	Hotelling's T^2 statistic	Univariate t statistic	Correlation
1	1403.9	18.6	−0.82
1'		3.5	
2	1400.6	17.2	0.78
2'		−7.6	
3	1174.1	−18.8	0.61
3'		11.4	

Table 20.3 shows Hotelling's T^2 and related statistics for the top 3 pairs of genes. Figure 20.2 shows that genes 1' and 2' have small t values but have high correlations with genes of large t values. Genes 1, 2, and 3 in Table 20.3 are contained in the top 5 genes of Section 20.3.2 found by DQDA and the univariate t statistic.

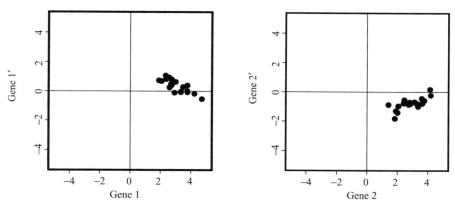

Figure 20.2   Scatter plots of two pairs of genes detected by Hotelling's T^2 statistic in Table 20.3. Each dot represents an ordered pair of log intensity ratios for two genes.

This result implies that single gene-based analyses may not detect interesting information. One of the explanations of this observation is that tumor and normal tissues are well separated in a higher dimension, whereas this separation is not realized when we make a projection of the higher-dimensional gene profile into each gene coordinate. Pairs of this kind will not be detected by a standard univariate method since one of the genes may have a small absolute t value.

20.3.4   A t-based statistic t_3

To detect a DE gene on the basis of a univariate t statistic we propose the following t_3 statistic as a means of pooling matched pair and two independent data sets. Following the notation in Table 20.2, we define $D_i = X_i - Y_i, i = 1, \ldots, n_1$. Let S_D^2, S_U^2 and S_V^2 be sample variances based on $\{D_i\}_{i=1}^{n_1}$, $\{U_j\}_{j=1}^{n_2}$, and $\{V_t\}_{t=1}^{n_3}$, respectively. Then, under the hypothesis that a specific gene is not differentially expressed, the following t_3 statistic has an approximate $N(0,1)$ distribution for large n_1, n_2 and n_3.

$$t_3 = \frac{n_1 \overline{D} + n_H (\overline{U} - \overline{V})}{\sqrt{n_1 S_D^2 + n_H^2 \left[\frac{1}{n_2} S_U^2 + \frac{1}{n_3} S_V^2\right]}} \tag{20.1}$$

where the 'bar' notation denotes the sample mean and n_H is the harmonic mean of n_2 and n_3. The prediction accuracy gained by pooling the matched pair and two independent data sets will be presented in a separate communication.

20.4   DISCUSSION

Once a small set of differentially expressed genes is identified from gene expression data, it is important to verify the significance of these genes at the transcriptional

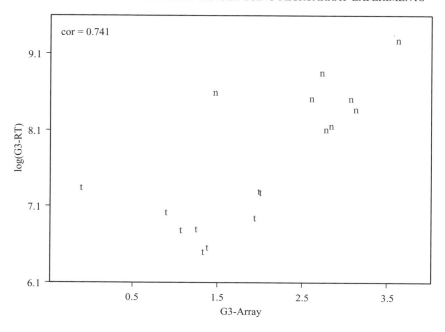

Figure 20.3   Scatter plot of real-time RT PCT versus microarray gene expression levels (log scale). 'n' and 't' stand for normal tissue and tumor, respectively.

level through real-time RT PCR or at the translational level with a tissue microarray. We performed real-time RT PCR assays on the top six genes based on 17 mRNA specimens (nine tumors and eight normal tissues) and obtained 'reasonable' concordance between two assays. Figure 20.3 shows a plot of real-time RT PCR measurements and gene expression levels both on the log scale for gene 3. Statistical analyses on the concordance between two assays will be reported in a separate communication.

The missing observations in Table 20.2 occurred primarily due to insufficient RNA extractions from specimens. One can consider pooling mRNA from several different specimens and then running technical replicates of the pool. It is unclear how to analyze the gene expression data which consist of unpooled and pooled mRNA extractions. Pooling – in particular, whether pooling improves efficiency even when it is not necessary – is a controversial issue. Kendziorsky et al. (2003) indicates that under certain circumstances pooling may lead to a gain efficiency. But the gain attained by pooling may not outweigh the loss of ability to observe the biological variability (Yang and Speed, 2003).

Recently Pepe et al. (2003) described an elegant piece of work of identifying genes using the receiver operating characteristic (ROC) curve for the development of biomarkers of ovarian cancers that can be used for population screening. Their data consist of independent observations whereas ours include paired observations.

The extension of Pepe *et al.*'s ROC curve method to our data set is a matter requiring further research.

In employing Hotelling's T^2 statistic in the present work, we did not have a formal test procedure. The development of a formal test procedure for detecting DE genes in terms of Hotelling's T^2 statistic or its robust version (Willems *et al.*, 2001) requires further research. We considered Hotelling's T^2 statistic for a pair of genes, denoted by $T^2_{(2)}$. Before extending it to $T^2_{(k)}$ for $k \geq 3$ genes, which requires intensive computation, it needs to be confirmed that this multivariate approach really does lead to gains in some important aspects that the univariate approach misses.

ACKNOWLEDGEMENTS

B.S. Kim's research was supported by a grant from the Korea Health 21 R&D Project, Ministry of Health and Welfare, Republic of Korea (02-PJ1-PG3-10411-00-03). S.H. Lee's work was supported by grant R04-203-000-10145-0 from the Basic Research Program of the Korea Science and Engineering Foundation. H.C. Chung and S.Y. Rha's work was supported by the Korea Science and Engineering Foundation (KOSEF) through the Cancer Metastasis Research Center (CMRC) at Yonsei University College of Medicine.

CHAPTER 21

Optimal Experimental Designs for Prediction of Morbidity after Lung Resection

Jesus F. López Fidalgo, Sandra A. Garcet Rodríguez
and Gonzálo Varela

University of Salamanca

21.1 MEDICAL PROBLEM

Pulmonary resection can be safely performed in patients with compromised pulmonary function if they are selected appropriately. Apart from simple preoperative pulmonary function tests, more sophisticated studies of cardiopulmonary function have been recommended to predict both postoperative mortality and morbidity. Exercise testing in the preoperative risk evaluation of lung resection candidates provides an integrated view of fitness of the respiratory and cardiovascular systems. There are some techniques that provide good indicators, but they are rather expensive and not available in many centers. Simple exercise tests have been advocated for years but some of them, such as walking and stair-climbing tests, lack standardization. Recently, it has been claimed that standardized preoperative exercise oximetry predicts postpneumonectomy outcome (Ninan *et al.*, 1997). Rao *et al.* (1995) establish that exercise oximetry is more accurate than preoperative forced expiratory volume in the first second (FEV1) to predict outcome in high-risk cases.

Recent Advances in Quantitative Methods in Cancer and Human Health Risk Assessment
Edited by L. Edler and C. Kitsos © 2005 John Wiley & Sons, Ltd

On the other hand, Kearney *et al.* (1994) found that desaturation on exercise is not a good predictor of cardiorespiratory risk after lung resection.

Varela *et al.* (2001) evaluated whether desaturation on standardized exercise can be used as an independent variable to predict postoperative cardiorespiratory morbidity when the effects of other potential risk factors are controlled by multivariate analysis. They worked with a population of 112 lung carcinoma patients scheduled for pulmonary resection. Patients who underwent exploratory or staging procedures or pulmonary resection performed by a video-assisted technique without thoracotomy and patients unable to perform a preoperative exercise test were excluded. The remaining 81 cases were included in a prospective observational clinical study. The selection criteria for operation included the absence of major co-morbidity refractory to medical therapy, PO_2 at rest over 50 mmHg, PCO_2 under 46 mmHg and predicted postoperative FEV1% (ppoFEV1) over 30 % of the standard value, measured as a percentage of the expected values for sex, age and height. Calculation of the ppoFEV1% was based on the number of non-obstructed pulmonary segments to be resected. Smoker patients were asked to stop smoking two weeks before surgery to avoid errors in estimating O_2 saturation. The absence of significant levels of blood carboxyhemoglobin was assessed by invasive arterial gasometry before admission. The day before operation, patients were asked to perform an incremental cycle ergometer protocol to exhaustion. Exercise started at 35 W and the power increased by 35 W every 3 min. Patients were encouraged to maintain a constant cycling cadence of 60/min. The test was interrupted after 12 min or before if the patient presented extreme dyspnea or fatigue, bradycardia, hypotension, electrocardiogram (ECG) ischemic changes or angina. Finger oximetry (by means of a calibrated Nonin 8600 pulse oximeter) and ECG were continuously monitored during the test and the occurrence of desaturation (cut-off value 90 %) at any time was recorded.

The independent variables included in the analysis were: age of the patient, body-mass index (BMI), presence or absence of cardiovascular co-morbidity, ppoFEV1 value (percentage of the expected values specific for sex, age and height) and presence or absence of desaturation during exercise test. The outcome considered was the occurrence of cardiorespiratory morbidity after surgery. Any of the following postoperative events were considered: pulmonary atelectasis or pneumonia, respiratory or ventilatory insufficiency at discharge (PO_2 under 60 mmHg or PCO_2 over 45 mmHg), need of mechanical ventilation at any time after extubation in the operating room, pulmonary thromboembolism, arrhythmia, myocardial ischemia or infarct and clinical cardiac insufficiency. Risk calculations (odds ratio with 95 % confidence interval) were carried out. Seventy-one cases were male and 10 were female. A lobectomy was performed in 62 cases, a pneumonectomy in 16 and a segmentectomy in 3. The mean age of patients was 63.6 years (standard deviation (SD) 10.3), the mean BMI was 25.9 (SD 4.9), and the mean ppoFEV1% was 64.1 (SD 20.4). Thirty-five patients presented cardiovascular co-morbidity: abnormal ECG (16 cases), hypertension (15 cases), cardiac arrhythmia (10 cases), coronary disease (4 cases), peripheral arterial disease (3 cases), previous pulmonary embolism or stroke (2 cases each) or cardiac insufficiency (1 case). Desaturation during exercise was found in 14 cases and was not related to low ppoFEV1%. In no case was the test stopped because of cardiocirculatory symptoms or ECG abnormalities. Thirty-two patients presented one or more cardiopulmonary complications. Respiratory insufficiency occurred in 12 patients (one needed mechanical ventilation), seven patients presented one or more episodes of atelectasis, another seven had clinical cardiac insufficiency (one with pulmonary edema), six patients were diagnosed with postoperative arrhythmia and five patients had a nosocomial pneumonia. The overall mortality was 6.1 %. On univariate analysis the probability of cardiorespiratory postoperative morbidity was higher in patients having low ppoFEV1% (odds ratio 7.1, $p < 0.001$) while an advanced age, high BMI, co-morbidity and exercise desaturation were unrelated to postoperative cardiorespiratory morbidity.

The design used by Varela *et al.* (2001) was unable to find significance in the exercise desaturation in order to predict postoperative cardiorespiratory morbidity. A better design would confirm whether this exercise is useful for making the decision to do surgery in a particular patient.

The motivation of this chapter is the utility of finding a good experimental design to predict cardiopulmonary morbidity after lung resection with standardized exercise oximetry. It will be shown that this design could save significant numbers of patients, while obtaining the same or better results. Three kinds of variables are considered: variables under the control of the experimenter, variables not under the control of the practitioner and with known values before the experiment is performed, and variables not under the control of the practitioner and with values unknown before the experiment is realized. An iterative algorithm is proposed for constructing optimal designs for a logistic morbidity prediction model for a cardiopulmonary problem.

21.2   PREDICTION MODEL AND ADVANTAGE OF DESIGNING THE EXPERIMENT

The main variables considered in Varela *et al.* (2001) are the 'percentage of maximum volume of expired air' (x_1), 'oxygen desaturation during the test' (x_2) and the 'exercise time in minutes' (x_3). Variable x_3 is completely under the control of the experimenter, in the sense that he or she can choose the exercise time for each patient. Variable x_1 is not subject to control, but its values are known before the exercise test is performed. As a matter of fact there is already a sample and the respiratory function is measured on each patient. Variable x_2 is not under control and is observed only during the exercise test. This means that in order to choose an exercise time for each patient the respiratory function can be taken into account, but not the desaturation measured after the exercise. From a statistical point of view this variable has to be treated carefully in order to produce correct results. The main objective was to predict cardiorespiratory morbidity after lung resection in surgery. This outcome was considered as a binary response variable Y since its presence or absence is clinically associated to mortality, the most important outcome in major surgical procedures. The results obtained from this study would be useful when a decision about possible surgery is to be made. A logistic model was considered for the probability of having complications after surgery:

$$p(Y = 1; x, \theta) = \frac{1}{1 + e^{-(\theta_1 x_1 + \theta_2 x_2 + \theta_3 x_3)}}.$$

This probability is a measure of the risk of surgery in a particular patient from his or her percentage of maximum volume of expired air, oxygen desaturation during the test and exercise time in minutes.

As mentioned above, an important point is to provide optimal exercise times for each patient in order to predict cardiopulmonary morbidity after lung resection with standardized exercise oximetry. Three kinds of surgery can be performed, depending on the amount of lung resected: lobectomy, pneumonectomy and segmentectomy. The kind of resection is decided during surgery. In the Varela *et al.* (2001) study, no correlation was found between postoperative morbidity and the age of the patient, BMI, and co-morbidity.

Then the logistic model provides a tool to measure the risk of complications after surgery and making the decision to perform surgery or not. Figure 21.1 shows an example of the risk logistic probability for values of ppoFEV1, using

$$p(Y = 1; x) = \frac{1}{1 + e^{-0.34 + 0.022 FEV1}}.$$

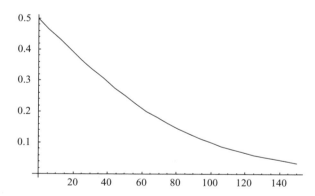

Figure 21.1 Logistic probability of morbidity after lung resection against percentage of respiratory function.

21.3 OPTIMAL EXPERIMENTAL DESIGN APPROACH

Let $f'(x) = (f_1(x), \ldots, f_m(x))$ denote a vector of m linearly independent continuous functions on some compact space X. A single observation consists of selecting an x in X and observing a random variable Y at x with regression function $E(Y|x) = \beta_1 f_1(x) + \ldots + \beta_m f_m(x)$ and constant variance σ^2. The function f is assumed known and σ unknown. An *(exact) experimental design* is a collection of n points $x_1, x_2, \ldots, x_m$, some of them eventually repeated. These n points are the experimental conditions at which the experiments are being performed. It is useful from a computational point of view to consider an experimental design as a probability measure ξ on X *(approximate experimental design)*. The set of all experimental designs will be denoted by Ξ. This idea comes from the fact that an exact design may be seen as a set of different points of the design jointly with the proportions of responses observed at each point $\xi(x_i) = n_i/n$, where n_i is the number of repetitions of x_i in the design. An exact design specifies that the experimenter has to take n_i observations at x_i, $\Sigma_i n_i = n$. From a practical point of view only designs with finite support are allowed. In this paper approximate designs with finite support will be considered.

If uncorrelated observations can be assumed, the covariance matrix of the least-squares estimate of θ is $\sigma^2 n^{-1} \mathbf{M}^{-1}(\xi)$, where $\mathbf{M}(\xi) = \Sigma_{x \in \chi} f(x) f'(x) \xi(x)$ is the *information matrix*. Let M be the compact set of information matrices. The superscript $+$ in any set will refer to the nonsingular information matrices. The *support* of a design, S_ξ, is the set of points of X with positive masses.

The objective is to find optimal designs making the inverse of the information matrix 'small'. Many different criterion functions $\Phi[M(\xi)]$ have been defined in the set of information matrices. A Φ-optimal design ξ^* will be a design minimizing $\Phi[M(\xi)]$. If the criterion is positive homogeneous, defined as $\Phi(\lambda M) = (1/\lambda)\Phi(M)(\lambda > 0)$, the so-called Φ-*efficiency* $\text{eff}_\Phi[M(\xi)] = \Phi[M(\xi^*)]/\Phi[M(\xi)]$ gives a measure of the goodness of a design. For instance, an efficiency of 85 % means a saving of 15 % of the observations when using the optimal design. One of the most popular criteria is D-optimality, based on the determinant of the inverse of the information matrix. This is equivalent to minimize the volume of the confidence ellipsoid of the parameters.

Computing optimal designs is not, in general, an easy task. The so-called *equivalence theorem* provides a powerful tool for checking whether a specific design is optimal or not. Moreover, the equivalence theorem gives the key for stating algorithms to compute optimal designs. It is important to say that this theorem is only valid for approximate designs.

In the general optimal design theory it is assumed that all of the explanatory variables are under the control of the experimenter, who may set these variables in the realization of the experiment. However, in practice there exist limitations. The problem of finding an optimal design among a class of designs satisfying some specific conditions has been considered only rarely in statistical design literature. Ardanuy and López-Fidalgo (1992) consider D-optimal designs seeking minimal weights at some points of the design support, for example when the experimenter already has the results of some experiments. Cook and Fedorov (1995) consider the problem of optimal designs with constraints on the total cost of the experiment, the location of the supporting point or the value of the auxiliary objective functions. Sahm and Schwabe (2000) give the theory for bounded designs. In all those cases a particular version of the equivalence theorem was provided.

If R is a particular restriction over the designs such that $\Xi_R = \{\xi \in \Xi | \xi \text{ satisfies } R\}$ is a convex set, then $M_R = \{M(\xi) | \xi \in \Xi_R\}$ is also a convex set. A restricted Φ-optimal design will be a design ξ^* such that

$$\Phi[M(\xi^*)] = \min_{\xi \in \Xi_R} \Phi[M(\xi)].$$

An equivalence theorem may be established in this case.

Cook and Thibodeau (1980) considered the particular case where some variables in the model can be controlled and others not, with values fixed and known before the experiment is realized. In this case the known values of the uncontrolled variables cause a restriction in the set of designs. Only designs with a marginal distribution on the uncontrolled variable, coincident with the values already obtained, can be taken into account. This is known as the marginally restricted (MR) design theory.

In the particular case considered in this chapter, there are also variables included in the model that are uncontrolled with unknown values before the experiment is performed. Let us clarify this concept for the case of the prognosis of lung cancer of a sample of 92 patients. The 'percentage of maximum volume of expired air' (variable x_1) is measured in all patients. We are in the situation of the MR theory since x_1 is not under the experimenter's control and its values are known in advance. When performing carrying out an investigation on those patients, one can examine oxygen desaturation during the test (x_2), for example during a cycling exercise. This information can then also be used for morbidity risk prediction before surgery. Notice, however, that this experiment can be performed under different exercise times (variable x_3). The experimenter may decide on the exercise time for each patient separately. Then the variable x_3 is completely under control. The variable x_2 is not subject to control and its values are not known before the exercise test is performed. The three variables may be considered in one model since all of them may provide information on morbidity. In this situation, new methods providing an equivalence theorem and algorithms for computing optimal designs for this very real situation are required (López-Fidalgo and Garcet-Rodríguez, 2004).

The situation involving the two variables x_2 and x_3 is referred to as a conditionally restricted (CR) optimal design problem since it is assumed that the experimenter may provide a conditional distribution of the probability of desaturation/no desaturation for different exercise times. The three-variables case is referred to as a marginally conditionally restricted (MCR) optimal design problem. In that case the experimenter should provide a conditional distribution of desaturation/no desaturation for different exercise times and values of the respiratory function of the patients.

The design space is now $X = X_1 \times X_2 \times X_3$ corresponding to uncontrolled variables with known and unknown values and the controlled variables, respectively. The MR and the CR designs will be denoted respectively as $\tilde{\xi}_1(x_1)$ and $\tilde{\xi}_{2|13}(x_2 | x_1, x_3)$. Next, a particular equivalence theorem is established for MCR D-optimality. A design ξ^* is MCR D-optimal if and only if

$$\sum_{x_1 \in \chi_1} \max_{x_3 \in \chi_3} \sum_{x_2 \in \chi_2} x' M^{-1}(\xi^*) x \tilde{\xi}_{2|13}(x_2 | x_1, x_3) \tilde{\xi}_1(x_1) = m.$$

The following algorithm is derived from this equivalence theorem for D-optimality:

1. An initial design $\xi^{(0)} \in \Xi_R^+$ is set up.

2. From $\xi^{(n)} \in \Xi_R^+$, let $x_3^{(n)}(x_1)$ be the point where the maximum of $\sum_{x_2 \in \chi_2} x' M^{-1}$
   $(\xi^{(n)}) x \tilde{\xi}_{2|13}(x_2|x_1, x_3)$ is reached.

3. A new conditional design is determined,

$$\xi_{3|1}^{(n+1)}(x_3|x_1) = \left(1 - \frac{1}{n+1}\right)\xi_{3|1}^{(n)}(x_3|x_1) + \frac{1}{n+1}\mathbf{1}_{x_3^{(n)}(x_1)}(x_3),$$

   where $\mathbf{1}_{x_3^{(n)}(x_1)}$ is a one-point design at $x_3^{(n)}(x_1)$.

4. The new joint design is given by

$$\xi^{(n+1)}(x) = \tilde{\xi}_1(x_1)\tilde{\xi}_{2|13}(x_2|x_1, x_3)\xi_{3|1}^{(n+1)}(x_3|x_1).$$

5. The procedure stops when

$$2 - \frac{1}{m}\sum_{(x_1, x_2) \in \chi_1 x \chi_2} x^{(n)'} M^{-1}(\xi^{(n)}) x^{(n)} \tilde{\xi}_{2|13}(x_2|x_1, x_3^{(n)}(x_1))\tilde{\xi}_1(x_1) \geq \delta,$$

where $0 < \delta < 1$ is a lower bound for the efficiency and $x^{(n)} = (x_1, x_2, x_3^{(n)}(x_1))$.

21.4   SOLUTION

The methods of the foregoing section have been applied to the nonlinear logistic model. It is well known that for nonlinear models the inverse of the Fisher information matrix is asymptotically proportional to the covariance of the maximum likelihood estimates under regularity conditions, satisfied here. This matrix depends on the parameter θ. The Fisher information matrix for this model is

$$M(\xi, \theta) = \sum_x x'x \left(\frac{1}{1 + e^{-\theta'x}}\right)^2.$$

If nominal values are available for the parameters, for example from retrospective studies, then the optimal design theory for linear models can be applied, in this case to $f(x) = (1 + e^{-\theta'x})^{-1}x$. The design space, the nominal values of the parameters, and the restrictions can be taken from Varela *et al.* (2001). In particular, $X_1 = \{0, 1\}$, with zero meaning a bad respiratory function (RF ≤ 52, corresponding to the 25th percentile); $X_2 = \{0, 1\}$, where zero means that desaturation does not appear, with a cut-off value of 90 %; and $X_3 = \{12, 18\}$, 12 and 18 minutes being the standard times for the exercise.

The estimates of $\hat{\theta}_1 = 1.7829$, $\hat{\theta}_2 = 0.2902$ and $\hat{\theta}_3 = -0.3810$ will be considered as the nominal values for computing the optimal design. The marginal for

Table 21.1   Conditional probability of desaturation given x_1 and x_3.

Respiratory function/ exercise time	12	18
0	0.3634	0.45
1	0.0857	0.10

x_1 means that about 24 % of the patients in the sample had a low respiratory function. Table 21.1 shows the probability of desaturation given low or high respiratory function and carrying out the exercise for 12 or 18 minutes. Since the 18 minute exercise was not considered in the original experiment, the corresponding conditional designs were set up based on expert experience. For 12 minutes the conditional design comes from the sample.

Using the theory given in Section 21.3, the MCR D-optimal design to be performed in practice is as follows. The 18 minute exercise will be performed with about 92.3 % of the patients chosen at random among the patients with high respiratory function, The remaining 7.7 % of the patients with high respiratory function should carry out the 12 minutes exercise. On the other hand, all the patients with low respiratory function will exercise for 18 minutes.

The D-efficiency of the design actually used in Varela et al. (2001) is about 65.9 %, meaning that the D-optimal design requires 34.1 % fewer patients to get the same statistical results. The efficiency of the Varela design is even lower if the design space is an interval of times, for example from 0 to 18 minutes. This makes the algorithmic implementation more complex.

In order to use these designs in practice an interesting question arises with respect to the exact optimal design theory. The design $\tilde{\xi}_1$ is usually an exact design used with the sample the practitioner has in advance. Meanwhile, the design $\tilde{\xi}_{2|13}$ does not need to be exact, since it is only a distribution of what might happen. On the other hand, the designs to be used in practice must be exact, even though the joint

Table 21.2   Actual design used in practice and D-optimal design to be applied for 92 patients. Given particular values of the Respiratory Function (RF) the table shows the distribution of the number of patients for the two different values of Exercise Time (T).

If RF	then T	Actual design	Optimal
≤ 52	12	22	0
> 52	12	70	6
≤ 52	18	0	22
> 52	18	0	64

design is not exact for a specific sample size. In the lung cancer case, the sample is divided into two groups, one with about 24 % of the patients with low respiratory function (RF ≤ 52) and the other group with about 76 % of the patients with high respiratory function (RF > 52); see Table 21.2. The desaturation column corresponds to the real data for the actual design and for the predicted data in the optimal design.

CHAPTER 22

Logistic Regression Methods and their Implementation

Vassiliki K. Kotti and Alexandros G. Rigas

Demokritos University of Thrace

22.1 INTRODUCTION

Logistic regression is one of the most popular statistical methods, which is used when the response variable has only two possible outcomes. Assume that we have a set of independent variables to be used for predicting (1) whether an earthquake is going to occur in a specific area, (2) whether a company is going bankrupt or (3) whether a person is likely to develop heart disease. Notice that with each of these scenarios the response can either be present or not. This situation occurs very often in medical and health-related studies, where the logistic regression method has been proved a very powerful tool for the assessment of risk factors. Annila *et al.* (1997) have used logistic regression to evaluate the influence of potential risk factors upon systemic honeybee sting reactions in beekeepers. A contemporary field is the investigation of polymorphisms and their role in the etiology of lung cancer; see Dally *et al.* (2003). In this chapter we apply logistic regression methods to the identification of the muscle spindle under the influence of a motoneuron and we investigate risk factors for the response of the system.

A great advantage of using logistic regression is that one can draw the practical inferences from the estimated model coefficients. Consider a logistic regression model that involves a response variable Y (occurrence of event), denoting for example whether a person suffers from lung cancer, and a binary explanatory variable X (exposure), denoting for example whether a person is a smoker. This simple case provides the framework for other situations. The conditional probability that a person suffers from lung cancer is $\pi(x) = \Pr(Y = 1|x)$, where x is the value of the exposure. The probabilities for all the possible outcomes are displayed in the 2×2 contingency table shown in Table 22.1.

Recent Advances in Quantitative Methods in Cancer and Human Health Risk Assessment
Edited by L. Edler and C. Kitsos   © 2005 John Wiley & Sons, Ltd

Table 22.1 Possible outcomes and their probabilities for a dichotomous exposure-outcome scenario modeled by logistic regression.

		Exposure to risk		
		$x = 1$	$x = 0$	Total
Occurrence of event	$y = 1$	$\pi(1) = \dfrac{e^{\beta_0 + \beta_1}}{1 + e^{\beta_0 + \beta_1}}$	$\pi(0) = \dfrac{e^{\beta_0}}{1 + e^{\beta_0}}$	1
	$y = 0$	$1 - \pi(1) = \dfrac{1}{1 + e^{\beta_0 + \beta_1}}$	$1 - \pi(0) = \dfrac{1}{1 + e^{\beta_0}}$	1
	Total	1	1	

The odds that the event occurs when there is exposure to the risk are defined as $\pi(1)/[1 - \pi(1)]$. This ratio is known as the odds of 'success'. Similarly, the odds that the event occurs when there is no exposure to the risk is defined as $\pi(0)/[1 - \pi(0)]$. The odds ratio is defined as the ratio of the odds for $x = 1$ to the odds for $x = 0$:

$$\psi = \frac{\pi(1)/[1 - \pi(1)]}{\pi(0)/[1 - \pi(0)]}. \tag{22.1}$$

By substituting into (22.1) the expressions in Table 22.1, the odds ratio can be written as

$$\psi = \exp(\beta_1). \tag{22.2}$$

The log-odds ratio is then given by $\ln(\psi) = \beta_1$. The main reason for the widespread use of logistic regression is the ease of interpretation of these coefficients related through equations (22.1) and (22.2). It is clear that the odds ratio can be estimated either from the entries of the 2×2 table through (22.1), or from the coefficients of the logistic regression model through (22.2). The odds ratio is useful because it depicts how much more likely it is for the outcome to be present among those with $x = 1$ than among those with $x = 0$. For example, $\psi = 2$ indicates that a disease occurs twice as often among exposed than among non-exposed persons. Furthermore, a confidence interval can be employed to provide additional information. This is obtained by calculating the endpoints of a confidence interval for the estimated coefficient $\hat{\beta}_1$ and then taking these values into the exponent. Generally, the $100(1 - a)\%$ confidence interval for the odds ratio is given by:

$$\exp[\hat{\beta}_1 \pm z_{a/2} \times \text{SE}(\hat{\beta}_1)], \tag{22.3}$$

where $z_{a/2}$ denotes the standard normal deviate with a tail area of $a/2$.

If the logistic regression model includes more than one explanatory variable, the estimated coefficients can be interpreted as increasing or decreasing the log-odds of 'success' and they show what happens to the log-odds if all the other explanatory variables are held constant. Values of ψ greater than 1 indicate an increase, and values of ψ less than 1 a decrease of the odds of 'success'. This corresponds to coefficient values $\beta > 0$ and $\beta < 0$, respectively.

The method which is usually employed for the estimation of the coefficients of a logistic regression model is the maximum likelihood estimation method (MLE). It is based on an iterative algorithm and performs very well for large data sets where it provides asymptotically unbiased estimates. However, for small, or large but sparse, data sets the method fails to converge or produces very poor results for the parameters estimates and their standard errors. Obviously, these results should not be used for drawing conclusions, especially in medical applications for which a bad decision could have serious consequences. Exact logistic regression (ELR) can be used as an alternative, which may result in very good estimates, albeit at the cost of more intensive computation.

22.2 NEUROPHYSIOLOGICAL EXAMPLE

The investigation of neurophysiological systems is an area of great importance when exploring the neural system. Many different approaches have been suggested, including the cross-correlation approach and the use of spectral analysis techniques. In this chapter we provide an alternative method based on logistic regression models. This allows the formulation of more flexible models with biologically interpretable parameters which can also be used for risk assessment. In this example, we examine the firing of a neurophysiological system under the effect imposed by a neuron.

Let Y_t describe the firing process of the system. By choosing the sampling interval h, the observations of the output can be written as follows:

$$y_t = \begin{cases} 1, & \text{when a spike occurs in } (t, t+h], \\ 0, & \text{otherwise,} \end{cases}$$

where $t = h, \ldots, Nh$ and $T = Nh$ is the time interval in which the process is observed. We usually choose $h = 1\,\text{ms}$. The input X_t imposed by the neuron on the system consists of the observations x_t defined similarly.

22.2.1 System description

The neurophysiological system we will examine is the muscle spindle, which is part of the skeletal muscles and which is responsible for the initiation of movement and the maintenance of muscle posture. Most skeletal muscles contain a number of these receptors, which lie parallel to extrafusal fibers. They consist of a number of specialized fibers lying parallel to each other and which are partially contained within a fluid-filled capsule of connective tissue. The fibers within a muscle spindle, known as intrafusal fibers, are considerably shorter than the extrafusal fibers. An excellent discussion of the structure of the muscle spindle and its functional role can be found in Matthews (1981). The effects of stimuli applied to the intrafusal muscle fibers are transmitted to the spinal cord by the axons of sensory nerves closely associated with the muscle spindle. The terminal branches of the sensory axons form spirals around the central region of the intrafusal muscle fibers.

In the absence of any input, the discharge of the sensory axons of the muscle spindle, known as Ia response, generates nerve action potentials at relatively constant rates. The output, which occurs under these conditions, is referred to as the spontaneous discharge of the muscle spindle. The action potential is a localized voltage change that occurs across the membrane, surrounding the nerve cell and axon, with an amplitude of approximately 100 mV and a duration of 1 ms. The discharge of the fine terminals of the sensory axons is also modified by action potentials carried by the axons of a group of cells called motoneurons. The bodies of these cells lie inside the spinal cord, while their long axons innervate the intrafusal fibers of the muscle spindles. We are interested in two cases: (a) discharge in the presence of a gamma motoneuron; and (b) discharge in the presence of an alpha motoneuron.

The experiments analyzed below used the tenuissimus muscle in anesthetized cats and recorded the responses of single sensory axons in dorsal root filaments. Gamma and alpha motoneuron axons isolated in ventral root filaments were stimulated by sequences of pulses at twice threshold. The distribution of intervals between pulses was approximately exponential. Fifteen-second sequences of the Ia response were recorded in the cases (a) and (b) defined above. The histograms of the input and output interspike intervals for the two data sets are shown in Figure 22.1. In case (a) the input and output data files consist of 1010 and 538 spikes respectively, while in case (b) they consist of 259 and 356 spikes respectively, recorded at time intervals of 15 870 ms.

22.2.2   System modeling

In this section we develop the logistic regression model that can be used for the identification of the system under the influence of the gamma or alpha motoneuron. This model was suggested by Brillinger (1988, 1992) for the identification of neuronal firing systems. The firing of the system occurs when the potential of the membrane that surrounds the sensory axon exceeds a critical level called the threshold. The membrane's potential at the trigger zone is influenced both by internal and external processes.

The internal processes are responsible for the spontaneous firing of the system. This is an ability of the system to produce a series of nerve pulses on its own, by increasing the resting potential to the level of the threshold. After the occurrence of a spike, the membrane potential resets to the resting level. In this case the system can be described by the threshold and the recovery function. We model the threshold potential level θ_t at the trigger zone at time t by $\theta_t = \theta_0 + \varepsilon_t$, where ε_t is the noise process that includes contributions of unmeasured terms that influence the firing of the system and θ_0 represents an unknown constant threshold. Other forms of threshold models can be considered that allow the threshold to vary with

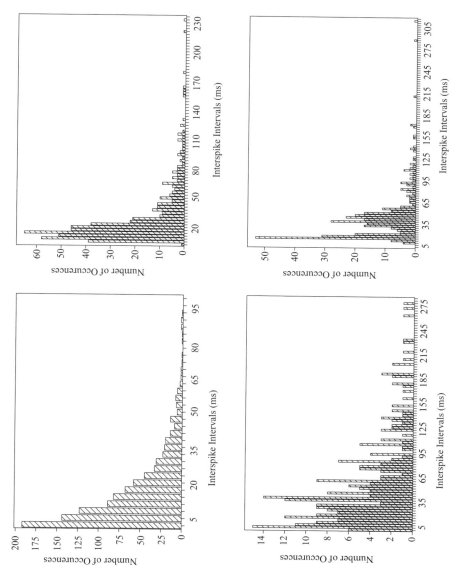

Figure 22.1 Histograms for the input and the output in the case of the gamma motoneuron (upper panel) and the alpha motoneuron (lower panel).

time (Kotti and Rigas, 2003a). Let V_t represent the recovery function described by a polynomial function of order k,

$$V_t = \sum_{i=1}^{k} \theta_i \gamma_t^i,$$

where γ_t is the time elapsed since the system last fired.

External processes are responsible for the firing of the system when it is affected by external parameters such as the presence of a motoneuron. The function representing the effect of a motoneuron on the muscle spindle at any given time t is based on a summation described by a set of coefficients $\{a_u\}$. The summation function is defined by

$$SF_t = \sum_{u \leq t} a_u x_{t-u},$$

where x_{t-u} is the observation of the input at time $t - u$.

The logistic regression model that describes the effect of the covariates incorporated in the recovery and the summation function at any given time t is expressed as

$$\log\left(\frac{p_t}{1 - p_t}\right) = \sum_{u \leq t} a_u x_{t-u} + \sum_{i=1}^{k} \theta_i \gamma_t^i - \theta_0 \qquad (22.4)$$

where p_t is the probability of an output spike to occur. The unknown parameters are the coefficients $\{a_u\}$, the recovery function parameters θ_i and the constant threshold θ_0. More details about the logistic model and the covariates included can be found in Kotti and Rigas (2002).

22.3   LOGISTIC REGRESSION

The purpose of this section is to provide an overview of the logistic regression models and the methods which are commonly applied for estimating the unknown parameters: maximum likelihood estimation and exact logistic regression.

22.3.1   Definitions

Consider that for each experimental unit, the response, Y, can take only one of two possible values, 0 and 1. We logically let $Y_i = 0$ when the unit does not possess the characteristic that the response represents, and $Y_i = 1$ when the unit does possess the characteristic. Associated with each individual experimental unit is a vector of covariates or explanatory variables $X = (x_1, x_2, \ldots, x_p)$, which can be either discrete or continuous or a combination of the two. The response probability is defined as

$$P(Y = 1|X) = \pi(x_1, x_2, \ldots, x_p) = E(Y = 1|x_1, x_2, \ldots, x_p).$$

The simple logistic regression model describes the relationship between the response probability and the explanatory variables and can be written in the form

$$P(Y = 1|X) = \pi(x_1, x_2, \ldots, x_p) = \frac{\exp(\beta_0 + \Sigma_{i=1}^{p} \beta_i x_i)}{1 + \exp(\beta_0 + \Sigma_{i=1}^{p} \beta_i x_i)}. \tag{22.5}$$

Equivalently, the logistic regression model can be written in terms of the log-odds of a positive response as:

$$\log\left[\frac{P(Y = 1|X)}{1 - P(Y = 1|X)}\right] = \beta_0 + \beta_1 x_1 + \beta_2 x_2 + \cdots + \beta_p x_p. \tag{22.6}$$

The method applied for the estimation of the unknown parameters $\beta_0, \beta_1, \ldots, \beta_p$ is crucial, since a misleading result could lead to false decisions.

22.3.2 Maximum likelihood estimation

The likelihood function is defined as the joint probability function of the random variables whose realizations constitute the sample. The observations $(y_1, y_2, \ldots, y_n)$ in a sample of size n are considered as realizations of the random variables $(Y_1, Y_2, \ldots, Y_n)$. The probability density function of Y_i,

$$P\{Y_i = y_i\} = \pi_i^{y_i}(1 - \pi_i)^{1-y_i}, \qquad y_i = 0, 1,$$

describes the contribution to the likelihood function of every single observation. Since the observations are assumed to be independent, the likelihood function is the joint probability

$$L_0 = P(Y_1 = y_1, Y_2 = y_2, \ldots, Y_n = y_n) = \prod_{i=1}^{n} \pi_i^{y_i}(1 - \pi_i)^{1-y_i}, \tag{22.7}$$

where $\pi_i = \pi(x_{1i}, x_{2i}, \ldots, x_{pi})$ is the conditional probability that Y_i equals 1, given x_i. It may be more convenient to use the log of the likelihood function

$$l(y_i, \pi_i) = \log L_0 = \sum_{i=1}^{n} \left[y_i \log\left(\frac{\pi_i}{1 - \pi_i}\right) + \log(1 - \pi_i) \right]. \tag{22.8}$$

The probability π_i is related to the unknown parameters $\beta_0, \beta_1, \ldots, \beta_p$ through (22.5) and thus the likelihood function is considered as a function of the unknown parameters. The maximum likelihood estimates of the unknown parameters are obtained by maximizing the log-likelihood function given by (22.8). More details on maximum likelihood estimation can be found in McCullagh and Nelder (1989).

22.3.3 Fallacies of asymptotic maximum likelihood estimation

Maximum likelihood is the most widely used estimation method in statistics. Its virtue lies in its good performance for large samples. It provides asymptotically unbiased estimates, which are known to be asymptotically normally distributed, irrespective of the distribution from which the original data were drawn. Furthermore, it is a very practical estimation procedure from a computational point of view, since an iterative algorithm is used which is implemented in almost every statistical package. For small samples, however, the estimates may be seriously biased, unless the sample data obey the normal distribution. If not, the parameter estimates can be poor and estimates of the standard errors invalid. These problems are caused by certain structures in the data, occurring when rare events are modeled, for example, when the data set is small or sparse. The most common numerical problem occurs with maximum likelihood estimation MLE when a collection of covariates separates the outcome space such that there is no overlap in the distribution of the covariates between the two possible outcome values. This phenomenon is called complete or quasi-complete separation. In these cases maximum likelihood estimates do not exist; see Albert and Anderson (1984) and Santner and Duffy (1986).

In the case of a continuous covariate X, complete separation happens when the X-values that correspond to $Y = 1$ exceed all the X-values that correspond to $Y = 0$. Quasi-complete separation occurs when one or more X-values correspond to both $Y = 0$ and $Y = 1$. A simple example presented by Hosmer and Lemeshow (1989) illustrates the problem. Suppose we have 12 (x, y) pairs of a covariate and an outcome, namely (1,0), (2,0), (3,0), (4,0), (5,0), ($x = 5.5$, or 6.0, or 12.0, $y = 0$), (6,1), (7,1), (8,1), (9,1), (10,1), and (11,1). The results of fitting a simple logistic regression model and letting x in the sixth pair take on one of the values 5.5, 6.0, or 12.0 are given in Table 22.2. When we use $x = 5.5$ we have complete separation, and when we use $x = 6.0$ we have quasi-complete separation. All the estimated parameters and standard errors are huge, since the maximum likelihood estimates do not exist. When we use $x = 12.0$, there is overlap and the estimated parameters

Table 22.2   The results obtained for the Hosmer and Lemeshow example by performing MLE and ELR. Note that for $x = 5.5$ the data are completely separated and for $x = 6.0$ they are quasi-completely separated. In these two cases the maximum likelihood estimates and their standard errors are extraordinary but the MUEs provided by performing exact logistic regression are reasonable. In the case $x = 12.0$ there is overlap, the maximum likelihood estimates exist and they are very close to the CMLE. NA: not available.

Estimates	$x = 5.5$	$x = 6.0$	$x = 12.0$
Maximum likelihood estimation			
x (SE)	20.6 (22.7)	7.2 (15.8)	0.32 (0.21)
Constant (SE)	−118.3 (130.2)	−43.3 (95.0)	−2.12 (1.51)
Exact logistic regression			
x (SE)	1.52 (NA)	0.99	0.29 (0.19)
95 % CI	(0.27, INF)	(0.20, INF)	(−0.07, 0.78)
Constant (SE)	−2.02 (NA)	−2.27 (NA)	−1.91 (1.42)
95 % CI	(−∞, 0.31)	(−∞, 0.10)	(−6.50, 1.25)

and standard errors become more reasonable. Complete or quasi-complete separation can be detected easily in the case of a single covariate X by ordering its values and comparing them with the Y-values. In the case of more than one covariate, an algorithm has been proposed by Santner and Duffy (1986) that can be used to determine whether the maximum likelihood estimates exist. Complete or quasi-complete separation does not arise very often in real data sets, since its occurrence almost exclusively requires dichotomous covariates. However, the probability of the occurrence of separation is not negligible when for small or sparse data sets many parameters are estimated in the regression.

In the case of a dichotomous covariate, the detection of separation can be achieved through the analysis of the corresponding contingency table. The neurophysiological example presented above illustrates this situation. We wish to determine the predictors of the muscle spindle's firing under the influence of a motoneuron. The covariates of interest are included in the summation and the recovery function. The effect of each of these covariates on the firing of the system can be studied simultaneously through the logistic regression model given by (22.4). In the case of the alpha motoneuron data set, most of the commonly used software packages fail, because the maximum likelihood estimates do not exist. This happens because all the observations of the covariate X_{t-13} with $x_{t-13} = 1$ occur when the output spike is absent, $Y = 0$. This is illustrated in the contingency table (Table 22.4). Notice that the cell with $X_{t-13} = 1$ and $Y = 1$ is empty. The existence of a single cell with a frequency of zero indicates the existence of quasi-complete separation. This situation causes problems for maximum likelihood, which uses X_{t-13} as a perfect predictor and attempts to set the estimate for a_{13} to $-\infty$, shown in Table 22.3. The problem becomes obvious through extreme estimates and very large standard errors; see Section 22.4.

22.3.4 Exact logistic regression

Exact logistic regression, proposed by Cox (1970), bases parameter estimation on the elimination of parameters remaining in the likelihood function, and by conditioning on their sufficient statistics. The likelihood function given by (22.7) can be written as

$$P(Y_1 = y_1, Y_2 = y_2, \ldots, Y_n = y_n) = \frac{\exp(\sum_{s=0}^{p} \beta_s t_s)}{\prod_{i=1}^{n} (1 + \exp(x_i \beta))}, \qquad (22.9)$$

where

$$t_s = \sum_{i=1}^{n} x_{is} y_i \qquad (22.10)$$

is the observed value of the random variable $T_s = \sum x_{is} Y_i$. The sufficient statistics $t_0, t_1, \ldots, t_p$ are subtotals of the columns of the matrix formed by the n rows x_i, the elements summed corresponding to the rows in which successes occur. The

Table 22.3   Results obtained for the neurophysiological example in the case of the alpha motoneuron by performing MLE and ELR. The estimated coefficients a_{13}, a_{19}, a_{25}, a_{31}, and a_{37} denote a problematic area on the summation function, caused by the extreme values of the maximum likelihood estimates and their standard errors. The MUE prove that these coefficients are statistically significant and they inhibit the response of the system. The lower 95 % exact confidence interval is $-\infty$, indicating that the likelihood function cannot be maximized. The maximum likelihood estimates are obtained by Genstat. The CMLE and the MUE are obtained by LogXact. NA: not available.

Logistic regression coefficients	Maximum likelihood estimate	SE	CMLE or MUE	SE	95 % Exact CI Lower	Upper
θ_0	3.4186	0.1307	3.4493 (CMLE)	0.2297	2.9905	3.9435
θ_1	0.0967	0.0105	0.0986 (CMLE)	0.0183	0.0629	0.1351
a_1	0.2168	0.2447	0.2134 (CMLE)	0.4238	−0.7897	1.0618
a_7	1.7565	0.1722	1.7414 (CMLE)	0.2994	1.0975	2.3617
a_{13}	−7.7503	6.6326	−2.2142 (MUE)	NA	−∞	−0.4818
a_{19}	−7.8191	6.7208	−2.2480 (MUE)	NA	−∞	−0.5272
a_{25}	−8.1085	6.6810	−2.5503 (MUE)	NA	−∞	−0.8199
a_{31}	−8.1542	6.7425	−2.5838 (MUE)	NA	−∞	−0.8594
a_{37}	−8.2998	6.6745	−2.7224 (MUE)	NA	−∞	−0.9879
a_{43}	−2.7278	0.7167	−2.4404 (MUE)	NA	−∞	−0.6608
a_{49}	−0.3193	0.2464	−0.3413 (CMLE)	0.4330	−1.3670	0.5291

distribution of $T_0, T_1, \ldots, T_p$ follows from summing (22.10) over all binary sequences that generate the particular values $t_0, t_1, \ldots, t_p$. We have

$$P(T_0 = t_0, T_1 = t_1, \ldots, T_p = t_p) = \frac{c(t_0, t_1, \ldots, t_p) \exp(\sum_{s=0}^{p} \beta_s t_s)}{\prod_{i=1}^{n} (1 + \exp(x_i \beta))}. \quad (22.11)$$

Suppose we are interested in one of the regression parameters, regarding the remainder as nuisance. Without loss of generality let us choose the parameter of interest to be β_p. To find the conditional distribution of T_p given $T_0 = t_0$, $T_1 = t_1, \ldots, T_{p-1} = t_{p-1}$, we have

$$P(T_p = t_p | T_0 = t_0, T_1 = t_1, \ldots, T_{p-1} = t_{p-1}) = \frac{P(T_0 = t_0, T_1 = t_1, \ldots, T_p = t_p)}{P(T_0 = t_0, T_1 = t_1, \ldots, T_{p-1} = t_{p-1})}.$$

The numerator is given by (22.11) and the denominator by summing (22.11) all over possible t_p. Thus, the conditional likelihood is given by

$$f(t_p | \beta_p) = \frac{c(t_0, t_1, \ldots, t_p) \exp(\beta_p t_p)}{\sum_u c(t_0, t_1, \ldots, t_{p-1}, u) \exp(\beta_p u)} \quad (22.12)$$

where the summation in the denominator is over all values of u for which $c(t_0, t_1, \ldots, t_{p-1}, u) \geq 1$. The conditional maximum likelihood estimate (CMLE) of β_p is obtained by maximizing (22.12). If however, either $t_p = t_{min}$ or $t_p = t_{max}$, where t_{min} and t_{max} are the smallest and largest possible values of t_p, the CMLE of β_p

is undefined. In this case a median unbiased estimate (MUE) of β_p can be obtained, which is always defined, even at the extreme points of the sample space. The MUE satisfies the condition $f(t_p|\beta_p) = 0.5$. More details about exact logistic regression can be found in Mehta and Patel (1995).

22.3.5 Advantages of exact logistic regression

The advantage of ELR is the existence of the estimates in the cases of small or sparse data sets, when it is possible to face the problem of the complete or quasi-complete separation. In the maximum likelihood approach, the log-likelihood increases monotonically by choosing larger and larger values for the coefficients and thus the method does not converge. For the ELR, the distribution of the sufficient statistics does exist, and exact confidence intervals and exact p-values can be obtained for the MUE. When the sample size grows or the data become less sparse, the asymptotic results will converge to the exact results.

The exact results for the Hosmer and Lemeshow example are given in Table 22.2. In the case of complete separation $(x = 5.5)$ and quasi-complete separation $(x = 6.0)$ the MUE and the exact confidence intervals are reasonable. The standard errors are not available and the estimated 95 % confidence intervals range up to ∞, which indicates that maximum likelihood method did not converge. In the case of overlap, the CMLE exists and it is very close to the maximum likelihood estimate. The problem of quasi-complete separation described in Section 22.3.3 is countered by applying exact methods. The MUE and the 95 % exact confidence interval for the coefficient a_{13} are shown in Table 22.3. More details about the interpretation of the estimated coefficients are provided in Section 22.4 below.

A disadvantage of ELR arises when the remaining covariates are continuous. In this case the conditional distribution of the sufficient statistics could degenerate to a single value. In this case no inference is possible. This condition does not arise very often and can be avoided by discretizing one or more of the continuous covariates.

22.3.6 Numerical aspects

Maximum likelihood enjoys widespread use because the estimates of the model coefficients can easily be obtained numerically by maximizing the likelihood function. These algorithms can be implemented easily and they are available on every statistical package (e.g. Genstat, SAS). When the problems discussed in Section 22.3.3 arise, the estimates either do not converge or are held at a limit. This situation can be identified by inflated estimates and standard errors of the unknown parameters.

ELR requires the enumeration of all possible permutations of the vector of binomial responses (y-vector) that meet certain criteria imposed by the observed data. We often refer to the collection of all these y-vectors as the 'reference set'. Each additional explanatory variable that is included in the logistic regression model imposes one additional constraint on the reference set. Generating and storing the reference set of y-vectors can consume a considerable amount of memory and computing time. In fact, the initial theory for ELR proposed by Cox (1970) was considered computationally infeasible for many years until the development of fast algorithmic methods that have been suggested by Tritchler (1984) and Hirji *et al.* (1987).

ELR is implemented in the program package LogXact, a statistical software package that specializes in exact methods. LogXact accepts up to 30 covariates for exact inference, but it is unlikely that it will solve a problem with so many covariates. The difficulty of solving a problem is determined by several characteristics of the data such as the number of responses, the imbalance between groups, and the spacing between values of continuous variables. More details about these numerical aspects can be found in LogXact User Manual (Cytel Software Corp., 2002).

22.4 NEUROPHYSIOLOGICAL EXAMPLE REVISITED

In the case of the gamma motoneuron, the maximum likelihood estimates are depicted in Figure 22.2. The estimated coefficients of the summation function are positive and far from zero in the interval 11–30 ms. This implies that the covariates $X_{t-11}, \ldots, X_{t-30}$ can be considered as risk factors because they significantly

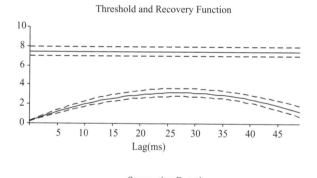

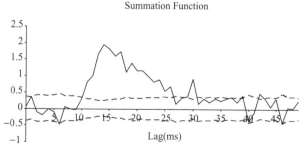

Figure 22.2 Estimates for the threshold, recovery and summation functions by performing maximum likelihood estimation. The dotted lines correspond to 95 % confidence intervals. The recovery function is represented by a second-order polynomial, which does not cross the estimated threshold level. This indicates that the system does not fire spontaneously. The summation function indicates an excitatory behavior, which occurs from 11 to 30 ms. During this time interval the estimated summation function is outside the confidence interval.

increase the odds of an output spike. The overall behavior of the summation function is *excitatory*, which means that the input spikes from a gamma motoneuron accelerate the firing of the system. The recovery function is described by a second-order polynomial since $\hat{\theta}_i, i \geq 3$ are not statistically significant. The form of the recovery function indicates that there is no spontaneous activity, because it does not cross the estimated threshold level. In other words, the presence of the gamma motoneuron destroys completely the spontaneous activity and therefore the recovery function cannot be considered as a significant risk factor. These results are in agreement with previous work where a Volterra-type stochastic model is used and the estimates of the parameters are obtained by employing spectral analysis techniques for stationary point processes (Rigas, 1996). More details about the methods applied in this case and the results obtained can be found in Kotti and Rigas (2002, 2003b).

A first comparison of the data sets collected in the case of the gamma and alpha motoneuron imposed on the muscle spindle, reveals that the input and output inter-spike intervals, in the case of the alpha motoneuron, are less frequent and if present then larger. This is a preliminary indication that this data set is sparse. A first step in dealing with this problem is to resample the data set using a sampling interval of 3 ms, instead of 1 ms, which was initially used for both cases. Resampling, the maximum likelihood estimate fails completely on the alpha motoneuron data set. The estimates are held at a limit and this is a clear indication that one or more of the parameters may then need to be infinite to maximize the likelihood. A solution in this case is to perform ELR. The logistic model, however, involves too many parameters and a very large set of observations, raising serious computational problems for the implementation of ELR. The number of parameters can be reduced by omitting some of the summation function covariates from the logistic regression model. The size of the sample space can be significantly reduced if we apply the ELR on three non-overlapping subsets of almost equal length.

The asymptotic and exact results in the case of the alpha motoneuron are presented in Table 22.3. The maximum likelihood estimates and the standard errors of the estimated coefficients $a_{13}, a_{19}, \ldots, a_{37}$ are very large compared with the rest, and they highlight a *problematic area* in the summation function. This occurs because of a zero frequency cell in the corresponding contingency tables, illustrated in Table 22.4 for X_{t-13} versus Y. This means that all observations of the response Y are gathered at the extreme 0 level of the covariate X_{t-13}. In other words X_{t-13} separates the sample space and does not allow any overlap. The same situation applies for all the covariates of the *problematic area* and it causes the maximum likelihood method to diverge. The estimates obtained by performing ELR seem to be more reasonable. The lower confidence bound for the problematic estimates is $-\infty$, which indicates that the data set contains observations at the extreme points of the sample space. The same, however, applies for the estimated coefficient a_{43}, which was not included in the *problematic area* according to maximum likelihood. This is caused by the separation of the sample space into three almost equal subsets, which splits the two observations of the (1,1) cell into three intervals. Therefore, the estimate is again defined at the extreme points of the sample space.

Table 22.4 Contingency tables for the covariates X_{t-7}, X_{t-13}, X_{t-43} and the response Y, in the case of the alpha motoneuron. Note the zero cell in the second contingency table, which is the responsible for the extreme estimate and standard error of the coefficient a_{13}.

		Y	
		0	1
X_{t-7}	0	4738	295
	1	196	61
X_{t-13}	0	4677	356
	1	257	0
X_{t-43}	0	4679	354
	1	255	2

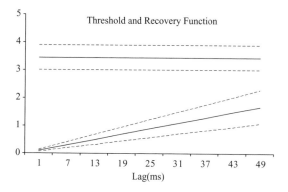

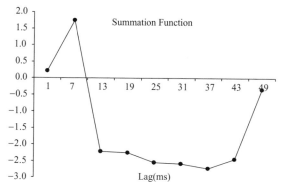

Figure 22.3 Estimates for the threshold, recovery and summation functions by performing ELR. The dotted lines correspond to the 95 % exact confidence intervals. The recovery function is represented by a first-order polynomial, which tends to cross the estimated threshold level. This may indicate that the system fires spontaneously. The summation function shows an inhibitory behavior, which occurs from 11 to 50 ms.

The estimates of the threshold, the recovery and the summation function obtained by performing ELR are depicted in Figure 22.3. The estimated coefficients of the summation function are positive for the first 10 ms and the covariate X_{t-7} significantly increases the probability of the system's firing. However, in the interval between 11 and 50 ms the probability of firing is reduced, as it is obvious from the negative values of the estimated coefficients. This means that the potential risk factors $X_{t-13}, \ldots, X_{t-43}$ decrease the odds of an output spike. The behavior of the summation function in this area is *inhibitory* which means that the occurrence of an input spike imposed by an alpha motoneuron blocks the response of the system in the interval between 11 and 50 msec. The recovery function is denoted by a first-order polynomial. The odds ratio of the estimated coefficient θ_1 is 1.1036, with a 95 % confidence interval (1.0647, 1.1439). Although the odds ratio is not dramatically high, the diagrammatic representation of the threshold and the recovery function shows an increase in the recovery, which tends to cross the threshold level. This fact indicates a simmering spontaneous activity of the system. Using spectral analysis techniques, Rigas and Liatsis (2000) came to the same conclusions about the behavior of the system in the presence of an alpha motoneuron.

22.5 DISCUSSION

This chapter has been concerned with methods of estimation used in logistic regression. These include maximum likelihood estimation and exact logistic regression. Although the former is computationally very desirable, sometimes it fails to converge and the estimates obtained can be misleading for the assessment of risk factors. In this case, exact logistic regression can be applied, which succeeds in finding estimates, but the computational cost is very heavy. An alternative method that can be used to avoid infinite regression coefficients arising under complete or quasi-complete separation is based on penalized maximum likelihood (Heinze and Schemper, 2002).

Two experimental conditions for muscle spindle are provided, where logistic regression is used for the assessment of the system's behavior. In the case of the gamma motoneuron the summation function significantly increases the occurrence of an output spike in the interval 11–30 ms, but the recovery function cannot be considered as significant risk factor. In the case of the alpha motoneuron, there is an increase in the probability of the system to fire for a very short period around 7 ms, but afterwards the firing probability decreases significantly in the interval 11–50 ms. There is also an indication that the system may fire spontaneously.

CHAPTER 23

The use of Logistic Regression, Discriminant Analysis and Classification Trees in Predicting Persisting Remission in Childhood Leukemia

Małgorzata Ćwiklińska-Jurkowska, Piotr Jurkowski and Andrzej Kołtan

Nicolaus Copernicus University

23.1 INTRODUCTION

Leukemia is the most frequent malignant disease in childhood. It constitutes about 35 % of all cancer cases under the age of 15 years. Approximately 80 % of childhood leukemia is acute lymphoblastic leukemia (ALL), from immature cells stemming from the lymphoid line. More than 95 % of children with ALL obtain remission with initial chemotherapy and about 70 % are cured after treatment. Another type of leukemia, not as common as ALL but more difficult to treat, is acute myelogenous leukemia (AML), stemming from the myeloid line.

Leukemia cells multiply in the bone marrow and slow down the production of normal blood cells, so that patients with acute leukemia frequently have a low number of red blood cells and platelets. Some of the frequent symptoms of ALL are: fever, fatigue, infections, paleness or pallor, bleeding, bruising, petechiae, or pain in the bones or joints. Very often the onset of leukemia shows symptoms similar to ordinary viral infection. The abnormal cells can gather in the central nervous

Recent Advances in Quantitative Methods in Cancer and Human Health Risk Assessment
Edited by L. Edler and C. Kitsos © 2005 John Wiley & Sons, Ltd

system (CNS) and the testes – 'sanctuary' sites for leukemic cells – making treatment by antineoplastic drugs very difficult.

Known risk factors of ALL are gender (male), age (between 2 and 5 years), race (white), higher socioeconomic status, ionizing radiation (*in utero*), therapeutic postnatal ionizing, and some genetic syndromes (e.g., Down syndrome, Bloom syndrome). Other factors are, for example, high birth weight (over 4000 g), maternal age (over 35 years), first born child or only child, maternal smoking prior to and during pregnancy, postnatal use of chloramphenicol, exposure to an electromagnetic field. Parental occupational exposure to hazardous substances is also a suspected risk factor of ALL (see Ross *et al.*, 1994).

The number of white blood cells (WBCs) at the moment of diagnosis of ALL is an important and independent prognostic factor of this disease (Poplack *et al.*, 1993; Pui *et al.*, 1990). Other features indicating a good or a bad prognosis, depending on the leukemia's type, are age (Poplack *et al.*, 1993), area of enlarged lymph nodes and the immunophenotype of the cells (Cortes and Kantarjian, 1995), gender (Cortes and Kantarjian, 1995; Poplack *et al.*, 1993; Pui *et al.*, 1990), cytogenetic disorders (Pui *et al.*, 1990), presence of some cells surface antigens (e.g., CD10 or CD34; Cortes and Kantarjian, 1995), response to steroid treatment (Reiter *et al.*, 1994; Cortes and Kantarjian, 1995), presence of leukemic infiltration in mediastinum or in the CNS (Poplack *et al.*, 1993), enlarged lymph nodes (Burke *et al.*, 1995), nonmyeloid localizations (Poplack *et al.*, 1993) and hemoglobin concentration (Poplack *et al.*, 1993). Some of those features were used to construct a prognostic score, indicating risk groups, and influencing the type of therapeutic scheme administered, such as the NOPHO Group Score (Schmiegelow *et al.*, 1995) or the BFM (Berlin–Frankfurt–Münster Group) risk score (Reiter *et al.*, 1994). In our investigations, reported below, we have included these factors.

The evaluation of the prognostic importance of the features described above is more frequently based on a one-dimensional statistical analysis (i.e., based on one variable after the other) than on the usage of multivariate statistical methods, although the authors often underline the importance of a multivariate analysis. The statistical procedure most often used to analyze prognostic factors is Cox's proportional hazards regression (Kleinbaum, 1997). Dördelmann *et al.* (2000) showed that the best predictor of a treatment result in children's ALL is response to prednisone therapy. This was confirmed by other investigations using the BFM risk score. Other prognostic factors for the course of ALL, found by multivariate methods, were the presence of Philadelphia chromosome, translocations associated with chromosome 11q23, an acute unclassified leukemia, mixed lineage leukemia, WBC count greater than or equal to 5×10^9 cells/l, and male gender (Horibe *et al.*, 2000). The presence or absence as well as the level of residual disease after the induction of remission is one of the best prognostic factors of a relapse in childhood ALL (Cave *et al.*, 1998). Multivariate methods were more often used to identify predictive features for children's AML. For example, vascular endothelial growth factor secretion and age (de Bont *et al.*, 2002), age greater than or equal to 8 years, WBC count greater than or equal to 10×10^9 cells/l (Katano *et al.*, 1997), high platelet count at the moment of diagnosis, absence of hepatomegaly, and less than

15 % bone marrow blasts on the 14th day after induction are prognostic factors of complete remission (Wells *et al.*, 2002).

The goal of our study, reported below, is to support the doctors' prognostic estimate using multivariate methods. Therefore, we aim, using different multivariate statistics, to select those variables (features) that are most predictive for the results of childhood ALL treatment. We compare the efficiency and usefulness of logistic regression, discriminant analysis and classification trees to predict persisting remission in childhood leukemia. Therefore, we studied a data set of 114 acute leukemia child patients with 21 explanatory variables. Since the medical data set examined was incomplete, casewise deletion and multiple imputation EM were used to fill in missing data. Different multivariate selection methods of the most discriminating variables (e.g., Bayesian discriminant methods, classification trees and logistic regression) aided the prediction of childhood leukemia's outcome and provided minimal subsets of prognostic variables, containing most often blood group, time until remission and presence of CD10 antigen on leukemic cell. These variables were also the ones that were prognostic for survival. On the basis of the selected variables we compare the effectiveness of linear, quadratic and kernel discriminant methods, CART and QUEST classification trees and also logistic regression.

23.2 PATIENTS

The data were collected at the clinic of Pediatric Hematology and Oncology of the Ludwik Rydygier Medical University in Bydgoszcz from a group of 114 newly diagnosed leukemic children (43 girls and 71 boys) aged between 6 months and 15.5 years.

Thirty-three patients had been stratified into two BFM risk groups (standard risk = SR, high risk = HR). Treatment for the SR group consisted of steroid prophase (prednisone – PRED) and methotrexate (MTX) intrathecal injection. In the first phase of remission induction PRED, vincristine (VCR), daunorubicine (DAUNO) and L-asparaginase (L-Asp) were used. Next 6-mercaptopurin (6-MP), cyclophosphamide (CTX) and cytarabine (ARA-C) were applied. As CNS prophylaxis, MTX intrathecal injections and CNS irradiations were used. For the HR group additional reinduction with dexamethasone (DEXA), VCR, adriablastine (ADR), L-Asp, CTX, thioguanine (6-TG), and ARA-C was conducted. The follow-up time varied between 0 and 3121 days (median = 1154 days). Event-free survival (EFS) varied from 0 to 3088 days (median = 935 days). EFS rate after 8 years was 0.51.

The remaining 81 patients were stratified by NOPHO criterion into three risk groups (SR, intermediate = IR, and HR). Patients from the SR group were treated with PRED, VCR, ADR and L-Asp, and in consolidation median range doses of MTX (MD-MTX) were administered. CNS prophylaxis consisted of MTX intrathecal injections, but CNS irradiations were not used. The IR group children were treated similarly, but with DAUNO instead of ADR, and the induction was prolonged with four series of ARA-C and two doses of MTX intrathecal injections.

In consolidation, instead of MTX 1 g/m^2 per day, 4 doses of MTX 0.5 g/m^2 per day were used. In this group, CNS irradiation was used. In the HR group PRED, DEXA, CTX, teniposide (VM-26), ARA-C and MTX intrathecal injections were used. CNS irradiation was more intensive than in the IR group (up to 24 Gy). The time of treatment in the IR and HR group was a maximum 2 years. Observation time for children stratified by NOPHO score was 4 to 7052 days (median = 3428 days). EFS was 0 to 7015 days (median = 2221days). EFS rate after 8 years was 0.5.

Table 23.1   Number, name and explanation of the explanatory variables used for the classification. Variables 2, 8 and 13 are quantitative, all others are qualitative. An asterisk denotes the most discriminating variables (see Section 23.4).

No	Feature	Explanation	No. of reported values
1	SEX	Gender (0 = female; 1 = male)	114
2	AGE	Age	114
3	NODES	Largest dimension of enlarged lymph nodes(in cm)	114
4	HEPAR	Hepatomegaly (cm under ribs)	114
5	SPLEEN	Splenomegaly (cm under ribs)	114
6	MEDIASTIN	Presence of leukemic infiltration in mediastinum (0 = no; 1 = yes)	111
7	CNS*	Presence of leukemic infiltration in CNS (0 = no; 1 = yes)	103
8	HB	Hemoglobin concentration	114
9	LEUKOC	WBC/leukocyte count	114
10	BLASTS	Immature WBC (blasts) count	114
11	PLT*	Platelets/Thrombocyte count	114
12	GR BLOOD*	Blood group (1, O+; 2, O−; 3, A+; 4, A−; 5, B+; 6, B−; 7, AB+, 8, AB−)	114
13	RF	Risk score counted as 0.2 log (blasts count)+0.06 (the part of HEPAR under costal margin in cm)+0.04 (the part of SPLEEN under costal margin in cm)	114
14	BFMGR	BFM risk group (SR = 1;HR = 0; score on the basis of WBC, MEDIASTIN, CNS and lymph node infiltration, age)	114
15	NOPHOGR	NOPHO risk group (SR = 1; IR = 2; HR = 3) score on the basis of WBC, MEDIASTIN and CNS infiltration, age, and the phenotype of leukemia)	114
16	STERID	Response to steroid treatment during induction (1 = good; 0 = bad)	114
17	TIMETOREM*	Time until reaching remission	114
18	FAB	FAB type of leukemic cells(1 = L$_1$; 2 = L$_2$; 3 = L$_3$)	68
19	PHENOT	Phenotype of leukemic cells (1 = T; 2 = B; 3 = non-T non-B)	57
20	CD10*	Presence of CD10 antigen on leukemic cells (1 = yes; 2 = no)	54
21	MYELO14	Myelogram on 14th day of treatment (1 = M1; 2 = M2; 3 = M3)	55

In our investigations, the treatment outcome was called 'good' if a child had achieved complete remission (without a relapse and without death) lasting until the end of observation time; all other cases were called 'bad'. In the following we consider three types of classification of each patient: classification A into two groups,

A1   alive and relapse-free ($n_{A1} = 63$),

A2   died or relapse ($n_{A2} = 51$);

classification B into three groups,

B1   died before first remission ($n_{B1} = 13$),

B2   died during first remission ($n_{B2} = 17$),

B3   alive ($n_{B3} = 84$);

and classification C into two groups (combining B1 and B2),

C1   died ($n_{C1} = 30$),

C2   alive during first remission ($n_{C2} = 84$).

We considered 21 predicting variables (features); see Table 23.1.

23.3   METHODS

Different multivariate statistical methods were applied, combined with classification and discriminant analysis methods as well as with different methods of handling incomplete data.

23.3.1   Selection of variables

The stepwise mixed (forward–backward) and forward search for the variables with the greatest discriminative power was based on minimizing Wilks's lambda (λ) statistic (Morrison, 1976). Small values of λ indicate good discriminant power of a subset of variables. At each step of the forward selection one enters the variable that adds most to the discriminatory power of the model as measured by Wilks's λ. In mixed forward–backward stepwise selection one analyses the model at each step as follows: if the variable in the model that contributes least to the discriminatory power by Wilks's λ fails to meet the criterion, that variable is eliminated; otherwise, of those variables not currently in the model, the one that most improves the discriminatory power of the model is entered.

For logistic regression we considered sets of variables selected stepwise using the residual chi-square statistic. We assessed the model fit by the Schwarz criterion

(Schwarz, 1978) and by the significance using minus twice the log-likelihood. The latter has a chi-square distribution under the null hypothesis that all coefficients of explanatory variables in the model are zero. The Schwarz criterion is a modified version of Akaike's information criterion (AIC). They both adjust the minus twice the log-likelihood statistic by the number of observations and the number of variables. Lower values are obtained for the better-fitting model. The Wald chi-square statistic was used to check the significance of an individual parameter. For classification trees we used predictor importance ranking.

23.3.2   Classification procedures

A discriminant analysis procedure is designed to develop a set of discriminating functions which can help predict the classifying result ('response', 'grouping') based on the values of other explanatory ('predicting') variables. Linear and quadratic discrimination (Morrison, 1976; Krzanowski, 1988; McLachlan, 1992) as well as kernel methods (Habbema et al., 1978) with normal kernel function, and the covariance matrix both pooled from different groups' covariance matrices and not pooled (using different covariance matrices in groups) were employed on the subset of the most discriminating variables selected. For the kernel method the radius was determined experimentally to achieve optimal leave-one-out classification.

We used classification trees such as the CART (Classification and Regression Trees) method of Breiman et al. (1984) and the novel QUEST (Quick, Unbiased, Efficient Statistical Tree) method of Loh and Shih (1997). We also applied logistic regression (Anderson, 1972), which is appropriate for mixed models.

23.3.3   Assessment of classification errors

The data set examined was not big enough to be divided into a learning and a testing sample. Thus, to measure the effectiveness of new patients' classification, we used cross-validation and we determined the leave-one-out error. For classification trees three random subsamples were used for cross-validation. For all methods examined we also computed the resubstitution error. For classification trees we used Statistica 5.0 for Windows (Statsoft) and for discriminant analysis and logistic regression we used SAS version 8.2 (SAS Institute Inc, Cary, NC).

23.3.4   Approaches to missing values

To perform discriminant analysis and logistic regression, values of all variables for each case are required. When data for some variables were missing we applied casewise deletion, obtaining smaller data sets. To manage the problem of missing values we also employed the multiple imputation method of filling in missing data with plausible values. We made use of the method of multiple imputation, EMis (expectation–maximization with importance resampling) by King et al. (2001), applying AMELIA: The Program for Imputing Missing Data. The number of imputed data sets was equal to 5.

23.4   RESULTS

Missing data can either be substituted by the group mean of the respective predicting variable, by case-wise deletion, or by imputation. In the latter case, a filled-in set of simulated data is created where the missing values are completed on the basis of an analysis of all information available from the original data. Our data set contained missing values not only for quantitative but also for qualitative variables. For this reason, we could not substitute missing values by means. Furthermore, this method would have led to bias and would have been admissible only when the number of missing data points was very small (i.e., less than 5 %). Since the proportions of missing values were substantial for some of the variables – even approaching 50 % (variables 18–21 of Table 23.1) – we used two kinds of analyses. At first, a case-wise deletion of missing data was performed, that is, a case was deleted from the analysis if it had missing data for at least one of the selected variables. In this way, a smaller set of patients without missing values remained for the analysis of many variables. For example, 54 patients were available for the six most discriminating variables selected ($\lambda_A = 0.67$) for classification A {variables 12, 20, 2, 4, 1, 21}, and 54 patients remained for the five most discriminating variables selected ($\lambda_C = 0.42$) for classification C {variables 12, 17, 7, 11, 20}. These five variables are the ones marked with an asterisk in Table 23.1. For all 21 variables we had only 44 patients (aged between 0.5 and 15.5 years) with full information ($\lambda_C = 0.29$, $\lambda_A = 0.41$), but for three variables {4, 12, 17}, selected by logistic regression and classification C, we have the full set of 114 patients without missing values ($\lambda_C = 0.74$).

Alternatively, we could have reduced the number of variables by removing those which were the most incomplete. Instead, we chose another type of analysis. We left all variables in the model and performed multiple imputation, obtaining five sets with all 21 variables and all 114 cases. Then we performed the discriminant methods five times and pooled the results of those five classifications. We computed means of the classification errors with their variation (not presented in classification summaries' tables).

For the two levels of classification A we were able to obtain only one canonical discriminant function. From Figure 23.1 one can see the good discrimination between groups A1 and A2 ($\lambda_A = 0.49$). For the three groups of patients B1, B2 and B3 we obtained two canonical discriminant functions with very good separation. This is confirmed by the relatively small value of Wilks's $\lambda_B = 0.26$. In order to increase the sizes of the groups we combined groups B1 and B2 into one group (C1: 'death') and performed the two-level classification C.

23.4.1   Classification C

We selected a subset of variables using stepwise selection. The criterion for goodness of discrimination was again Wilks's λ. Stepwise forward selection for classification C, without filling in missing values, gave a set of nine most discriminating variables variables: {12, 17, 7, 11, 20, 1, 8, 5, 6}; $\lambda_C = 0.34$). The same result

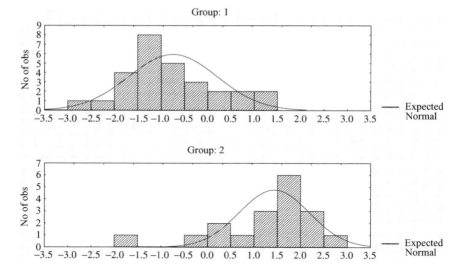

Figure 23.1 Classification A. Histogram of canonical discriminant function on the basis of 10 best discriminating original variables {12, 20, 2, 4, 1, 21, 16, 7, 15, 10}.

was obtained for mixed selection. The most meaningful reduction in Wilks's λ was achieved for variables chosen first. For example, for the five prime variables we obtained $\lambda_C = 0.42$. Those were variables 12, 17, 7, 11, 20: GRBLOOD, TIMETORE, CNS, PLT, CD10; see Table 23.1. On the basis of these five variables we estimated the classification error of different discriminant methods (Table 23.2).

Table 23.2 Results of classification C. Error rate of different discriminant methods on the basis of the five most discriminating variables {12, 17, 7, 11, 20}, selected by stepwise method on Wilks's λ and the best classification tree.

Method	Case-wise deletion ($n = 54$)		Multiple imputation (5 sets; $n = 114$)	
	Resubstitution	Cross-validation	Mean resubstitution	Mean cross-validation
Linear	0.019	0.11	0.19	0.2
Quadratic	0.056	0.11	0.15	0.22
Kernel pooled covariance (radius $r = 1.0$)	0.056	0.093	0.147	0.21
Kernel non-pooled covariance (radius $r = 1.0$)	0.037	0.093	0.147	0.18
Classification tree (QUEST FACT $F = 0.05$) using variables No. 12, 17, 18, 20	0.04	0.27	0.15	0.27

For five data sets, completed by multiple imputation, the subsets of most discriminating variables were all nearly the same as those obtained above. We performed a discriminant analysis on this subset of variables. Table 23.2 compares the results for the original data set with that of the pooled results for the five completed data sets, for the different methods on the basis of the five variables. The best results (smallest errors) are underlined in each column.

The results of the discriminant analysis were investigated using equal prior (EP) probabilities as well as prior probabilities proportional to group size (PP). Notice that the numbers of patients in the two groups of classification C differed considerably ($n = 30$ versus $n = 84$). Consequently, the EP results were worse than the PP results. Table 23.2 shows the PP results only. Kernel radius r, chosen as the most optimal by leave-one-out classifications, was 1.0 in all examined cases. The results of the best classification tree are presented in the last row of Table 23.2. Figure 23.2 shows the result of the QUEST classification tree with five splits and six nodes on the basis of four most important variables {12, 17, 18, 21}. We observed a large difference between the resubstitution (0.04) and the global cross-validation error (0.27). This indicates that the tree is 'overfitted'. Most important variables were GRBLOOD and TIMETOREM {12, 17}. These variables were also chosen by stepwise logistic regression (see Table 23.3) where several subsets of variables were found. All these subsets are significant at a level smaller than 0.01 using the minus

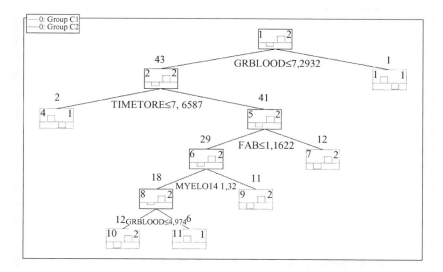

Figure 23.2 Classification C. Tree for predicting alive patients with QUEST, FACT = 0.05. Resubstitution error = 0.04; global cross-validation error = 0.27. Numbers near the branches of the tree (line segments) show the number of patients from the learning sample. Numbers in the upper left-hand corner denote the following node number. Numbers in the upper right-hand corner specify the group to which the patient is classified, when satisfying the condition of this node written below the node.

twice the log-likelihood statistic. Significant coefficients for each explanatory variable confirmed by the Wald statistic are marked by an asterisk. The subset of the five variables is exactly the same as that obtained with the stepwise mixed method and the forward selection method using Wilks's λ. Logistic regression was no more efficient than other methods. Most efficient were nonparametric methods with normal kernels, both for the original and the imputed data sets. For the imputed data sets with all 21 variables we obtained the best results for kernel with PP (leave-one-out mean error $= 0.13$, not presented in this paper).

One can use a simple linear discriminant function to classify a new patient x as

$$\text{LDF}_C(x) = 6.288 \times \text{CNS} - 0.00001 \times \text{PLT} + 1.28 \times \text{GRBLOOD} - 0.18 \\ \times \text{TIMETORE} - 3.39 \times \text{CD10} - 0.51.$$

If $\text{LDF}_C(x)$ is bigger than 0, we classify the new patient x to group C1 else to group C2 with resubstitution error $= 0.019$ and leave-one-out error $= 0.11$. The easy to use classification tree (see Figure 23.2) has a considerably larger cross-validation error. The errors for the original data set ($n = 54$ cases) and the data set completed by multiple imputation ($n = 114$) are compared in Tables 23.2 and 23.3.

Table 23.3 Results of Classification C. Error rate of logistic regression for variables selected stepwise on the basis of residual chi-square statistic (an asterisk denotes a coefficients significant at level 0.05)

Number of variables	Variables	Standardized parameter estimate	Odds ratio	Case-wise deletion ($n = 54$) Resubstitution error	Multiple imputation (5 sets; $n = 114$) Mean resubstitution error
3	4	0.483^*	1.507		
	12	0.195^*	2.804	0.21	0.22
	17	-1.475^*	0.858		
4	17	-0.266^*	0.758		
	7	2.02^*	16983		
	12	2.4^*	7.993	0.12	0.18
	20	-0.33	0.185		
5	12	2.014^*	5.684		
	17	-2.277^*	0.79		
	7	1.83^*	7093	0.11	0.17
	11	-0.339	1.0		
	20	-1.37	0.153		
6	6	1.239	0.000006		
	7	2.052	16317		
	11	0.32	1.0	0.11	0.21
	12	3.189	15.653		
	17	-2.59	0.734		
	20	-1.637	0.00025		

23.4.2   Classification A

The stepwise mixed forward–backward method and also the forward method provide the six variables {20, 12, 7, 8, 5, 9} with $\lambda_A = 0.67$. With this set of features we performed the same classification set as shown in Table 23.2 for classification C. We can again recommend the use of kernel functions. For imputed data sets and all 21 variables we obtained the highest effectiveness for kernel PP (average leave-one-out error $= 0.2$). The classification trees with the smallest cross-validation errors were once again overfitted. Logistic regression was again not as efficient as other methods. In this analysis the most important variables were blood group and CD10 {12, 20}.

The linear discriminant function for classifying a new patient x into groups A1 and A2 is given as

$$\text{LDF}_A(x) = -0.3974 \times \text{GRBLOOD} + 2.8 \times \text{CD10} - 0.788 \times \text{CNS} + 0.09$$
$$\times \text{HB} - 0.05 \times \text{SPLEEN} - 0.73.$$

If this value is bigger than 0 we can classify a new patient x to group A1 else to group A2 (resubstitution error $= 0.18$ and leave-one-out error $= 0.35$). In general, the errors were larger than for classification C, which can be explained easily by the values of Wilks's λ.

23.4.3   Classification B

The most discriminating variables, chosen by the mixed (forward–backward) selection procedure on the basis of Wilks's λ_A, are {7, 12, 17, 20, 21}. The best satisfying results were obtained likewise for nonparametric kernel methods.

23.5   DISCUSSION

The subset of variables selected by the stepwise procedure does not always lead to the best possible model and Wilks's λ need not be the best measure of discriminatory power. Though this method is best when the data of the groups are multivariate normally distributed with equal covariance matrices, it is often used also for variables not fulfilling those assumptions. We should emphasize that our data do not satisfy this assumption. However, when connecting the selection of the model with knowledge of the data and the leave-one-out procedure for assessing the error, this selection procedure can be valuable. Subsets of variables obtained in tree classification and in other classification methods were more consistent for classification C. The better results obtained for classification C than for classification A are explicable by a smaller value of Wilks's λ. For all 21 variables considered, $\lambda_C = 0.295$; and $\lambda_A = 0.41$, and for the five or six most discriminating variables $\lambda_C = 0.42$ and $\lambda_A = 0.67$.

Variables {12, 17, 20} – GRBLOOD, TIMETOREM and CD10 – proved to be important in all three classifications. For all three classifications, the variable selections for data sets completed by multiple imputations were nearly the same as for the original data set with case-wise deletion. For all three classifications, blood group (variable 12) was the first (or second) among most sets of discriminating variables, and it was present in all subsets. We are not aware of other work where blood group was a prognostic factor of child ALL. However, blood group H was associated with bad prognosis in patients with AML in Marosi *et al.* (1992) and it probably also was with B-cell precursor ALL (Fink *et al.*, 1993).

Logistic regression has a simple underlying linear structure and is more popular and more available than kernel discrimination. The smallest resubstitution error obtained for logistic regression was not substantially inferior to other classification methods. Classification trees are flexible and have become very common for classification. Their ability to display the results graphically in an easily understandable way and their ease of interpretation make this method very suitable in aiding medical diagnosis. However, for our data we struggled with overfitted trees.

We should emphasize that for all classification problems examined the most effective cross-validation result of all discriminant classifiers considered was obtained for the kernel normal discrimination both for the incomplete original data and for data sets after multiple imputation. Worse results for sets after multiple imputation may be explained by a change in the sizes of groups analyzed. Other investigators concluded that multiple imputation is robust and may forgive departures from the imputation model (Schafer *et al.*, 1998; Kott, 1995). The method can be applied even if the data are not missing at random (MAR). One should, however, remark that the MAR assumption is not testable, at least not without additional assumptions. The validity of inferences from multiple imputations has also been discussed (see Fay, 1992; Schafer *et al.*, 1996).

23.6 CONCLUDING REMARKS

Different methods of selection of the most discriminating variables (discriminant methods, classification trees and logistic regression) for aiding prediction of outcome of childhood leukemia resulted in similar sets of prognostic variables. The prognostic value of the variables determined in this analysis could be confirmed by an evaluation of overall survival and event-free survival (work in progress). Blood group is the most important or second most important variable for all classification problems considered. Additionally, for predicting patient survival during the first remission, the second most important variable is the time until remission, and for predicting outcome without event (relapse or death) the most important variable is the presence of CD10 antigen on leukemic cells.

Classification trees are flexible, easy to use and understood by doctors, but the classification error for a new patient/trial by cross-validation was less satisfying. Although the resubstitution error was small, the best trees obtained appeared to be overfitted.

We obtained an increase in classification errors for sets after multiple imputations. For our data, for all classification problems, the most effective results were achieved by nonparametric Bayesian discrimination with normal kernels.

CHAPTER 24

Non-melanoma Skin and Lung Cancer Incidence in Relation to Arsenic Exposure: 20 Years of Observation

Vladimír Bencko, Petr Franěk and Jiří Rameš

Charles University Prague

Elenóra Fabiánová

Regional Institute of Health Banská Bystrica

Miloslav Götzl

District Hospital of Bojnice

24.1 INTRODUCTION

The trace element contents of coal show marked geographic variations (Thornton and Farago, 1997). In a previous study (Bencko, 1997; Bencko *et al.*, 2001) we examined the ecological as well as the human health hazards (e.g., neuro- and immunotoxicity) of environmental pollution due to exhausts emitted from a power plant burning local coal with high arsenic content. At the time of their recruitment, all human subjects included in that study had been living and/or working in the area surrounding the power plant. The population studied was followed up longitudinally over a period of 20 years to examine the trend in the incidence of non-melanoma skin cancer (NMSC) and lung cancer, the malignancies most frequently related to exposure to arsenic (Agency for Toxic Substances and Disease Registry, 2000;

Recent Advances in Quantitative Methods in Cancer and Human Health Risk Assessment
Edited by L. Edler and C. Kitsos © 2005 John Wiley & Sons, Ltd

World Health Organization, 2000; Pleško *et al.*, 2000). We summarize the data we gathered during this 20-year follow-up period.

Our database of 1503 NMSC cases (756 in men and 747 in women) and 1117 lung cancer cases (1007 in men and 110 in women) was collected over a period from 1977 through 1996 from a region polluted by emissions of a power plant that had been burning local coal with high arsenic content (ranging from 900 to 1500 g per tonne dry weight) since the mid 1950s.

24.2 MATERIAL AND METHODS

24.2.1 Study base

The cohorts studied were assembled over a 20-year period beginning in 1977. During the study period, a population-based survey was conducted in the central Slovakian district of Prievidza. The aim of the survey was to study the trend in the incidence of all types of malignant diseases. Furthermore, we created a local cancer register for the entire administrative region, with a population of about 125 000. During the study period, the actual size of population in Prievidza district remained more or less stable, as was evident during several censuses conducted by the government.

As part of the study, any patient diagnosed or suspected as having a malignant lesion was referred to the district oncologist for final diagnosis and treatment. In all subjects included, the diagnosis of cancer was confirmed by histological examinations of tissue samples obtained by biopsy or at autopsy. Structured questionnaires were used for collecting and recording data pertaining to the subjects' personal data, and residential, family and occupational histories. The data thus obtained were stored in a central database.

Our study base represents 1 335 000 man-years and 1 337 000 woman-years from a population of approximately 125 000 inhabitants.

24.2.2 Statistics

In the case of suspected residential exposure to arsenic, the size of the population at risk was estimated according to Breslow and Day (1987) using census data, and the estimated figures closely parallel those released by the Slovak Statistical Bureau.

Estimation of demographic data was as follows. Denote by A_i^{1970}, A_i^{1980} and A_i^{1991} the known sizes of the ith age group of population A obtained from census data. Partially linear estimations of person-years in time periods were calculated as follows: for 1977–1981,

$$C_1 = \sum_{i=1977}^{1980} \left(A_i^{1970} + (i - 1970) \frac{A_i^{1980} - A_i^{1970}}{1980 - 1970} \right) + \left(A_i^{1980} + \frac{A_i^{1991} - A_i^{1980}}{1991 - 1980} \right)$$

$$= 3 A_i^{1970} + 2 A_i^{1980} + \frac{12}{5} \left(A_i^{1980} - A_i^{1970} \right) + \frac{1}{11} \left(A_i^{1991} - A_i^{1980} \right)$$

for 1982–1986,

$$C_2 = \sum_{i=1982}^{1986} \left(A_i^{1980} + (i - 1980) \frac{A_i^{1991} - A_i^{1980}}{1991 - 1980} \right) = 5A_i^{1980} + \frac{20}{11} \left(A_i^{1991} - A_i^{1980} \right)$$

and for 1987–1991,

$$C_3 = \sum_{i=1987}^{1991} \left(A_i^{1980} + (i - 1980) \frac{A_i^{1991} - A_i^{1980}}{1991 - 1980} \right) = 5A_i^{1980} + \frac{45}{11} \left(A_i^{1991} - A_i^{1980} \right).$$

Incomplete census data were available for the exposed villages and the Prievidza district in the years 1992, 1993, 1994, 1995, 1996 and 1997 – for some of the villages only total numbers of men and women (or total numbers of inhabitants) were available for years 1992, 1993 and 1994. Unfortunately, the age categories 0–4, 5–9, ..., 30–34 were joined into one age group in these additional census data. In order to maintain consistency with the calculations in the previous periods the aggregate number A in the combined category 0–34 in the particular area (i.e. village or Prievidza district) observed in the particular year 1995 and 1996 in the case of the villages, and 1992–1996 in the case of the Prievidza district) was divided into the categories 0–4, 5–9, ..., 30–34 as follows:

$$A_i = A \frac{A_i^{1980} + A_i^{1991}}{A^{1980} + A^{1991}},$$

where A^{1980} and A^{1991} are sums of the observed headcounts in the categories 0–4, 5–9, ..., 30–34 in the census years 1980 and 1991 and A_i^{1980} and A_i^{1991}, $i = 0$–4, 5–9, ..., 30–34, are the observed headcounts from these years. Hence the aggregate value A was divided according to the historically observed structure. The average of the years 1980 and 1991 was used so as not to copy the situation observed in 1991 in full.

Having the values in the required age categories in the years 1991 (census data) and 1994 (census data combined with the estimation described above), the 1992, 1993 and 1994 values in the different age and sex categories were calculated using linear interpolation as described for the first three periods. The approximated values were then multiplied by appropriate constants to match the known totals for men and women in these years.

In the case of suspected occupational exposure to arsenic, the size of the population at risk was estimated using data recorded in the employees' registry maintained by the power plant authority. A complete set of numbers of employees of the power station were available divided into the required age categories for all observed years. Although no benchmark figure was available, it is unlikely that there remained any differential contamination in our estimates of the sizes of the various cohorts included in our study.

The age-adjusted incidence rates (AIRs) in different groups were evaluated using direct standardisation methodology. The world standard population was used as a standard population. The study subjects were stratified into different age groups by decade intervals (0–9, ..., 60–69, 70+). For two-by-two comparisons of AIRs in different groups (defined by a combination of smoking and exposure status), the ratio of rates (RR) was evaluated for two particular groups and its 95 % confidence interval calculated as already described (Breslow and Day, 1987; Boyle and Parkin, 1991). Both direct and indirect standardisations were used to cross-verify the results (Kahn, 1989). Not unexpectedly, the results of all three methods correspond well to one another as long as each group thus compared contained a reasonable number of persons-years. While this was the case in residential exposure, the variances of AIRs were very large in power plant employees, presumably due to the small number of person-years.

Accordingly, the results of the three different methods used varied in this subset of population. However, their statistical interpretations remained the same. Standard statistical software (MS Access 2000 and MS Excel 2000 Applications) was used for all statistical analyses.

24.2.3   Exposure assessment

Exposure assessment of the local non-occupationally exposed general population of the district was based on biological monitoring of arsenic in hair and urine samples obtained from groups of 20–25 ten-year-old boys from different localities situated up to a distance of 30 km from the local power plant. The district of exposure was divided into two areas marked off by a circle of radius 7.5 km around the power plant. The criterion for higher exposure included a mean arsenic concentration in excess of 3 µg per gram of hair. Close to 20 % of the study subjects lived within 7.5 km of the exposed region, and the rest living in other parts of the district served as "control" population.

Although not free of problems, hair appears to be the most readily obtainable biological specimen for determining arsenic exposure. Our data lend further credence to the idea of using hair arsenic concentrations for monitoring environmental pollution due to arsenic. As the levels of arsenic in various biological specimens show marked individual variations, groupwise comparison of arsenic levels proved to be more meaningful (Bencko, 1995). The levels of arsenic in urine reflect the amount of arsenic that an individual has recently inhaled or ingested. Although not universally accepted, an arsenic level in excess of 3 µg per gram of hair should be considered as abnormally high, while values up to 1 µg/g may not indicate high exposure to arsenic (Bencko, 1995; World Health Organization, 2000).

24.3   RESULTS

The age-adjusted incidence of histologically confirmed NMSC in non-occupational settings ranged from 43.7 to 92.0 per 100 000 population in men and from 34.6 to 79.1 in women. The age-adjusted incidence of histologically confirmed lung cancer ranged from 10.9 to 89.8 per 100 000 population in men and from 1.3 to 10.1 in women.

Table 24.1 Non-melanoma skin cancer incidence in the population living in the vicinity of the power plant burning coal of high arsenic content and in the rest of the district.

(a) Males only

	1977–1981		1982–1986		1987–1991		1992–1996	
	Exp. cases (p-years)	Reference cases (p-years)	Exp. cases (p-years)	Reference cases (p-years)	Exp. cases (p-years)	Reference cases (p-years)	Exp. cases (p-years)	Reference cases (p-years)
Absolute number	44	125	32	134	30	142	27	222
Expected number	23.8		20.8		18.6		24.7	
Non-standardized rate	98.4	45.8	77.6	46.5	81.9	46.9	78.2	70.9
Age standardized rate	93.9	45.9	66.9	45.9	65.2	46.0	57.8	65.7
Statistical parameters (95 % confidence interval)								
SMR	2.05		1.46		1.42		0.88	
Mantel–Haenszel estimate	2.02	(1.43–2.85)	1.46	(0.99–2.15)	1.39	(0.94–2.05)	0.88	(0.59–1.31)
Probability	<0.01	S	0.05	S	0.10	NS	0.54	NS

Table 24.1 (*Continued*)

(b) Females only

	1977–1981		1982–1986		1987–1991		1992–1996	
	Exp. cases (p-years)	Reference cases (p-years)	Exp. cases (p-years)	Reference cases (p-years)	Exp. cases (p-years)	Reference cases (p-years)	Exp. cases (p-years)	Reference cases (p-years)
Absolute number	46	118	32	134	22	165	25	205
Expected number	22.7		20.1		20.1		23.4	
Non-standardized rate	104.9	43.3	78.3	46.3	59.7	53.9	70.9	65.9
Age standardized rate	81.4	34.6	54.4	37.4	39.8	42.7	37.5	56.1
Statistical parameters (95 % confidence interval)								
SMR	2.35		1.45		0.93		0.67	
Mantel–Haenszel estimate	2.25	(2.23–2.27)	1.47	(1.45–1.48)	0.88	(0.88–0.90)	0.70	(0.46–1.06)
Probability	<0.01	S	0.05	S	0.59	NS	0.09	NS

Table 24.2 Non-melanoma skin and lung cancer incidence in workers (males only) of the power plant burning coal of high arsenic content and in the rest of the district population.

(a) Non-melanoma skin cancer

	1977–1981		1982–1986		1987–1991		1992–1996	
	Exp. cases (p-years)	Reference cases (p-years)	Exp. cases (p-years)	Reference cases (p-years)	Exp. cases (p-years)	Reference cases (p-years)	Exp. cases (p-years)	Reference cases (p-years)
Absolute number	3	166	7	159	9	163	11	238
Expected number	3.5		3.7		3.7		4.5	
Non-standardized rate	45.0	53.3	95.0	49.3	123.6	49.0	173.3	69.7
Age standardized rate	44.6	68.4	355.5	61.0	10 317	59.7	7 357	63.8
Statistical parameters (95 % confidence interval)								
SMR	0.65		5.83		172.00		115.24	
Mantel–Haenszel estimate	0.83	(0.26–2.62)	2.70	(1.27–5.75)	3.55	(1.81–6.95)	4.49	(2.47–8.14)
Probability	<0.75	NS	0.01	S	<0.01	S	<0.01	S

Table 24.2 (*Continued*)

(b) Lung cancer

	1977–1981		1982–1986		1987–1991		1992–1996	
	Exp. cases (p-years)	Reference cases (p-years)	Exp. cases (p-years)	Reference cases (p-years)	Exp. cases (p-years)	Reference cases (p-years)	Exp. cases (p-years)	Reference cases (p-years)
Absolute number	3	208	6	235	7	300	4	244
Expected number	4.4		5.4		6.6		4.5	
Non-standardized rate	45.0	66.8	81.3	72.9	96.1	90.3	63.0	71.4
Age standardized rate	44.7	87.8	204.4	92.1	1368.3	112.8	3666.5	65.5
Statistical parameters (95 % confidence interval)								
SMR	0.51		2.22		12.13		1.67	
Mantel–Haenszel estimate	0.56	(0.18–1.75)	1.19	(0.53–2.68)	1.28	(0.61–2.69)	1.73	(0.66–4.53)
Probability	<0.31	NS	0.67	NS	0.52	NS	0.26	NS

The prime objective of the present study was to examine whether environmental pollution due to arsenic would have any effect on the incidence of NMSC and lung cancer. The data presented here did, in fact, show that over the first 10-year period there had been a dramatic increase in the incidence of NMSC in the most polluted region of Prievidza district (Tables 24.1 and 24.2). This upward trend gradually reversed during the next five-year period. In our opinion, this downward trend in the incidence of NMSC is most likely attributed to the measures taken by the plant authority to reduce the levels of arsenic emissions from the plant. We feel strongly that the downward trend in the incidence of NMSC following reduction in the arsenic emissions from the power plant may suggest a dose–effect relationship between the degree of environmental pollution due to arsenic and NMSC incidence. The biological plausibility of such a notion is understandable, considering the fact that arsenic is a known inducer of *p53* mutations in basal cells (Seidl *et al.*, 2001).

24.4   DISCUSSION

The incidence of skin cancer showed an upward trend during the last five years of the study in the regions considered to be less polluted. Understandably, the individuals living in this area had been exposed to lower levels of arsenic over a prolonged period of time. These data suggest that arsenic may have a cumulative effect on the incidence of NMSC.

We did not observe any sex-related bias in the incidence of NMSC in our study population. The incidence of NMSC appeared to have been markedly influenced by exposure to arsenic in occupational settings (Table 24.3a). This may not be surprising, as a recent study has noted that the levels of arsenic still often exceed the permissible levels in such industrial operations as maintenance and boiler cleaning. An expected difference in lung cancer incidence in environmental settings is demonstrated in Table 24.3. In occupational settings the development of lung cancer incidence follows a dramatically different pattern. The small numbers of cases represent a significant problem.

Since industrial safety measures have been markedly improved as compared to those in place in the 1960s and 1970s, we are currently focusing our attention on the long-term effects of arsenic exposure on human health in those occupational settings (Buchancová *et al.*, 1998; Fabiánová *et al.*, 2000).

We carefully evaluated the history of smoking habits of all study subjects in both environmental and occupational settings. This provided us an opportunity to examine the potential interaction between arsenic exposure and cigarette smoking in the induction of malignant lesions in the lungs as well as in other body sites (Welch, 1982; Jarup and Pershagen, 1991; Hertz-Picciotto *et al.*, 1992). We have also considered the smoking habits of the general population and their relevance to the population we studied. Hitherto we have not found reliable statistical tools and data to perform a relevant analysis enabling us to assess the share of arsenic and smoking in our lung cancer cases database. The problem in this context is the difficulty of comparing our smoking habit data, collected carefully in a standard

Table 24.3 Lung cancer incidence in population living in the vicinity of the power plant burning coal of high arsenic content and in the rest of the district.

(a) Males only

	1977–1981		1982–1986		1987–1991		1992–1996	
	Exp. cases (p-years)	Reference cases (p-years)	Exp. cases (p-years)	Reference cases (p-years)	Exp. cases (p-years)	Reference cases (p-years)	Exp. cases (p-years)	Reference cases (p-years)
Absolute number	37	174	41	200	36	271	5	243
Expected number	29.7		30.2		33.1		24.6	
Non-standardized rate	82.7	63.7	99.4	69.4	98.3	89.5	14.5	77.5
Age standardized rate	77.7	66.1	85.1	69.9	78.5	89.8	10.8	73.2
Statistical parameters (95 % confidence interval)								
SMR	1.17		1.22		0.87		0.15	
Mantel–Haenszel estimate	1.19	(0.84–1.70)	1.24	(0.88–1.73)	0.87	(0.61–1.23)	0.15	(0.06–0.36)
Probability	0.33	NS	0.21	NS	0.42	NS	<0.01	S

Table 24.3 (*Continued*)

(b) Females only

	1977–1981		1982–1986		1987–1991		1992–1996	
	Exp. cases (p-years)	Reference cases (p-years)	Exp. cases (p-years)	Reference cases (p-years)	Exp. cases (p-years)	Reference cases (p-years)	Exp. cases (p-years)	Reference cases (p-years)
Absolute number	4	18	6	28	2	28	1	23
Expected number	3.1		4.2		3.2		2.4	
Non-standardized rate	9.1	6.6	14.7	9.7	5.4	9.1	2.8	7.2
Age standardized rate	5.3	5.8	10.1	7.5	3.1	7.3	1.1	6.0
Statistical parameters (95 % confidence interval)								
SMR	0.92		1.34		0.43		0.33	
Mantel–Haenszel estimate	1.25	(0.42–3.67)	1.31	(0.54–3.15)	0.48	(0.11–2.01)	0.33	(0.04–2.45)
Probability	0.67	NS	0.55	NS	0.30	NS	0.25	NS

manner, with 'soft' data from the general population available for only a limited part of our study period.

Although debatable, cigarette smoking is not considered as an important risk factor for NMSC (Nieuwenhuijsen *et al.*, 2001; Pesch *et al.*, 2002). The possibility that the study cohorts differed in terms of the exposure to ultraviolet radiation (Rossman, 1999; Seidl *et al.*, 2001) is considered extremely unlikely as the study populations in the more as well as less polluted areas comprise almost equal proportions of villagers and city dwellers.

24.5 CONCLUSION

Our data demonstrate a positive correlation between human cumulative exposure to arsenic and incidence of NMSC. This adds further confirmation to the long clinical and epidemiological experience corroborating NMSC and exposure to arsenic. Due to the almost equal likelihood of ultraviolet lilght exposure of the populations residing in more and less polluted areas of the study region, this confounding variable might not have any effect on the differences in incidence of NMSC as noted between these populations. A less pronounced relationship was noted between arsenic exposure and incidence of lung cancer. This is most likely to be due to the presence of such confounding variables as cigarette smoking.

ACKNOWLEDGEMENTS

This study was supported by EC INCO COPERNICUS EXPASCAN grant ERBBIC 15 CT98-0325. Statistical analysis was carried out in collaboration with EuroMISE Centre Cardio, supported by project LN00B107 of the Ministry of Education of the Czech Republic.

CHAPTER 25

Thyroid Cancer Incidence Rates in Zaragoza

Milagros Bernal

University of Zaragoza

25.1 INTRODUCTION

Thyroid cancer is a disease with an incidence that is generally constant in a population (Yamashita *et al.*, 1997). In Europe the incidence rate is about 2.22 per 100 000 inhabitants. This rate shows changes over time in certain geographical zones due to substantial changes in the environment, almost always related to radiation. Examples are radiation exposures in Hiroshima and Nagasaki as a consequence of the atomic bomb, and most recently in Belarus, Russia and Ukraine as a consequence of the Chernobyl accident in 1986 when large amounts of radiation were emitted into the environment. Changes were also recorded in a large part of the rest of Europe (World Health Organization, 1996). The problem was that the actual geographical zone that suffered the impact from the radiation was not known at that time and that the radioactive cloud could have migrated from one geographical zone to another which would subsequently suffer from the environmental impact of that radiation and would have an increased cancer risk due to radiation.

The Spanish district of Zaragoza was not heavily exposed to radiation as a result of the Chernobyl accident. However, there had been concerns among the Spanish public about the health consequences even from low exposure levels and the small increase in radiation in the area after the accident. Therefore, the authorities of the Zaragoza district were interested in investigating the changes in thyroid cancer incidence and thyroid cancer mortality in the years following the accident. Before 1986, the thyroid cancer incidence rate in Spain varied between 1.8 and 2.0 new cases per 100 000 inhabitants. After 1986 thyroid cancer incidence data were collected to investigate hypotheses as to the possible consequences of the Chernobyl accident in this area of Spain. Those hypotheses were highly important for the discussion of the future of energy production policy in Europe, in particular, when it was discussed whether the nuclear energy production should be maintained or abandoned.

From a physical point of view it seems rather improbable that the radiation levels detected in Spain exceeded normal levels as a consequence of the Chernobyl accident. It is also improbable that exposure after the accident was increased by imports of contaminated food from affected zones or that in the future the radiation from Chernobyl could have a carcinogenic or toxic effect on humans. On the other hand, according to some authors, the increase of radioactive contamination in, for example, cheese and some types of vegetables could have been large enough to affect the thyroid system, and these effects could then be related to an increase in thyroid cancer incidence, especially in women, causing a special histopathological type of papillary carcinoma in the thyroid.

This study aims to describe thyroid cancer incidence in Zaragoza after the Chernobyl accident and to establish a relationship between low radiation exposure after Chernobyl and thyroid cancer. We give a descriptive evaluation of thyroid cancer incidence ratios and examine how thyroid cancer incidence varied over the last ten years.

25.2   MATERIAL AND METHODS

A representative sample of 300 000 inhabitants was identified in part of the province of Zaragoza located in the Ebro valley in the Northwest of Spain. From a demographic point of view, this area can be characterized by the results of the population censuses of the years 1986, 1991 and 1996. Extrapolating the years between censuses provides the yearly data (Carreter, 1996).

Thyroid cancer incidence rates in this area from 1989 until 1998 were obtained from global annual incidence rates (World Health Organization, 1971) and were calculated using the method of cumulative incidence rates. The diagnosis of patients with thyroid cancer was based on clinical and pathological criteria (Isselbacher, 1994). Included were all cases of thyroid cancer that occurred between 1989 and 1998 in Health District III of the province of Zaragoza, comprising about 300 000 inhabitants. The 10-year period was further divided into two sections of five years each to test for any statistically significant effects using the Wilcoxon test. Linear regression was applied to annual incidence rates for the years studied and the slope parameter was calculated to estimate the yearly increase in incidence rates throughout this period. This analysis was adjusted for confounders through an analysis of variance. Specific rates of thyroid cancer were adjusted for gender using the direct method.

Spontaneous thyroid cancers in the investigated area were not considered as cases when those persons had earlier undergone radiotherapy for some previous neoplastic disease or other causes.

25.3 RESULTS

Among the 300 000 inhabitants of Health District III of the province of Zaragoza were found a total of 131 thyroid cancer cases between 1989 and 1998; 30 (23 %) in men and 101 (77 %) in women. The annual incidence per 100 000 inhabitants was therefore 4.3 (adjusted 3.25). It was higher in women (6.73, adjusted 4.4) than in men (2.14, adjusted 1.61). The specific crude rates as well as the adjusted rates by gender are shown in Table 25.1.

Table 25.1 Thyroid cancer incidence in Zagaroza.

(a) Males only Year	Cases	Rate	95 % confidence limits	Adj. Rate
1989	1	0.63	0.1–1.87	0.37
1990	6	3.76	1.38–8.2	2.21
1991	1	0.63	0.1–1.87	0.37
1992	3	1.90	0.38–5.5	1.25
1993	1	0.63	0.1–1.87	0.37
1994	4	2.50	0.68–6.4	1.97
1995	4	2.50	0.68–6.4	1.97
1996	4	2.50	0.68–6.4	1.97
1997	5	3.44	2.9–11.4	2.31
1998	1	0.63	0.1–1.87	0.37

(b) Females only Year	Cases	Rate	95 % confidence limits	Adj. Rate
1989	11	6.86	3.44–12.35	5.33
1990	8	4.99	1.82–9.15	4.28
1991	12	7.48	3.95–12.72	5.26
1992	10	6.24	2.9–11.4	5.09
1993	8	4.99	1.82–9.15	4.28
1994	10	6.24	2.9–11.4	5.09
1995	9	6.06	2.57–10.6	4.57
1996	9	6.06	2.57–10.6	4.57
1997	10	6.24	2.9–11.4	5.09
1998	14	8.73	5.24–14.4	6.76

The most frequent histopathologic type was papillary carcinoma (84 cases, 64.1 %), followed by follicular (18 cases, 13.7 %) and unclassified carcinoma (17 cases, 12.9 %). To a lesser extent were observed medullar and anaplasic carcinoma (4 cases each, 3.1 %) and one case of Hürthle's carcinoma.

Most of those diagnosed cases were found in the limited disease condition (101 cases, 77 %). In 24 patient (18 %) there were metastases in regional ganglia, and in 6 patients (4.5 %) metastasis had spread. The geographical distribution was as follows: 81 cases (61.1 %) lived in urban and 50 persons (38.8 %) in rural areas.

Linear regression of the variation of the incidence rate throughout the 10 years showed no statistically significant increase of the slope (s) during this time either in women, $s = 0.19$ ($p = 0.15$), or in men, $s = 0.07$ ($p = 0.47$). The corresponding confidence intervals were $(-0.08, 3.5)$ and $(-0.06, 3.95)$, respectively. Therefore, it is concluded that incidence rates have remained practically constant in this part of Western Europe.

Furthermore, the logit model gave no statistically significant increase in the slope during this time either in women, $s = 0.62$ ($p = 0.10$), or in men, $s = 0.55$ ($p = 0.14$). The corresponding confidence intervals were $(-0.73, 5.96)$ and $(0.85, 4.77)$, respectively.

25.4 DISCUSSION

Worldwide there are an estimated 5 cases of thyroid cancer per 100 000 inhabitants. This rate is higher than the incidence observed in our study. In the area studied the incidence rates of thyroid cancer were 0.70 (adjusted 0.62) in men and 3.85 (adjusted 3.37) in women before 1986 (Bernal and De Frutos, 1994). It is notable that in 1998, in Health District III of the province of Zaragoza, the rate of incidence of thyroid cancer appeared to be 9.3 (adjusted 7.3) per 100 000 inhabitants (men and women combined). A follow-up study of the cancer incidence in this area is now of great importance.

A comparison of the incidence rates of the two 5-year periods of this study showed, however, no significant differences (Wilcoxon test: $p = 0.76$). Within the first half of the decade studied the rates showed more variations than in the second half. Regression showed that the increase in the slope was not statistically significant, either overall or in men. In women we observed a slight increasing trend. Similar effects have been observed by others (O'Hanlon et al., 1997; Ballivet et al., 1995). One cause of this increase could have been the improvement of techniques to diagnose thyroid cancer. The possibility that improved techniques would have increased the ability to detect cancerous nodule biopsies from 29 % to 42 % has been discussed. Increased thyroid cancer incidence rates in zones of high exposure have been reported by others (Carson et al., 1996).

An exhaustive study showed increased thyroid cancer incidence rates in Bulgaria, Austria, Greece and Romania. Increases from 3.07 in 1957 to 7.8 in 1994 were described for Tyrol in Austria (Parshkov et al., 1997). These figures can be compared with those obtained in Connecticut after the accident at the Millstone nuclear plant which showed an increase from 1.30 to 5.78 in women and from 0.30 to 2.77 in men (Lukacs et al., 1997).

In our study, there was no increase in thyroid cancer in children: the rates remained the same. Thyroid cancer in children is estimated at 0.5 cases per million per year worldwide. It is increased in areas affected by the Chernobyl accident (Zheng et al., 1996).

Thyroid sarcomas are extremely rare but have been described in persons living in nuclear disaster areas (Jacob et al., 1998). The cases described are not only more frequent, but also more severe, although no histopathologic information has been given. No sarcomas were observed in our study.

Other studies described an increase in thyroid cancer incidence in adolescents (aged 10–14 years) closely related to radiation. We found two cases within this age group. The much larger incidence of thyroid cancer in women than in men conforms with other findings in Europe (Sichel et al., 1996; Danese et al., 1997).

Individuals previously irradiated were not included in this study. Thus we cannot compare our results with other studies that compared the growth of thyroid cancer in relation to posterior radiation of the nose, throat, head or neck.

Iodine deficit may be related to follicular carcinomas, and excessive consumption of certain types of cheese and vegetables was related to papillary cancer (Galanti et al., 1997b). Based on histopathological information it was pointed out that economically developed countries most frequently encounter the papillary type of thyroid cancer, followed by follicular and other histophatological types (Galanti et al., 1997a). We should remark that a slight increase in papillary type cancers has been observed in the region studied. But with economic improvements and better links, Spanish nutritional habits have changed substantially, and one can assume an increase in the consumption of cheeses and vegetables. Therefore, a change of the histopathologic type of thyroid cancer at the expense of the follicular variety has to be considered (Fahey et al., 1995; Ertürk et al., 1996).

There is a need to combine clinical, genetic, epidemiological and pharmacological research so as to create models that could explain these differences in thyroid cancer incidence within and between countries. At the moment one can only speculate on genetic factors or susceptibilities as yet unknown.

References

Aaltonen, L. A., Peltomäki, P., Leach, F. S., Sistonen, P., Pylkkänen, L., Mecklin, J.-P., Järvinen, H., Powell, S. M., Jen, J., Hamilton, S. R., Peterson, G. M., Kinzler, K. W., Vogelstein, B. and de la Chapelle, A. (1993). Clues to the pathogenesis of familiar colorectal cancer. *Science* **260**, 812–816.

Abdelbasit, K. M. and Plackett, R. L. (1982). Experimental design for joint action. *Biometrics* **38**, 171–179.

Abraham, K., Krowke, R. and Neubert, D. (1988). Pharmacokinetics and biological activity of 2,3,7,8-tetrachlorodibenzo-*p*-dioxin. *Archives of Toxicology* **62**, 359–368.

Agency for Toxic Substances and Disease Registry (2000). *Toxicological Profile for Arsenic (update)*. Atlanta, GA: Department of Health & Human Services, USA, p. 428.

Albert, A. and Anderson, J. A. (1984). On the existence of maximum likelihood estimates in logistic models. *Biometrika* **71**, 1–10.

Albert, A., Gertman, P. M. and Louis, T. A. (1978a). Screening for the early detection of cancer. I. The temporal history of a progressive disease state. *Mathematical Biosciences* **40**, 1–59.

Albert, A., Gertman, P. M., Louis, T. A. and Liu, S. I. (1978b). Screening for the early detection of cancer. II. The impact of the screening on the natural history of the disease. *Mathematical Biosciences* **40**, 61–109.

Albertini, R. J. (2001). Developing sustainable studies on environmental health. *Mutation Research* **480–481**, 317–331.

Alexandrov, K., Cascorbi, I., Rojas, M., Bouvier, G., Kriek E. and Bartsch, H. (2002). *CYP1A1* and *GSTM1* genotypes affect benzo[*a*]pyrene DNA adducts in smokers' lung: comparison with aromatic/hydrophobic adduct formation. *Carcinogenesis* **23**, 1969–1977.

Alitalo, K., Schwab, M., Lin, C. C., Varmus, H. E. and Bishop, J. M. (1983). Homogeneously staining chromosomal regions contain amplified copies of an abundantly expressed cellular oncogene (*c-myc*) in malignant neuroendocrine cells from a human colon carcinoma. *Proceedings of the National Academy of Sciences of the USA* **80**, 1707.

Alitalo, K., Winqvist, R., Lin, C. C., de la Chapelle, A., Schwab, M. and Bishop, J. M. (1984). Aberrant expression of an amplified *c-myb* oncogene in two cell lines from a colon carcinoma. *Proceedings of the National Academy of Sciences of the USA* **81**, 4534.

Alizadeh, A. A., Eisen, M. B., Davis, R. E., Ma, C., Lossos, I. S., Rosenwald, A., Boldrick, J. C., Sabet, H., Tran, T., Yu, X., Powell, J. I., Yang, L., Marti, G. E., Moore, T., Hudson, J. Jr., Lu, L., Lewis, D. B., Tibshirani, R., Scherlock, G., Chan, W. C., Greiner, T. C., Weisenburger, D. D., Armitage, J. O., Warnke, R., Levy, R., Wilson, W., Grever, M. R., Bryd, J. C., Botstein, D., Brown, P. O. and Staudt, L. M. (2000). Distinct types of diffuse large B-cell lymphoma identified by gene expression profiling. *Nature* **403**, 503–511.

Amaral Mendes, J. J. (2002). The endocrine disrupters: A major medical challenge. *Food and Chemical Toxicology* **40**, 781–788.

Amaral Mendes, J. J. and Pluygers, E. (1999). Use of biochemical and molecular biomarkers for cancer risk assessment in humans. In *Perspectives on Biologically Based Cancer Risk Assessment*, V. J. Cogliano, E. G. Luebeck and G. A. Zapponi (eds), 81–182. New York: Kluwer Academic/Plenum Publishers.

Andersen, M. E. (2003). Toxicokinetic modeling and its applications in chemical risk assessment. *Toxicology Letters* **138**, 9–27.

Andersen, M. E., Birnbaum, L. S., Barton, H. A. and Eklund, C. R. (1997a). Regional hepatic CYP1A1 and CYP1A2 induction with 2,3,7,8-tetrachlorodibenzo-*p*-dioxin evaluated with a multicompartment geometric model of hepatic zonation. *Toxicology & Applied Pharmacology* **144**, 145–155.

Andersen, M. E., Eklund, C. R., Mills, J. J., Barton, H. A. and Birnbaum, L. S. (1997b). A multicompartment geometric model of the liver in relation to regional induction of cytochrome P450s. *Toxicology & Applied Pharmacology* **144**, 135–144.

Andersen, M. E., Mills, J. J., Gargas, M. L., Kedderis, L., Birnbaum, L. S., Neubert, D. and Greenlee, W. F. (1993). Modeling receptor-mediated processes with dioxin: implications for pharmacokinetics and risk assessment. *Risk Analysis* **13**, 25–36.

Andersen, M. E., Yang, R. S., French, C. T., Chubb, L. S. and Dennison, J. E. (2002). Molecular circuits, biological switches, and nonlinear dose-response relationships. *Environmental Health Perspectives* **110**, 971–978.

Anderson, J. A. (1972). Separate sample logistic discrimination. *Biometrika* **59**, 19–35.

Anderson, T. W. (2003). *An Introduction to Multivariate Statistical Analysis*, 3rd edition. New York: Wiley.

Annila, I. T., Annila, P. A. and Morsky, P. (1997). Risk assessment in determining systemic reactivity to honeybee stings in beekeepers. *Annals of Allergy Asthma & Immunology* **78**, 473–477.

Anonymous (2000). Consultation on assessment of the health risk of dioxins; reevaluation of the tolerable daily intake (TDI): Executive summary. *Food Additives and Contaminants* **17**, 223–240.

Ardanuy, R. and López Fidalgo, J. (1992). Optimal design with constraint support. *Revista de Matemática e Estatística* **10**, 193–205.

Arends, J. W. (2000). Molecular interactions in the Vogelstein model of colorectal carcinoma. *Journal of Pathology* **190**, 412.

Armitage, P. and Doll, R. (1954). The age distribution of cancer and a multistage theory of carcinogenesis. *British Journal of Cancer* **8**, 1–12.

Armitage, P. and Doll, R. (1957). A two-stage theory of carcinogenesis in relation to the age distribution of human cancer. *British Journal of Cancer* **11**, 161–169.

Arms, A. D. and Travis, C. C. (1988). *Reference Physiological Parameters in Pharmacokinetic Modeling*. Washington, DC: United States Enviromental Protection Agency.

Ashford, N. A. and Miller, C. S. (1996). Low-level chemical sensitivity: current perspectives. *International Archives of Occupational and Environmental Health* **68**, 367–376.

Ashford, N. A. and Miller, C. S. (1998). Low-level chemical exposures: a challenge for science and policy. *Viewpoint* **32**, 508–509.

Ashton-Rickardt, P. G., Dunlop, M. G., Nakamura, Y., Morris, R. G., Purdie, C. A., Steel, C. M., Evans, H. J., Bird, C. C. and Wylie, A. H. (1989). High frequency of APC loss in sporadic colorectal carcinoma due to breaks clustered in 5q21–22. *Oncogene* **4**, 1169.

Atkinson, A. C. and Bailey, R. A. (2001). One hundred years of the design of experiments on and off the pages of Biometrika. In *Biometrika: One Hundred Years*, D. M. Titterington and D. R. Cox (eds). Oxford: Oxford University Press.

Atkinson, N. E., Bartoszyński, R., Brown, B.W. and Thompson, J. R. (1983). On estimating the growth function of tumors. *Mathematical Biosciences* **67**, 145–166.

Atkinson, N. E., Brown, B. W. and Thompson, J. R. (1987). On the lack of concordance between primary and secondary tumor growth rates. *Journal of the National Cancer Institute* **78**, 425–435.

Aylward, L. L., Hays, S. M., Karch, N. J. and Paustenbach, D. J. (1996). Relative susceptibility of animals and humans to the cancer hazard posed by 2,3,7,8-tetrachlorodibenzo-*p*-dioxin using internal measures of does. *Enviromental Science & Technology* **30**, 3534–3543.

Bagdonavičius, V. and Nikulin, M. (1997). Semiparametric estimation in the generalized additive multiplicative model. In *Probability and Statistics, 2*, I. A. Ibragimov and V. A. Sudakov (eds), 7–27. St Petersburg: Proceedings of the Steklov Mathematical Institute.

Bagdonavičius, V. and Nikulin, M. (1999a). On semiparametric estimation of reliability from accelerated data. In *Statistical and Probabilistic Models in Reliability*, N. Ionescu and N. Limnios (eds), 75–89. Boston: Birkhäuser.

Bagdonavičius, V. and Nikulin, M. (1999b). Generalized proportional hazards model based on modified partial Likelihood. *Lifetime Data Analysis* **5**, 329–350.

Bagdonavičius, V. and Nikulin, M. (2000). On semiparametric estimation of reliability from accelerated data. In *Statistical and Probabilistic Models in Reliability*, N. Ionescu and N. Limnios (eds), 75–89. Boston: Birkhäuser.

Bagdonavičius, V. and Nikulin, M. (2002). *Accelerated Life Models: Modeling and Statistical Analysis*. Boca Raton, FL: Chapman & Hall.

Bagdonavičius, V. and Nikulin, M. (2004). Stochastical modelling in survival analysis and its influence on duration analysis. In *Advances in Survival Analysis*, N. Balakrishnan and C. R. Rao (eds), vol. 23. Amsterdam: North-Holland.

Bagdonavičius, V., Hafdi, M., El Himdi, K. and Nikulin, M. (2002a). Statistical analysis of the generalised linear proportional hazards model. *Proceedings of the Steklov Mathematical Institute, **294**, 5–18.

Bagdonaviccius, V., Hafdi, M. and Nikulin, M. (2002b). The generalized proportional hazards model and its application for statistical analysis of the Hsieh model. In *Proceedings of the Second Euro-Japanese Workshop on Stochastic Risk Modelling for Finance, Insurance, Production and Reliability*, T. Dohi, N. Limnios and S. Osaki (eds), 42–53. Chamonix, France.

Bagdonavičius, V., Hafdi, M. and Nikulin, M. (2004a). Analysis of survival data with cross-effects of survival functions, *Biostatistics* **5**, 415–425.

Bagdonavičius, V., Levuliene, R. and Nikulin, M. (2004b). Tests d'égalité contre alternative de croissement de deux functions de survie. *Comptes Rendus de l'Academie des Sciences de Paris*, Ser. I **339**, 425–428.

Baker, S. G., Erwin, D., Kramer, B. S. and Prorok, P. C. (2003). Using observational data to estimate an upper bound on the reduction in cancer mortality due to periodic screening. *BMC Medical Research Methodology*, **3**, 4.

Baker, S. J., Fearon, E. R., Nigro, J. M., Hamilton, S. R., Preisinger, A. C., Jessup, J. M., VanTuinen, P., Ledbetter, D. H., Barker, D. F. and Nakamura, Y. (1989). Chromosome 17 deletions and *p53* gene mutations in colorectal carcinomas. *Science* **244**, 217–221.

Ballivet, S., Salmi, L. R., Dubourdieu, D. and Bach, F. (1995). Incidence of thyroid cancer in New Caledonia, South Pacific, during 1985–1992. *American Journal of Epidemiology* **8**, 741–746.

Balmain, A. and Harris, C. C. (2000). Carcinogenesis in mouse and human cells: parallels and paradoxes. *Carcinogenesis* **21**, 371.

Bannasch, P. (1996). Pathogenesis of hepatocellular carcinoma: sequential cellular, molecular, and metabolic changes. *Progress in Liver Diseases* **14**, 161–191.

Barlow, S. M., Greig, J. B., Bridges, J. W., Carere, A., Carpy, A. J. M., Galli, C. L., Kleiner, J., Knudsen, I., Koeter, H. B. W. M., Levy, L. S., Madsen, C., Mayer, S., Narbonne, J.-F., Pfannkuch, F., Prodanchuk, M. G., Smith, M. R. and Steinberg, P. (2002). Hazard identification by methods of animal-based toxicology. *Food and Chemical Toxicology* **40**, 145–191.

Barnes, D. G., Daston, G. P. *et al.* (1995). Benchmark dose workshop – criteria for use of a benchmark dose to estimate a reference dose. *Regulatory Toxicology and Pharmacology* **21**, 296–306.

Barrett, M. T., Sanchez, C. A., Prevo, L. J., Wong, D. J., Galipeau, P. C., Paulson, T. G., Rabinovitch, P. S. and Reid, B. J. (1999). Evolution of neoplastic cell lineages in Barrett's oesophagus. *Nature Genetics* **22**, 106–109.

Bartoszyński, R. (1987). A modeling approach to metastatic progression of cancer. In *Cancer Modeling*, J. R. Thompson and B. W. Brown (eds), 237–267. New York: Marcel Dekker.

Bartoszyński, R., Edler, L., Hanin, L., Kopp-Schneider, A., Pavlova, L., Tsodikov, A., Zorin, A. and Yakovlev, A. (2001). Modeling cancer detection: Tumor size as a source of information on unobservable stages of carcinogenesis. *Mathematical Biosciences* **171**, 113–142.

Bartsch, H., Nair, U., Risch, A., Rojas, M., Wikman, H. and Alexandrov, K. (2000). Genetic polymorphism of CYP genes, alone or in combination, as a risk modifier of tobacco-related cancers. *Cancer Epidemiology Biomarkers & Prevention* **9**, 3–28.

Bates, D. M. and Watts, D. G. (1988) *Nonlinear Regression Analysis and Its Applications.* Edinbrugh: Oliver and Boyd.

Baxevanis, A. D. (2003). The Molecular Biology Database Collection: 2003 update. *Nucleic Acids Research* **31**, 1–12.

Becher, H., Flesch-Janys, D., Gurn, P. and Steindorf, K. (1998). *Krebsrisikoabschätzung für Dioxine.* Forschungsbericht 293 62 111, UBA FB 97–110 im Auftrag des Umweltbundesamts. Berlin: Erich Schmidt Verlag.

Bedford, T. and Cook, R. (2001). *Probabilistic Risk Analysis – Foundations and Methods.* Cambridge: Cambridge University Press.

Begg, C. B. and Berwick, M. (1997). A note on the estimation of relative risks of rare genetic susceptibility markers. *Cancer Epidemiology Biomarkers & Prevention* **6**, 99–103.

Behrens, J., Jerchow, B. A., Würtele, M., *et al.* (1998). Functional interaction of an axin homolog, conductin, with beta-catenin, APC and GSK3beta. *Science* **280**, 596.

Bencko, V. (1995). Use of human hair as a biomarker in the assessment of exposure to pollutants in occupational and environmental settings. *Toxicology* **101**, 29–39.

Bencko, V. (1997). Health aspects of burning coal with a high arsenic content: the Central Slovakia experience. In *Arsenic: Exposure and Health Effects*, C. O. Abernathy, R. L. Calderon and W. R. Chappell (eds), 84–92. London: Chapman & Hall.

Bencko, V., Rames, J. and Götzl, M. (2001). Preliminary analysis of lung cancer incidence in arsenic exposed population. In *Arsenic Exposure and Health Effects*, C. O. Abernathy, R. L. Calderon and W. R. Chappell (eds), 185–192. New York: Chapman & Hall.

Benhamou, S., Lee, W. J., Alexandrie, A. K., Boffetta, P., Bouchardy, C., Butkiewicz, D., Brockmöller, J., Clapper, M. L., Daly, A., Dolzan, V., Ford, J., Gaspari, L., Haugen, A., Hirvonen, A., Husgafvel-Pursiainen, K., Ingelman-Sundberg, M., Kalina, I., Kihara, M., Kremers, P., Le Marchand, L., London, S. J., Nazar-Stewart, V., Onon-Kihara, M., Rannug, A., Romkes, M., Ryberg, D., Seidegard, J., Shields, P., Strange, R. C., Stucker, I., To-Figueras, J., Brennan, P. and Taioli, E. (2002). Meta- and pooled analyses of the effects of glutathione S-transferase M1 polymorphisms and smoking on lung cancer risk. *Carcinogenesis* **23**, 1343–1350.

Benjamini, V. and Hochberg, V. (1995). Controlling the false discovery rate: a practical and powerful approach to multiple testing. *Journal of the Royal Statistical Society B* **57**, 289–300.

Berenbaum, M. C. (1977). Synergy, additivism and antogonism in immunosuppression. *Clinical and Experimental Immunology* **28**, 1–18.

Berenbaum, M. C. (1981). Criteria for analyzing interactions between biologically active agents. *Advances in Cancer Research* **35**, 269–335.

Berenbaum, M. C. (1985). The expected effect of a combination of agents: the general solution. *Journal of Theoretical Biology* **114**, 413–431.

Berenbaum, M. C. (1990). What is synergy? *Pharmacological Reviews* **47**, 93–141.

Bernal, M. and De Frutos, A. (1994). Epidemiología del cáncer de tiroides en Zaragoza (1989–1991). *Oncología* **17**, 367–370.

Bernardo, J. M. and Smith, A. F. M. (1994). *Bayesian Theory*. New York: Wiley.

Bernillon, P. and Bois, F. Y. (2000). Statistical issues in toxicokinetic modeling: a Bayesian perspective. *Environmental Health Perspectives* **108**, 883–893.

Berwick, M. and Vineis, P. (2000). Markers of DNA repair and susceptibility to cancer in humans: an epidemiologic review. *Journal of the National Cancer Institute* **92**, 874–897.

Bisgaard, S. (1994). A note on the definition of resolution for blocked 2^{k-p} designs. *Technometrics* **36**, 308–311.

Bliss, C. I. (1934). The methods of probits. *Science* **79**, 38–39.

Bliss, C. I. (1939). The toxicity of poisons applied jointly. *Annals of Applied Biology* **26**, 585–615.

Blumenson, L. E. (1976). When is screening effective in reducing the death rate? *Mathematical Biosciences* **30**, 273–303.

Blumenson, L. E. (1977). Detection of disease with periodic screening: Transient analysis and application to mammography examination, *Mathematical Biosciences* **33**, 73–106.

Bogdanffy, M. S., Sarangapani, R. *et al.* (1999). A biologically based risk assessment for vinyl acetate-induced cancer and noncancer inhalation toxicity. *Toxicological Sciences* **51**, 19–35.

Bois, F. Y. (1999). Analysis of PBPK models for risk characterization. *Annals of the New York Academy of Sciences* **895**, 317–337.

Bois, F. Y. (2000a). Statistical analysis of Clewell *et al.* PBPK model of trichloroethylene kinetics. *Environmental Health Perspectives* **108**(2), 307–316.

Bois, F. Y. (2000b). Statistical analysis of Fisher *et al.* PBPK model of trichloroethylene kinetics. *Environmental Health Perspectives* **108**(2), 275–282.

Bois, F. Y. (2001). Applications of population approaches in toxicology. *Toxicology Letters* **120**, 385–394.

Boland, C. R., Sato, J., Appelman, H. D., Bresalier, R. S. and Feinberg, A. P. (1995). Microallelotyping defines the sequence and tempo of allelic losses at tumour suppressor gene loci during colorectal cancer progression. *Nature Medicine* **1**, 902–909.

Boland, C. R., Thibodeau, S. N., Hamilton, S. R., Sidransky, D., Eshleman, J. R., Burt, R. W. *et al.* (1998). A National Cancer Institute workshop on microsatelite instability for cancer detection and familial predisposition: development of international criteria for the determination of microsatelite instability in colorectal cancer. *Cancer Research* **58**, 5248.

Bonassi, S. and Au, W. W. (2002). Biomarkers in molecular epidemiology studies for health risk prediction. *Mutation Research* **511**, 73–86.

Bonissone, P. P. (1990). Summarizing and propagating uncertain information with triangular norms. In *Readings in Uncertain Reasoning,* G. Shafer and J. Pearl (eds), 239–253. San Mateo, CA: Morgan Kaufmann.

Bonkhoff, H., Fixemer, T. and Remberger, K. (1998). Relation between Bcl-2, cell proliferation and the androgen receptor status in prostate tissue and precursors of prostate cancer. *Prostate* **34**, 251.

Bos, J. L., Fearon, E. R., Hamilton, S. R., Verlaan-de Vries, M., van Boom, J. H., van der Eb, A. J. and Vogelstein, B. (1987). Prevalence of ras gene mutations in human colorectal cancer. *Nature* **327**, 293.

Bosland, M. C. (1992). Animal models for the study of prostate carcinogenesis. *Journal of Cellular Biochemistry*, Suppl. **16H**, 89.

Bostwick, D. G., Qian, J. and Frankel, K. (1995). The incidence of high grade prostatic intraepithelial neoplasia in needle biopsies. *Journal of Urology* **154**, 1791–1794.

Boucher, K. M. and Kerber, R. A. (2001). The shape of the hazard function for cancer incidence. *Mathematical and Computer Modeling* **33**, 1361–1376.

Bova, G. S., Carter, B. S., Bussemakers, M. J. G., Emi, M., Fujiwara, Y., Kyprianou, N., Jacobs, S. C., Robinson, J. C., Epstein, J. I., Walsh, P. C. and Isaacs, W. B. (1993). Homozygous deletion and frequent allelic loss of chromosome 8q22 loci in prostate cancer. *Cancer Research* **53**, 3869.

Box, G. E. P. and Draper, N. R. (1987). *Empirical Model-Building and Response Surfaces*. New York: Wiley.

Boyd, J. and Risinger, J. I. (1991). Analysis of oncogene alterations in human endometrial carcinoma: prevalence of *ras* mutations. *Molecular Carcinogenesis* **4**, 189.

Boyle, P. and Parkin, D. M. (1991) Statistical methods for registries. In *Cancer Registration: Principles and Methods*, IARC Scientific Publications No. 95, 126–158. Lyon: International Agency for Research on Cancer.

Braithwaite, E., Wu, X. and Wang, Z. (1999). Repair of DNA lesions: mechanisms and relative repair efficiencies. *Mutation Research* **424**, 207–219.

Breiman, L., Friedman, J. H., Olshen, R. A. and Stone, C. H. (1984). *Classification and Regression Trees*. Belmont, CA: Wadsworth.

Breslow, N. E. and Day, N. E. (1980). *Statistical Methods in Cancer Research. Volume 1: The Analysis of Case–Control Studies*. Lyon: International Agency for Research on Cancer.

Breslow, N. E. and Day, N. E. (1987). *Statistical Methods in Cancer Research* (Vol. II). New York: Oxford University Press.

Brillinger, D. R. (1988). The maximum likelihood approach to the identification of neuronal firing systems. *Annals of Biomedical Engineering* **16**, 3–16.

Brillinger, D. R. (1992). Nerve cell spike train data analysis: a progression of technique. *Journal of the American Statistical Association* **87**, 260–271.

Broadwater, R. P., Shaalan, H. E. *et al.* (1994). Decision evaluation with interval mathematics: a power distribution system case study. *IEEE Transactions on Power Delivery* **9**, 59–65.

Brookmeyer, R. and Day, N. (1987). Two-stage model for the analysis of cancer screening data. *Biometrics* **43**, 657–669.

Brown, B. W., Atkinson, N. E., Bartoszyński, R. and Montague E. D. (1984). Estimation of human tumor growth rate from distribution of tumor size at detection. *Journal of the National Cancer Institute* **72**, 31–38.

Brown, C. C. and Koziol, J. A. (1983). Statistical aspects of the estimation of human risk from suspected environmental carcinogens. *SIAM Review* **25**, 151–181.

Brown, R. P., Delp, M. D., Lindstedt, S. L., Rhomberg, L. R. and Beliles, R. P. (1997). Physiological parameter values for physiologically based pharmacokinetic models. *Toxicology and Industrial Health* **13**, 407–484.

Buchancová, J., Klimentová, G., Knižková, M., Meško, D., Gáliková, E., Kubík, J., Fabiánová, E. and Jakubis, M. (1998). Health status of workers of a thermal power station exposed for prolonged periods to arsenic and other elements from fuel. *Central European Journal of Public Health* **6**, 29–36.

Burkart, W. and Jung, T. (1998). Health risks from combined exposures: mechanistic considerations on deviations from additivity. *Mutation Research* **411**, 119–128.

Burke, G. W., Cirocco, R., Markou, M., Temple, J. D., Allouch, M., Roth, D., Nery, J. and Miller, J. (1995). Early development of acute myelogenous leukemia following kidney transplantation: possible role of multiple serum cytokines. *Leukemia and Lymphoma* **19**, 173–80.

Burkholder, I. and Kopp-Schneider, A. (2002). Incorporating phenotype-dependent growth rates into the color-shift model for preneoplastic hepatocellular lesions. *Mathematical Biosciences* **179**, 145–160.

Burney, T. L., Rockove, S., Eiseman, J. L., Jacobs, S. C. and Kyprianou, N. (1994). Partial growth suppression of human prostate cancer cells by the *Krev-1* suppressor gene. *Prostate* **25**, 177.

Burns, P. A., Kemp, C. J., Gannon, J. V., Lane, D. P., Bremner, R. and Balmain, A. (1991). Loss of heterozygosity and mutational alterations of the *p53* gene in skin tumours of interspecific hybrid mice. *Oncogene* **6**, 2363.

Butt, J. (1980). *Reaction Kinetics and Reactor Design.* Englewood Cliffs, NJ. Prentice Hall.

Caduff, R. F., Svoboda-Neumann, S. M., Johnston, C. M., Bartos, R. E. and Frank, T. S. (1997). Molecular analysis in endometrial cancer. *Verhandlungen der Deutschen Gesellschaft für Pathologie* **81**, 219.

Cahill, D. P., Lengauer, C., Yu J., Riggins, G. J., Willson, J. K., Markowitz, S. D., Kinzler, K.W. and Vogelstein, B. (1998). Mutations of mitotic checkpoint genes in human cancers. *Nature* **392**, 300–303.

Cahill, D. P., Kinzler, K. W., Vogelstein, B. and Lengauer, C. (1999). Genetic instability and Darwinian selection in tumours. *Trends in Cellular Biology* **9**, 57–60.

Calabrese, E. J. (1978). *Methodological Approaches to Deriving Environmental and Occupational Health Standards.* New York: Wiley.

Calabrese, E. J. (ed.) (1992). *Biological Effects of Low Level Exposures to Chemicals and Radiation.* Boca Raton, FL: Lewis Publishers.

Calabrese, E. J. (1993). *Principles of Animal Extrapolation.* New York: Wiley.

Calabrese, E. J. (2001a). Over-compensation stimulation: a mechanism for hormetic effects. *Critical Reviews in Toxicology* **31**, 425–470.

Calabrese, E. J. (2001b). The future of hormesis: where do we go from here? *Critical Reviews in Toxicology* **31**, 637–648.

Calabrese, E. J. and Baldwin, L. A. (1997a). *Perspectives on Chemical Hormesis. Quotations by Researchers over the Past Century.* Amherst: University of Massachusetts.

Calabrese, E. J. and Baldwin, L. A. (1997b). A quantitatively-based methodology for the evaluation of chemical hormesis. *Human and Ecological Risk Assessment* **3**, 545–554.

Calabrese, E. J. and Baldwin, L. A. (1997c). The dose determines the stimulation (and poison): development of a chemical hormesis database. *International Journal of Toxicology* **16**, 545–559.

Calabrese, E. J. and Baldwin, L. A. (1998a). A general classification of U-shaped dose-response relationships in toxicology and their mechanistic foundations. *Human of Experimental Toxicology* **17**, 353–364.

Calabrese, E. J. and Baldwin, L. A. (1998b). Can the concept of hormesis be generalized to carcinogenesis? *Regulatory Toxicology and Pharmacology* **28**, 230–241.

Calabrese, E. J. and Baldwin, L. A. (1998c). Hormesis as a biological hypothesis. *Environmental Health Perespectives* **106**, Suppl. 1.

Calabrese, E. J. and Baldwin, L. A. (1998d). Hormesis as a default parameter in RfD derivation. *Human of Experimental Toxicology* **17**, 444–447.

Calabrese, E. J. and Baldwin, L. A. (1999a). Chemical hormesis: its historical foundations as a biological hypothesis. *Toxicologic Pathology* **27**(2), 195–196.

Calabrese, E. J. and Baldwin, L. A. (1999b). Radiation hormesis: its historical foundations as a biological hypothesis. *BELLE Newsletter* **8**(2), December.

Calabrese, E. J. and Baldwin, L. A. (1999c). The marginalization of hormesis, *Toxicologic Pathology* **27**, 184–194.

Calabrese, E. J. and Baldwin, L. A. (2000a). Radiation hormesis: the demise of a legitimate hypothesis. *Human & Experimental Toxicology* **19**, 76–84.

Calabrese, E. J. and Baldwin, L. A. (2000b). Reevaluation of the fundamental dose-response relationship. A new database suggests that the U-shaped, rather than the signoidal, curve predominates. *BioScience* **49**, 725–732.

Calabrese, E. J. and Baldwin, L. A. (2000c). Tales of two similar hypotheses: the rise and fall of chemical and radiation hormesis. *Human & Experimental Toxicology* **19**, 85–97.

Calabrese, E. J. and Baldwin, L. A. (2001a). Agonist concentration gradients as a generalized regulatory implementation strategy. *Critical Reviews in Toxicology* **31**, 471–473.

Calabrese, E. J. and Baldwin, L. A. (2001b). Hormesis: a generalized and unifying hypothesis. *Critical Reviews in Toxicology* **31**, 353–424.

Calabrese, E. J. and Baldwin, L. A. (2001c). Hormesis: U-shaped dose-response response and their centrality toxicology. *Trends in Pharmacological Science* **22**, June.

Calabrese, E. J. and Baldwin, L. A. (2001d). The frequency of U-shaped dose-response in toxicologic pathology. *Toxicological Sciences* **62**, 330–338.

Calabrese, E. J. and Baldwin, L. A. (2001e). U-shaped dose-responses in biology, toxicology and public health. *Annual Review of Public Health* **22**, 15–33.

Calabrese, E. J. and Baldwin, L. A. (2003a). The hormetic dose-response model is more common then the threshold model in toxicology. *Toxicological Sciences* **71**, 246–250.

Calabrese, E. J. and Baldwin, L. A. (2003b). Toxicology rethinks its central belief. Hormesis demands for a reappraisal of the way risks are assessed. *Nature* **421**, 691–692.

Calabrese, E. J., Baldwin, L. A. and Holland C. (1999). Hormesis: a highly generalizable and reproducible phenomenon with important implications for risk assessment. *Risk Analysis* **19**.

Calabretta, B., Kaczmarek, L., Ming, P. L., Au, F. and Ming, S. (1985). Expression of *c-myc* and other cell cycle-dependent genes in human colon neoplasia. *Cancer Research* **45**, 6000.

Calvert, P. M. and Frucht, H. (2002). The genetics of colorectal cancer. *Annals of Internal Medicine*, **137**, 603.

Cancré, N., Bois, F. Y., *et al.* (1999). Screening blood donations for hepatitis C in central Africa: analysis of a risk- and cost-based decision tree. *Medical Decision Making* **19**, 296–306.

Cardone, M. H., Roy, N., Stennicke, H. R., *et al.* (1998). Regulation of cell death protease caspase-9 by phosphorylation. *Science* **282**, 1318.

Carreter, C. (1996). *Estructura Demográfica de la Provincia de Zaragoza*. Zaragoza: Gabinete de Insalud.

Carson, H. J., Castelli, M. J. and Gattuso, P. (1996). Incidence of neoplasia in Hashimoto's thyroiditis: a fine-needle aspiration study. *Diagnostic Cytopathology* **1**, 38–42.

Cascorbi, I., Henning, S., Brockmöller, J., Gephart, J., Meisel, C., Müller, J. M., Loddenkemper, R. and Roots, I. (2000). Substantially reduced risk of cancer of the aerodigestive tract in subjects with variant -463A of the myeloperoxidase gene. *Cancer Research* **60**, 644–649

Cassee, F. R., Groten, J. P. and Feron V. J. (1996). Changes in nasal epithelium of rats exposed by inhalation to mixtures of formaldehyde, acetaldehyde, and acrolein. *Fundamental and Applied Toxicology* **29**, 208–218.

Cassee, F. R., Groten, J. P. and Van Bladeren, P. J. (1998). Toxicological evaluation and risk assessment of chemical mixtures. *Critical Reviews in Toxicology* **28**, 73–101.

Cauffiez, C., Lo-Guidice, J. M., Quaranta, S., Allorge, D., Chevalier, D., Cenee, S., Hamdan, R., Lhermitte, M., Lafitte, J. J., Libersa, C., Colombel, J. F., Stucker, I. and Broly, F. (2004). Genetic polymorphism of the human cytochrome CYP2A13 in a French population: implication in lung cancer susceptibility. *Biochemical and Biophysical Research Communications* **317**, 662–669.

Cave, H., Van der Werff-ten Bosch, J., Suciu, S., Guidal, C., Waterkeyn, C., Otten, J., Bakkus, M., Thielemans, K., Grandchamp, B. and Vilmer, E. (1998). Clinical significance of minimal residual disease in childhood acute lymphoblastic leukemia. European Organization for Research and Treatment of Cancer – Childhood Leukemia Cooperative Group. *New England Journal of Medicine* **339**, 591–598.

Ceci, C. and Mazliak, L. (2002). Optimal design in nonparametric life testing. Laboratoire de Probabilités et Modèles Aléatoires, Universités de Paris V et VII, Paris.

CFR (1998). *Code of Federal Regulations*, 40, 180.3, July 1.

Chan, K. S. and Ledolter, J. (1995). Monte Carlo EM estimation for time series models involving counts. *Journal of the American Statistical Association* **90**, 242–252.

Chang, J. C., Wooten, E. C., Tsimelzon, A., Hilsenbeck, S. G., Gutierrez, M. C., Elledge, R., Mohsin, S., Osborne, C. K., Chamness, G. C., Allred, D. C. and O'Connell, P. (2003). Gene expression profiling for the prediction of therapeutic response to docetaxel in patients with breast cancer. *Lancet* **362**, 362–369.

Chapman, P. M. (2001). Reflections on the future of hormesis. *Critical Reviews in Toxicology* **31**, 649–651.

Chappell, W. R. and Mordenti, J. (1991). Extrapolation of toxicological and pharmacological data from animals to humans. *Advances in Drug Research* **20**, 116.

Charles, D. (1999). *Chemical Hormesis: Beneficial Effects at Low Exposures, Adverse Effects at High Exposures*. College Station: Texas A&M University.

Chaudhuri, S., Cariappa, A., Tang, M., Bell, D., Haber, D. A., Isselbacher, K. J., Finkelstein, D., Forcione, D. and Pillai, S. (2000). Genetic susceptibility to breast cancer: HLA DQB*03032 and HLA DRB1*11 may represent protective alleles. *Proceedings of the National Academy of Sciences of the USA* **97**, 11 451–11 454.

Chen, C. (2000). Biologically based dose-response model for liver tumor induced by trichloroethylene. *Environmental Health Perspectives*, Suppl. **108**, 335–342.

Chen, C. and Farland, W. (1991). Incorporating cell proliferation in quantitative cancer risk assessment: approaches, issues, and uncertainties. In B. Butterworth, T. Slaga, W. Farland and M. McClain (eds), *Chemically Induced Cell Proliferation: Implication for Risk Assessment*, pp. 481–499. New York: Wiley-Liss.

Chen, C. and Oberdoster, G. (1996). Selection of models for assessing dose-response relationships for particle-induced lung cancer. *Inhalation Toxicology* **8**, 259–278.

Chen, C., Gibb, H. and Moini, A. (1991). A model for analyzing data initiation-promotion studies. *Environmental Health Perspectives* **90**, 287–292.

Chen, H. H., Duffy, S. W. and Tabar, L. (1996). A Markov chain method to estimate the tumor progression rate from preclinical to clinical phase, sensitivity and positive predictive value for mammography in breast cancer screening. *The Statistician* **45**, 307–317.

Chen, J. J. and Gaylor, D. W. (1992). Dose response modeling of quantitative response data for risk assessment. *Communications in Statistics – Theory and Methods* **21**, 2367–2381.

Chen, J. J., Hass, B. S. and Heflich, R. H. (1989). A response-additive model for analyzing mixtures of two chemicals in the Salmonella reversion assay. *Biometrical Journal* **31**, 495–503.

Chen, J. J., Kodell, R. L. and Gaylor, D. W. (1996a). Risk assessment for nonquantal toxic effects. In *Toxicology and Risk Assessment: Principles, Methods, and Applications*, A. Fan and L. S. Chang (eds), 503–513. New York: Marcel Dekker.

Chen, J. J., Li, L.-A. and Jackson, C. D. (1996b). Analysis of quantal response data from mixtures experiments. *Environmetrics* **7**, 503–512.

Chen, J. J., Chen, Y.-J., Rice, G., Teuschler, L. K., Hamernik, K., Protzel, A. and Kodell, R. L. (2001). Using dose addition to estimate cumulative risks from exposures to multiple chemicals. *Regulatory Toxicology and Pharmacology* **34**, 35–41.

Chen, J. J., Chen, Yi-Ju, Rice, G., Teuschler, L. K., Hamernik, K., Protzel, A. and Kodell, R. L. (2003). Cumulative risk assessment for quantitative response data. *Environmetrics* **14**, 339–353.

Chernoff, H. (1953). Locally optimal designs for estimating parameters. *Annals of Mathematical Statistics* **24**, 586–602.

Chien, J. Y., Thummel, K. E. and Slattery, J. T. (1997). Pharmacokinetic consequences of induction of CYP2E1 by ligand stabilization. *Drug Metabolism and Disposition* **25**, 1165–1175.

Christofori, G. and Semb, H. (1999). The role of cell-adhesion molecule E-cadherin as a tumor suppressor gene. *Trends Biochemical Sciences* **24**, 73.

Chu, K. (1985). Multievent model of carcinogenesis: a mathematical model for cancer causation and prevention. In *Carcinogenesis: A Comprehensive Survey*, Vol. 8, 411–421. New York: Raven Press.

Chyczewski, L., Niklinski, J. and Pluygers, E. (eds) (2002). *Endocrine Disruptors and Carcinogenic Risk Assessment*. NATO Science Series I, Vol 340. Amsterdam: IOS Press.

Cipra, B. (1993). Engineers look to Kalman filtering for guidance. *SIAM News*, **26**(5).

Clark, A. J. (1937). *Handbook of Experimental Pharmacology*. Berlin: Springer.

Clayton, D. and Schifflers, E. (1987). Models for temporal variation in cancer rates. II: Age-period-cohort models. *Statistics in Medicine* **6**, 469–481.

Clewell, H. J., Gentry, P. R., Covington, T. R. and Gearhart, J. M. (2000). Development of a physiologically based pharmacokinetic model of trichloroethylene and its metabolites for use in risk assessment. *Environmental Health Perspectives* **108**, 283–305.

Coffey, D. S. (1993). Prostate cancer. An overview of an increasing dilemma. *Cancer* **71**, 880.

Cogliano, V. J., Kroese, E. D., Zapponi, G. A., Attins, L. and Marcello, I. (1999a). Introduction. In *Perspectives on Biologically Based Cancer Risk Assessment*, V. J. Cogliano, E. G. Luebeck and G. A. Zaponi (eds), 1–20. New York: Kluwer.

Cogliano, V. J., Luebeck, E. G. and Zapponi, G. (eds) (1999b). *Perspectives on Biologically-Based Cancer Risk Assessment*, NATO Challenges of Modern Society, Vol 23, Kluwer Academic/Plenum Publishers.

Cogliano, V. J., Caldwell, J. C. and Scott, C. S. (2002). Risk assessment and the risk management in the European Community and in the United States. In *Endocrine Disrupters and Carcinogenic Risk Assessment*, L. Chyczewski, J. Niklinski and E. Pluygers (eds), NATO Science Series I, Vol 340, 9–14. IOS Press and Kluwer Academic Press.

Connell, D. W., Braddock, R. D. and Mani, S. V. (1993). Prediction of the partition coefficient of lipophilic compounds in the air-mammal tissue system. *Science of the Total Environment*, **Suppl.** (Pt 2), 1383–1396.

Conolly, R. B. and Lutz, W. K. (2004). Non-monotonic dose-response relationships: Mechanistic basis, kinetic modeling, and implications for risk assessment. *Toxicological Sciences* **77**, 151–157.

Cook, R. D. and Fedorov, V. (1995). Constrained optimization of experimental design. *Statistics* **26**, 129–178.

Cook R. D. and Thibodeau, L. A. (1980). Marginally restricted D-optimal designs. *Journal of the American Statistical Association* **75**, 366–371.

Cornell, J. A. (1990). *Experiments with Mixtures. Designs, Models and the Analysis of Mixture Data*, 2nd edn. New York: Wiley.

Cortes, J. E. and Kantarjian, H. M. (1995). Acute lymphoblastic leukemia. A comprehensive review with emphasis on biology and therapy. *Cancer* **76**, 2393–2417.

Coussens, L. M. and Werb, Z. (1996). Matrix metalloproteinases and the development of cancer. *Chemistry & Biology* **3**, 895.

Cox, D. R. (1970). *Analysis of Binary Data*. New York: Chapman & Hall.

Cox, D. R. (1972). Regression models and life tables. *Journal of the Royal Statistical Society*, Series B **34**, 187–220.

Cox, L. A. (2001). *Risk Analysis: Foundations, Models and Methods*. New York: Kluwer.

Coyle, D. (2003). Who's better not best: appropriate probabilistic uncertainty analysis. *International Journal of Technology Assessment in Health Care* **19**, 540–545.

Cronin, K. A., Legler, J. M. and Etzioni, R. D. (1998). Assessing uncertainty in microsimulation modelling with application to cancer screening interventions. *Statistics in Medicine* **17**, 2509–2523.

Crump, K. (1994). Limitations of biological models of carcinogenesis for low-dose extrapolation. *Risk Analysis* **14**, 883–886.

Crump, K. S. (1984). A new method for determining allowable daily intakes. *Fundamental and Applied Toxicology* **4**, 854–871.

Crump, K. (2001). Evaluating the evidence for hormesis: a statistical perspective. *Critical Reviews in Toxicology* **31**, 669–679.

Crump, K., Hoel, D., Langley, C. R. and Peto, R. (1976). Fundamental carcinogenic processes and their implications for low dose risk assessment. *Cancer Research* **36**, 2973–2979.

Currie, D. J. (1982). Estimating Michaelis–Menten parameters: bias, variance and experimental design. *Biometrics* **38**, 907–919.

Cytel Software Corp. (2002). LogXact 5 User Manual. Cytel.

Dally, H., Gassner, K., Jäger, B., Schmezer, P., Spiegelhalder, B., Edler, L., Drings, P., Dienemann, H., Schulz, V., Kayser, K., Bartsch, H. and Risch, A (2002). Myeloperoxidase (MPO) genotype and lung cancer histologic types: The MPO -463 A allele is associated with reduced risk for small cell lung cancer in smokers. *International Journal of Cancer* **102**, 530–535.

Dally, H., Edler L., Jäger B., Schmezer, P., Spiegelhalder, B., Dienemann, H., Drings, P., Schulz, V., Kayser, K., Bartsch, H. and Risch, A. (2003). The CYP3A4*1B allele increases risk for small cell lung cancer: effect of gender and smoking dose. *Pharmacogenetics* **13**, 607–618.

Dally, H., Bartsch, H., Jäger, B., Edler, L., Schmezer, P., Spiegelhalder, B., Dienemann, H., Drings, P., Kayser, K., Schulz, V. and Risch, A. (2004) Genotype relationships in the CYP3A locus in Caucasians. *Cancer Letters* **207**, 95–99.

Danese, D., Gardini, A., Farsetti, A., Sciacchitano, S., Andreoli, M., Pontecorvi, A. (1997). Thyroid carcinoma in children and adolescents. *European Journal of Pediatrics* **156**, 190–194.

Davidson, S. (2000) Research suggests importance of haplotypes over SNPs. *Nature Biotechnology* **18**, 1134–1135.

Davidson, I. W. F., Parker, J. C. and Beliles, R. P. (1986). Biological basis for extrapolation across mammalian species. *Regulatory Toxicology and Pharmacology* **6**, 211–237.

Davies, B. D. and Morris, T. (1993). Physiological parameters in laboratory animals and humans. *Pharmaceutical Research* **10**(7), 1093–1095.

Davis, J. M. and Svendsgaard, D. J. (1992). U-shaped dose-response curves: their occurrence. *Journal of Toxicology and Environmental Health* **30**, 71–83.

Day, N. E., Walter, S. D. (1984). Simplified models of screening for chronic disease. Estimation procedures from mass screening programs. *Biometrics* **40**, 1–14.

DeAngelo, A. (1996). Dichloroacetic acid case study, presented to Expert Panel to Evaluate EPA's Proposed Guidelines for Cancer Risk Assessment Using Chloroform and Dichloroacetate as Case Studies. Workshop, September 10–12, at ILSI Health and Environmental Sciences Institute, Washington, DC.

de Bont, E. S., Fidler, V., Meeuwsen, T., Scherpen, F., Hahlen, K. and Kamps, W. A. (2002). Vascular endothelial growth factor secretion is an independent prognostic factor for relapse-free survival in pediatric acute myeloid leukemia patients. *Clinical Cancer Research* **8**, 2856–2861.

D'Emilia, J., Bulovas, K., D'Erole, K., Wolf, B., Steele, G. and Summerhayes, I. C. (1989). Expression of the c-erbB-2 gene product (P185) at different stages of neoplastic progression in the colon. *Oncogene* **4**, 1233.

Dempster, A. P. (1968). A generalization of Bayesian inference, with discussion. *Journal of the Royal Statistical Society*, Series B **30**, 205–247.

Dette, H. and Biedermann, S. (2003). Robust and efficient designs for the Michaelis–Menten model. *Journal of the American Statistical Association* **88**, 679–686.

Dewanji, A., Venzon, D. J. and Moolgavkar, S. H. (1989). A stochastic two-stage model for cancer risk assessment: II. The number and size of premalignant clones. *Risk Analysis* **9**, 179–187.

Diamandis, E. P. (2004). Mass spectrometry as a diagnostic and a cancer biomarker discovery tool: Opportunities and potential limitations. *Molecular & Cellular Proteomics* **3**, 367–378.

Dirven, H. A. M, van den Broek, P. H. H. and Jongeneelen, F. J. (1990). Effect of di(2-ethylhexyl)phthalate on enzyme activity levels in liver and serum of rats. *Toxicology* **65**, 199–207. Erratum in *Toxicology* (1991) **67**, 127.

Dobrev, I. D., Andersen, M. E. and Yang, R. S. (2002). In silico toxicology: simulating interaction thresholds for human exposure to mixtures of trichloroethylene, tetrachloroethylene, and 1,1,1-trichloroethane. *Environmental Health Perspectives* **110**, 1031–1039.

Dong, J-T., Lamb, P. W., Rinker-Schaeffer, C. W., Vukanovic, J., Ichikawa, T., Isaacs, J. T. and Barrett, J. C. (1995). *KAI1Science* **268**, 884.

Dördelmann, M., Reiter, A., Borkhardt, A., Wolf-Dieter, L., Götz, N., Viehmann, S., Gadner, H., Riehm, H. and Schrappe, M. for the ALL-BFM Group (2000). Prednisone response is the strongest predictor of treatment outcome in infant acute lymphoblastic leukemia. *Blood* **94**, 1209–1217.

Dresler, C. M., Fratelli, C., Babb, J., Everley, L., Evans, A. A. and Clapper, M. L. (2000). Gender differences in genetic susceptibility for lung cancer. *Lung Cancer* **30**, 153–160.

Druckrey, H. (1967). Quantitative aspects in chemical carcinogenesis. In *Potential Carcinogenic Hazards from Drugs*, UICC Monograph No. 7., R. Truhaut (ed.), 60–78. Berlin: Springer.

Dubois, D. and Prade, H. (1990). An introduction to possibilistic and fuzzy logics. In *Readings in Uncertain Reasoning,* G. Shafer and J. Pearl (eds), 742–761. San Mateo, CA: Morgan Kaufmann.

Dudoit, S., Fridlyand, J. and Speed, T. P. (2002a). Comparison of discrimination methods for the classification of tumors using gene expression data. *Journal of the American Statistical Association* **97**, 77–87.

Dudoit, S., Yang, Y. H., Callow, M. J. and Speed, T. P. (2002b). Statistical methods for identifying differentially expressed genes in replicated cDNA microarray experiments. *Statistica Sinica* **2**, 111–139.

Duffy, S.W., Chen, H. H., Tabar, L. and Day, N. E. (1995). Estimation of mean sojourn time in breast cancer screening using a Markov chain model of both entry to and exit from the preclinical detectable phase. *Statistics in Medicine* **14**, 1531–1543.

Duggleby, R. G. (1979). Experimental designs for estimating the kinetic parameters for enzyme-catalysed reactions. *Journal of Theoretical Biology* **81**, 671- 684.

Dunlop, M. G., Farrington, S. M., Carothers, A. D. *et al.* (1997). Cancer risk associated with germline DNA mismatch repair gene mutations. *Human Molecular Genetics* **6**, 105.

Dunning, A. M., Healey, C. S., Pharoah, P. D., Teare, M. D., Ponder, B. A. and Easton, D. F. (1999). A systematic review of genetic polymorphisms and breast cancer risk. *Cancer Epidemiology Biomarkers & Prevention* **8**, 843–854.

Dybing, E., Doe, J., Groten, J., Kleiner, J., O'Brien, J., Renwick, A. G., Schlatter, J., Steinberg, P., Tritscher, A., Walker, R. and Younes, M. (2002). Hazard characterization of chemicals in food and diet: dose response, mechanisms and extrapolation issues. *Food and Chemical Toxicology* **40**, 237–282.

Dyrskjot, L., Thykjaer, T., Kruhoffer, M., Jensen, J. L., Marcussen, N., Hamilton-Dutoit, S., Wolf, H. and Orntoft, T. F. (2003). Identifying distinct classes of bladder carcinoma using microarrays. *Nature Genetics* **33**, 90–96.

Eddy, D. M. (1983). A mathematical model for timing repeated medical tests. *Medical Decision Making* **3**, 34–62.

Edler, L. (1992). Statistical methods for short-term tests in genetic toxicology: the first fifteen years. *Mutation Research* **277**, 11–33.

Edler, L. (1999). Statistische Konzepte und Modelle zur Behandlung multipler Einwirkungen. Presented on occasion of the retirement of Prof. Dr. Johannes Konietzko, University of Mainz, 30 June.

Edler, L. and Kopp-Schneider, A. (1998). Statistical models for low dose exposure. *Mutation Research* **405**(2), 227–236.

Edler, L. and Portier, C. J. (1992). Uncertainty in physiological pharmacokinetic modeling and its impact on statistical risk estimation of 2,3,7,8-TCDD. *Chemosphere* **25**, 239–242.

Edler, L., Portier, C. J. and Kopp-Schneider, A. (1994). Zur Existenz von Schwellenwerten: Wissenschaftliche Methode oder statistische Artefakte in der Risikoabschätzung. *Zentralblatt für Arbeitsmedizin* **44**, 16–21.

Edler, L., Poirier, K., Dourson, M., Kleiner, J., Mileson, B., Nordmann, H., Renwick, A., Slob, W., Walton, K. and Würtzen, G. (2002). Mathematical modelling and quantitative methods. *Food and Chemical Toxicology* **40**, 283–326.

Eisenbrand, G., Pool-Zobel, B., Baker, V., Balls, M., Blaauboer, B. J., Boobis, A., Carere, A., Kevekordes, S., Lhugenot, J. C., Pieters, R. and Kleiner, J. (2002). Methods of in vitro toxicology. *Food and Chemical Toxicology* **40**, 193–236.

El-Masri, H. A., Thomas, R. S., Benjamin, S. A. and Yang, R. S. H. (1995). Physiologically based pharmacokinetic/pharmacodynamic modeling of chemical mixtures and possible applications in risk assessment. *Toxicology* **105**, 275–282.

El-Masri, H. A., Reardon, K. F. and Yang, R. S. H. (1997). Integrated approaches for the analysis of toxicologic interactions of chemical mixtures. *Critical Reviews in Toxicology* **27**, 175–197.

Elashoff, R. M., Fears, T. R. and Schneiderman, M. A. (1987). Statistical analysis of a carcinogen mixture experiment. I. Liver carcinogens. *Journal of the National Cancer Institute* **79**(3), 509–525.

Emmert-Buck, M. R., Vocke, C. D., Pozzatti, R. O., Duray, P. H., Jennings, S. B., Florence, C. D., Zhuang, Z., Bostwick, D. G., Liotta, L. A. and Linehan, W. M. (1995). Allelic loss on chromosome 8p12–21 in microdissected prostatic intraepithelial neoplasia. *Cancer Research* **55**, 2959.

Endrenyi, L. and Chan, F. Y. (1981). Optimal design of experiments for the estimation of precise hyperbolic kinetic and binding parameters. *Journal of Theoretical Biology* **90**, 241–263.

Enzmann, H., Edler, L. and Bannasch, P. (1987). Simple elementary method for the quantification of focal liver lesions induced by carcinogens. *Carcinogenesis* **8**, 231–235.

Eppert, K., Scherer, S. W., Ozcelik, H., *et al.* (1996). MADR2 maps to 18q21 and encodes a TGFbeta-regulated MAD-related protein that is functionally mutated in colorectal carcinoma. *Cell* **86**, 543.

Ertürk, E., Tuncel, E., Yerci, Ö., Gürsoy, N., İmamoğlu, Ş., Korun, N. and Arinik, A. (1996). A retrospective analysis of thyroid cancer. *Journal of Environmental Pathology, Toxicology and Oncology*, **15**, 245–249.

Ewens, J. W. and Grant, R. G. (2002). *Statistical Methods in Bioinformatics*. New York: Springer.

Fabiánová, E., Hettychová, L., Hrubá, F., Koppová, K., Marko, M., Maroni, M., Grech, G. and Bencko, V. (2000). Health risk assessment for inhalation exposure to arsenic. *Central European Journal of Public Health* **8**, 28–32.

Fahey, T. J. 3rd, Reeve, T. S. and Delbridge, L. (1995). Increasing incidence and changing presentation of thyroid cancer over a 30-year period. *British Journal of Surgery* **4**, 518–520.

Fay, R. (1992). When are inferences from multiple imputations valid? In *Proceedings of the Survey Research Methods Section*, 227–232. Alexandria, VA: American Statistical Association.

Fearnhead, N. S., Britton, M. P. and Bodmer, W. F. (2001). The ABC of APC. *Human Molecular Genetics* **10**, 721–733.

Fearon, E. R. and Vogelstein, B. (1990). A genetic model for colorectal tumorigenesis. *Cell* **61**, 7589.

Fechner, G. T. (1860). *Elemente der Psychophysik*. Leipzig: Breitkopf und Hartel.

Fehr, E. and Fischbacher, U. (2003). The nature of human altruism. *Nature* **425**, 785–791.

Feigelson, H. S., Coetzee, G. A., Kolonel, L. N., Ross, R. K. and Henderson, B. E. (1997). A polymorphism in the *CYP17* gene increases the risk for breast cancer. *Cancer Research* **57**, 1063–1065.

Feldstein, M. and Zelen, M. (1984). Inferring the natural time history of breast cancer: implications for tumor growth rate and early detection. *Breast Cancer Research and Treatment* **4**, 3–10.

Feron, V. J. Woutersen, R. A., Arts, J. H. E., Cassee, F. R., De Vrijer, F. and van Bladeren, P. J. (1995). Safety evaluation of the mixture of chemicals at a specific workplace: theoretical considerations and a suggested two-step procedure. *Toxicology Letters* **76**, 47–55.

Feyler, A., Voho, A., Bouchardy, C., Kuokkanen, K., Dayer, P., Hirvonen, A. and Benhamou, S. (2002). Point: myeloperoxidase $-463G \rightarrow$ A polymorphism and lung cancer risk. *Cancer Epidemiology Biomarkers & Prevention* **11**, 1550–1554.

Filipsson, A. F. and Victorin, K. (2003). Comparison of available benchmark dose softwares and models using trichloroethylene as a model substance. *Regulatory Toxicology and Pharmacology* **37**, 343–355.

Filser, J. G., Johanson, G., Kessler, W., Kreuzer, P. E., Stei, P., Baur, C. and Csanady, G. A. (1993). A pharmacokinetic model to describe toxicokinetic interactions between 1,3-butadiene and styrene in rats: predictions for human exposure. *IARC Scientific Publications* **127**, 65–78.

Fingerhut, M. A., Halperin, W. E., Marlow, D. A., Piacitelli, L., Honchar, P. A., Sweeny, M. H., Griefe, A. L., Dill, P. A., Steenland, K. and Suruda, H. (1991). Cancer mortality in workers exposed to 2,3,7,8-tetrachlorodibenzo-*p*-dioxin. *New England Journal of Medicine* **324**, 212–218.

Fink, F., Koller, U., Mayer, H., Haas, O. A., Grumayer-Panzer, E. R., Urban, C., Dengg, K., Mutz, I., Tuchler, H. and Gatterer-Menz, I. (1993). Prognostic significance of myeloid-associated antigen expression on blast cells in children with acute lymphoblastic leukemia. The Austrian Pediatric Oncology Group. *Med. and Pediatr. Oncol.*, **21**, 340–346.

Finkel, A. M. (1990). *Confronting Uncertainty in Risk Management*. Washington, DC: Center for Risk Management.

Finney, D. J. (1971). *Probit Analysis*, 3rd edn. Cambridge: Cambridge University Press.

Finney, D. J. (1947). The estimation from original records of the relationship between dose and quantal response. *Biometrika* **34**, 320–334.

Fiserova-Bergerova, V. (1995). Extrapolation of physiological parameters for physiologically based simulation models. *Toxicology Letters* **79**, 77–86.

Fiserova-Bergerova, V. and Diaz, M. L. (1986). Determination and prediction of tissue-gas partition coefficients. *International Archives for Occupational and Environmental Health* **58**, 75–87.

Fisher, J. W., Gargas, M. L., Allen, B. C. and Andersen, M. E. (1991). Physiologically based pharmacokinetic modeling with trichloroethylene and its metabolite, trichloroacetic acid, in the rat and mouse. *Toxicology and Applied Pharmacology* **109**, 183–195.

Fisher, J. W., Whittaker, T. A, Taylor, D. H., Chlewell, H. J. III and M. E. Andersen (1989). Physiologically based pharmacokinetic modeling of the pregnant rat: A multiroute exposure model for trichloroethylene and its metabolite, trichloracetic acid. *Toxicology and Applied Pharmacology,* **99**, 395–414.

Flehinger, B. J. and Kimmel, M. (1987). The natural history of lung cancer in a periodically screened population. *Biometrics* **43**, 127–144.

Flehinger, B. J. and Kimmel, M. (1991). Screening for cancer in relation to the natural history of the disease. In *Mathematical Population Dynamics*, O. Arino, D. E. Axelrod and M. Kimmel (eds), 383–390. New York: Marcel Dekker.

Flehinger, B. J., Kimmel, M. and Melamed, M. R. (1988). The natural history of adenocarcinoma/large cell carcinoma of lung: conclusions from screening programs in New York and Baltimore. *Journal of the National Cancer Institute* **80**, 337–344.

Flehinger, B. J., Kimmel, M., Polyak, T. and Melamed, M. R. (1993). Screening for lung cancer. The Mayo lung project revisited. *Cancer* **72**, 1573–1580.

Fodde, R. (2002). The *APC* gene in colorectal cancer. *European Journal of Cancer* **38**, 867–871.

Fodde, R., Kuipers, J., Rosenberg, C., Smits, R., Kielman, M., Gaspar, C., van Es J. H., Breukel, C., Wiegant, J., Giles, R. H. and Clevers, H. (2001). Mutations in the *APC* tumour suppressor gene cause chromosomal instability. *Nature Cell Biology* **3**, 433–438.

Ford, I., Kitsos, C. P. and Titterington, D. M. (1989). Recent advances in nonlinear experimental design. *Technometrics* **31**, 49–60.

Forrester, K., Almoguera, C., Han, K., Grizzle, W. E. and Perucho, M. (1987). Detection of high incidence of *K-ras* oncogenes during human colon tumorigenesis. *Nature* **327**, 298–303.

Fowles, J. R., Alexeeff, G. V., *et al.* (1999). The use of benchmark dose methodology with acute inhalation lethality data. *Regulatory Toxicology and Pharmacology* **29**, 262–278.

Fraser, T. R. (1872). The antagonism between the actions of active substances. *British Medical Journal* **2**, 485.

Frederick, C. B., Gentry, P. R., Bush, M. L., Lomax, L. G., Black, K. A., Finch, L., Kimbell, J. S., Morgan, K. T., Subramaniam, R. P., Morris, J. B. and Ultman, J. S. (2001). A hybrid computational fluid dynamics and physiologically based pharmacokinetic model for comparison of predicted tissue concentrations of acrylic acid and other vapors in the rat and human nasal cavities following inhalation exposure. *Inhalation Toxicology* **13**, 359–376.

Frei, W. (1913). Versuche über Kombination von Desinfektionsmitteln. *Zeitschrift für Hygiene und Infektionskrankheiten* **75**, 433–496.

Fuhr, U. (2000). Induction of drug metabolising enzymes: pharmacokinetic and toxicological consequences in humans. *Clinical Pharmacokinetics* **38**(6), 493–504.

Fukuchi, T., Sakamoto, M., Tsuda, H., *et al.* (1998). Beta-catenin mutation in carcinoma of the uterine endometrium. *Cancer Research* **58**, 3526.

Fullman, R. L. (1953). Measurement of particle sizes in opaque bodies. *Transactions of the AIME* **197**, 447–452.

Furberg, A. H. and Ambrosone, C. B. (2001) Molecular epidemiology, biomarkers and cancer prevention. *Trends in Molecular Medicine* **7**, 517–521.

Fusenig, N. E., Amer, S. M., Boukamp, P. and Worst, P. K. (1978). Characteristics of chemically transformed mouse epidermal cells in vitro and in vivo. *Bulletin du Cancer* **65**, 271.

Fusenig, N. E., Drazlieva Petrusevska, R. T. and Breitkreutz, D. (1985). Phenotypic and cytogenetic characteristics of different stages during spontaneous transformation of mouse keratinocytes in vitro. *Carcinogenesis: A Comprehensive Survey*, **9**, 293.

Gaddum, J. H. (1933). *Reports on Biological Standards. III. Methods of Biological Assay Depending on a Quantal Response.* Special Report Series, 183. London: Medical Research Council.

Galanti, M. R., Ekbom, A., Grimelius, L. and Yuen, J. (1997a). Parental cancer and risk of papillary and follicular thyroid carcinoma. *British Journal of Cancer* **3**, 451–456.

Galanti, M. R., Hansson, L., Bergstrom, R., Wolk, A., Hjartaker, A., Lund, E., Grimelius, L. and Ekbom, A. (1997b). Diet and the risk of papillary and follicular thyroid carcinoma: a population-based case-control study in Sweden and Norway. *Cancer Causes Control* **2**, 205–214.

Galipeau, P. C., Paulson, T. G., Rabinovitch, P. S. and Reid B. J. (1999). Evolution of neoplastic cell lineages in Barrett's oesophagus. *Nature Genetics* **22**, 106–109.

Gao, X., Honn, K. V., Grignon, D., Sakr, W. and Chen, Y. Q. (1993). Frequent loss of expression and loss of heterozygosity of the putative tumor suppressor gene *DCC* in prostatic carcinomas. *Cancer Research* **53**, 2723.

Gao, X., Porter, A. T. and Honn, K. V. (1997). Involvement of the multiple tumor suppressor genes and 12-lipoxygenase in human prostate cancer. Therapeutic implications. *Advances in Experimental Medicine and Biology* **407**, 41.

Gao, X., Zacharek, A., Salkowski, A., Grignon, D. J., Sakr, W., Porter, A. T. and Honn, K. V. (1995). Loss of heterozygosity of the *BRCA1* and other loci on chromosome 17q in human prostate cancer. *Cancer Research* **55**, 1002.

Gargas, M. L., Burgess, R. J., Voisard, D. E., Cason, G. H. and Andersen, M. E. (1989). Partition coefficients of low-molecular-weight volatile chemicals in various liquids and tissues. *Toxicology and Applied Pharmacology* **98**, 87–99.

Gart, J. J., Krewski, D., Lee, P. N., Tarone, R. E. and Wahrendorf, J. (1986). *Statistical Methods in Cancer Research: The Design and Analysis of Long-Term Animal Experiments.* Lyon: IARC Scientific Publications.

Gaylor, D. W. (1989). Quantitative risk analysis for quantal reproductive and developmental effects. *Environmental Health Perspectives* **79**, 243–246.

Gaylor, D. O. and Zheng, Q. (1996). Risk assessment of nongenotoxic carcinogens based on cell proliferation/death rates in rodents. *Risk Analysis* **16**, 221–225.

Gaylor, D. W., Lutz, W. K. and Conolly, R. B. (2004). Statistical analysis of non-monotonic dose-response relationships: Research design and analysis of nasal cell proliferation in rats exposed to formaldehyde. *Toxicological Sciences* **77**, 158–164.

Ge, Y., Dudoit, S. and Speed, T. P. (2003). Resampling-based multiple testing for microarray data analysis. Tech. report, Dept. of Statistics, University of California, Berkeley.

Gehring, P. J., Watanabe, P. G. and Park, C. N. (1978). Resolution of dose-response toxicity data for chemicals requiring metabolic activation. Example – vinyl chloride. *Toxicology and Applied Pharmacology* **44**, 581–591.

Geisler, I. and Kopp-Schneider, A. (2000). A model for hepato-carcinogenesis with clonal expansion of three successive phenotypes of preneoplastic cells. *Mathematical Biosciences* **168**, 167–185.

Gelman, A., Bois, F. Y., *et al.* (1996). Physiological pharmacokinetic analysis using population modeling and informative prior distributions. *Journal of the American Statistical Association* **91**, 1400–1412.

Gelman, A. and Rubin, D. B. (1996). Markov chain Monte Carlo methods in biostatistics. *Statistical Methods in Medical Research* **5**, 339–355.

Gelman, A., Carlin, J. B., Stern, H. S. and Rubin, D. B. (1995). *Bayesian Data Analysis.* London: Chapman & Hall.

Gennings, C. (1995). An efficient experimental design for detecting departure from additivity in mixtures of many chemicals. *Toxicology* **105**, 189–197.

Gennings, C. and Carter, W. H. Jr. (1995). Utilizing concentration-response data from individual components to detect statistically significant departures form additivity in chemical mixtures. *Biometrics* **51**, 1264–1277.

Gennings, C., Dawson, K. S., Carter, W. and Myers, R. H. (1990). Interpreting plots of a multidimensional dose-response surface in a parallel coordinate system. *Biometrics* **46**, 719–735.

Gephart, L. A., Salminen, W. F., *et al.* (2001). Evaluation of subchronic toxicity data using the benchmark dose approach. *Regulatory Toxicology and Pharmacology* **33**, 37–59.

Gershwin, M. E. and Smith, N. T. (1973). Interaction between drungs using three dimensional isobo; ographic interpretation. *Archives Internationales de Pharmacodynamie et de Therapie* **201**, 154–161.

Gibaldi, M. and Perrier, D. (1982). *Pharmacokinetics.* New York: Marcel Dekker.

Gilberg, F., Urfer, W. and Edler, L. (1999). Heteroscedastic nonlinear regression. Models with random effects and their application to enzyme kinetic data. *Biometrical Journal* **41**, 543–557.

Gilks, W. R., Richardson, S. and Spiegelhalter, D. J. (1996). Introducing Markov chain Monte Carlo. In *Markov Chain Monte Carlo in Practice*, W. R. Gilks, S. Richardson and D. J. Spiegelhalter (eds). London: Chapman & Hall.

Giltinan, D. M., Capizzi, T. P. and Malani, H. (1988). Diagnostic tests for similar action of two compounds. *Applied Statistics* **37**, 39–50.

Godschalk, R. W., van Schooten, F. J. and Bartsch, H. (2003). A critical evaluation of DNA adducts as biological markers for human exposure to polycyclic aromatic compounds. *Journal of Biochemistry and Molecular Biology* **36**, 1–11.

Goldstein, N. S., Bhanot, P., Odish, E. and Hunter, S. (2003). Hyperplastic-like colon polyps that preceded microsatellite-unstable adenocarcinomas. *American Journal of Clinical Pathology* **119**, 778–796.

Golub, T. R., Slonim, D. K., Tamayo, P., Huard, C., Gaasenbeek, M., Mesirov, J. P., Coller, H., Loh, M. L., Downing, J. R., Caligiuri, M. A., Bloomfield, C. D. and Lander, E. S. (1999). Molecular classification of cancer: class discovery and class prediction by gene expression monitoring. *Science* **286**, 531–537.

Gordon, J. and Shortliffe, E. H. (1990). The Dempster–Shafer theory of evidence. In *Readings in Uncertain Reasoning*, G. Shafer and J. Pearl (eds), 529–539. San Mateo, CA: Morgan Kaufmann.

Gorlova, O. Y., Amos, C., Henschke, C., Lei, L., Spitz, M., Wei, Q., Wu, X. and Kimmel, M. (2003). Genetic susceptibility for lung cancer: interactions with gender and smoking history and impact on early detection policies. *Human Heredity* **56**, 139–145.

Gorlova, O. Y., Kimmel, M. and Henschke, C. (2001). Modeling of long-term screening for lung carcinoma. *Cancer* **92**, 1531–1540.

Gorlova, O., Peng, B., Yankelevitz, D., Henschke, C. and Kimmel, M. (2005). Estimating the growth rates of primary lung tumours from samples with missing measurements. *Statistics in Medicine*, to appear, Published online: 29 Nov 2004.

Grady, W. M., Rajput, A., Myeroff, L., Liu, D. F., Kwon, K., Willis, J. and Markowitz, S. (1998). Mutation of the type II transforming growth factor-beta receptor is coincident with the transformation of human colon adenomas to malignant carcinomas. *Cancer Research* **58**, 3101–3104.

Grana, X. and Reddy, E. P. (1995). Cell cycle control in mammalian cells: role of cyclins, cyclin-dependent kinases, growth suppressor genes and cyclin-dependent kinase inhibitors. *Oncogene* **11**, 211.

Greenland, S. (2000). Principles of multilevel modelling. *International Journal of Epidemiology* **29**, 158–167.

Greenland, S. (2001). Sensitivity analysis, Monte Carlo risk analysis, and Bayesian uncertainty assessment. *Risk Analysis* **21**, 579–583.

Greenwood, P. E. and Nikulin, M. (1996). *A Guide to Chi-squared Testing*. New York: Wiley.

Gregori, G., Hanin, L., Luebeck, G., Moolgavkar, S. and Yakovlev, A. (2001). Testing goodness of fit with stochastic models of carcinogenesis. *Mathematical Biosciences* **175**, 13–29.

Grewal, M. and Andrews, A. (2001). *Kalman Filtering: Theory and Practice*. New York: Wiley.

Groten, J. P., Schoen, E. D. and Feron, V. J. (1996). Use of factorial designs in combination toxicity studies. *Food and Chemical Toxicology* **34**, 1083–1089.

Groten, J. P., Sinkeldam, E. J., Muys, T., Lutten, J. B. and Van Bladeren, P. J. (1991). Interaction of dietary Ca, P, Mg, Mn, Cu, Fe, Zn and Se with the accumulation and oral toxicity of cadmium in rats. *Food and Chemical Toxicology* **29**, 249–258.

Guillemette, C., De Vivo, I., Hankinson, S. E., Haiman, C. A., Spiegelman, D., Housman, D. E. and Hunter, D. J. (2001). Association of genetic polymorphisms in UGT1A1 with breast cancer and plasma hormone levels. *Cancer Epidemiology Biomarkers & Prevention* **10**, 711–714.

Guillemette, C., Millikan, R. C., Newman, B. and Housman, D. E. (2000). Genetic polymorphisms in uridine diphospho-glucuronosyltransferase 1A1 and association with breast cancer among African Americans. *Cancer Research* **60**, 950–956.

Gyorffy, B., Kocsis, I. and Vasarhelyi, B. (2004). Biallelic genotype distributions in papers published in *Gut* between 1998 and 2003: altered conclusions after recalculating the Hardy–Weinberg equilibrium. *Gut* **53**, 614–615.

Haag-Gronlund, M., Franssonsteen, R., *et al.* (1995). Application of the benchmark method to risk assessment of trichloroethene. *Regulatory Toxicology and Pharmacology* **21**, 261–269.

Haaland, P. D. and O'Connell, M. A. (1995). Inference for contrast-saturated fractional factorials. *Technometrics* **37**, 92–93.

Habbema, J. D. F., Hermans, J. and Reme, J. (1978). Variable kernel density estimation in discriminant analysis. In *Compstat 1978*, L. C. A. Corsten and J. Hermans (eds), 178–185. Vienna: Physica.

Haber, L. T., Allen, B. C., *et al.* (1998). Non-cancer risk assessment for nickel compounds: issues associated with dose-response modeling of inhalation and oral exposures. *Toxicological Sciences* **43**, 213–229.

Hachiya, T., Kuriaki, Y., Ueoka, Y., Nishida, J., Kato, K. and Wake, N. (1999). WAF1 genotype and endometrial cancer susceptibility. *Gynecology and Oncology* **72**, 187–192.

Haddad, S., Tardif, R., Charest-Tardif, G. and Krishnan, K. (1999). Physiological modeling of the toxicokinetic interactions in a quaternary mixture of aromatic hydrocarbons. *Toxicology and Applied Pharmacology* **161**, 249–257.

Haddad, S., Charest-Tardif, G., Tardif, R. and Krishnan, K. (2000). Validation of a physiological modeling framework for simulating the toxicokinetics of chemicals in mixtures. *Toxicology and Applied Pharmacology* **167**, 199–209.

Haddad, S., Beliveau, M., Tardif, R. and Krishnan, K. (2001). A PBPK modeling-based approach to account for interactions in the health risk assessment of chemical mixtures. *Toxicological Sciences* **63**, 125–31.

Haddow, S., Fowlis, D. J., Parkinson, K., Akhurst, R. J. and Balmain, A. (1991). Loss of growth control by TGF-beta occurs at a late stage of mouse skin carcinogenesis and is independent of *ras* gene activation. *Oncogene* **6**, 1465.

Hames, Y. Y. (1998). *Risk Modeling, Assessment and Management.* New York: Wiley.

Hanahan, D. and Folkman, J. (1996). Patterns and emerging mechanisms of the angiogenic switch during tumorigenesis. *Cell* **86**, 353.

Hanahan, D. and Weinberg, R. A. (2000). The hallmarks of cancer. *Cell* **100**, 57–70.

Hanash, S. (2003). Disease proteomics. *Nature* **422**, 226–232.

Hanin, L. G. (2002). Identification problem for stochastic models with application to carcinogenesis, cancer detection and radiation biology. *Discrete Dynamics in Nature and Society* **7**, 177–189.

Hanin, L. G. and Yakovlev, A. Y. (1996). A nonidentifiability aspect of the two-stage model of carcinogenesis. *Risk Analysis* **16**(5), 711–715.

Hanin, L. G. and Yakovlev, A. Y. (2004), Multivariate distributions of clinical covariates at the time of cancer detection. *Statistical Methods in Medical Research.* **13**, 457–489.

Hanin, L. G., Tsodikov, A. D. and Yakovlev, A. Y. (2001). Optimal schedules of cancer surveillance and tumor size at detection. *Mathematical and Computer Modelling* **33**, 1419–1430.

Hanin, L. G., Miller, A., Zorin, A. V. and Yakovlev, A. Y. (2004). The University of Rochester model of breast cancer detection and survival. In *NCI Monograph Series*, to appear.

Hann, B. and Balmain, A. (2001). Building 'validated' mouse models of human cancer. *Current Opinion in Cell Biology* **13**, 778.

Hare, L. B. (1974). Mixture designs applied to food formulation. *Food Technology* **28**, 50–62.

Harrison, M. C. (2001). A possible path forward for hormesis. *Critical Reviews in Toxicology* **31**, 653–654.

Hart, R. W. and Frome, L. T. (1996). Toxicological defense mechanisms and how they may affect the nature of the dose-response relationship. *BELLE Newsletter* **5**, 1–16.

Hastie, T. and Tibshirani, R. (1984). Generalized additive models. *Statistical Science* **1**, 297–309.

Hattori, S. (2000). Harmonization of radiation for human life. Summary report of radiation hormesis research. In *Proceedings of the 10th International Congress of the International Radiation Protection Association*, May 14–19, Hiroshima, Japan, P-2a-91.

Hazelton, W. D., Luebeck, E. G., Heidenreich, W. F. and Moolgavkar, S. H. (2001). Analysis of a cohort of Chinese tin miners with arsenic, radon, cigarette and pipe smoke exposures using the biologically-based two-stage clonal expansion model. *Radiation Re*search **156**, 78–94.

He, T. C., Sparks, A. B., Rago, C., *et al.* (1998). Identification of *c-myc* as a target of the APC pathway. *Science* **281**, 1509.

Heidenreich, W. F. (1996). On the parameters of the clonal expansion model. *Radiation and Environmental Biophysics* **35**, 127–129.

Heidenreich, W. F., Luebeck, E. G. and Moolgavkar, S. H. (1997). Some properties of the hazard function of the two-mutation clonal expansion model. *Risk Analysis* **17**, 391–399.

Heidenreich, W. F., Luebeck, E. G. and Moolgavkar, S. H. (2004). Effects of exposure uncertainties in the TSCE model and application to the Colorado miners data. *Radiation Research* **161**, 72–81.

Heinze, G. and Schemper, M. (2002). A solution to the problem of separation in logistic regression. *Statistics in Medicine* **21**, 2409–2419.

Henschke, C. I., McCauley, D. I., Yankelevitz, D. F., Naidich, D. P., McGuinness, G., Miettinen, O. S., Libby, D. M., Pasmantier, M. W., Koizumi, J., Altorki, N. K. and Smith, J. P. (1999). Early Lung Cancer Action Project: Overall design and findings from baseline screening. *Lancet* **354**, 99–105.

Henschke, C. I., Naidich, D. P., Yankelevitz, D. F., Mirtcheva, R., McGuinness, G., McCauley, D. I., Smith, J. P., Libby, D., Pasmantier, M., Koizumi, J., Flieder, D., Vazquez, M., Altorki, N. and Miettinen, O. S. (2001). Early Lung Cancer Action Project: Initial results of annual repeat screening. *Cancer* **92**, 153–159.

Henschke, C. I., Yankelevitz, D. F., Mirtcheva, R., McGuinness, G., McCauley, D. and Miettinen, O. S. (2002a). CT screening for lung cancer: frequency and significance of part-solid and nonsolid nodules. *American Journal of Radiology* **178**, 1053–1057.

Henschke, C. I., Yankelevitz, D. F., Smith, J. P. and Miettinen, O. S. (2002b). Screening for lung cancer: The Early Lung Cancer Action approach. *Lung Cancer* **35**, 143–148.

Henschke, C. I., Wisnivesky, J. P., Yankelevitz, D. F. and Miettinen, O. S. (2003a). Screen-diagnosed small stage I cancers of the lung: genuineness and curability. *Lung Cancer* **39**, 327–330.

Henschke, C. I., Yankelevitz, D. F. and Kostis, W. J. (2003b). CT screening for lung cancer: Bias, shift and controversies. In *Multidetector-Row CT of the Thorax*, U. J. Schoepf (ed.). Berlin: Springer.

Henschke, C. I., Yankelevitz, D. F., Naidich, D., McCauley, D. I., McGuinness, G., Libby, D. M., Smith, J. P., Pasmantier, M. W. and Miettinen, O. S. (2004a). CT screening for lung cancer: suspiciousness of nodules at baseline according to size. *Radiology* **231**, 164–168.

Henschke, C. I., Yankelevitz, D. F, Wisnivesky, J. P., Smith, J. P., Libby, D. and Pasmantier, M. (2005). CT Screening for lung cancer: The diagnostic-prognostic approach. In *Lung Cancer: Principles and Practice*, 3rd edn, H. I. Pass, D. P. Carbone, D. H. Johnson, J. D. Minna and A. T. Turrisi (eds). Lippincott: Williams and Wilkins. In press.

Henschler, D., Bolt, H. M., Jonker, D., Pieters, M. N. and Groten, J. P. (1996). Experimental designs and risk assessment in combination toxicology: panel discussion. *Food and Chemical Toxicology* **34**, 1183-1185.

Herrero-Jimenez, P., Thilly, G., Southam, P. J., Tomita-Mitchell, A., Morgenthaler, S., Furth, E. E. and Thilly, W. G. (1998). Mutation, cell kinetics, and subpopulations at risk for colon cancer in the United States. *Mutation Research* **400**, 553–578.

Hertz-Picciotto, I., Smith, A. H., Holtzman, D., Lipsett, M. and Alexeeff, G. (1992). Synergism between occupational arsenic exposure and smoking in the induction of lung cancer. *Epidemiology* **3**, 23–31.

Herzig, M. and Christofori, G. (2002). Recent advances in cancer research: mouse models of tumorigenesis. *Biochimica et Biophysica Acta,* **1602**, 97.

Hirji, K. F., Mehta, C. R. and Patel, N. R. (1987). Computing distributions for exact logistic regression. *Journal of the American Statistical Association* **82**, 1110–1117.

Hodgson, E. and Levi, P. E. (1987). *A Textbook of Modern Toxicology.* New York: Elsevier.

Hoeting, J. A., Madigan, D., *et al.* (1999). Bayesian model averaging: a tutorial. *Statistical Science* **4**, 382–417.

Hogue, C. (2003). Genes, computers & chemicals. *Chemical and Engineering News* **81**(41), 50–53.

Holford, T. R. (1991). Understanding the effects of age, period, and cohort on incidence and mortality rates. *Annual Review of Public Health* **12**, 425–457.

Holford, T. R. (1992) Analyzing the temporal effects of age, period and cohort. *Statistical Methods in Medical Research* **1**, 317–337.

Holland, N. T., Smith, M. T., Eskenazi, B. and Bastaki, M. (2003). Biological sample collection and processing for molecular epidemiological studies. *Mutation Research* **543**, 217–234.

Holmquist, G. P. (1998). Chronic low-dose lesion equilibrium along genes: measurement, molecular epidemiology, and theory of the minimal relevant dose. *Mutation Research* **405**, 155–159.

Horibe, K., Hara, J., Yagi, K., Tawa, A., Komada, Y., Oda, M., Nishimura, S., Ishikawa, Y., Kudoh, T. and Ueda, K. (2000). Prognostic factors in childhood acute lymphoblastic leukemia in Japan. Japan Association of Childhood Leukemia Study. *International Journal of Hematology* **72**, 61–68.

Hornhardt, S., Jung, T. and Burkart, W. (2000). Radiation in complex exposure situations: assessing health risks at low levels from concomitant exposures to radiation and chemicals. In *Proceedings of the 10th International Congress of the International Radiation Protection Association*, May 14–19, Hiroshima, Japan, T-20(2)-2, P-2a-97.

Hosmer, D. W. and Lemeshow, S. (1989). *Applied Logistic Regression.* New York: Wiley.

Hothorn, L. and Lehmacher, W. (1991). A simple testing procedure 'control versus k treatments' for one-sided ordered alternatives, with application in toxicology. *Biometrical Journal* **33**, 179–189.

Hsieh, F. (2001). On heteroscedastic hazards regression models: theory and application. *Journal of the Royal Statistical Society*, Series B **63**, 63–79.

Hu, P. and Zelen, M. (1997). Planning clinical trials to evaluate early detection programmes. *Biometrika* **84**, 817–829.

Hudmon, K. S., Honn, S. E., Jiang, H., Chamberlain, R. M., Xiang, W., Ferry, G., Gosbee, W., Hong, W. K. and Spitz, M. R. (1997). Identifying and recruiting healthy control subjects from a managed care organization: a methodology for molecular epidemiological case–control studies of cancer. *Cancer Epidemiology Biomarkers & Prevention* **6**, 565–571.

Hussain, S. P. and Harris, C. C. (2000). Molecular epidemiology and carcinogenesis: endogenous and exogenous carcinogens. *Mutation Research* **462**, 311–322.

Hussain, S. P., Hofseth, L. J. and Harris, C. C. (2001). Tumor suppressor genes: at the crossroads of molecular carcinogenesis, molecular epidemiology and human risk assessment. *Lung Cancer* **34**, 7–15.

Ilyas, M. and Tomlinson, I. P. M. (1997). The interactions of APC, E-cadherin and beta-catenin in tumor development and progression. *Journal of Pathology* **182**, 128.

Imaida, K., Tatematsu, M., Kato, T., Tsuda, H. and Ito, N. (1989). Advantages and limitations of stereological estimation of placental glutathione S-transferase-positive rat-liver cell foci by computerized 3-dimensional reconstruction. *Japanese Journal of Cancer Research* **80**, 326–330.

Iman, R. L. and Helton, J. C. (1988). An investigation of uncertainty and sensitivity analysis techniques for computer models. *Risk Analysis* **8**, 71–90.

Ingelman-Sundberg, M., Ronis, M. J., Lindros, K. O., Eliasson, E. and Zhukov, A. (1994). Ethanol-inducible cytochrome P4502E1: regulation, enzymology and molecular biology. *Alcohol Suppl.* **2**, 131–139.

Ings, R. M. (1990). Interspecies scaling and comparisons in drug development and toxicokinetics. *Xenobiotica* **20**(11), 1201–1231.

International Agency for Research on Cancer (1997). *Polychlorinated Dibenzo-para-dioxins and Dibenzofurans.* IARC Monographs on the Evaluation of the Carcinogenic Risk to Humans, Vol. 69. Lyon: IARC.

Inoue, M. (2001). Current molecular aspects of the carcinogenesis of the uterine endometrium. *International Journal of Gynecological Cancer* **11**, 339.

International Human Genome Sequencing Consortium (2001). Initial sequencing and analysis of the human genome. *Nature* **409**, 860–921.

International Life Science Institute (ILSI) (1995). *Low-Dose Extrapolation of Cancer Risk. Issues and Perspectives.* Washington, DC: ILSI Press.

IPCS (2002). *Environmental Health Criteria 228: Principles and Methods for the Assessment of Risk from Essential Trace Elements.* Geneva: World Health Organization, International Programme on Chemical Safety (IPCS).

Isaacs, W. B. (1995). Molecular genetics of prostate cancer. *Cancer Surveys* **25**, 357.

Issaq, H. J., Veenstra, T. D., Conrads, T. P. and Felschow D. (2002). The SELDI-TOF MS approach to proteomics: Protein profiling and biomarker identification. *Biochemical and Biophysical Research Communications*, **292**, 587–592.

Isselbacher, K. J., *et al.* (eds) (1994). *Harrison's Principles of Internal Medicine* Vol. II (13th edition). New York: McGraw-Hill.

Ittrich, C., Deml, E., Oesterle, D., Küttler, K., Mellert, W., Enzmann, H., Bannasch, P., Haertel, T., Mönnikes, O., Schwarz, M. and Kopp-Schneider, A. (2003). Prevalidation of a rat liver foci bioassay (RLFB) based on results from 1600 rats: a study report. *Toxicologic Pathology* **31**, 60–79.

Iverson, S. and Arley, N. (1950). On the mechanism of experimental carcinogenesis. *Acta Path. Microbiol. Scand.*, **27**, 773–803.

Jacob, P., Goulko, G., Heidenreich, W. F., Likhtarev, I., Kairo, I., Tronko, N. D., Bogdanova, T. I., Kenigsberg, J., Buglova, E., Drozdovitch, V., Golovneva, A., Demidchik, E. P., Balonov, M., Zvonova, I. and Beral, V. (1998). Thyroid cancer risk to children calculated. *Nature* **392**, 31–32.

Jarup, L. and Pershagen, G. (1991). Arsenic exposure, smoking and lung cancer in smelter workers – a case control study. *American Journal of Epidemiology* **134**, 545–551.

Jass, J. R. (2003). Hyperplastic-like polyps as precursors of microsatellite-unstable colorectal cancer. *American Journal of Clinical Pathology* **119**, 773–775.

Jen, J., Powell, S. M., Papadopoulos, N., Smith, K. J., Hamilton, S. R., Vogelstein, B. and Kinzler, K. W. (1994). Molecular determinants of dysplasia in colorectal lesions. *Cancer Research* **54**, 5523–5526.

Jepson, G. W., Hoover, D. K., Black, R. K., McCafferty, J. D., Mahle, D. A. and Gearhart, J. M. (1994). A partition coefficient determination method for nonvolatile chemicals in biological tissues. *Fundamental and Applied Toxicology* **22**, 519–524.

Jonas, W. B. (2001). The future of hormesis: what is the clinical relevance to hormesis? *Critical Reviews in Toxicology* **31**, 655–658.

Josang, A. (2001). A logic for uncertain probabilities. *International Journal of Uncertainty, Fuzziness and Knowledge-Based Systems* **9**, 279–311.

Jung, D. and Konietzko, J. (1994). Polychlorierte Dibenzo-papa-dioxine und Dibenzofurane. In J. Konietzko and H. Dupuis (eds), *Handbuch der Arbeitsmedizin. Arbeitsphysiologie – Arbeitspathologie – Prävention.* Landsberg a. L.: ecomed, pp. 1–20.

Kahn, H. A. (1989). *Statistical Methods in Epidemiology.* New York: Oxford University Press.

Kalbfleisch, J. D. and Prentice, R. L. (1980). *The Statistical Analysis of Failure Time Data.* New York: Wiley.

Kalliomaa, K., Haag-Gronlund, M., *et al.* (1998). A new model function for continuous data sets in health risk assessment of chemicals using the benchmark dose concept. *Regulatory Toxicology and Pharmacology* **27**, 98–107.

Kalman, R. (1960). A new approach to linear filtering and prediction poblem. *Transactions of the ASME – Journal of Basic Engineering* **82**, 34–45.

Kalman, R. (1961). New methods and results in linear prediction and filtering theory. In *Proceedings of the Symposium in Engineering Applications of Random Function Theory and Probability.* New York: Wiley.

Kaltz-Wittmer, C., Klenk, U., Glaessgen, A., Aust, D. E., Diebold, J., Lohrs, U. and Baretton, G. B. (2000). FISH analysis of gene aberrations (MYC, CCND1, ERBB2, RB and AR) in advanced prostatic carcinomas before and after androgen deprivation therapy. *Laboratory Investigation* **80**, 1455.

Kamlet, M. J., Doherty, R. M., Fiserova-Bergerova, V., Carr, P. W., Abraham, M. H. and Taft, R. W. (1987). Solubility properties in biological media: Prediction of solubility and partition of organic nonelectrolytes in blood and tissues from solvatochromic parameters. *Journal of Pharmaceutical Sciences* **76**, 14–17.

Kantarci, O. H., Lesnick, T. G., Yang, P., Meyer, R. L., Hebrink, D. D., McMurray, C. T. and Weinshenker, B. G. (2002). Myeloperoxidase -463 (G $\rightarrow$ A) polymorphism associated with lower risk of lung cancer. *Mayo Clinic Proceedings* **77**, 17–22.

Kantorovich, L. V. and Akilov, G. P. (1982). *Functional Analysis*, 2nd edn. New York: Pergamon Press.

Kapitanovic, S., Radosevic, S., Kapitanovic, M., Andelinovic, S., Ferencic, Z., Tavassoli, M., Primorac, D., Sonicki, Z., Spaventi, S., Pavelic, K. and Spaventi, R. (1997). The expression of p185 (HER-2/neu) correlates with the stage of disease and survival in colorectal cancer. *Gastroenterology* **112**, 1103–1113.

Kaplan, K. B., Burds, A. A., Swedlow, J. R., Bekir, S. S., Sorger, P. K. and Nathke, I. S. (2001). A role for the adenomatous polyposis coli protein in chromosome segregation. *Nature Cell Biology* **3**, 429–432.

Karp, J. E., Chiarodo, A., Brawley, O. and Kelloff, G. J. (1996). Prostate cancer prevention: investigational approaches and opportunities. *Cancer Research* **56**, 5547.

Katano, N., Tsurusawa, M., Hirota, T., Horikoshi, Y., Mimaya, J., Yanai, M., Tsuji, Y. and Fujimoto, T. (1997). Treatment outcome and prognostic factors in childhood acute myeloblastic leukemia: a report from the Japanese Children's Cancer and Leukemia Study Group (CCLSG). *International Journal of Hematolology* **66**, 103–110.

Katsanakis, K. D., Gorgoulis, V., Papavassiliou, A. and Zoumpourlis, V. (2002). The progression in the mouse skin carcinogenesis model correlates with ERK1/2 signaling. *Molecular Medicine* **8**, 624.

Kavlock, R. J., Schmid, J. E., *et al.* (1996). A simulation study of the influence of study design on the estimation of benchmark doses for developmental toxicity. *Risk Analysis* **16**, 399–410.

Kawajiri, K. (1999). CYP1A1. In *Metabolic Polymorphisms and Susceptibility to Cancer*, IARC Scientific Publication No. 148, P. Vineis N. Malats, M. Lang, A. d'Errico, N. Caporaso, J. Cuzick and P. Boffetta (eds), 159–172. IARC, Lyon: International Agency for Research on Cancer.

Kearney D. J., Lee T. H., Reilly J. J., DeCamp M. M. and Sugarbaker D. J. (1994). Assessment of operative risk in patients undergoing lung resection. *Chest* **105**, 753–759.

Kedderis, G. L. (1997). Extrapolation of in vitro enzyme induction data to humans in vivo. *Chemico-biological Interactions* **107**, 109–121.

Kelly, C. and Rice, J., (1990). Monotone smoothing with application to dose-response curves and the assessment of synergism. *Biometrics* **46**, 1071–1085.

Kendall, D.G. (1948). On the generalized birth-and-death process. *Annals of Mathematical Statistics* **19**, 1–15.

Kendall, D. G. (1960). Birth-and-death processes, and the theory of carcinogenesis. *Biometrika* **47**, 13–21.

Kendziorsky, C. M., Zhang, Y., Lan, H. and Attie, A. D. (2003). The efficiency of pooling mRNA in microarray experiments. *Biostatistics* **4**, 465–477.

Kenigsberg, J. (2000). Problem of the low doses in radiation protection for workers and members of the public. In *Proceedings of the 10th International Congress of the International Radiation Protection Association*, May 14–19, Hiroshima, Japan, P-2b-111.

Khuder, S. A. (2001). Effect of cigarette smoking on major histological types of lung cancer: a meta-analysis. *Lung Cancer* **31**, 139–148.

Kibel, A. S., Suarez, B. K., Belani, J., Oh, J., Webster, R., Brophy-Ebbers, M., Guo, C., Catalona, W. J., Picus, J. and Goodfellow, P. J. (2003). CDKN1A and CDKN1B polymorphisms and risk of advanced prostate carcinoma. *Cancer Research* **63**, 2033–2036.

Kihara, C., Tsunoda, T., Tanaka, T., Yamana, H., Furukawa, Y., Ono, K., Kitahra, O., Zembutsu, H., Yanagawa, R., Hirata, K., Takagi, T. and Nakamura, Y. (2001). Prediction of sensitivity of esophageal tumors to adjuvant chemotherapy by cDNA microarray analysis of gene-expression profiles. *Cancer Research* **61**, 6474–6479.

Kim, A. H., Kohn, M. C., *et al.* (2002). Impact of physiologically based pharmacokinetic modeling on benchmark dose calculations for TCDD-induced biochemical responses. *Regulatory Toxicology and Pharmacology* **36**, 287–296.

Kimmel, M. and Flehinger, B. J. (1991). Nonparametric estimation of the size–metastasis relationship in solid cancers. *Biometrics* **47**, 987–1004.

King, G., Honaker, J., Joseph, A. and Scheve, K. (2001). Analysing incomplete political science data: An alternative for multiple imputation. *American Political Science Review* **95**, 49–69.

Kinzler, K. W. and Vogelstein, B. (1997). Gatekeepers and caretakers. *Science* **386**, 761–763.

Kirch, R. and Klein, M. (1974). Surveillance schedules for medical examinations. *Management Science* **20**, 1403–1409.

Kitagawa, G. (1998). A self-organizing state-space model. *Journal of the American Statistical Association* **93**, 443.

Kitsos, C. P. (1986). Design and inference in nonlinear problems. PhD thesis, University of Glasgow, UK.

Kitsos, C. P. (1989). Fully sequential procedures in nonlinear design problems. *Computational Statistics and Data Analysis* **8**, 13–19.

Kitsos, C. P. (1992). Adopting sequential procedures for biological based experiments. In *MODA-3 (Model Oriented Data Analysis)*, W. Muller, H. Wynn and A. Zhigljavsky (eds), 3–9. Heidelberg: Physica.

Kitsos, C. P. (1995). On the support points of D-optimal nonlinear experimental designs for chemical kinetics. In *MODA4 – Advances in Model-Oriented Data Analysis*, C. P. Kitsos and W. G. Muller (eds), 71–76. Heidelberg: Physica.

Kitsos, C. P. (1998). The role of covariates in experimental carcinogenesis. *Biometrical Letters* **35**, 95–106.

Kitsos, C. P. (1999). Optimal designs for estimating the percentiles of the risk in multistage models in carcinogenesis. *Biometrical Journal* **41**, 33–43.

Kitsos, C. P. (2001). Design aspects for the Michaelis–Menten model. *Biometrical Letters* **38**, 53–66.

Kitsos, C. P., Titterington, D. M. and Torsney, B. (1988). An optimal design problem in rhythmometry. *Biometrics* **44**, 657–671.

Klein, M. and Bartoszyński, R. (1991). Estimation of growth and metastatic rates of primary breast cancer. In *Mathematical Population Dynamics*, O. Arino, D. E. Axelrod and M. Kimmel (eds), 397–412. New York: Marcel Dekker.

Klein, M. T., Hou, G., Quann, R. J., Wei, W., Liao, K. H., Yang, R. S. H, Campain, J. A., Mazurek, M. A. and Broadbelt, L. J. (2002). BioMOL: a computer-assisted biological modeling tool for complex chemical mixtures and biological processes at the molecular level. *Environmental Health Perspectives* **110**(6), 1025–1029.

Klein, J. P. and Moeschberger, M. L. (1997). *Survival Analysis: Techniques for Censored and Truncated Data*. New York: Springer.

Kleinbaum, D. G. (1997). *Survival Analysis: A Self-Learning Text*. New York: Springer.

Klir, J. G. and Yuan, B. (1995). *Fuzzy Sets and Fuzzy Logic: Theory and Applications*. Englewood Cliffs, NJ: Prentice Hall.

Knaak, J. B., Al-Bayati, M. A. and Raabe, O. G. (1995). Development of partition coefficients, V_{max} and K_m values, and allometric relationships. *Toxicology Letters* **79**, 87–98.

Knudson, A. G. (1971). Mutation and cancer: statistical study of retinoblastoma. *Proceedings of the National Academy of Sciences* **68**, 820–823.

Knudson, A. G. Jr. (1985). Hereditary cancer, oncogenes and antioncogenes. *Cancer Research* **45**, 1437.

Kodell, R. L. and West, R. W. (1993). Upper confidence limits on excess risk for quantitative responses. *Risk Analysis* **13**, 177–182.

Koeneman, K. S., Pan, C. X., Jin, J. K., Pyle, J. M. 3rd, Flanigan, R. C., Shankey, T. V. and Diaz, M. O. (1998). Telomerase activity, telomere length and DNA ploidy in prostatic intraepithelial neoplasia (PIN). *Journal of Urology* **160**, 1533.

Kogevinas, M., Becher, H., Benn, T., Bertazzi, P. A., Boffetta, P., Bueno-de-Mesquita, H. B., Coggon, D., Colin, D., Flesch-Janys, D., Fingerhut, M., Green, L., Kauppinen, T., Littorin, M., Lynge, E., Mathews, J. D., Neuberger, M., Pearce, N. and Saracci, R. (1997). Cancer mortality in workers exposed to phenoxy herbicides, chlorophenols, and dioxins. An expanded and updated international cohort study. *American Journal of Epidemiology* **145**, 1061–1075.

Kohn, M. C. (1997). The importance of anatomical realism for validation of physiological models of disposition of inhaled toxicants. *Toxicology and Applied Pharmacology* **147**, 448–458.

Kohn, M. C. (2000). Current directions in physiological modeling for environmental health sciences: an overview. *Environmental Health Perspectives* **108**, 857–859.

Kohn, M. C., Lucier, G. W., Clark, G. C., Sewall, C., Tritscher, A. and Portier, C. J. (1993). A mechanistic model of effects of dioxin on gene expression in the rat liver. *Toxicology & Applied Pharmacology* **120**, 138–153.

Kohn, M. C., Sewall, C. H., Lucier, G. W. and Portier C. J. (1996). A mechanistic model of effects of dioxin on thyroid hormones in the rat. *Toxicology & Applied Pharmacology* **136**, 29–48.

Kohn, M. C., Walker, N. J., Kim, A. H. and Portier, C. J. (2001). Physiological modeling of a proposed mechanism of enzyme induction by TCDD. *Toxicology* **162**, 193–208.

Kopp-Schneider, A. (1997). Carcinogenesis models for risk assessment. *Statistical Methods in Medical Research* **6**, 317–340.

Kopp-Schneider, A. (2003). Biostatistical analysis of focal hepatic preneoplasia. *Toxicologic Pathology* **31**, 121–125.

Kopp-Schneider, A. and Portier, C. J. (1991). Distinguishing between models of carcinogenesis: the role of clonal expansion. *Fundamental and Applied Toxicology* **17**, 601–613.

Kopp-Schneider, A., Portier, C. J. and Sherman, C. D. (1994). The exact formula for tumor incidence in the two-stage model. *Risk Analysis* **14**, 1079–1080.

Kopp-Schneider, A., Portier, C. J. and Bannasch, P. (1998). A model for hepatocarcinogenesis treating phenotypical changes in focal hepatocellular lesions as epigenetic events. *Mathematical Biosciences* **148**, 181–204.

Kopp-Schneider, A., Geisler, I. and Edler, L. (2002). Complex mechanistic carcinogenicity modeling. In *Endocrine Disrupters and Carcinogenic Risk Assessment*, J. Chyczewsli, E. Nikliniski, E. Pluygers (eds), 317–328. Amsterdam: IOS Press.

Koshinsky, H. A. and Khachatourians, G. G. (1992a). Trichothecene synergism, additivity and antagonism: the significance of the maximally quiescent ratio. *Natural Toxins* **1**, 38–47.

Koshinsky, H. A. and Khachatourians, G. G. (1992b). Bioassay for deoxynivalenol based on the interaction of T-2 toxin with trichothecene mycotoxins. *Bulletin of Environmental Contamination and Toxicology* **49**, 246–251.

Kott, P. S. (1995). A paradox of multiple imputation. In *Proceedings of the Survey Research Methods Section*, 380–383. Alexandria VA: American Statistical Association.

Kotti, V. K. and Rigas, A. G. (2002). Identification of a stochastic neuroelectric system using the maximum likelihood approach. In *Proceedings of the 6th International Conference on Signal Processing,* B. Yuan and X. Tang (eds.), 1492–1495. Beijing: IEEE Press.

Kotti, V. K. and Rigas, A. G. (2003a). A nonlinear stochastic model used for the identification of a biological system. In *Mathematical Modeling & Computing in Biology and Medicine*, V. Capasso (ed.), 587–592. Bologna: The Miriam Project Series, Progetto Leonardo, Escapulario Co.

Kotti, V. K. and Rigas, A. G. (2003b). Identification of a complex neurophysiological system using the maximum likelihood approach. *Journal of Biological Systems* **11**, 189–204.

Krewski, D. and van Ryzin, J. (1981). Dose response models for quantal response toxicity data. In M. Csörgö, D. Dawson, J. N. K. Rao and E. Saleh (eds), *Current Topics in Probability and Statistics*, pp. 201–231. Amsterdam: North Holland.

Krishnan, K., Haddad, S., Béliveau, M. and Tardif, R. (2002). Physiological modeling and extrapolation of pharmacokinetic interactions from binary to more complex chemical mixtures. *Environmental Health Perspectives* **110**, 989–994.

Kroes, R., Renwick, A. G., Cheeseman, M., Kleiner, J., Mangelsdorf, I., Piersma, A., Schilter, B., Schlatter, J., van Schothorst, F., Vos, J. G. and Würtzen, G. (2004). Structure-based Thresholds of Toxicological Concern (TTC): Guidance for application to substances present at low levels in the diet. *Food and Chemical Toxicology* **42**, 65–83.

Krzanowski, W. J. (1988). *Principles of Multivariate Analysis, A User's Perspective*. Clarendon: Oxford University Press.

Kulesz-Martin, M., Kilkenny, A. E., Holbrook, K. A., Digernes, V. and Yuspa, S. H. (1983). Properties of carcinogen altered mouse epidermal cells resistant to calcium-induced terminal differentiation. *Carcinogenesis* **4**, 1367.

Lagarda, H., Catasus, L., Arguelles, R., *et al.* (2001). *K-ras* mutations in endometrial carcinomas with microsatellite instability. *Journal of Pathology* **193**, 193.

Laurent-Puig, P., Blons, H. and Cugnenc, P.-H. (1999). Sequence of molecular genetic events in colorectal tumorigenesis. *European Journal of Cancer Prevention* **8**, S39–S47.

Lax, S. F., Kendall, B., Tashiro, H., *et al.* (2000). The frequency of *p53*, *K-ras* mutations, and microsatellite instability differs in uterine endometrioid and serous carcinoma: evidence of distinct molecular genetic pathways. *Cancer* **88**, 814.

Leavens, T. L. and Bond, J. A. (1996). Pharmacokinetic model describing the disposition of butadiene and styrene in mice. *Toxicology* **113**, 310–313.

Lee, S. J. and Zelen, M. (1998). Scheduling periodic examinations for the early detection of disease: applications to breast cancer. *Journal of the American Statistical Association* **93**, 1271–1281.

Lee, W. H., Morton, R. A., Epstein, J. I., Brooks J. D., Campbell, P. A., Bova, G. S., Hsieh, W. S., Isaacs, W. B. and Nelson, W. G. (1994). Cytidine methylation of regulatory sequences near the pi-class glutathione S-transferase gene accompanies human prostatic carcinogenesis. *Proceedings of the National Academy of Sciences USA* **91**, 11 733.

Lehman, A. J. and Fitzhugh, O. G. (1954). 100-fold margin of safety. *Association Food Drug Office U.S. Q. Bulletin* **18**, 33–35.

Lehmann, E. L. (1986). *Testing Statistical Hypotheses*, 2nd edn. New York: Wiley.

Leung, H. W., Ku, R. H., Paustenbach, D. J. and Andersen, M. E. (1988). A physiologically based pharmacokinetic model for 2,3,7,8-tetrachlorodibenzo-*p*-dioxin in C57BL/6J and DBA/2J mice. *Toxicology Letters* **42**, 15–28.

Leung, H. W., Paustenbach, D. J., Murray, F. J. and Andersen, M. E. (1990). A physiological-based pharmacokinetic description of the tissue distribution and enzyme inducing properties of 2,3,7,8-tetrachlorodibenzo-*p*-dioxin in the rat. *Toxicology and Applied Pharmacology* **103**, 399–410.

Levine, D. S. (1994). Barrett's esophagus. *Scientific American Science & Medicine* **1**, 16–25.

Levine, D. S. (1995). Barrett's esophagus and other premalignant conditions. *Current Opinion in Gastroenterology* **11**, 359–365.

Levine, R. L., Cargile, C. B., Blazes, M. S., *et al.* (1998). PTEN mutations and microsatellite instability in complex atypical hyperplasia, a precursor lesion to uterine endometrioid carcinoma. *Cancer Research* **58**, 3254.

Liao, K. H., Dobrev, I. D., Dennison Jr., J. E., Andersen, M. E., Reisfeld, B., Reardon, K. F., Campain, J. A., Wei, W., Klein, M. T., Quann, R. J. and Yang, R. S. H. (2002). Application of biologically based computer modeling to simple or complex mixtures. *Environmental Health Perspectives* **110**, 957–963.

Lin, J. H. and Lu, A. Y. (1998). Inhibition and induction of cytochrome P450 and the clinical implications. *Clinical Pharmacokinetics* **35**, 361–390.

Liteplo, R. G. and Meek, M. E. (2001). N-nitrosodimethylamine: Hazard characterization and exposure-response analysis. *Journal of Environmental Science and Health Part C. Environmental Carcinogenesis & Ecotoxicology Reviews* **19**, 281–304.

Little, J., Bradley, L., Bray, M. S., Clyne, M., Dorman, J., Ellsworth, D. L., Hanson, J., Khoury, M., Lau, J., O'Brien, T. R., Rothman, N., Stroup, D., Taioli, E., Thomas, D., Vainio, H., Wacholder, S. and Weinberg, C. (2002a). Reporting, appraising, and integrating data on genotype prevalence and gene–disease associations. *American Journal of Epidemiology* **156**, 300–310.

Little, M. and Wright, E. (2003). A stochastic carcinogenesis model incorporating genomic instability fitted to colon cancer data. *Mathematical Biosciences* **183**, 111–134.

Little, M. P., Haylock, R. G. and Muirhead, C. R. (2002b). Modelling lung tumour risk in radon-exposed uranium miners using generalizations of the two-mutation model of Moolgavkar, Venzon and Knudson. *International Journal of Radiation Biology* **78**, 49–68.

Liu, J. and Chen, R. (1998). Sequential Monte Carlo methods for dynamic systems. *Journal of the American Statistical Association* **93**, 1032–1044.

Liu, J., Neuwald, A. and Lawrence, C. (1997). Markov structures in biological sequence alignments. Technical report, Stanford University.

Liu, S.-Z. (2003). Nonlinear dose-response relationship in the immune system following exposure to ionizing radiation: Mechanisms and Implications, nonlinearity in biology. *Toxicology and Medicine* **1**, 71–92.

Loda, M., Cukor, B., Tam, S. W., *et al.* (1997). Increased proteasome-dependent degradation of the cyclin-dependent kinase inhibitor p27 in aggressive colorectal carcinomas. *Nature Medicine* **3**, 231.

Loeb, K. R. and Loeb, L. A. (2000). Significance of multiple mutations in cancer. *Carcinogenesis* **21**, 379–385.

Loeb, L. A. (1998). Cancer cells exhibit a mutator phenotype. *Advances in Cancer Research* **72**, 25–56.

Loeb, L. A. (2001). A mutator phenotype in cancer. *Cancer Research* **61**, 3230–3239.

Loewe, S. (1928). Die quantitativen Probleme der Pharmakologie. *Ergebnisse der Physiologie, biologischen Chemie und experimentellen Pharmakologie* **27**, 47–187.

Loewe, S. (1953). The problem of synergism and antagonism of combined drugs. *Arzneimittel Forschung* **3**, 285–290.

Loewe, S. and Muischnek, H. (1926). Über Kombinationswirkungen. *Archiv für experimentelle Pathologie und Pharmakologie* **114**, 313–326.

Loh, W. Y. and Shih, Y. S. (1997). Split selection methods for classification trees. *Statistica Sinica* **7**, 815–840.

Lönnstedt, I. and Speed, T. P. (2002). Replicated microarray data. *Statistica Sinica* **12**, 31–46.

López-Fidalgo, J. and Garcet-Rodríguez, S. (2004). Optimal experimental designs when some independent variables are not subject to control. *Journal of the American Statistical Association* **99**, 1190–1199.

Louis, T., Albert, A. and Heghinian, S. (1978). Screening for the early detection of cancer. III. Estimation of disease natural history. *Mathematical Biosciences* **40**, 111–144.

Lucier, G. W., Portier, C. J. and Gallo, M. A. (1993). Receptor mechanisms and dose-response models for the effects of dioxins. *Environmental Health Perspectives* **101**, 36–44.

Luebeck, E. G. and Moolgavkar, S. H. (2002). Multistage carcinogenesis and the incidence of colorectal cancer. *Proceedings of the National Academy of Sciences* **99**, 15 095–15 100.

Luebeck, E. G., Curtis, S., Cross, F. and Moolgavkar, S. (1996). Two-stage model of radon-induced malignant lung tumors in rats: effects of cell killing. *Radiation Research* **145**, 163–173.

Luebeck, E. G., Heidenreich, W. F., Hazelton, W. D., Paretzke, H. G. and Moolgavkar, S. H. (1999a). Biologically-based analysis of the data for the Colorado plateau uranium miners cohort: age, dose, and dose-rate effects. *Radiation Research* **152**, 339–351.

Luebeck, E. G., Watanabe, K. and Travis, C. (1999b). Biologically based models of carcinogenesis. In *Perspectives on Biologically Based Cancer Risk Assessment*, V. J. Cogliano, E. G. Luebeck and G. A. Zapponi (eds), 205–241. New York: Kluwer Academic/Plenum Publishers.

Lukacs, G. L., Szakall, S., Kozma, I., Gyory, F. and Balazs, G. (1997). Changes in the epidemiological parameters of radiation-induced illnesses in East Hungary 10 years after Chernobyl. *Langenbecks Archiv für Chirurgie Suppl. Kongressb.* **114**, 375–377.

Lutz, W. K. (1990). Dose-response relationship and low dose extrapolation in chemical carcinogenesis. *Carcinogenesis* **11**(8), 1243–1247.

Lutz, W. K. (1998). Dose response relationships in chemical carcinogenesis: superposition of different mechanisms of action, resulting in linear-sublinear curves, practical thresholds, J-shapes. *Mutation Research* **405**, 117–124.

Lutz, R. J., Dedrick, R. L. and Zaharko, D. S. (1980). Physiological pharmacokinetics: an *in vivo* approach to membrane transport. *Pharmacology and Therapeutics* **11**, 559–592.

Macgregor, P. F. (2003). Gene expression in cancer: the application of microarrays. *Expert Reviews in Molecular Diagnosis* **3**, 185–200.

Mahadevia, P. J., Fleisher, L. A., Frick, K. D., Eng, J., Goodman, S. N. and Powe, N. R. (2003). Lung cancer screening with helical computed tomography in older adult smokers: a decision and cost-effectiveness analysis. *Journal of the American Medical Association* **289**, 313–322.

Malliri, A., Kammen, R. A., Clark, K., Valk, M., Michiels, F. and Collard, J. G. (2002). Mice deficient in the Rac activator Tiam1 are resistant to Ras-induced skin tumours. *Nature* **417**, 867.

Mandard, A. M., Hainaut, P. and Hollstein, M. (2000). Genetic steps in the development of squamous cell carcinoma of the esophagus. *Mutation Research* **462**, 335–342.

Mandel, J. S., Church, T. R., Bond, J. H., Ederer, F., Geisser, M. S., Mongin, S. J., Snover, D. C. and Schuman, L. M. (2000). The effect of fecal occult-blood screening on the incidence of colorectal cancer. *New England Journal of Medicine* **343**, 1603–1607.

Mantel, N. and Bryan, W. R. (1961). 'Safety' testing of carcinogenic agents. *Journal of the National Cancer Institute* **27**, 455–470.

Mantel, N. and Haenszel, W. (1959). Statistical aspects of the analysis of data from retrospective studies of disease. *Journal of the National Cancer Institute* **22**, 719–748.

Manz, A., Berger, J., Dwyer, J. H., Flesh-Janys, D., Nagel, S. and Waltsgott, H. (1990). Cancer mortality among workers in a chemical plant contaminated with dioxin. *Lancet* **338**, 959–964.

Mao, J. H. and Balmain, A. (2003). Genomic approaches to identification of tumor-susceptibility genes using mouse models. *Current Opinion in Genetics & Development* **13**, 14.

Marcus, P. M., Bergstrahl, E. J., Fagerstrom, R. M., Williams, D. E., Fontana, R., Taylor, W. F. and Prorok, P. C. (2000). Lung cancer mortality in the Mayo Lung Project: impact of extended follow-up. *Journal of the National Cancer Institute* **92**, 1308–1316.

Marks, F. and Fürstenberger, G. (1987). From the normal cell to cancer. The multistep process of skin carcinogenesis. In *Concepts and Theories in Carcinogenesis*, A. P. Maskens, P. Ebbesen and A. Burny (eds), 169–184. Amsterdam: Exerpta Medica.

Marosi, C., Koller, U., Koller-Weber, E., Schwarzinger, I., Schneider, B., Jager, U.,Vahls, P., Nowotny, H., Pirc-Danoewinata, H. and Steger, G. (1992). Prognostic impact of karyotype and immunologic phenotype in 125 adult patients with de novo AML. *Cancer Genetics and Cytogenetics* **61**, 14–25.

Matias-Guiu, X., Catasus, L., Bussaglia, E., *et al.* (2001). Molecular pathology of endometrial hyperplasia and carcinoma. *Human Pathology*, **32**, 569.

Matthews, P. B. C. (1981). Review lecture: Evolving views on the internal operation and functional role of the muscle spindle. *Journal of Physiology* **320**, 1–30.

Mauderly, J. L. (1993). Toxicological approaches to complex mixtures. *Environmental Health Perspectives* Suppl. **101**(4), 155–165.

McCullagh, P. and Nelder, J. A. (1989). *Generalized Linear Models*, 2nd edn. London: Chapman & Hall.

McDorman, K. S. and Wolf, D. C. (2002). Use of the spontaneous Tsc2 knockout (Eker) rat model of hereditary renal cell carcinoma for the study of renal carcinogens. *Toxicologic. Pathology* **30**, 675–680.

McLachlan, G. J. (1992). *Discriminant Analysis and Statistical Pattern Recognition.* New York: Wiley.

McLachlan, G. J. and Krishnan T. (1997). *The EM Algorithm and Extensions.* New York: Wiley.

Medinsky, M. A. and Klaassen, C. D. (1996). Toxicokinetics. In C. D. Klaassen (ed.), *Casarett & Doull's Toxicology: The Basic Science of Poisons*, pp. 187–198. New York: McGraw-Hill.

Medinsky, M. A., Sabourin, P. J., Lucier, G., Birnbaum, L. S. and Henderson, R. F. (1989). A physiological model for simulation of benzene metabolism by rats and mice. *Toxicology and Applied Pharmacology* **99**, 193–206.

Meek, M. E. B. (1999). Application of uncertainty factors in the priority substances program and international harmonization. *Human and Ecological Risk Assessment* **5**, 1013–1022.

Mehlen, P. and Fearon, E. R. (2004). Role of the dependence receptor DCC in colorectal cancer pathogenesis. *Journal of Clinical Oncology* **16**, 3420.

Mehta, C. R. and Patel, N. R. (1995). Exact logistic regression: Theory and examples. *Statistics in Medicine* **14**, 2143–2160.

Meng, Z. and Zhang, L. (2000). Cytogenetic adaptive response induced by pre-exposure in human lymphocytes and marrow cells of mice. In *Proceedings of the 10th International Congress of the International Radiation Protection Association*, May 14–19, Hiroshima, Japan, P-2b-69.

Mestiri, S., Bouaouina, N., Ahmed, S. B., Khedhaier, A., Jrad, B. B., Remadi, S. and Chouchane, L. (2001). Genetic variation in the tumor necrosis factor-alpha promoter region and in the stress protein hsp70–2: susceptibility and prognostic implications in breast carcinoma. *Cancer* **91**, 672–678.

Michaelis, L. and Menten, M. L. (1913). Kinetics for intertase action. *Biochemische Zeitung* **49**, 333–369.

Mileson, B. E., Chambers, J. E., Chen, W. L., Dettbarn, W., Ehrich, M., Eldefrawi, A. T., Gaylor, D. W., Hamernik, K., Hodgson, E., Karczmar, A., Padilla, S., Pope, C., Richardson, R. J., Saunders, D. R., Sheets, L. P., Sultatos, L. G. and Wallace, K. B. (1998). Common mechanism of toxicity: A case study of organophosphorus pesticides. *Toxicological Sciences* **41**, 8–20.

Mitchel, R. E. J. and Borham, D. R. (2000). Radiation Protection in the world of modern radiobiology: time for a new approach. In *Proceedings of the 10th International Congress of the International Radiation Protection Association*, May 14–19, Hiroshima, Japan, PS-1-2, P-2a-87.

Mollerup, S., Ryberg, D., Hewer, A., Phillips, D. H. and Haugen, A. (1999). Sex differences in lung CYP1A1 expression and DNA adduct levels among lung cancer patients. *Cancer Research* **59**, 3317–3320.

Montironi, R., Hamilton, P. W., Scarpelli, M., Tompson, D. and Bartels, P. H. (1999). Subtle morphological and molecular changes in normal-looking epithelium in prostates with prostatic intraepithelial neoplasia or cancer. *European Urology* **35**, 468.

Moolgavkar, S. H. (1994). Biological models of carcinogenesis and quantitative cancer risk assessment. *Risk Analysis* **14**, 879–882.

Moolgavkar, S. H. and Knudson, A. (1981). Mutation and cancer: A model for human carcinogenesis. *Journal of the National Cancer Institute* **66**, 1037–1052.

Moolgavkar, S. H. and Luebeck, E. G. (1990). Two-event model for carcinogenesis: Biological, mathematical and statistical considerations. *Risk Analysis* **10**, 323–341.

Moolgavkar, S. H. and Luebeck, E. G. (1992a). Multistage carcinogenesis: population-based model for colon cancer. *Journal of the National Cancer Institute* **84**, 610–618.

Moolgavkar, S. H. and Luebeck, E. (1992b). Interpretation of labeling indices in the presence of cell death. *Carcinogenesis* **13**, 1007–1010.

Moolgavkar, S. H. and Luebeck, E.G. (2002). Dose-response modeling for cancer risk assessment. In *Human and Ecological Risk Assessment: Theory and Praxis*, D. J. Paustenbach (ed), 151–188. New York: Wiley.

Moolgavkar, S. H. and Stevens, R. G. (1981). Smoking and cancers of bladder and pancreas: risks and temporal trends. *Journal of the National Cancer Institute* **67**, 15–23.

Moolgavkar, S. H. and Venzon, D. J. (1979). Two-event models for carcinogenesis: incidence curves for childhood and adult tumors. *Mathematical Biosciences* **47**, 55–77.

Moolgavkar, S. H., Luebeck, E. G., de Gunst, M., Port, R. E. and Schwarz, M. (1990). Quantitative analysis of enzyme-altered foci in rat hepato-carcinogenesis experiments I: single agent regimen. *Carcinogenesis* **11**, 1271–1278.

Moolgavkar, S. H., Luebeck, E.G. and Anderson, E. L. (1998). Estimation of unit risk for coke oven emissions. *Risk Analysis*, **18**, 813–825.

Moolgavkar, S., Krewski, D., Zeise, L., Cardis, E. and Moller, H. (eds) (1999). *Quantitative Estimation and Prediction of Human Cancer Risks.* IARC Scientific Publication No 131. Lyon: International Agency for Research on Cancer.

Mordenti, J. (1986). Man versus beast: pharmacokinetic scaling in mammals. *Journal of Pharmaceutical Sciences* **75**, 1028–1040.

Morgan, B. J. T. (1992). *Analysis of Quantal Response Data.* London: Chapman & Hall.

Morris, R. W. (1989) Testing statistical hypotheses about rat liver foci. *Toxicologic Pathology* **17**, 569–578.

Morrison, D. F. (1976). *Multivariate Statistical Methods.* New York: McGraw-Hill.

Mortazavi, S. M. J. (2000). *An Introduction to Radiation Hormesis*, 612–852. Kyoto: Biology Division, Kyoto University of Education.

Mortazavi, J. M. J., Ikushima, T., Mozdarani, H. and sharafi, A. A. (2000). Synergistic effect versus radioadaptive response: possible implications of such response in the estimation of risks of low-level radiation can be more problematical. In *Proceedings of the 10th International Congress of the International Radiation Protection Association*, May 14–19, Hiroshima, Japan, T-7-5, P-2b-70.

Mortazavi, J. M. J. and Mozdarani, H. (2000). The dependence of the magnitude of induced adaptive response on the dose of pre-irradiation of cultured human lymphocytes under the optimum irradiation time scheme. In *Proceedings of the 10th International Congress of the International Radiatioin Protection Association*, May 14–19, Hiroshima, Japan, T-7-5, P-2b-71.

Morton, R. S., Ewing, C. M., Nagafuchi, A., Tsukita, S. and Isaacs, W. B. (1993). Reduction in E-cadherin levels and deletion of the alpha-catenin gene in human prostate cancer cells. *Cancer Research* **53**, 3585.

Mumtaz, M. M., Sipes, G., Clewell, H., J. and Yang, R. S. H. (1993). Risk assessment of chemical mixtures: biologic and toxicologic issues. *Fundamental and Applied Toxicology* **21**, 258–269.

Murphy, J. E., Janszen, D. B. and Gargas, M. L. (1995). An in vitro method for determination of tissue partition coefficients of non-volatile chemicals such as 2,3,7,8-tetrachlorodi-benzo-*p*-dioxin and estradiol. *Journal of Applied Toxicology* **15**, 147–152.

Murrell, J. A., Portier, C. J., *et al.* (1998). Characterizing dose-response I: Critical assessment of the benchmark dose concept. *Risk Analysis* **18**, 13–26.

Mutter, G. L., Lin, M. C., Fitzgerald, J. T., *et al.* (1992). Altered PTEN expression as a diagnostic marker for the earliest endometrial precancers. *Journal of the National Cancer Institute* **92**, 924.

Narotsky, M. G., Weller, E. A., Chinchilli, V. M. and Kevlock, R. J. (1995). Non-additive developmental toxicity in mixtures of trichloroethylene di(2-ethylhexyl)phthalate and heptachlor in a $5 \times 5 \times 5$ design. *Fundamental and Applied Toxicology* **27**, 203–216.

National Academy of Sciences USA (1989). *Biologic Markers in Pulmonary Toxicology.* Washington, DC: National Academy Press.

National Research Council (1983). *Risk Assessment in the Federal Government: Managing the Process.* Washington, DC: National Academy Press.

National Research Council (1988). *Complex Mixtures: Methods for In Vivo Toxicity Testing.* Washington, DC: National Academy Press.

National Research Council (1980). *Principles of Toxicological Interactions Associated with Multiple Chemical Exposures.* Washington, DC: National Academy Press.

National Research Council (1994). *Science and Judgment in Risk Assessment.* Washington, DC: National Academy Press.

Nestorov, I. (2001). Modelling and simulation of variability and uncertainty in toxicokinetics and pharmacokinetics. *Toxicology Letters* **120**, 411–420.

Nestorov, I. (2003). Whole body pharmacokinetic models. *Clinical Pharmacokinetics* **42**(10), 883–908.

Neyman, J. and Scott, E. (1967). Statistical aspects of the problem of carcinogenesis. In *Proceedings of the 5th Berkeley Symposium on Mathematical Statistics and Probability,* L. Le Cam and J. Neyman (eds.), 745–776. Berkeley: University of California Press.

Nguyen, D. V., Arpat, A. B., Wang, N. and Carroll, R. J. (2002). DNA microarray experiments: biological and technological aspects. *Biometrics* **58**, 701–717.

Nicholson, J. K. and Wilson, I. D. (2003). Opinion: understanding 'global' systems biology: metabonomics and the continuum of metabolism. *Nature Reviews Drug Discovery* **2**, 668–676.

Nicholson, J. K., Lindon, J. C. and Holmes, E. (1999). Metabonomics: understanding the metabolic responses of living systems to pathophysiological stimuli via multivariate statistical analysis of biological NMR spectroscopic data. *Xenobiotica* **29**, 1181–1189.

Nieuwenhuijsen, M. J., Rautiu, R., Ranft, U., *et al.* (2001). Exposure to arsenic and cancer risk in central and east Europe. Final report, Project EXPASCAN IC 15 CT98 0325. Brussels: European Union.

Ninan, M., Sommers, E., Landreneau, R. J., Weyant, R., Tobias, J., Luketich J., Ferson, P. and Keenan R. J. (1997). Standardized exercise oximetry predicts postpneumonectomy outcome. *Annals of Thoracic Surgery* **64**, 328–333.

Nordling, C. O. (1953). A new theory of the cancer inducing mechanism. *British Journal of Cancer* **7**, 68–72.

Nowak, M. A., Komarova, N. L., Sengupta, A., Jallepalli, P. V., Shih, I. M., Vogelstein, B. and Lengauer, C. (2002). The role of chromosomal instability in tumor initiation. *Proceedings of the National Academy of Sciences* **99**, 16 226–16 231.

Oehler, M. K., Brand, A. and Wain, G. V. (2003). Molecular genetics and endometrial cancer. *Journal of the British Menopause Society* **9**, 27.

O'Hagan, A. (1994). *Kendall's Advanced Theory of Statistics, Vol 2B: Bayesian Inference.* London: Edward Arnold.

O'Hanlon D. M., Little, M. P., Given, H. F. and Quill, D. S. (1997). Thyroid disease in the West of Ireland: an atypical incidence of neoplasia. *Irish Journal of Medical Science* **2**, 70–71.

Ohnishi, T., Takahashi, A. and Ohnishi, K. (2000). Tumor suppressor p53 response is blunted by low-dose-rate radiation. In *Proceedings of the 10th International Congress of the International Radiation Protection Association,* May 14–19, Hiroshima, Japan, P-2b-73.

Ohser, J. and Lurz, U. (1994). *Quantitative Gefügeanalyse: Theoretische Grundlagen und Anwendungen.* Freiberger Forschungshefte B274. Deutscher Verlag f. Grundstoffindustrie.

Ohser, J. and Sandau, K. (2000). Considerations about the estimation of size distribution in Wicksell's corpuscle problem. In *Statistical Physics and Spatial Statistics,* K. Mecke and D. Stoyan (eds). Heidelberg: Springer.

Oien, K. A., Vass, J. K., Downie, I., Fullarton, G. and Keith, W. N. (2003). Profiling, comparison and validation of gene expression in gastric carcinoma and normal stomach. *Oncogene* **22**, 4287–4300.

Okabe, H., Satoh, S., Kato, T., Kitahara, O., Yanagawa, R., Yamaoka, Y., Tsunoda, T., Furukawa, Y. and Nakamura, Y. (2001). Genome-wide analysis of gene expression in human hepatocellular carcinomas using cDNA microarray: identification of genes involved in viral carcinogenesis and tumor progression. *Cancer Research* **61**, 2129–2137.

Olin, S., Farlad, W., Rhomberg, L., Scheuplein, R., Starr, T. and Wilson, J. (1995). *Low-Dose Extrapolation of Cancer Risk: Issues and Perspectives*. Washington, DC: ILSI Press.

Olsen, O. and Gotzsche, P. C. (2001). Cochrane review on screening for breast cancer with mammography. *Lancet* **358**, 1340–1342.

Olson, H. M., Kadyszewski, E. and Beierschmitt, W. (2001). Hormesis – a pharmaceutical industry perspective. *Critical Reviews in Toxicology* **31**, 659–661.

Otori, K., Konishi, M., Sugiyama, K., Hasebe, T., Shimoda, T., Kikuchi-Yanoshita, R., Mukai, K., Fukushima, S., Miyaki, M. and Esumi, H. (1998). Infrequent somatic mutation of the adenomatous polyposis coli gene in aberrant crypt foci of human colon tissue. *Cancer* **83**, 896–900.

Ott, M. and G., Zober, A. (1996). Cause specific mortality and cancer incidence among employees exposed to 2,3,7,8-TCDD after a 1953 reactor accident. *Occupational & Environmental Medicine* **53**, 606–612.

Palmero, I., Pantoja, C. and Serrano, M. (1998). p19^{arf} links the tumor suppressor *p53* to *Ras*. *Nature* **395**, 125–126.

Pantuck, E. J., Pantuck, C. B., Ryan, D. E. and Conney, A. H. (1985). Inhibition and stimulation of enflurane metabolism in the rat following a single dose or chronic administration of ethanol. *Anesthesiology* **62**, 255–262.

Papathoma, A. S., Zoumpourlis, V., Balmain, A. and Pintzas, A. (2001). Role of matrix metalloproteinase-9 in progression of mouse skin carcinogenesis. *Molecular Carcinogenesis* **31**, 74.

Parc, Y. R., Halling, K. C., Wang, L., Christensen, E. R., Cunningham, J. M., French, A. J., *et al.* (2000). HMSH6 alterations in patients with microsatelite instability-low colorectal cancer. *Cancer Research* **60**, 2225.

Parham, F. M. and Portier, C. J. (1998). Using structural information to create physiologically based pharmacokinetic models for all polychlorinated biphenyls. II. Rates of metabolism. *Toxicology & Applied Pharmacology* **151**, 110–116.

Park, B. K. and Kitteringham, N. R. (1990). Assessment of enzyme induction and enzyme inhibition in humans: toxicological implications. *Xenobiotica* **20**, 1171–1185.

Park, I. W., Wistuba, I. I., Maitra, A., Milchgrub, S., Virmani, A. K., Minna, J. D. and Gazdar, A. F. (1999). Multiple clonal abnormalities in the bronchial epithelium of patients with lung cancer. *Journal of the National Cancer Institute* **91**, 1863–1868.

Parkinson, A. (1996). Biotransformation of xenobiotics. In *Casarett and Doull's Toxicology: The Basic Science of Poisons*, C. D. Klaassen (ed), 113–186. New York: McGraw-Hill.

Parmigiani, G. (1991). On optimal screening schedules. *Biometric Bulletin* **8**(3), 21.

Parmigiani, G. (1992). *Optimal scheduling of fallible inspections*. ISDS 92, Duke University.

Parmigiani, G. (1993). On optimal screening ages. *Journal of the American Statistical Association* **88**, 622–628.

Parmigiani, G. (1997). Timing medical examinations via intensity functions. *Biometrika* **84**, 803–816.

Parmigiani, G. and Kamlet, M.S. (1993). A cost-utility analysis of alternative strategies in screening for breast cancer. In *Bayesian Statistics in Science and Technology: Case Studies*, C. Gatsonis, J. Hodges, R. E. Kass and N. Singpurwalla (eds), 390–402. New York: Springer.

Parmigiani, G., Garrett, E. S., Irizarry, R. A. and Zeger, S. L. (eds) (2003). *The Analysis of Gene Expression Data, Methods and Software*. New York: Springer.

Parshkov, E. M., Chebotareva, I. V., Solokov, V. A. and Dallas, C. E. (1997). Additional thyroid dose factor from transportation sources in Russia after the Chernobyl disaster. *Environmental Health Perspectives* Suppl., 1491–1496.

Parthasarathy, K. S. (1998). *Radiation Hormesis.* AERB Newsletter, Quarterly Publication from the Indian Atomic Energy Regulation Board.

Pastino, G. M., Flynn, E. J. and Sultatos, L. G. (2000). Genetic polymorphisms in ethanol metabolism: issues and goals for physiologically based pharmacokinetic modeling. *Drug & Chemical Toxicology* **23**, 179–201.

Paustenbach, D.J. (2002). *Human and Ecological Risk Assessment: Theory and Practice.* New York: Wiley.

Payne, S. (2001) 'Smoke like a man, die like a man'?: A review of the relationship between gender, sex and lung cancer. *Social Science & Medicine* **53**, 1067–1080.

Peltomäki, P., Aaltonen, L. A., Sistonen, P., Pylkkönen, L., Mecklin, J-P, Järvinen, H., Green, J. S., Jass, J. R, Weber, J. L., Leach, F. S., Petersen, G. M., Hamilton, S. R., de la Chapell, A. and Vogelstein B. (1993). Genetic mapping of a locus predisposing to human colorectal cancer. *Science* **260**, 810–812.

Peltomäki, P. and de la Chapelle, A. (1997). Mutations predisposing to hereditary nonpolyposis colorectal cancer. *Advances in Cancer Research* **71**, 93–119.

Pepe, M. S., Longton, G., Anderson, G. L. and Schummer, M. (2003). Selecting differentially expressed genes from microarray experiments. *Biometrics* **59**, 133–142.

Perbellini, L., Brugnone, F., Caretta, D. and Maranelli, G. (1985). Partition coefficients of some industrial aliphatic hydrocarbons (C5-C7) in blood and human tissues. *British Journal of Industrial Medicine* **42**, 162–167.

Perera, F. P. and Weinstein, I. B. (1982). Molecular epidemiology and carcinogen-DNA adduct detection: new approaches to studies of human cancer causation. *Journal of Chronic Diseases* **35**, 581–600.

Perou, C. M., Sorlie, T., Eisen, M. B., Van de Rijn, M., Jeffrey, S. S., Rees, C. A., Pollack, J. R., Ross, D. T., Johnsen, H., Akslen, L. A., Fluge, O., Pergamenschikov, A., Williams, C., Zhu, S. X., Lonning, P. E., Borresen-Dale, A. L., Brown, P. O. and Botstein, D. (2000). Molecular portraits of human breast tumours. *Nature* **406**, 747–752.

Persson, L. (2000). Effects of low-dose ionising radiation. In *Proceedings of the 10th International Congress of the International Radiation Protection Association*, May 14–19, Hiroshima, Japan, P-2a-89.

Pesch, B., Ranft, U., Jakubis, P., Nieuwenhuijsen, M. J., Hergemoller, A., Unfried, K., Jakubis, M., Miskovic, P. and Keegan, T. (2002). Environmental arsenic exposure from a coal-burning power plant as a potential risk factor for non-melanoma skin carcinoma: results from a case–control study in the district of Prievidza, Slovakia. *American Journal of Epidemiology,* **155**, 798–809.

Petricoin, E. F., Ardekani, A. M., Hitt, B. A., Levine, P. J., Fusaro, V. A., Steinberg, S. M., Mills, G. B., Simone, C., Fishman, D. A., Kohn, E. C. and Liotta, L. A. (2002). Use of genomic patterns in serum to identify ovarian cancer. *Lancet* **359**, 572–577.

Pettersson, M., Bylund, M. and Alderborn, A. (2003). Molecular haplotype determination using allele-specific PCR and pyrosequencing technology. *Genomics*, **82** 390–396.

Pflug, G. C. (1996). *Optimization of Stochastic Models: The Interface between Simulation and Optimization.* Boston: Kluwer.

Piantadosi, S. (1997). *Clinical Trials: A Methodologic Perspective.* New York: Wiley.

Piegorsch, W. W. and Bailer, A. J. (1997). *Statistics for Environmental Biology and Toxicology. Interdisciplinary Statistics.* London: Chapman & Hall.

Pierce, L. M., Sivaraman, L., Chang, W., Lum, A., Donlon, T., Seifried, A., Wilkens, L. R., Lau, A. F. and Le Marchand, L. L. (2000). Relationships of TP53 codon 72 and HRAS1 polymorphisms with lung cancer risk in an ethnically diverse population. *Cancer Epidemiology Biomarkers & Prevention* **9**, 1199–1204.

Pietra, G. G. (1990). The pathology of carcinoma of the lung. *Seminars in Roentgenology* **25**, 25–33.

Pike, M. C. (1966). A method of analysis of a certain class of experiments in carcinogenesis. *Biometrics* **22**, 142–161.

Pinsky, P. F. (2001). Estimation and prediction for cancer screening models using deconvolution and smoothing. *Biometrics* **57**, 389–395.

Pitot, H. C., Goldsworth, T. L., Campbell, H. A. and Poland, A. (1980). Quantitative evaluation of the promotion by TCDD of hepatogenesis and diethylnitrosamine. *Cancer Research* **40**, 3616.

Placket, R. L. and Hewlett, P. S. (1948). Statistical aspects of the independent joint action of poisons, particulary insecticides. I. The toxicity of a mixture of poisons. *Annals of Applied Biology* **35**, 347–358.

Pleško, I., Severi, G., Obšitníková, A. and Boyle, P. (2000). Trends in the incidence of non-melanoma skin cancer in Slovakia, 1978–95. *Neoplasma* **47**, 137–142.

Polyak, K. and Higgins, G. J. (2001). Gene discovery using the serial analysis of gene expression technique: implications for cancer research. *Journal of Clinical Oncology* **19**, 2948.

Poole, D. and Raftery, A. E. (2000). Inference for deterministic simulation models: the Bayesian melding approach. *Journal of the American Statistical Association* **95**, 1244–1255.

Poplack, D. G., Kum, L. E., Magrath, I. T. and Pizzo, P. A. (1993). Leukemias and lymphomas of childhood. In *Cancer Principles Practice of Oncology*, 4th edn, V. T. de Vita (ed.), 1792–1818. Philadelphia: Lippincott.

Pories, S. E., Ramchurren, N., Summerhayes, J. and Steele, G. (1993). Animal models for colon carcinogenesis. *Archives of Surgery* **128**, 647.

Pories, S. E., Summerhayes, J. C. and Steele, G. O. (1991). Oncogene-mediated transformation. *Archives of Surgery* **126**, 1387.

Portier, C. (1987). Statistical properties of a two-stage model of carcinogenesis. *Environmental Health Perspectives* **76**, 125–139.

Portier, C. and Bailer, A. (1989). Two-stage models of tumor incidence for historical control animals in the NTP carcinogenesis experiments. *Journal of Toxicology and Environmental Health* **27**, 21–45.

Portier, C. and Hoel, D. (1983). Low-dose rate extrapolation using the multistage model. *Biometrics* **39**, 897–906.

Portier, C., Tritscher, A., Kohn, M., Sewall, C., Clark, G., Edler, L., Hoel, D. and Lucier, G. (1993). Ligand/receptor binding for 2,3,7,8-TCDD. Implications for risk assessment. *Fundamental & Applied Toxicology* **20**, 48–56.

Portier, C. J., Sehrman, C. D., Kohn, M., Edler, L., Kopp-Schneider, A., Maronpot, R. M. and Lucier, G. (1996). Modeling the number and size of hepatic focal lesions following exposure to 2,3,7,8-TCDD. *Toxicology & Applied Pharmacology* **138**, 20–30.

Portier, C. J., Edler, L., Jung, D., Needham, L., Masten, S., Parham, F. and Lucier, G. (1999). Half-lives and body burdens for dioxin and dioxin-like compounds in humans estimated from an occupational cohort in Germany. *Organohalogen Compounds* **42**, 129–138.

Potten, C. S. and Loeffler, M. (1990). Stem cells: attributes, cycles, spirals, pitfalls and uncertainties. Lessons for and from the crypt. *Development* **110**, 1001–1020.

Potter, J. D. (1999). Colorectal cancer: molecules and populations. *Journal of the National Cancer Institute* **91**, 916–932.

Poulin, P. and Krishnan, K. (1995). An algorithm for predicting tissue: blood partition coefficients of organic chemicals from n-octanol: water partition coefficient data. *Journal of Toxicology and Environmental Health* **46**(1), 117–129.

Powell, S. M., Zilz, N., Beazer-Barclay, Y., Bryan, T. M., Hamilton, S. R., Thibodeau, S. N., Vogelstein, B. and Kinzler, K. W. (1992). APC mutations occur early during colorectal tumorigenesis. *Nature* **359**, 235–237.

Prevo, L. J., Sanchez, C. A., Galipeau, P. C. and Reid, B. J. (1999) p53-mutant clones and field effects in Barrett's esophagus. *Cancer Research* **59**, 4784–4787.

Prorok, P. C. (1976a). The theory of periodic screening I: Lead time and proportion detected. *Advances in Applied Probability* **8**, 127–143.

Prorok, P. C. (1976b). The theory of periodic screening II: Doubly bounded recurrence times and mean lead time and detection probability estimation. *Advances in Applied Probability* **8**, 460–476.

PSD (1999). *Methodology for the Toxicological Assessment of Exposures from Combinations of Cholinesterase Inhibiting Compounds.* Medical and Toxicology Panel, Advisory Committee on Pesticides, Pesticides Safety Directorate, UK Ministry of Agriculture, Fisheries and Food, April 19.

Psichari, E., Balmain, A., Plows, D., Zoumpourlis, V. and Pintzas, A. (2002). High activity of serum response factor in the mesenchymal transition of epithelial tumor cells is regulated by RhoA Signaling. *Journal of Biological Chemistry* **277**, 29 490–29 495.

Pugh, T. D., King, J. H., Koen, H., Nychka, D., Chover, J. and Wahba, G. (1983). Reliable stereologiocal method for estimating the number of microscopic hepatocellular foci from their transections. *Cancer Research* **43**, 1261–1268.

Pui, C. H., Carroll, A. J., Head, D., Raimondi, S. C., Shuster, J. J., Crist, W. M., Link, M. P., Borowitz, M. J., Behm, F. G., Land, V. J., *et al.* (1990). Near-triploid and near-tetraploid acute lymphoblastic leukemia of childhood. *Blood* **76**, 590–596.

Pulford, D. J., Falls, J. G., Killian, J. K. and Jirtle, R. L. (1999). Polymorphisms, genomic imprinting and cancer susceptibility. *Mutation Research* **436**, 59–67.

Puri, P. S. (1967). A class of stochastic models of response after infection in the absence of defense mechanism. In *Proceedings of the Fifth Berkeley Symposium on Mathematical Statistics and Probability*, L. Le Cam and J. Neyman (eds), Vol. 4, 511–535. Berkeley: University of California Press.

Puri, P.S. (1971). A quantal response process associated with integrals of certain growth processes. In *Mathematical Aspects of Life Sciences*, Queen's Papers in Pure and Applied Mathematics No. 26, M. T. Wasan (ed.). Kingston, Ontario, Canada: Queen's University.

Puri, P. S. and Senturia, J. (1972). On a mathematical theory of quantal response assays. In *Proceedings of the Sixth Berkeley Symposium on Mathematical Statistics and Probability*, L. Le Cam, J. Neyman and E. L. Scott (eds), Vol. 4, 231–247. Berkeley: University of California Press.

Quick, D. J. and Shuler, M. L. (1999). Use of in vitro data for construction of a physiologically based pharmacokinetic model for naphthalene in rats and mice to probe species differences. *Biotechnology Progress* **15**, 540–555.

Quintanilla, M., Brown, K., Ramsden, M. and Balmain, A. (1986). Carcinogen-specific mutation and amplification of Ha-ras during mouse skin carcinogenesis. *Nature* **322**, 78–80.

Raabe, O. G. (2000). Evidence supporting nonlinear effective threshold dose-response relationships for radiation carcinogenesis. In *Proceedings of the 10th International Congress of the International Radiation Protection Association*, May 14–19, Hiroshima, Japan, P-2a-86.

Rasty, G., Murray, R., Lu, L., *et al.* (1998). Expression of *HER-2/neu* oncogene in normal, hyperplastic and malignant endometrium. *Annals of Clinical and Laboratory Science* **28**, 138.

Rattan, S. I. (2001). Hormesis in biogerontology. *Critical Reviews in Toxicology* **31**, 663–664.

Rao, V., Todd, T. R. J., Kuus, A., Buth, K. J. and Pearson, F. G. (1995). Exercise oximetry versus spirometry in the assessment of risk prior to lung resection. *Annals of Thoracic Surgery* **60**, 603–609.

Reiter, A., Schrappe, M., Ludwig, W. D., Hiddemann, W., Sauter, S., Henze, G., Zimmermann, M., Lampert, F., Havers, W., Niethammer, D., *et al.* (1994). Chemotherapy in 998 unselected childhood acute lymphoblastic leukemia patients. Results and conclusions of the multicenter trial ALL-BFM 86. *Blood* **84**, 3122–3133.

Renwick, A. G., Barlow, S. M., Hertz-Picciotto, I., Boobis, A. R., Dybing, E., Edler, L., Eisenbrand, G., Greig, J. B., Kleiner, J., Lambe, J., Müller, D. J. G., Smith, M. R., Tritscher, A., Tuijtelaars, S., van den Brandt, P. A., Walker, R. and Kroes, R. (2003). Risk charcterization of chemiocals in food and diet. *Food and Chemical Toxicology* **41**, 1211–1271.

Rhyu, M. S. (1995). Telomeres, telomerase and immortality. *Journal of the National Cancer Institute* **87**, 884.

Ries, L. A. G., Eisner, M. P., Kosary C. L., Hankey, B. F., Miller, B. A., Clegg, L. and Edwards, B. K. (eds) (2001). *SEER Cancer Statistics Review, 1973–1998.* Bethesda, MD: National Cancer Institute.

Rigas, A. G. (1996). Stochastic modeling of a complex physiological system. In *Proceedings of the International Conference on Differential Equations and Their Applications to Biology and Industry,* 409–415. Singapore: World Scientific.

Rigas, A. G. and Liatsis P. (2000). Identification of a neuroelectric system involving a single input and a single output. *Signal Processing* **80**, 1833–1894.

Risch, A., Wikman, H., Thiel, S., Schmezer, P., Edler, L., Drings, P., Dienemann, H., Kayser, K., Schulz, V., Spiegelhalder, B. and Bartsch, H. (2001) Glutathione-S-transferase M1, M3, T1 and P1 polymorphisms and susceptibility to non-small-cell lung cancer subtypes and hamartomas. *Pharmacogenetics* **11**,757–764.

Risinger, J. I., Hayes, A. K., Berchuck, A. and Barrett, J. C. (1997). PTEN/MMAC1 mutations in endometrial cancers. *Cancer Research* **57**, 4736.

Robles, A. I., Rodriquez-Puebla, M. L., Glick, A. B., *et al.* (1998). Reduced skin tumor development in cyclin D1-deficient mice highlights the oncogenic *ras* pathway in vivo. *Genes and Development* **12**, 2469.

Rojas, M., Alexandrov, K., Cascorbi, I., Brockmöller, J., Likhachev, A., Pozharisski, K., Bouvier, G., Auburtin, G., Mayer, L., Kopp-Schneider, A., Roots, I. and Bartsch, H. (1998). High benzo[*a*]pyrene diol-epoxide DNA adduct levels in lung and blood cells from individuals with combined *CYP1A1 MspI/MspI-GSTM1*0/*0* genotypes. *Pharmacogenetics* **8**, 109–118.

Rojas, M., Godschalk, R., Alexandrov, K., Cascorbi, I., Kriek, E., Ostertag, J., van Schooten, F.J. and Bartsch, H. (2001). Myeloperoxidase-463A variant reduces benzo[*a*]pyrene diol epoxide DNA adducts in skin of coal tar treated patients. *Carcinogenesis* **22**, 1015–1018.

Rosenwald, A., Wright, G., Chan, W. C., Connors, J. M., Campo, E., Fisher, R. I., Gascoyne, R. D., Muller-Hermelink, H. K., Smeland, E. B. and Staudt, L. M. (2002). The use of molecular profiling to predict survival after chemotherapy for diffuse large B-cell lymphoma. *New England Journal of Medicine* **346**, 1937–1947.

Ross, J. A., Davies, S. M., Potter, J. D. and Robison, L. L. (1994). Epidemiology of childhood leukemia, with a focus on infants. *Epidemiological Review,* **16**, 243–272.

Rossman, T. G. (1999). Arsenic genotoxicity may be mediated by interference with DNA damage-inducible signaling. In *Arsenic Exposure and Health Effects,* C. O. Abernathy, R. L. Calderon and W. R. Chappell (eds), 233–241. New York: Elsevier.

Rostami Hodjegan, A., Lennard, M.S., Woods, H.F. and Tucker, G.T. (1998). Meta-analysis of studies of the CYP2D6 polymorphism in relation to lung cancer and Parkinson's disease. *Pharmacogenetics* **8**, 227–238.

Rothman, N., Wacholder, S., Caporaso, N. E., Garcia-Closas, M., Buetow, K. and Fraumeni Jr., J. F. (2001). The use of common genetic polymorphisms to enhance the epidemiologic study of environmental carcinogens. *Biochimica et Biophysica Acta* **1471**, C1-C10.

Sahm, M. and Schwabe R. (2000). A note on optimal bounded designs. In *Optimun Design, A. Atkinson, B. Bogacka and A. Zhigljavsky (eds), 131–140. Dordrecht: Kluwer.*

Sand, S., Filipsson, A. F., *et al.* (2002). Evaluation of the benchmark dose method for dichotomous data: Model dependence and model selection. *Regulatory Toxicology and Pharmacology* **36**, 184–197.

Sandberg, A. A. (1992). Chromosomal abnormalities and related events in prostate cancer. *Human Pathology* **23**, 368.

Santin, A. D., Bellone, S., Gokden, M., *et al.* (2002). Overexpression of *HER-2/neu* in uterine serous papillary cancer. *Clinical Cancer Research* **8**, 1271.

Santner, T. J. and Duffy, D. E. (1986). A note on A. Albert's and J.A. Anderson's conditions for the existence of maximum likelihood estimates in logistic regression models. *Biometrika* **73**, 755–758.

Sasaki, H., Nishii, H., Takahashi, H., *et al.* (1993). Mutation of the *Ki-ras* protooncogene in human endometrial hyperplasia and carcinoma. *Cancer Research* **53**, 1906.

Sato, A. and Nakajima, T. (1979). Partition coefficients of some aromatic hydrocarbons and ketones in water, blood and oil. *British Journal of Industrial Medicine* **36**, 231–234.

Sawyer, C., Peto, R., Bernstein, L. and Pike, M. C. (1984). Calculation of carcinogenic potency from long-term animal carcinogenesis experiments. *Biometrics* **40**, 27–40.

Schafer, J. L. and Olsen, M. K. (1998). Multiple imputation for multivariate missing-data problems: a data analyst's perspective. *Multivariate Behavioral Research* **33**, 545–571.

Schafer, J. L., Ezzatti-Rice, T. M., Johnson, W., Khare, M., Little, R. J. A. and Rubin, D. B. (1996). The NHANES III multiple imputation project. In *Proceedings of the Survey Research Methods Section*, 28–37. Alexandria, VA: American Statistical Association.

Scheffé, H. (1958). Experiments with mixtures. *Journal of Royal Statistical Society*, Series B **21**, 344–360.

Scheffé, H. (1963). The simplex-centroid design for experiments with mixtures. *Journal of Royal Statistical Society*, Series B **25**, 235–265.

Scher, H. I., Sarkis, A., Reuter, V., Cohen, D., Netto, G., Petrylak, D., Lianes, P., Fuks, Z., Mendelsohn, J. and Cordon-Cardo, C. (1995). Changing pattern of expression of the epidermal growth factor and transforming growth factor alpha in the progression of prostatic neoplasms. *Clinical Cancer Research* **1**, 545.

Schmiegelow, K., Yssing, M., Hertz, H., Scherling, B., Holm, K. and Schmiegelow, M. (1995). Akut lymfoblastaer leukaemi hos born. En retrospektiv opgorelse: 1970–1991. (Acute lymphoblastic leukemia in children. A retrospective study: 1970–1991). *Ugeskr Laeger*, **157**(1), 41–46.

Schneiderman, M. A., Decoufle, P. and Brown, C. C. (1979). Thresholds for environmental cancer: biologic and statistical considerations. *Annals of the New York Academy of Sciences* **329**, 92–130.

Schulte, P. A. and Perera, F. P. (1997). Transitional studies. In *Application of Biomarkers in Cancer Epidemiology*, P. Toniolo, P. Boffetta, D. E. G. Shuker, H. Rothman, B. Hulka and N. Pearce (eds). IARC Scientific Publications No 142. Lyon: International Agency for Cancer Research.

Schulz, H. (1988). Über Hefegifte. *Pflügers Archiv European Journal of Physiology*, **42**, 517.

Schwartz, M. (1978a). A mathematical model used to analyze breast cancer screening strategies. *Operations Research* **26**, 937–955.

Schwartz, M. (1978b). An analysis of the benefits of serial screening for breast cancer based upon a mathematical model of the disease. *Cancer* **41**, 1550–1564.

Schwarz, G. (1978), Estimating the dimension of a model. *Annals of Statistics* **6**, 461–464.

Scientific Committee of the Food Safety Council (1978). *Proposed System for Food Safety Assessment. Report of the Scientific Committee of the Food Safety Council.* Columbia, MD.

Seber, C. A. F. and Wild, C. J. (1989). *Nonlinear Regression.* New York: Wiley.

Segel, I. H. (1993). *Enzyme Kinetics Behavior and Analysis of Rapid Equilibrium and Steady-State Enzyme Systems.* New York: Wiley.

Seidl, H., Kreimer-Erlacher, H., Back, B., Soyer, H. P., Hofler, G., Kerl, H. and Wolf, P. (2001). Ultraviolet exposure as the main initiator of p53 mutations in basal cell carcinomas from psoralen and ultraviolet A-treated patients with psoriasis. *Journal of Investigative Dermatology* **117**, 365–370.

Sellers, T. A. and Yates, J. R. (2003). Review of proteomics with applications to genetic epidemiology. *Genetic Epidemiology* **24**, 83–98.

Shafer, G. (1976). *A Mathematical Theory of Evidence.* Princeton, NJ: Princeton University Press.

Shahani, A. K. and Crease, D. M. (1977). Towards models of screening for early detection of disease. *Advances in Applied Probability* **9**, 665–680.

Shen, Y. and Zelen, M. (1999). Parametric estimation procedures for screening programmes: Stable and nonstable disease models for multimodality case finding. *Biometrika* **86**, 503–515.

Shen, Y. and Zelen, M. (2001). Screening sensitivity and sojourn time from breast cancer early detection clinical trials: mammograms and physical examinations. *Journal of Clinical Oncology* **19**, 3490–3499.

Shih, I. M., Zhou, W., Goodman, S. N., Lengauer, C., Kinzler, K. W. and Vogelstein, B. (2001). Evidence that genetic instability occurs at an early stage of colorectal tumorigenesis. *Cancer Research* **61**, 818–822.

Sichel, J. Y., Wygoda, M., Dano, I., Osin, P. and Elidan, J. (1996). Fibrosarcoma of the thyroid in a man exposed to fallout from the Chernobyl accident. *Annals of Otology Rhinology and Laryngoloy* **10**, 832–834.

Silvey, S. D. (1980). *Optimal Design.* London: Chapman & Hall.

Simmons, J. E. (1995). Chemical mixtures: Challenge for toxicology and risk assessment. *Toxicology* **105**, 111–119.

Simon, R. and Sauter, G. (2002). Tissue microarrays for miniaturized high-throughput molecular profiling of tumors. *Experimental Hematology* **30**, 1365–1372.

Slob, W. (1999). Thresholds in toxicology and risk assessment. *International Journal of Toxicology* **18**, 259–268.

Slob, W. (2002). Dose-response modelling of continuous endpoints. *Toxicological Sciences* **66**, 298–312.

Smelt, V. A., Mardon, H. J. and Sim, E. (1998). Placental expression of arylamine N-acetyltransferases: evidence for linkage disequilibrium between NAT1*10 and NAT2*4 alleles of the two human arylamine N-acetyltransferase loci NAT1 and NAT2. *Pharmacology and Toxicology* **83**, 149–157.

Smith, A. and Gelfand, A. (1992). Bayesian statistics without tears: a sampling–resampling perspective. *American Statistician* **46**, 84–89.

Smith, A. F. M. and Roberts, G. O. (1993). Bayesian computation via the Gibbs sampler and related Markov chain Monte Carlo methods. *Journal of the Royal Statistical Society Series B* **55**, 3–23.

Sørlie, T., Perou, C. M, Tibshirani, R., Aas, T., Geisler, S., Johnsen, H., Hastie, T., Eisen, M. B., Van de Rijn, M., Jeffrey, S. S., Thorsen, T., Quist, H., Matese, J. C, Brown, P. O., Botstein, D., Lønning, P. E. and Børresen-Dale, A. L. (2001). Gene expression patterns of breast carcinomas distinguish tumor subclasses with clinical implications. *Proceedings of the National Academy of Sciences* **98**, 10 869–10 874.

Southam, C. M. and Ehrlich, (1943). Effects of extracts of western red-cedar heartwood on certain wood-decaying fungi in culture. *Phytopathology* **33**, 517–524.

Sparks, A. B., Morin, P. J., Vogelstein, B. and Kinzler, K. W. (1998). Mutational analysis of the APC/beta-catenin/Tcf pathway in colorectal cancer. *Cancer Research* **58**, 1130–1134.

Speed, T. (ed.) (2003). *Statistical Analysis of Gene Expression Microarray Data.* Boca Raton, FL: Chapmann & Hall/CRC.

Spiegelhalter, D., Thomas, A. and Best, N. (2003). WinBUGS user manual, Version 1.4. Cambridge University.

Stablein, D. and Koutrouvelis, I. A. (1985). A two sample test sensitive to crossing hazards in uncensored and singly censored data. *Biometrics* **41**, 643–652.

Stayner, L., Bailer, A. J., Smith, R., Gilbert, S., Rice, F. and Kuempel, E. (1999). Sources of uncertainty in dose-response modeling of epidemiological data for cancer risk assessment. *Annals of the New York Academy of Sciences* **895**, 212–222.

Stebbing, A.R. D. (1981). The kinetics of growth control in a colonial hydroid. *Journal of the Marine Biology Association of the United Kingdom* **61**, 35–63.

Steel, G. G. and Peckham, M. J. (1979). Exploitable mechanisms in combined radiotherapy-chemotherapy: the concept of additivity. *International Journal of Radiation Oncology, Biology and Physics* **5**, 85–91.

Stephens, J. C., Schneider, J. A., Tanguay, D. A., Choi, J., Acharya, T., Stanley, S. E., Jiang, R., Messer, C. J., Chew, A., Han, J. H., Duan, J., Carr, J. L., Lee, M. S., Koshy, B., Kumar, A. M., Zhang, G., Newell, W. R., Windemuth, A., Xu, C., Kalbfleisch, T. S., Shaner, S. L., Arnold, K., Schulz, V., Drysdale, C. M., Nandabalan, K., Judson, R. S., Ruano, G. and Vovis, G.F. (2001). Haplotype variation and linkage disequilibrium in 313 human genes. *Science* **293**, 489–493.

Stern, M. C., Umbach, D. M., van Gils, C. H., Lunn, R. M. and Taylor, J. A. (2001). DNA repair gene XRCC1 polymorphisms, smoking and bladder cancer risk. *Cancer Epidemiology Biomarkers & Prevention* **10**, 125–131.

Stevens, R.G. and Moolgavkar, S.H. (1984). A cohort analysis of lung cancer and smoking in British males. *American Journal of Epidemiology* **119**, 624–641.

Storm, J. E. and Rozman, K. K. (1997). Evaluation of alternative methods for establishing safe levels of occupational exposure to vinyl halides. *Regulatory Toxicology and Pharmacology* **25**, 240–255.

Stoyan, D., Kendall, W. S. and Mecke, J. (1995). *Stochastic Geometry and Its Applications*, 2nd edition. Chichester: Wiley.

Strohman, R. (1992). Maneuvering in the complex path from genotype to phenotype. *Science* **296**(26), 701–703.

Svendsgaard, D. J. and Hertzberg, R. C. (1994). Statistical methods for the toxicological evaluation of the additivity assumption as used in the environmental protection agency chemical mixture risk assessment guideline. In *Toxicology of Chemicals Mixtures*, R. S. H. Yang (ed.). San Diego: Academic Press.

Takayama, T., Katsuki, S., Takahashi, Y., Ohi, M., Nojiri, S., Sakamaki, S., Kato, J., Kogawa, K., Miyake, H. and Niitsu, Y. (1998). Aberrant crypt foci of the colon as precursors of adenoma and cancer. *New England Journal of Medicine* **339**, 1277–1284.

Tan, W. Y. (1991). *Stochastic Models of Carcinogenesis.* New York: Marcel Dekker.

Tan, W. Y. (2002). *Stochastic Models with Applications to Genetics, Cancers, and Aids and Other Biomedical Systems*. Singapore: World Scientific.

Tan, W. and Chen, C. (1995). A nonhomogeneous stochastic model of carcinogenesis for assessing risk of environmental agents. In O. Arino, D. Axelrod, and M. Kimmel (eds), *Mathematical Population Dynamics* Vol. 3, Section 1, Chapter 5, pp. 49–67. Winnipeg: Wuerz.

Tan, W. Y. and Chen, C. (1998). Stochastic modeling of carcinogenesis: some new insight. *Mathematical and Computer Modelling* **28**, 49–71.

Taningher, M., Malacarne, D., Izzotti, A., Ugolini, D. and Parodi, S. (1999). Drug metabolism polymorphisms as modulators of cancer susceptibility. *Mutation Research* **436**, 227–261.

Tardif, R., Charest-Tardif, G., Brodeur, J. and Krishnan, K. (1997). Physiologically based pharmacokinetic modeling of a ternary mixture of alkyl benzenes in rats and humans. *Toxicology and Applied Pharmacology* **144**, 120–134.

Tardif, R., Lapare, S., Charest-Tardif, G., Brodeur, J. and Krishnan, K. (1995). Physiologically-based pharmacokinetic modeling of a mixture of toluene and xylene in humans. *Risk Analysis* **15**, 335–342.

Tashiro, H., Lax, S. F., Gaudin, P. B., *et al.* (1997). Microsatelite instability is uncommon in uterine serous carcinoma. *American Journal of Pathology* **150**, 75.

Terakawa, N., Kigawa, J., Taketani, Y., Yoshikawa, H., Yajima, A., Noda, K., Okada, H., Kato, J., Yakushiji, M., Tanizawa, O., Fujimoto, S., Nozawa, S., Takahashi, T., Hasumi, K., Furihashi, N., Aono, T., Sakamoto, A. and Furusato, M. (1997). The behavior of endometrial hyperplasia: a prospective study. Endometrial Hyperplasia Study Group. *Journal of Obstetrics and Gynaecology Research* **23**, 223.

Terse, P. S., Madhyastha, M. S., Zurovac, O., Stringfellow, D., Maquardt, R. R. and Kemppainen, W. (1993). Comparison of *in vitro* and *in vivo* biological activity of mycotoxins. *Toxicon* **31**, 913–919.

Texas Institute for Advancement of Chemical Technology. (1999). What are the facts? – Chemical hormesis: Beneficial effects at low exposures, adverse effects at high exposures. College Station: Texas A&M University.

Thall, P. F. and Russel, K. (1998). A strategy for dose-dinding and safety monitoring based on efficacy and adverse outcomes in phase I/II clinical trials. *Biometrics* **54**, 251–264.

Thiagalingam, S., Lengauer, C., Leach, F. S., *et al.* (1996). Evaluation of candidate tumor suppressor genes on chromosome 18 in colorectal cancers. *Nature Genetics* **13**, 343.

Thier, R., Bruning, T., Roos, P.H. and Bolt, H. M. (2002a) Cytochrome P450 1B1, a new keystone in gene–environment interactions related to human head and neck cancer? *Archives of Toxicology* **76**, 249–256.

Thier, R., Golka, K., Bruening, T., Ko, Y. and Bolt, H. M. (2002b). Genetic susceptibility to environmental toxicants: the interface between human and experimental studies in the development of new toxicological concepts. *Toxicology Letters* **127**, 321–327.

Thomas, A., Sellers, T. A. and Yates, J. R. (2003). Review of proteomics with applications to genetic epidemiology. *Genetic Epidemiology* **24**, 83–98.

Thomassen, D. G. (2001). Commentary on white paper the future of hormesis: where do we go from here? *Critical Reviews in Toxicology* **31**, 665–667.

Thornton, I. and Farago, M. (1997). The geochemistry of arsenic. In *Arsenic, Exposure and Health Effects*. C. O. Abernathy, R. L. Calderon and W. R. Chappell (eds), 1–16. New York: Chapman & Hall.

Thorslund, T. W. (1987). Quantitative dose-response model for tumor-promoting activity of TCDD. Apendix A: A cancer risk specific dose estimate for 2,3,7,8-TCDD. EPA/600//6–88/007Ab.

Thorslund, T. W., Brown, C. C. and Charnley, G. (1986). Biologically motivated cancer risk models. *Risk Analysis* **7**, 109–119.

Toide, K., Yamazaki, H., Nagashima, R., Itoh, K., Iwano, S., Takahashi, Y., Watanabe, S. and Kamataki, T. (2003). Aryl hydrocarbon hydroxylase represents CYP1B1, and not CYP1A1, in human freshly isolated white cells: Trimodal distribution of Japanese population according to induction of CYP1B1 mRNA by environmental dioxins. *Cancer Epidemiology Biomarkers & Prevention* **12**, 219–222.

Tost, J., Brandt, O., Boussicault, F., Derbala, D., Caloustian, C. and Lechner, D. (2002) Molecular haplotyping at high throughput. *Nucleic Acids Research* **30**, e96.

Toyoshiba, H., Walker, N. J., Bailer, A. J. and Portier, C. J. (2004). Evaluation of toxic equivalency factors for induction of cytochromes P459 CYP1A1 and CYP1A2 enzyme activity by dioxin-like compounds. *Toxicology and Applied Pharmacology*, **194**, 156–168.

Tratnyek, P. G., Weber, E. J. and Schwarzenbach, R. P. (2003). Quantitative structure–activity relationships for chemical reductions of organic contaminants. *Environmental Toxicology and Chemistry* **22**, 1733–1742.

Travis, C. C. (ed.) (1989). *Biologically-based methods for cancer risk assessment.*

Travis, C. C., White, R. K. and Ward, R. C. (1990). Interspecies extrapolation of pharmacokinetics. *Journal of Theoretical Biology* **142**, 285–304.

Travis, W. D., Brambilla, E. H., Müller-Hermelink, K. and Harris, C. C. (eds) (2004). *Pathology and Genetics of Tumours of the Lung, Pleura, Thymus and Heart.* Lyon: International Agency for Research on Cancer.

Tritchler, D. (1984). An algorithm for exact logistic regression. *Journal of the American Statistical Association* **79**, 709–711.

Tsodikov, A. D. (1992). Screening under uncertainty. Games approach. *Journal of Mathematical Modelling and Simulation in System Analysis* **9**, 259–262.

Tsodikov, A. D. and Yakovlev, A. Y. (1991). On the optimal policies of cancer screening. *Mathematical Biosciences* **107**, 21–45.

Tsodikov, A. D., Yakovlev, A.Y. and Petukhov, L. (1991). Some approaches to screening optimization. In *Statistique des Processus en Milieu Medical.* B. Bru, C. Huber and B. Prum (eds), 1–48. Université Paris V, Paris.

Tsodikov, A. D., Asselain, B., Fourquet, A., Hoang, T. and Yakovlev, A.Y. (1995). Discrete strategies of cancer post-treatment surveillance. Estimation and optimization problems. *Biometrics* **51**, 437–447.

Tusher, V., Tibshirani, R. and Chu, G. (2001). Significance analysis of microarrays applied to transcriptional responses to ionizing radiation. *Proceedings of the National Academy of Sciences of the USA* **98**, 5116–5121.

Umbas, R., Isaacs, W. B., Bringuier, P. P., Shaafsma, H. E., Karthaus, H. F. M., Oosterhof, G. O. N., Debruyne, F. M. J. and Schalken, J. A. (1994). Decreased E-cadherin expression is associated with poor prognosis in patients with prostate cancer. *Cancer Research* **54**, 3929.

University of Connecticut Health Center (2004). Virtual Cell Modeling and Simulation Framework. National Center for Research Resources, National Institutes of Health. (http://www.nrcam.uchc.edu/index.html)

Unkelbach, H. D. and Wolf, T. (1984). Drug combinations – concepts and terminology. *Arzneimittel-Forschung* **34**, 935–938.

Unkelbach, H. D. and Wolf, T. (1985). Qualitative Dosis-Wirkungs-Analysen. Einzelsubstanzen und Kombinationen. In R. J. Lorenz and J. Vollmar (eds), *Biometrie.* Stuttgart: Fischer.

Upton, A. C. (2001). Radiation hormesis: data and interpretations. *Critical Reviews in Toxicology* **31**, 681–695.

US Environmental Protection Agency (1985): Health assessment document for polychlorinated dibenzo-*p*-dioxins. Final Report EPA/600/8–84/014F, EPA, Washington, DC.

US Environmental Protection Agency (1986a). Guidelines for the health risk assessment of chemical mixtures. *Federal Register*, **51**, 34 014–34 025.

US Environmental Protection Agency (1986b). Guidelines for carcinogen risk assessment. *Federal Register* **51**, 33 992–34 003. (http://www.epa.gov/ncea/raf)

US Environmental Protection Agency (1992a). Guidelines for exposure assessment. *Federal Register* **57**(104), 22 888–2 29 38. (http://cfpub2.epa.gov/ncea/cfm/recordisplay.cfm? deid=15263)

US Environmental Protection Agency (1992b). Draft report: a cross-species scaling factor for carcinogen risk assessment based on equivalence of mg/kg$^{3/4}$/day. *Federal Register* **57**(109), 24 152–24 173.

US Environmental Protection Agency (1994): Health assessment document for 2,3,7,8-tetrachlorodibenzo-*p*-dioxin (TCDD) and related compounds. External Review Draft EPA/600/BP-92/0001b, Volumes I–III, EPA Washington, DC.

US Environmental Protection Agency. (1996). Proposed guidelines for carcinogenic risk assessment, Notice - Part II. Federal Register 61. No. 79, 17 960–18 011, April 23.

US Environmental Protection Agency (1999). Guidelines for Carcinogenic Risk Assessment, EPA Washington, DC.

US Environmental Protection Agency (2000a): Health assessment document for 2,3,7,8-tetrachlorodibenzo-*p*-dioxin (TCDD) and related compounds. Final Review Draft (www. epa.gov/ncea/pdfs/dioxin/).

US Environmental Protection Agency (2000b). Supplementary Guidance for Conducting Health Risk Assessment of Chemical Mixtures. Office of Research and Development, Washington, D.C. EPA/630/R-00/002. (www.epa.gov/NCEA/raf/chem_mix.htm)

US Environmental Protection Agency (2001a). Help Manual for Benchmark Dose Software. Version 1.3.

US Environmental Protection Agency (2001b). Trichloroethylene health risk assessment: synthesis and characterization. Washington: EPA/600/P-01/002A. (http://cfpub2.epa.gov/ ncea/cfm/recordisplay.cfm?deid=23249)

US Environmental Protection Agency (2002). Guidance on Cumulative Risk Assessment of Pesticide Chemicals That Have a Common Mechanism of Toxicity. OPP, Washington, D.C. (http://www.epa.gov/oppfead1/trac/science/cumulative_guidance.pdf)

US Environmental Protection Agency (2003a). Draft Final Guidelines for Carcinogen Risk Assessment. Washington: EPA/630/P-03/001A. (http://www.epa.gov/ncea/raf/cancer2003. htm)

US Environmental Protection Agency (2003b). Supplemental guidance for assessing risks from early-life exposure to potential carcinogens. Washington: EPA/630/R-03/003. (http:// cfpub2.epa.gov/ncea/cfm/recordisplay.cfm?deid=55446)

US Environmental Protection Agency (2003c). Benchmark Dose Software.

US Environmental Protection Agency (2003d). A framework for a computational toxicology research program in ORD. Draft Conference Report, EPA/600/R-03/065.

US Environmental Protection Agency Risk Assessment Forum. (2000). Benchmark Dose Technical Guidance Document. External Review Draft. Washington, DC.

Vallander, S. S. (1973). Calculation of the Wasserstein distance between probability distributions on the line. *Theory of Probability and Its Applications* **18**, 784–786.

Van de Wetering, M., Sancho, E., Verweij, C., de Lau W., Oving, I., Hurlstone, A., van der Horn, K., Batlle, E., Coudreuse, D., Haramis, A. P., Tjon-Pon-Fong, M., Moerer, P., van den Born, M., Soete, G., Pals, S., Eilers, M., Medema, R. and Clevers, H. (2002). The beta-catenin/TCF-4 complex imposes a crypt progenitor phenotype on colorectal cancer cells. *Cell* **111**, 241–250.

Van den Akker-van Marle, M. E., Reep-van den Berch, C. M. M., Moral, A. D., Ascunce, N. and De Koning, H. J. (1997). Breast cancer screening in Navarra: Interpretation of a high detection rate at the first screening round and a low rate at the second round. *International Journal of Cancer*, **73**, 464–469.

Van den Berg, M., Birnbaum, L., Bosveld, A. T. C., Brunström, B., Cook, P., Feeley, M., Giesy, J. P., Hanberg, A., Hasegawa, R., Kennedy, S. W., Kubiak, T., Larsen, J. C., van Leeuwen, F. X. R., Liem, A. K. D., Nolt, C., Peterson, R. E., Poellinger, L., Safe, S., Schrenk, D., Tillitt, D., Tysklind, M., Younes, M., Waern, F. and Zacharewski, T. (1998). Toxic equivalency factors (TEFs) for PCBs, PCDDs, PCDFs for humans and wildlife. *Environmental Health Perspectives* **106**, 775–792.

Van den Brandt, P., Voorrips, L., Hertz-Picciotto, I., Shuker, D., Boeing, H., Speijers, G., Guittard, C., Kleiner, J., Knowles, M., Wolk, A. and Goldbohm, A. (2002). The contribution of epidemiology to risk assessment of chemicals in food and diet. *Food and Chemical Toxicology* **40**, 387–424.

Van Oortmarssen, G. (1995). *Evaluation of Mass Screening for Cancer: A Model-Based Approach*. Offsetdrukkerij, Alblasserdam, The Netherlands.

Van Ryzin, J. and Rai, K. (1987). A dose-response model incorporating non-linear kinetics. *Biometrics* **43**, 95–105.

Van Schooten, F. J., Boots, A. W., Knaapen, A. M., Godschalk, R. W., Maas, L. M., Borm, P. J., Drent, M. and Jacobs, J. A. (2004). Myeloperoxidase (MPO) $-463G \rightarrow A$ reduces MPO activity and DNA adduct levels in bronchoalveolar lavages of smokers. *Cancer Epidemiology Biomarkers & Prevention* **13**, 828–833.

Van't Veer, L. J., Dai, H., van de Vijver, M. J., He, Y. D., Hart, A. A. M., Mao, M., Peterse, H. L., van der Kooy, K., Marton, M. J., Witteveen, A. T., Schreiber, G. J., Kerkhoven, R. M., Roberts, C., Linsley, P. S., Bernards, R. and Friend, S. H. (2002). Gene expression profiling predicts clinical outcome of breast cancer. *Nature* **415**, 530–536.

Varela, G., Cordovilla, R., Jiménez, M. F. and Novoa, N. (2001). Utility of standarized exercise oximetry to predict cardiopulmonary morbidity after lung resection. *European Journal of Cardio-thoracic Surgery* **19**, 351–354.

Varner, J. A. and Cherish, D. A. (1996). Integrins and cancer. *Current Opinion in Cell Biology* **8**, 724.

Vasselli, J. R., Shih, J. H., Iyengar, S. R., Maranchie, J., Riss, J., Worrel, R., Torres-Cabala, C., Tablios, R., Mariotti, A., Stearman, R., Merino, M., Walther, M. M., Simon, R., Klausner, R. D. and Linehan, W. M. (2003). Predicting survival in patients with metastatic kidney cancer by gene-expression profiling in the primary tumor, *Proceedings of the National Academy of Sciences of the USA* **100**, 6958–6963.

Vaughan, T. L. (2002). Esophagus. In *Cancer Precursors*, E. L. Franco and T. E. Rohan (eds), 69–116. New York: Springer.

Venter, J. C. *et al.* (2001). The sequence of the human genome. *Science* **291**, 1304–1351.

Vider, B. Z., Zimber, A., Chastre, E., Prevot, S., Gespach, C., Estlein, D., Wolloch, Y., Tronick, S. R., Gazit, A. and Yaniv, A. (1996). Evidence for the involvement of the Wnt 2 gene in human colorectal cancer. *Oncogene* **12**, 153–158.

Vineis, P., Bartsch, H., Caporaso, N., Harrington, A. M., Kadlubar, F. F., Landi, M. T., Malaveille, C., Shields, P. G., Skipper, P., Talaska, G., *et al.* (1994). Genetically based N-acetyltransferase metabolic polymorphism and low-level environmental exposure to carcinogens. *Nature* **369**, 154–156.

Vineis, P., Malats, N., Lang, M., d'Errico, A., Caporaso, N., Cuzick, J. and Boffetta, P. (eds) (1999a). *Metabolic Polymorphisms and Susceptibility to Cancer.* IARC Scientific Publication No. 148. IARC, Lyon: International Agency for Research on Cancer.

Vineis, P., Malats, N., Porta, M. and Real, F. X. (1999b). Human cancer, carcinogenic exposures and mutation spectra. *Mutation Research* **436**, 185–194.

Vineis, P., Veglia, F., Benhamou, S., Butkiewicz, D., Cascorbi, I., Clapper, M. L., Dolzan, V., Haugen, A., Hirvonen, A., Ingelman-Sundberg, M., Kihara, M., Kiyohara, C., Kremers, P., Le Marchand, L., Ohshima, S., Pastorelli, R., Rannug, A., Romkes, M., Schoket, B., Shields, P., Strange, R. C., Stucker, I., Sugimura, H., Garte, S., Gaspari, L. and Taioli, E. (2003). CYP1A1 T3801 C polymorphism and lung cancer: A pooled analysis of 2451 cases and 3358 controls. *International Journal of Cancer* **104**, 650–657.

Vogelstein, B. and Kinzler, K. W. (1993). The multistep nature of cancer. *Trends in Genetics* **9**, 138–141.

Vogelstein, B. and Kinzler K.W. (eds) (2002). *The Genetic Basis of Human Cancer*, 2nd edn. New York: McGraw-Hill.

Vogelstein, B. and Kinzler, K.W. (2004). Cancer genes and the pathways they control. *Nature Medicine* **10**, 789.

Vose, D. (2000). *Risk Analysis*, 2nd edn. Chichester: Wiley.

Voutsinas, G. (2001). Mutagenesis, apoptosis, basic relation to carcinogenic models. *Folia Histochemica et Cytobiologica*, **39**, 56–57.

Wahrendorf, J., Zentgraf, R. and Brown, C. C. (1981). Optimal designs for the analysis of interactive effects of two carcinogens or other toxicants. *Biometrics* **37**, 45–54.

Wakefield, J. C. (1996). The Bayesian analysis of population pharmaco-kinetic models. *Journal of the American Statistical Association*, **91**, 62–75.

Walter, S. D. and Day, N. E. (1983). Estimation of the duration of a pre-clinical disease state using screening data. *American Journal of Epidemiology* **118**, 865–886.

Walter, S. D., Kubik, A., Parkin, D. M., Reissigova, J., Adamec, M. and Khlat, M. (1992). The natural history of lung cancer estimated from the results of a randomized trial of screening. *Cancer Causes Control* **3**, 115–123.

Wang, H., Tan, W., Hao, B., Miao, X., Zhou, G., He, F.and Lin, D. (2003) Substantial reduction in risk of lung adenocarcinoma associated with genetic polymorphism in CYP2A13, the most active cytochrome P450 for the metabolic activation of tobacco-specific carcinogen NNK. *Cancer Research* **63**, 8057–8061.

Ward, R., Meagher, A., Tomlinson, I., O'Connor, T., Norrie, M., Wu, R. and Hawkins, N. (2001). Microsatellite instability and the clinicopathological features of sporadic colorectal cancer. *Gut* **48**, 821–829.

Watanabe, J., Shimada, T., Gillam, E. M., Ikuta, T., Suemasu, K., Higashi, Y., Gotoh, O. and Kawajiri, K. (2000). Association of CYP1B1 genetic polymorphism with incidence to breast and lung cancer. *Pharmacogenetics* **10**, 25–33.

Watanabe, K. H., Bois, F. Y., Daisey, J. M., Auslander, D. M. and Spear, R. C. (1994). Benzene toxicokinetics in humans – bone marrow exposure to metabolites. *Occupational and Environmental Medicine* **51**(6), 414–420.

Weber, E. and Bannasch, P. (1994). Dose and time dependence of cellular phenotype in rat hepatic preneoplasia and neoplasia induced by continuous oral exposure to N-nitrosomorpholine. *Carcinogenesis* **15**, 1235–1242.

Wei, C. G. and Tanner, M. A. (1990). A Monte Carlo implementation of the EM algorithm and the poor man's data augmentation algorithms. *Journal of the American Statistical Association* **85**, 699–704.

Wei, Q., Cheng, L., Amos, C. I., Wang, L. E., Guo, Z., Hong, W. K. and Spitz, M. R. (2000). Repair of tobacco carcinogen-induced DNA adducts and lung cancer risk: a molecular epidemiologic study. *Journal of the National Cancer Institute* **92**, 1764–1772.

Weinberg, R. A. (1995). The retinoblastoma protein and cell cycle control. *Cell* **81**, 323.

Welch, K., Higgins, I., Oh, M. and Burchfield, C. (1982). Arsenic exposure, smoking and respiratory cancer in copper smelter workers. *Archives of Environmental Health*, **387**, 325–335.

Weller, E. A., Catalano, P. J., *et al.* (1995). Implications of developmental toxicity study design for quantitative risk assessment. *Risk Analysis* **15**, 567–574.

Wells, R. J., Arthur, D. C., Srivastava, A., Heerema, N. A., *et al.* (2002). Prognostic variables in newly diagnosed children and adolescents with acute myeloid leukemia: Children's Cancer Group Study 213. *Leukemia* **16**, 601–607.

West, M. (2003). Bayesian factor regression models in the "Large p, Small n" paradigm. In *Bayesian Statistics* 7, J. M. Bernardo, M. Bayarri, J. Berger, A. Dawid, D. Heckerman, A. Smith and M. West (eds) 723–732. Oxford: Oxford University Press.

Weston, A. and Godbold, J. (1997). Polymorphisms of H-ras-1 and p53 in breast cancer and lung cancer: a meta-analysis. *Environmental Health Pespectives* **105**, 919–926.

Whittemore, A. and Keller, J. B. (1978). Quantitative theories of carcinogenesis. *SIAM Review*, **20**, 1–30.

Wicksell, S. D. (1925). The corpuscle problem. A mathematical study of a biometrical problem. *Biometrika* **17**, 84–99.

Wikle, C. (2003). Hierarchical Bayesian models for predicting the spread of ecological processes. *Ecology* **82**, 1382–1394.

Wikman, H., Kettunen, E., Seppanen, J. K., Karjalainen, A., Hollmen, J., Anttila, S. and Knuutila, S. (2002). Identification of differentially expressed genes in pulmonary adenocarcinoma by using cDNA array. *Oncogene* **21**, 5804–5813.

Wikman, H., Thiel, S., Jäger, B., Schmezer, P., Spiegelhalder, B., Edler, L., Dienemann, H., Kayser, K., Schulz, V., Drings, P., Bartsch, H. and Risch, A. (2001). Relevance of N-acetyltransferase 1 and 2 (NAT1, NAT2) genetic polymorphisms in non-small cell lung cancer susceptibility. *Pharmacogenetics* **11**, 157–168.

Wild, C. P., Law, G. R. and Roman, E. (2002). Molecular epidemiology and cancer: promising areas for future research in the post-genomic era. *Mutation Research* **499**, 3–12.

Wilkinson, C. F., Christoph, G. R., Julien, E., Kelley, J. M., Kronenberg, J., McCarthy, J. and Reiss, R. (2000). Assessing the risks of exposures to multiple chemicals with a common mechanism of toxicity: How to cumulate? *Regulatory Toxicology and Pharmacology* **31**, 30–43.

Willems, B. A. T, Melnick, R. L., Kohn, M. C. and Portier, J. C. (2001). A physiologically based pharmacokinetic model for inhalation and intravenous administration of naphthalene in rats and mice. *Toxicology and Applied Pharmacology* **176**, 81–91.

Willems, G., Pison, G., Rousseeuw, P. J. and van Alest, S. (2002). A robust Hotelling test. *Metrika* **55**, 125–138

Williams, N. S., Gaynor, R. B., Scoggin, S., Verma, U., Gokaslan, T., Simmang, C., Fleming, J., Tavana, D., Frenkel, E. and Becerra, C. (2003). Identification and validation of genes involved in the pathogenesis of colorectal cancer using cDNA microarrays and RNA interference. *Clinical Cancer Research* **9**, 931–946.

Wisnivesky, J. P., Mushlin, A., Sicherman, N. and Henschke, C. I. (2003). Cost-effectiveness of baseline low-dose CT screening for lung cancer: preliminary results. *Chest* **124**, 614–621.

Wistuba, I. I., Behrens, C., Virmani, A. K., Mele, G., Milchgrub, S., Girard, L., Fondon, J. W. III, Garner, H. R., McKay, B., Latif, F., Lerman, M. I., Lam, S., Gazdar, A. F. and Minna, J. D. (2000). High resolution chromosome 3p allelotyping of human lung cancer and preneoplastic/preinvasive bronchial epithelium reveals multiple, discontinuous sites of 3p allele loss and three regions of frequent breakpoints. *Cancer Research* **60**, 1949–1960.

Wong, D. J., Paulson, T. G., Prevo, L. J., Galipeau, P. C., Longton, G., Blount, P. L. and Reid, B. J. (2001). p16(INK4a) lesions are common, early abnormalities that undergo clonal expansion in Barrett's metaplastic epithelium. *Cancer Research* **61**, 8284–8289.

World Health Organization (1971). *Annuaire de Statistiques Sanitaires Mondiales Mouvement de la Population et Causes de Décès I*. Geneva: WHO.

World Health Organization (1987). Air quality guidelines for Europe. WHO regional publications, European series No.23.

World Health Organization (1996). *International Conference: One Decade after Chernobyl*. European Commission International Atomic Energy Agency.

World Health Organization (2000). Arsenic. In: *Air Quality Guidelines for Europe*, 2nd edition. WHO Regional Publications, European Series No. 91.

World Medical Association (2002). World Medical Association Declaration of Helsinki: Ethical principles for medical research involving human subjects. *Journal of Postgraduate Medicine* **48**, 206–208.

Wosniok, W., Kitsos, C. and Watanabe, K. (1999). Statistical issues in the application of multistage and biologically based models. In *Perspectives on Biologically Based Risk Assessment*, by Cogliano V. J., Luebeck E. G. and Zapponi G. A.(eds), 243–274. New York: Kluwer Academic/Plenum Publishers.

Woutersen, R. A., Jonker, D., *et al.* (2001). The benchmark approach applied to a 28-day toxicity study with Rhodorsil Silane in rats: the impact of increasing the number of dose groups. *Food and Chemical Toxicology* **39**, 697–707.

Wu, H.-D. I. (2002). A partial score test for difference among heteroscedastic populations. Preprint of the School of Public Health, China Medical College, Taichung, Taiwan, 21 October.

Wu, H.-D. I. (2004). Effect of ignoring heterogeneity in hazards regression. In *Parametric and Semiparametric Models with Applications to Reliability, Survival Analysis, and Quality of Life*, 239–252. Boston: Birkhäuser.

Wu, X., Gu, J., Amos, C. I., Jiang, H., Hong, W. K. and Spitz, M. R. (1998). A parallel study of in vitro sensitivity to benzo[a]pyrene diol epoxide and bleomycin in lung carcinoma cases and controls. *Cancer* **83**, 1118–1127.

Wulfkuhle, J. D., Liotta, L. A. and Petricoin, E. F. (2003). Proteomic applications for the early detection of cancer. *Nature Reviews on Cancer* **3**, 267–275.

Xu, L. L., Liu, G., Miller, D. P., Zhou, W., Lynch, T. J., Wain, J. C., Su, L. and Christiani, D. C. (2002). Counterpoint: the myeloperoxidase $-463G \rightarrow A$ polymorphism does not decrease lung cancer susceptibility in Caucasians. *Cancer Epidemiology Biomarkers & Prevention* **11**, 1555–1559.

Yakovlev, A.Y. and Tsodikov, A.D. (1996). *Stochastic Models of Tumor Latency and Their Biostatistical Applications*. Singapore: World Scientific.

Yakovlev, A.Y., Asselain, B., Bardou, V.-J., Fourquet, A., Hoang, T., Rochefodiere, A. and Tsodikov, A.D. (1993). A simple stochastic model of tumor recurrence and its application to data on premenopausal breast cancer. In *Biometrie et Analyse de Donnés Spatio-Temporelles*, B. Asselain, M. Boniface, C. Duby, C. Lopez, J. P. Masson and J. Tranchefort (eds), 66–82. Rennes: Société Française de Biometrie, ENSA.

Yamashita, H., Noguchi, S., Watanabe, S., Uchino, S., Kawamoto, H., Toda, M., Murakami N. and Nakayama, I. (1997). Associated with adenomatous goiter: an analysis of the incidence and clinical factors. *Surgery Today*, **27**, 495–499.

Yang, C. P., Gallagher, R. P., Weiss, N. S., Band, P. R., Thomas, D. B. and Russell, D. A. (1989). Differences in incidence rates of cancers of the respiratory tract by anatomic subsite and histologic type: an etiologic implication. *Journal of the National Cancer Institute* **81**, 1828–1831.

Yang, G. and Chen, C. (1991). Stochastic two-stage carcinogenesis model: a new approach to computing probability of observing tumor in animal bioassays. *Mathematical Biosciences*, **104**, 247–258.

Yang, R. S. H. (1994a). Toxicology of chemical mixtures derived from hazardous waste sites or application of pesticides and fertilizers. In *Toxicology of Chemical Mixtures*, R. S. H. Yang (ed). San Diego, CA: Academic Press.

Yang, R. S. H. (1994b). Introduction to the toxicology of chemical mixtures. In *Toxicology of Chemical Mixtures*, R. S. H. Yang (ed.). San Diego, CA: Academic Press.

Yang, R. S. H. and Rauckman, E. J. (1987). Toxicological studies of chemical mixtures of environmental concern at the National Toxicology Program: health effects of ground-water contaminants. *Toxicology* **47**, 15–34.

Yang, R. S. H., Hong, H. L. and Boorman, G. A. (1989). Toxicology of chemical mixtures: experimental approaches, underlying concepts, and some results. *Toxicology Letters* **49**, 183–197.

Yang, R. S. H., El-Masri, H. A., Thomas, R. S., Constan, A. A. and Tessari, J. D. (1995). The application of physiologically based pharmacokinetic/ pharmacodynamic (PBPK/PD) modeling for exploring risk assessment approaches of chemical mixtures. *Toxicology Letters* **79**, 193–200.

Yang, Y. H., Dudoit, S., Luu, P., Lin, D. M., Peng, V., Ngai, J. and Speed, T. P. (2002). Normalization for cDNA microarray data: a robust composite method addressing single and multiple slide systematic variation. *Nucleic Acids Research* **30**, e15.

Yang, Y. H. and Speed, T. (2003). Design and analysis of comparative microarray experiments. In *Statistical Analysis of Gene Expression Microarray Data*, T. Speed (ed.), 35–91. New York: Springer.

Yeoh, E. J., Ross, M. E., Shurtleff, S. A., Williams, W. K, Patel, D., Mahfouz, R., Behm, F. G., Raimondi, S. C., Relling, M. V., Patel, A., Cheng, C., Campana, D., Wilkins, D., Zhou, X., Li, J., Liu, H., Pui, C. H., Evans, W. E., Naeve, C., Wong, L. and Downing, J. R. (2002). Classification, subtype discovery, and prediction of outcome in pediatric acute lympho-blastic leukemia by gene expression profiling. *Cancer Cell* **1**, 133–143.

Yonezawa, M., Takahashi, A., Ohnishi, K., Misonoh, J. and Ohnishi, T. (2000). Suppression of p53 and bax accumulation after X-irradiation by small dose preirradiation survival response of C57BL/6 mice. In *Proceedings of the 10th International Congress of the International Radiation Protection Association*, May 14–19, Hiroshima, Japan, P-2b-83.

Zeise, L., Wilson, R., *et al.* (1987). Dose-response relationships for carcinogens: a review. *Environmental Health Perspectives* **73**, 259–308.

Zelen, M. (1968). A hypothesis for the natural time history of breast cancer. *Cancer Research* **28**, 207–216.

Zelen, M. (1993). Optimal scheduling of examinations for the early detection of disease. *Biometrika* **80**, 279–293.

Zelen, M. and Feinleib, M. (1969). On the theory of screening for chronic disease. *Biometrika* **56**, 601–614.

Zhang, H., LeCulyse, E., Liu, L., Hu, M., Matoney, L., Zhu, W. and Yan, B. (1999). Rat pregnane X receptor: molecular cloning, tissue distribution, and xenobiotic regulation. *Archives of Biochemistry and Biophysics* **368**, 14–22.

Zhang, X., Su, T., Zhang, Q. Y., Gu, J., Caggana, M., Li, H. and Ding, X. (2002). Genetic polymorphisms of the human *CYP2A13* gene: identification of single-nucleotide polymorphisms and functional characterization of an Arg257Cys variant. *Journal of Pharmacology and Experimental Therapy* **302**, 416–423.

Zheng, Q. A. (1994). On the exact hazard and survival functions of the MVK stochastic carcinogenesis model. *Risk Analysis* **14**, 1081–1084.

Zheng, Q. A (1997a). A unified approach to a class of stochastic carcinogenesis models. *Risk Analysis* **17**, 617–624.

Zheng, T., Holford, T. R., Chen, Y., Ma, J. Z., Flannery, J., Liu, W., Russi, M. and Boyle P. (1996). Trend and age-period-cohort effect on incidence of thyroid cancer in Connecticut, 1935–1992. *International Journal of Cancer* **4**, 504–509.

Zhou, W., Liu, G., Thurston, S. W., Xu, L. L., Miller, D. P., Wain, J. C., Lynch, T. J., Su, L. and Christiani, D. C. (2002). Genetic polymorphisms in N-acetyltransferase-2 and microsomal epoxide hydrolase, cumulative cigarette smoking, and lung cancer. *Cancer Epidemiology Biomarkers & Prevention* **11**, 15–21.

Zhu, H., Xiong, S. and Chen, W. (2000). Radiation-induced progressive decreasing in the expression of reverse transcriptase gene of hEST2 and telomerase activity. In *Proceedings of the 10th International Congress of the International Radiation Protection Association*, May 14–19, Hiroshima, Japan, P-2b-59.

Zober, A., Messerer, P. and Huber, P. (1990). Thirty-four-year mortality follow-up of BASF employees exposed to 2,3,7,8-TCDD after the 1953 accident. *International Archives of Occupational and Environmental Health* **62**, 139–157.

Zocchi, S. S. and Atkinson, A. C. (1999). Optimum experimental designs for multinomial logistic models. *Biometrics* **55**, 437–444.

Zou, T. T., Selaru, F. M., Xu, Y., Shustova, V., Yin, J., Mori, Y., Shibata, D., Sato, F., Wang, S., Olaru, A., Deacu, E., Liu, T. C., Abraham, J. M. and Meltzer, S. J. (2002). Application of cDNA microarrays to generate a molecular taxonomy capable of distinguishing between colon cancer and normal colon. *Oncogene* **21**, 4855–4862.

Zoumpourlis, V., Papassava, P., Linardopoulos, S., Gillespie, D., Balmain, A. and Pintzas, A. (2000). High levels of phosphorylated c-Jun, Fra-1, Fra-2 and ATF-2 proteins correlate with malignant phenotypes in the multistage mouse skin carcinogenesis model. *Oncogene* **19**, 4011.

Zoumpourlis, V., Solakidi, S., Papathoma, A. and Papaevangeliou, D. (2003). Alterations in signal transduction pathways implicated in tumour progression during multistage mouse skin carcinogenesis. *Carcinogenesis* **24**, 1159–1165.

Index

WILEY SERIES IN PROBABILITY AND STATISTICS

ESTABLISHED BY WALTER A. SHEWHART AND SAMUEL S. WILKS

The *Wiley Series in Probability and Statistics* is well established and authoritative. It covers many topics of current research interest in both pure and applied statistics and probability theory. Written by leading statisticians and institutions, the titles span both state-of-the-art developments in the field and classical methods.

Reflecting the wide range of current research in statistics, the series encompasses applied, methodological and theoretical statistics, ranging from applications and new techniques made possible by advances in computerized practice to rigorous treatment of theoretical approaches.

This series provides essential and invaluable reading for all statisticians, whether in academia, industry, government, or research.

---

*Now available in a lower priced paperback edition in the Wiley Classics Library.

BENDAT and PIERSOL · Random Data: Analysis and Measurement Procedures, *Third Edition*
BERNARDO and SMITH · Bayesian Theory
BERRY, CHALONER, and GEWEKE · Bayesian Analysis in Statistics and
Econometrics: Essays in Honor of Arnold Zellner
BHAT and MILLER · Elements of Applied Stochastic Processes, *Third Edition*
BHATTACHARYA and JOHNSON · Statistical Concepts and Methods
BHATTACHARYA and WAYMIRE · Stochastic Processes with Applications
BILLINGSLEY · Convergence of Probability Measures, *Second Edition*
BILLINGSLEY · Probability and Measure, *Third Edition*
BIRKES and DODGE · Alternative Methods of Regression
BLISCHKE and MURTHY (editors) · Case Studies in Reliability and Maintenance
BLISCHKE and MURTHY · Reliability: Modeling, Prediction, and Optimization
BLOOMFIELD · Fourier Analysis of Time Series: An Introduction, *Second Edition*
BOLLEN · Structural Equations with Latent Variables
BOROVKOV · Ergodicity and Stability of Stochastic Processes
BOULEAU · Numerical Methods for Stochastic Processes
BOX · Bayesian Inference in Statistical Analysis
BOX · R. A. Fisher, the Life of a Scientist
BOX and DRAPER · Empirical Model-Building and Response Surfaces
*BOX and DRAPER · Evolutionary Operation: A Statistical Method for Process
Improvement
BOX, HUNTER, and HUNTER · Statistics for Experimenters: An Introduction to
Design, Data Analysis, and Model Building
BOX and LUCEÑO · Statistical Control by Monitoring and Feedback Adjustment
BRANDIMARTE · Numerical Methods in Finance: A MATLAB-Based Introduction
BROWN and HOLLANDER · Statistics: A Biomedical Introduction
BRUNNER, DOMHOF, and LANGER · Nonparametric Analysis of Longitudinal Data in
Factorial Experiments
BUCKLEW · Large Deviation Techniques in Decision, Simulation, and Estimation
CAIROLI and DALANG · Sequential Stochastic Optimization
CHAN · Time Series: Applications to Finance
CHATTERJEE and HADI · Sensitivity Analysis in Linear Regression
CHATTERJEE and PRICE · Regression Analysis by Example, *Third Edition*
CHERNICK · Bootstrap Methods: A Practitioner's Guide
CHERNICK and FRIIS · Introductory Biostatistics for the Health Sciences
CHILÈS and DELFINER · Geostatistics: Modeling Spatial Uncertainty
CHOW and LIU · Design and Analysis of Clinical Trials: Concepts and Methodologies, *Second Edition*
CLARKE and DISNEY · Probability and Random Processes: A First Course with Applications,
Second Edition
*COCHRAN and COX · Experimental Designs, *Second Edition*
CONGDON · Applied Bayesian Modelling
CONGDON · Bayesian Statistical Modelling
CONGDON · Bayesian Models for Categorical Data
CONOVER · Practical Nonparametric Statistics, *Second Edition*
COOK · Regression Graphics
COOK and WEISBERG · Applied Regression Including Computing and Graphics
COOK and WEISBERG · An Introduction to Regression Graphics
CORNELL · Experiments with Mixtures, Designs, Models, and the Analysis of Mixture Data,
Third Edition
COVER and THOMAS · Elements of Information Theory
COX · A Handbook of Introductory Statistical Methods
*COX · Planning of Experiments

*Now available in a lower priced paperback edition in the Wiley Classics Library.

CRESSIE · Statistics for Spatial Data, *Revised Edition*

CSÖRGŐ and HORVÁTH · Limit Theorems in Change Point Analysis

DANIEL · Applications of Statistics to Industrial Experimentation

DANIEL · Biostatistics: A Foundation for Analysis in the Health Sciences, *Sixth Edition*

*DANIEL · Fitting Equations to Data: Computer Analysis of Multifactor Data, *Second Edition*

DASU and JOHNSON · Exploratory Data Mining and Data Cleaning

DAVID and NAGARAJA · Order Statistics, *Third Edition*

*DEGROOT, FIENBERG, and KADANE · Statistics and the Law

DEL CASTILLO · Statistical Process Adjustment for Quality Control

DENISON, HOLMES, MALLICK, and SMITH · Bayesian Methods for Nonlinear Classification and Regression

DETTE and STUDDEN · The Theory of Canonical Moments with Applications in Statistics, Probability, and Analysis

DEY and MUKERJEE · Fractional Factorial Plans

DILLON and GOLDSTEIN · Multivariate Analysis: Methods and Applications

DODGE · Alternative Methods of Regression

*DODGE and ROMIG · Sampling Inspection Tables, *Second Edition*

*DOOB · Stochastic Processes

DOWDY and WEARDEN, and CHILKO · Statistics for Research, *Third Edition*

DRAPER and SMITH · Applied Regression Analysis, *Third Edition*

DRYDEN and MARDIA · Statistical Shape Analysis

DUDEWICZ and MISHRA · Modern Mathematical Statistics

DUNN and CLARK · Applied Statistics: Analysis of Variance and Regression, *Second Edition*

DUNN and CLARK · Basic Statistics: A Primer for the Biomedical Sciences, *Third Edition*

DUPUIS and ELLIS · A Weak Convergence Approach to the Theory of Large Deviations

EDLER and KITSOS (editors) · Recent Advances in Quantitative Methods in Cancer and Human Health Risk Assessment

*ELANDT-JOHNSON and JOHNSON · Survival Models and Data Analysis

ENDERS · Applied Econometric Time Series

ETHIER and KURTZ · Markov Processes: Characterization and Convergence

EVANS, HASTINGS, and PEACOCK · Statistical Distributions, *Third Edition*

FELLER · An Introduction to Probability Theory and Its Applications, Volume I, *Third Edition,* Revised; Volume II, *Second Edition*

FISHER and VAN BELLE · Biostatistics: A Methodology for the Health Sciences

*FLEISS · The Design and Analysis of Clinical Experiments

FLEISS · Statistical Methods for Rates and Proportions, *Second Edition*

FLEMING and HARRINGTON · Counting Processes and Survival Analysis

FULLER · Introduction to Statistical Time Series, *Second Edition*

FULLER · Measurement Error Models

GALLANT · Nonlinear Statistical Models

GELMAN and MENG (editors): Applied Bayesian Modeling and Casual Inference from Incomplete-data Perspectives

GHOSH, MUKHOPADHYAY, and SEN · Sequential Estimation

GIESBRECHT and GUMPERTZ · Planning, Construction, and Statistical Analysis of Comparative Experiments

GIFI · Nonlinear Multivariate Analysis

GLASSERMAN and YAO · Monotone Structure in Discrete-Event Systems

GNANADESIKAN · Methods for Statistical Data Analysis of Multivariate Observations, *Second Edition*

GOLDSTEIN and LEWIS · Assessment: Problems, Development, and Statistical Issues

GREENWOOD and NIKULIN · A Guide to Chi-Squared Testing

GROSS and HARRIS · Fundamentals of Queueing Theory, *Third Edition*

*Now available in a lower priced paperback edition in the Wiley Classics Library.

*Now available in a lower priced paperback edition in the Wiley Classics Library.

*Now available in a lower priced paperback edition in the Wiley Classics Library.

McLACHLAN and PEEL · Finite Mixture Models

McNEIL · Epidemiological Research Methods

MEEKER and ESCOBAR · Statistical Methods for Reliability Data

MEERSCHAERT and SCHEFFLER · Limit Distributions for Sums of Independent
Random Vectors: Heavy Tails in Theory and Practice

*MILLER · Survival Analysis, *Second Edition*

MONTGOMERY, PECK, and VINING · Introduction to Linear Regression Analysis,
Third Edition

MORGENTHALER and TUKEY · Configural Polysampling: A Route to Practical
Robustness

MUIRHEAD · Aspects of Multivariate Statistical Theory

MURRAY · X-STAT 2.0 Statistical Experimentation, Design Data Analysis, and
Nonlinear Optimization

MURTHY, XIE, and JIANG · Weibull Models

MYERS and MONTGOMERY · Response Surface Methodology: Process and Product
Optimization Using Designed Experiments, *Second Edition*

MYERS, MONTGOMERY, and VINING · Generalized Linear Models. With
Applications in Engineering and the Sciences

NELSON · Accelerated Testing, Statistical Models, Test Plans, and Data Analyses

NELSON · Applied Life Data Analysis

NEWMAN · Biostatistical Methods in Epidemiology

OCHI · Applied Probability and Stochastic Processes in Engineering and Physical Sciences

OKABE, BOOTS, SUGIHARA, and CHIU · Spatial Tesselations: Concepts and
Applications of Voronoi Diagrams, *Second Edition*

OLIVER and SMITH · Influence Diagrams, Belief Nets and Decision Analysis

PALTA · Quantitative Methods in Population Health: Extensions of Ordinary Regressions

PANKRATZ · Forecasting with Dynamic Regression Models

PANKRATZ · Forecasting with Univariate Box-Jenkins Models: Concepts and Cases

*PARZEN · Modern Probability Theory and It's Applications

PEÑA, TIAO, and TSAY · A Course in Time Series Analysis

PIANTADOSI · Clinical Trials: A Methodologic Perspective

PORT · Theoretical Probability for Applications

POURAHMADI · Foundations of Time Series Analysis and Prediction Theory

PRESS · Bayesian Statistics: Principles, Models, and Applications

PRESS · Subjective and Objective Bayesian Statistics, *Second Edition*

PRESS and TANUR · The Subjectivity of Scientists and the Bayesian Approach

PUKELSHEIM · Optimal Experimental Design

PURI, VILAPLANA, and WERTZ · New Perspectives in Theoretical and Applied Statistics

PUTERMAN · Markov Decision Processes: Discrete Stochastic Dynamic Programming

*RAO · Linear Statistical Inference and Its Applications, *Second Edition*

RAUSAND and HØYLAND · System Reliability Theory: Models, Statistical Methods and Applications,
Second Edition

RENCHER · Linear Models in Statistics

RENCHER · Methods of Multivariate Analysis, *Second Edition*

RENCHER · Multivariate Statistical Inference with Applications

RIPLEY · Spatial Statistics

RIPLEY · Stochastic Simulation

ROBINSON · Practical Strategies for Experimenting

ROHATGI and SALEH · An Introduction to Probability and Statistics, *Second Edition*

ROLSKI, SCHMIDLI, SCHMIDT, and TEUGELS · Stochastic Processes for Insurance and Finance

ROSENBERGER and LACHIN · Randomization in Clinical Trials: Theory and Practice

ROSS · Introduction to Probability and Statistics for Engineers and Scientists

*Now available in a lower priced paperback edition in the Wiley Classics Library.

*Now available in a lower priced paperback edition in the Wiley Classics Library.

WESTFALL and YOUNG · Resampling-Based Multiple Testing: Examples and
    Methods for *p*-Value Adjustment

WHITTAKER · Graphical Models in Applied Multivariate Statistics

WINKER · Optimization Heuristics in Economics: Applications of Threshold Accepting

WONNACOTT and WONNACOTT · Econometrics, *Second Edition*

WOODING · Planning Pharmaceutical Clinical Trials: Basic Statistical Principles

WOOLSON and CLARKE · Statistical Methods for the Analysis of Biomedical Data,
    Second Edition

WU and HAMADA · Experiments: Planning, Analysis, and Parameter Design Optimization

YANG · The Construction Theory of Denumerable Markov Processes

*ZELLNER · An Introduction to Bayesian Inference in Econometrics

ZELTERMAN · Discrete Distributions: Applications in the Health Sciences

ZHOU, OBUCHOWSKI, and McCLISH · Statistical Methods in Diagnostic Medicine

*Now available in a lower priced paperback edition in the Wiley Classics Library.